FREE Study Skills DVD Offer

Dear Customer,

Thank you for your purchase from Mometrix! We consider it an honor and privilege that you have purchased our product and want to ensure your satisfaction.

As a way of showing our appreciation and to help us better serve you, we have developed a Study Skills DVD that we would like to give you for <u>FREE</u>. **This DVD covers our "best practices" for studying for your exam, from using our study materials to preparing for the day of the test.**

All that we ask is that you email us your feedback that would describe your experience so far with our product. Good, bad or indifferent, we want to know what you think!

To get your **FREE Study Skills DVD**, email <u>freedvd@mometrix.com</u> with "FREE STUDY SKILLS DVD" in the subject line and the following information in the body of the email:

    a. The name of the product you purchased.

    b. Your product rating on a scale of 1-5, with 5 being the highest rating.

    c. Your feedback. It can be long, short, or anything in-between, just your impressions and experience so far with our product. Good feedback might include how our study material met your needs and will highlight features of the product that you found helpful.

    d. Your full name and shipping address where you would like us to send your free DVD.

If you have any questions or concerns, please don't hesitate to contact me directly.

Thanks again!

Sincerely,

Jay Willis
Vice President
<u>jay.willis@mometrix.com</u>
1-800-673-8175

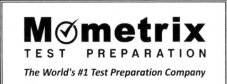

USMLE

Step 1 Preparation

SECRETS

Study Guide
Your Key to Exam Success

USMLE Exam Review for the
United States Medical Licensing
Examination Step 1

Published by
Mometrix Test Preparation
USMLE Exam Secrets Test Prep Team

Written and edited by the USMLE Exam Secrets Test Prep Staff

Printed in the United States of America

This paper meets the requirements of ANSI/NISO Z39.48-1992 (Permanence of Paper).

Mometrix offers volume discount pricing to institutions. For more information or a price quote, please contact our sales department at sales@mometrix.com or 888-248-1219.

USMLE® is a registered trademark of the Federation of State Medical Boards (FSMB) and the National Board of Medical Examiners® (NBME®), which were not involved in the production of, and do not endorse, this product.

ISBN 13: 978-1-61073-000-6
ISBN 10:1-61073-000-3

Dear Future Exam Success Story:

Congratulations on your purchase of our study guide. Our goal in writing our study guide was to cover the content on the test, as well as provide insight into typical test taking mistakes and how to overcome them.

Standardized tests are a key component of being successful, which only increases the importance of doing well in the high-pressure high-stakes environment of test day. How well you do on this test will have a significant impact on your future, and we have the research and practical advice to help you execute on test day.

The product you're reading now is designed to exploit weaknesses in the test itself, and help you avoid the most common errors test takers frequently make.

How to use this study guide

We don't want to waste your time. Our study guide is fast-paced and fluff-free. We suggest going through it a number of times, as repetition is an important part of learning new information and concepts.

First, read through the study guide completely to get a feel for the content and organization. Read the general success strategies first, and then proceed to the content sections. Each tip has been carefully selected for its effectiveness.

Second, read through the study guide again, and take notes in the margins and highlight those sections where you may have a particular weakness.

Finally, bring the manual with you on test day and study it before the exam begins.

Your success is our success

We would be delighted to hear about your success. Send us an email and tell us your story. Thanks for your business and we wish you continued success.

Sincerely,

Mometrix Test Preparation Team

Need more help? Check out our flashcards at: http://MometrixFlashcards.com/USMLE

TABLE OF CONTENTS

Top 20 Test Taking Tips

1. Carefully follow all the test registration procedures
2. Know the test directions, duration, topics, question types, how many questions
3. Setup a flexible study schedule at least 3-4 weeks before test day
4. Study during the time of day you are most alert, relaxed, and stress free
5. Maximize your learning style; visual learner use visual study aids, auditory learner use auditory study aids
6. Focus on your weakest knowledge base
7. Find a study partner to review with and help clarify questions
8. Practice, practice, practice
9. Get a good night's sleep; don't try to cram the night before the test
10. Eat a well balanced meal
11. Know the exact physical location of the testing site; drive the route to the site prior to test day
12. Bring a set of ear plugs; the testing center could be noisy
13. Wear comfortable, loose fitting, layered clothing to the testing center; prepare for it to be either cold or hot during the test
14. Bring at least 2 current forms of ID to the testing center
15. Arrive to the test early; be prepared to wait and be patient
16. Eliminate the obviously wrong answer choices, then guess the first remaining choice
17. Pace yourself; don't rush, but keep working and move on if you get stuck
18. Maintain a positive attitude even if the test is going poorly
19. Keep your first answer unless you are positive it is wrong
20. Check your work, don't make a careless mistake

General Principles

Deoxyribonucleic acid (DNA)

There are three components of DNA – the five-carbon sugar, deoxyribose, existing in the furanose form of a five-member ring, where one of the members is oxygen; four nucleic acids, or bases – adenine (A), guanine (G), cytosine (C), and thymine (T); and phosphoric acid residues (phosphates). Adenine and guanine are purines, molecules with double-ring structures rich in nitrogen hence their designation as bases. They are larger than the pyrimidines cytosine and thymine, which each have only one nitrogenous ring. DNA is a chainlike polymeric structure consisting of one base attached to one molecule of the sugar (a nucleoside) in turn anchored to the phosphate groups (becoming a nucleotide). Each segment polymerizes with the segment above and below it by phosphodiesterase bonds. The deoxyribose portion of the molecule has linkages on the third and fifth carbons, leading each chain to be organized with a 3′ carbon on one end and a 5′ carbon on the other end. The chains lie next to each other in a head-to-tail arrangement. The intrinsic molecular arrangement causes the structure to twist into a gentle coil, or helix. Because the bases have different sizes, the A, G, C, or T bases project outward like dissimilar teeth on a zipper. A complementary strand of DNA is formed such that A always pairs with T and G with C. Because the four letters can be repeated in any sequence, the coding possibilities are truly infinite. The principal intermolecular force holding the two strands of DNA together in the familiar double helix is hydrogen bonding.

When one strand of DNA is paired with a complementary strand of DNA, neither one can be used or read by the cellular machinery. Only the phosphorylated sugar surfaces are presented to the nucleoplasm, not the inside portion that codes for something. Think of DNA like the pages of a closed book, where both pages contain patches of useful information, and the equivalent place on the facing sheet mainly serves to protect those data. The covers of such a book are the histone proteins, which enclose and somewhat organize the structure of chromosomes. When the information is to be accessed, the histones must first disperse. Next, the appropriate portion of the book must be opened. It is not necessary to read the book from beginning to end; rather, the desired portion of DNA is exposed by the enzyme helicase, which cleaves the hydrogen bonds between the zipper-like strands. Next, the DNA must be uncoiled by the enzyme topoisomerase. There now exists in the nucleus of a cell a long, straightened segment of DNA that is open to reading while other segments remain closed. Like a real book, multiple regions of the DNA can be opened at any one time. DNA that is not being read appears as clumped chromatin in histologic preparations.

Mitosis

To make a copy of DNA, the double helix must first be unwound as described in the previous question. During DNA replication, two single-strand polymers are formed – one against the complementary "sense" template of DNA and another against its own complementary "antisense" strand. The enzyme that facilitates this process is DNA polymerase. The ability to use this enzyme in a laboratory setting has allowed significant advances in DNA technology. It is now possible to make large numbers of copies of DNA fragments by the polymerase chain reaction (PCR). These replicate copies can then be sorted by gel electrophoresis to establish various forms of information about the DNA source. The technique is useful in anthropology, criminology, and of course in clinical medical practice. For example, it is now possible to do PCR tests quite rapidly to test for specific infectious agents.

Epigenetics

Epigenetics (literally, "upon the gene," although that is not the exact origin of the word) describes a set of factors that regulate the final expression of the genetic code. One example is the alteration of histone proteins into forms that adhere more tightly to the DNA and "forbid" its reading, so to speak. Although almost any cell with a nucleus (recall that red blood cells expel their nuclei) has all the genes to make a complete individual – something desired when cloning is undertaken – many of these genes are permanently silenced. The ability to undo this silencing would allow the generation of pluripotent stem cells from almost any tissue. Methylation of DNA also affects transcription. Another example of an epigenetic issue is the post-transcriptional modification of proteins. Factors affecting epigenesis include aging, certain foods, and exposure to chemicals, including drugs. Epigenesis helps explain why some persons with genes related to cancer development, such as BRCA1 or BRCA2, never develop a malignancy, even though their relatives do. Thus, the genetic code remains unaltered *per se*, but epigenetic factors substantially affect what subsequently happens inside cells.

DNA exchange between organisms of the same and different species

Bacteria are able to transfer extrachromosomal pieces of DNA (plasmids) between members of the same species across a conjugation structure and through the process of transformation, they can acquire plasmids directly from their environment. This ability underlies the spread of antibiotic resistance. Although the exact concept of exchange is not operative in the situation where viruses incorporate their own DNA into a mammalian cell, the nature of lysogeny is nonetheless similar. Many genes of higher organisms probably arose in this manner. The ability to confer new abilities across species boundaries may lead to mutualistic relationships and even coevolution.

Transcription

The usual dictionary definition does not fully describe the reading process involving DNA. The first step toward the synthesis of a protein is transcription, which means copying the DNA into the new complementary language of ribonucleic acid (RNA). This is NOT translation. RNA has a structure very similar to DNA, except that the pyrimidine uracil is substituted for thymine.

The master plan of transcription is to make a strand of RNA that is complementary to DNA. Thus, an RNA adenine base will sit opposite a DNA thymine base, and wherever adenine appears in DNA, a uracil base will be organized opposite it. Thus, the new DNA-RNA pairing is as shown below:

DNA A C G T A C C G   original code
RNA U G C A U G G C   transcribed code

The enzyme that helps accomplish this assembly is *RNA polymerase II.*

Gene expression: translation, post-translational processing, modifications and disposition of proteins (degradation), including protein/glycoprotein synthesis, intra-/extracellular sorting, and processes/functions related to the Golgi complex and rough endoplasmic reticulum

Translation

The RNA that is assembled against the DNA template is referred to as messenger RNA (m-RNA). This long molecule – perhaps several thousand bases long – passes lengthwise through a pore in the nuclear membrane into the cytoplasm of the cell. In bacteria, ribosome pieces known as 30S (which is smaller) and a larger 50S component come together to form a large macromolecule with a channel on one side, into which one end of the m-RNA fits. The information coded by m-RNA is interpreted one *codon* at a time. A codon is an array of three bases, for example, UUC or AGC. The four letters can be arranged in groups of three in 64 ways ($4^3 = 64$). There are codes for "begin" and "stop" and codes for each of the 20 amino acids. Because there are 64 possible codes, there is considerable redundancy. For example, although there is only one code for methionine and for "start," there are four different codes for the amino acid leucine. A different type of RNA, transfer or t-RNA, is now brought into juxtaposition with the m-RNA. The t-RNA has a stereotypic shape, more or less like a cross, with three loops at tips of the two arms and at the foot of the cross. The foot region bears the anticodon, which is complementary to one of the m-RNA codons. The "crown" of this cross is the end of the t-RNA strand bearing a single amino acid, which is specific to the codon/anticodon arrangement. Sequentially, using guanine triphosphate as an energy source, one codon at a time is recognized and one t-RNA molecule brings one amino acid to a locus on the ribosome. As another amino acid is brought alongside by the next t-RNA, a molecule of water is removed between the amine ($-NH_2$) group of one amino acid and the carboxylic group ($-COOH$) of the other to form an amide (CONH) bond between the two. In this way, peptides are assembled, rather like beads on a string.

Intron and exon

Not all DNA is translated into proteins – in fact, much of it is not. That is not to say that it is entirely silent in cellular physiology. Introns are regions that are not ultimately translated into proteins. The m-RNA that is created against this portion of the DNA template is excised before protein synthesis. The part upon which protein is formatted is termed the exon (mnemonic: introns stay in the cell, and exons go out). A related but different concept is the formation of antisense m-RNA against some portions of the DNA strand. Although the function of these portions of m-RNA is controversial, it is likely that they code for ribosomal proteins or for some other regulatory steps.

Operon, repressor, inducer, promoter, silencer, enhancer, and terminator

A gene is more than just a simple DNA code that always says, "read me." It is accompanied by (and usually intimately surrounded by) other DNA regions that modify expression of the gene in question. The operon model, as studied in *Escherichia coli*, includes binding sites for factors that increase the output of a gene (enhancers and inducers), for molecules that downregulate the gene (repressors), and for factors that, in higher species, presumably permanently silence the function of genes, as occurs during embryogenesis. Note that some chemicals are said to "derepress" a chronically downregulated gene, by causing the repressor molecule to detach from the DNA. The terminator region usually creates a spontaneously folding m-RNA that prevents further enzymatic synthesis of m-RNA upon the DNA template. This is not to be confused with the terminator gene, which is an insert into certain genomic plants, allowing the normal single-generation function of the plant but rendering it sterile and therefore unable to produce another generation of seed crops.

Post-transcriptional modification of m-RNA

The m-RNA that was formed against a DNA template does not all code for useful proteins. These noncoding portions, or introns, must be excised. Usually, spliceosomes (a complex of RNA and protein) form at the front and back ends of this portion of m-RNA, fold it into a loop, and then facilitate the removal of this section from the chain. A second strategy for modifying the m-RNA involves increasing its half-life by protecting is from exonuclease enzyme degradation. Adding multiple adenosine units to the 3′ end (polyadenylation) achieves this purpose. Finally, modifications of the 5′ end also discourage enzymatic degradation of the RNA. Frank revision of the RNA code, a process termed RNA editing, occurs in viruses and may be very important in their ability to modify their virulence.

Example: A 65-year-old patient is noted to have silvery scalp hair, but his eyebrows are still dark brown. Explain how this can occur, using your knowledge of gene expression.

The man was able to express the genes for dark hair uniformly at a younger age. Hair pigmentation relates to a balance of melanin production and cellular peroxidation of the chemical. As seen in other animals, such as the family dog, graying of hair occurs gradually in some skin regions, but not others, due to the local tissue inability to produce enough melanin to escape oxidative degradation. Because this occurs in patchy distribution and later in life, it should be regarded as gene downregulation and it is *not* due to mosaicism of pigment genes. Genes can be turned entirely on or off, but more commonly they are regulated more subtly – up- or downregulated – rather like a rheostat, which brightens or dims lighting.

Intracellular protein degradation

Some proteins are quite stable, and others undergo rapid degradation to their constituent amino acids. In other cases, proteins experience limited reformatting by the cleavage of amide bonds to produce a functional protein and a short polypeptide residue. Obviously, the problem for the cell is to create wanted proteins and dispose of unwanted or damaged ones without having widespread proteolysis. This is accomplished in two ways. Some proteins are digested within lysosomes. Others are attached to one or more (often many) ubiquitin molecules. This new complex targets the protein for destruction by proteasomes, which can be found in the nucleus and the cytoplasm of cells. The ubiquitin is reused after proteolysis has been accomplished. The process uses ATP energy to hydrolyze amide bonds.

Post-translational modification of proteins

Proteins can be chemically altered during their ribosomal synthesis, in other words, along the rough endoplasmic reticulum. This process is termed cotranslational modification. Alternatively, post-translational modification occurs principally in the Golgi complex. Phosphorylation and sulfation of proteins can occur in this site, but the most important process is modification of the polypeptide chain itself. A good example of post-translational modification of a protein is the transformation of preproinsulin to proinsulin to the final insulin hexameric structure that is sequestered in granules, awaiting release. Endo- and exopeptidases are involved.

Glycoproteins

Glycosylated proteins are important in cell-cell interactions, particularly the process of recognition, and also structurally, in the adsorption of water molecules. Many proteins that are secreted undergo the attachment of sugar moieties, but this process also occurs in certain membrane-fixed proteins that project beyond the cell surface. The attachment can occur at the amino group in asparagine, or linkage can be established through the oxygen atom in the alcohol side chain of serine or threonine or the modified amino acids hydroxylysine or hydroxyproline. Multiple sugars can be involved, including simple sugars, fucose, xylose, neuraminic acid, glucosamine, galactosamine, and sialic acid. N-glycosylation occurs both co- and post-translationally (in the rough endoplasmic reticulum and in the Golgi apparatus), whereas O-glycosylation happens in the

Golgi organelle. Note that this is different from glycation, which is the nonenzymatic attachment of sugars to proteins; the latter process produces hemoglobin A1C.

Mechanisms used by cells to sort proteins

It is one thing to code for a protein, but an altogether different problem lies in getting the protein to its final destination. The concept of cell polarity (essentially, certain proteins moving toward the surface or being packaged for external release), scaffolding, and tagging or marking are all involved. Clathrins are a category of protein that self-assemble into polyhedral shapes reminiscent of viruses. The clathrin-adaptor protein complex is critical for directing proteins to certain membrane highly structured, but free-floating (glyco) sphingolipid components lead to significant tissue dysfunction. For example, in some of the many variants of retinitis pigmentosa, photoreceptor proteins are arranged incorrectly. Misalignment of cell surface proteins may also be involved in the loss of cell-cell contact that accompanies malignancy and metastasis.

Grouping amino acids by their chemical structure

The 20 amino acids are conveniently grouped into five chemical categories:
1. acidic (one extra carboxylic acid group) – aspartate and glutamate
2. basic (one or two extra amine group) – histidine, arginine, and lysine
3. aromatic – tyrosine, phenylalanine, and tryptophan
4. aliphatic and nonpolar – glycine, alanine, valine, leucine, isoleucine, and methionine
5. aliphatic and polar (contain hydroxyl or sulfhydryl groups) – serine, threonine, cysteine, proline, asparagines, and glutamine

Nine are essential – H I L L M P P T V.

Enzyme structure

Enzymes (E) are protein catalysts. As such, they have complex 3D shapes, typically being more or less globular. They have an active site (AS) where a substrate (S) binds. Substrates must be properly configured efficiently to fit into the AS. Think of a baseball glove; it is best configured to baseballs, although it is possible to catch golf, tennis, and perhaps softballs with it. Although a beach ball has the correct shape, it is too large to fit into the glove. When S binds to E, a new molecule, ES briefly exists. The enzyme changes shape and bends or stretches bonds in the substrate portion of the new ES molecule. This lowers the activation energy (E_a) required for a reaction (e.g., hydrolytic cleavage) to take place at a given temperature. When more than one S can bind at the AS, the substrates compete and competitively inhibit each other. When a cofactor, coenzyme, or toxin binds at a different site somewhere else on the protein molecule to change its shape and affect AS binding, the process is termed noncompetitive inhibition (or facilitation).

Protein structure

Proteins have four principal structural levels:
- Primary – This refers to the order of the constituent amino acids, e.g., alanine-tyrosine-alanine-glutamic acid-histidine. Each amino acid is referred to as a "residue."
- Secondary – The polypeptide chain arranges itself spontaneously either into an α helix or a β "pleated sheet." These are usually represented in 3D diagrams as a twisted ribbon or a straight line, respectively

- Tertiary – The polypeptide chain further folds into a space-conserving globular structure. Think of a conventional spiral telephone cord twisting into a ball.
- Quaternary – Some proteins are organized into polymeric units with identical protein monomers: dimers, trimers, and tetramers. Insulin is a hexamer. Metalloproteins – some proteins are organized around a metal ion; hemoglobin (iron) and insulin (zinc) are examples.

Vitamins

Vitamins have a wide variety of chemical structures; they are generally classified as fat soluble (A, D, E, and K) or water soluble (the various B vitamins and ascorbic acid, or vitamin C). Although patients taking large doses of the fat-soluble vitamins have the potential to develop overdosage conditions, these are obviously much less common with vitamins B and C. In fact, ascorbic acid is often taken as a cheap means of acidifying the urine. Most of the B vitamins function as coenzymes or cofactors; vitamin C typically acts either as an antioxidant or free-radical scavenger. Vitamin A is involved in the general maintenance of epithelial tissues such as the retina and the skin. Vitamin D has complex roles in calcium metabolism, vitamin E has protean roles in metabolism including the regulation of gene expression, and vitamin K helps modify some of the proteins involved in the coagulation system.

G6-PD deficiency

Glucose-6-phosphate dehydrogenase is the enzyme that converts 6-phosphoglucose into 6-phosphocglucono-δ-lactone, converting NADP into NADPH in the process. The NADPH is used to reduce glutathione, and this reduced compound is used to reduce the oxidative stresses inside erythrocytes. This pathway is the only source of reductive protection against free radicals and peroxidation in erythrocytes. The result is hemolytic anemia due to premature death of erythrocytes.

Glycogen generation

Plants store glucose as polymeric units of starch, with linkages at the 1 and 4 carbons of adjacent glucose molecules. The structure is linear. Animals make the branched carbohydrate glycogen where ordinary 1,4 linkages exist but also where 1,6 branches arise from the parent chain. The principal store of glycogen is in the liver, with some marginal reserve stores in skeletal muscle cells. The body has a very limited supply of glucose in the bloodstream – about 100 mg/100 ml, therefore, around 5 grams. In contrast, the glycogen stores may amount to about 20 to 25 times as much. Glycogen is used by hydrolytically snipping off glucose molecules one at a time, primarily at the 1,4 linkages. (A different enzyme is used to attack the branch points.) This process is stimulated by glucagon release from the α cells of pancreatic islets. Even so, body sources of glucose are relatively limited. Fat stores are normally burned next, reserving structural proteins for last in the process of starvation. It is hardly surprising that man and other large mammals must eat frequently.

Hexose monophosphate shunt

These reactions occur in the cytosol. The effect of this system is to generate the five-carbon sugar, ribose, which is a component of DNA and RNA. As well, it allows cells to initiate four-carbon sugar synthesis, which is the gateway to the production of the cyclic (aromatic) amino acids. During the oxidative phase, 6-phosphoglucose (a phosphorylated polyalcohol) is oxidized into 6-phosphogluconic acid, with the production of one NADPH molecule from NADP. A second step

- 7 -

cleaves off CO_2 and generates another molecule of NADPH with the attendant formation of 5-phosphoribose. Rather than just decomposing glucose for its bond energies, this process uses most of the molecule for alternate, anabolic steps.

Insulin

Insulin is a hormone that causes glucose to enter skeletal muscle, fat, and liver cells. In liver and muscle, the effect is ultimately to stimulate the production of glycogen, whereas in fat, it leads to the synthesis of fatty acids and then triglycerides. The active form of insulin consists of an A and a B chain linked by two disulfide bridges; an intermediate C chain (which also acts as a hormone) is cleaved before storage in a hexameric form. Beta cells in the pancreatic islets of Langerhans incorporate glucose by means of a transporter enzyme (GLUT2); a cascade of events ensues, involving glycolysis, increased permeability to potassium, and ultimately, calcium-dependent release of insulin from granules into capillaries. The blood glucose versus insulin level graph is the classic example of a feedback mechanism; low blood glucose levels cause insulin levels to fall, and vice versa. In the healthy state, blood glucose oscillates around a set point somewhere around 90 mg/100 ml blood.

Phosphorylation

Many carbohydrate molecules that are important in intermediary metabolism, even glucose, might be said to be dull or boring in isolation. Phosphorylating them often directs them onto metabolic pathways because of the great electron affinity afforded by multiple oxygen atoms in proximity to each other. It also prevents them from leaving the cell because transporter proteins no longer recognize the changed molecule. Just as important, if not more so, is the phosphorylation of proteins. Again, the addition of an inorganic phosphate (usually arising as the terminal phosphate group in adenosine triphosphate [ATP]) creates a highly hydrophilic zone on the polypeptide, inducing stereoconformational changes that are important in regulating the function of the proteins. This is particularly shown in a variety of schemata relating to membrane transport and signal transduction.

Fatty acid synthesis and degradation

Fatty acids with the general formula of $H_3C-(CH_2)_n-COOH$ are synthesized from two-carbon units in the form of acetyl-CoA and three-carbon units in the form of malonyl-CoA. The first step is the addition of each of these entities to a carrier protein (CP). The acetyl-CoA (only) is subsequently transferred to a different carrier, after which it undergoes condensation with the malonyl-CoA-CP complex. A molecule of carbon dioxide is released, and a four-carbon unit is formed. Three steps follow: NADPH-mediated reduction, a dehydration, and a second reduction reaction again using NADPH. The product is a four-carbon butyryl-CP complex. Six more additions of two-carbon units from malonyl-CoA-CP occur to produce the 16-carbon unit of palmitic acid. These lipogenic reactions occur in the cytosol. Degradation (beta-oxidation) requires that the fatty acids be transported into the mitochondrion using carnitine-palmityl transferase to get them across the outer mitochondrial membrane. Essentially, the reverse of the synthesis process occurs during breakdown, but here the hydrogen receptors are FAD and NAD. Two-carbon acetate moieties are cleaved off and enter the Krebs cycle; the driving force of $FADH_2$ and NADH is used to generate ATP.

Urea cycle

The urea cycle, sometimes called the ornithine cycle, uses energy to rid the body of ammonia (NH_3) by converting it to urea, $H_2N–CO–NH_2$. In the mitochondrion, ATP is used to add ammonia to the bicarbonate ion, resulting in the formation of carbamoyl phosphate, which in turn fuses with ornithine to make a molecule of citrulline. Three additional converting steps in the cytoplasm result in the production of arginine, which is split into urea and ornithine. The ornithine then enters the mitochondrion. Urea is water soluble and easily excreted by the kidney as a "safe" form of nitrogen. The process occurs mainly in liver cells and to a lesser extent in renal cells. Thus, liver failure results in ammonia accumulation, a highly toxic condition.

Synthesis of purines and pyrimidines

Purines (a short name, but they are two rings wide) are synthesized in a complicated set of steps beginning with the amination of ribose-5-phosphate. In other words, they are made by attachments to the sugar. Magnesium is a key requirement for all steps, and the ribotide known as inosine monophosphate is the resultant product. In the case of pyrimidines (long name, but only one ring wide), the ring is manufactured first by combining carbamoyl phosphate (1C, 1N) and aspartate (3C, 1N) into the pyrimidine ring and then attaching this to a molecule of ribose phosphate to produce uridine monophosphate.

Sodium/potassium pump

Cells must have a mechanism to deal with the inexorable leak of sodium ions from the outside, in and potassium ions from inside, out. The ATP-dependent sodium-potassium pump is the archetypal example of active transport. Here, three sodium ions are pumped out of the cell – against a chemical gradient *and* against an electrical gradient – by an ATP-dependent transporter protein. As soon as the transporter molecule undergoes conformational shift, it loses its affinity for the sodium ions and they enter the extracellular space. Two potassium ions now adhere to different binding sites. They enter the cell against a chemical gradient but with a very strong electrical gradient. As much as 2% or 3% of all metabolic expenditures is used to run this biological bilge pump.

Chylomicrons

Chylomicrons are relatively large, complicated, spherical fat assemblies that are packaged by enterocytes and transferred to the intestinal lymphatics – the lacteal system. They first pass through the cisterna chyli in the abdomen, then into the thoracic duct, and into the venous side of the circulation. They consist of small amounts of cholesterol and proteins and modest amounts of surface lipoproteins interspersed with various apolipoproteins. Their principal constituent is triglycerides (three fatty acids attached to glycerol). They allow transport of immiscible fats in the plasma compartment of blood.

Glycolysis

In glycolysis, a process that occurs in the cytosol, glucose is converted into pyruvate. Think "6 → 2 x 3," meaning that a six-carbon sugar is split into two three-carbon units. The first steps involve the phosphorylation of glucose, its conversion into phosphofructose, and then a second phosphorylation into 1,6-diphosphofructose. So far, two molecules of ATP have been consumed. The diphosphofructose is then split into two molecules of glyceraldehyde-3-phosphate. In a rare example of the use of inorganic phosphate, this molecule is next loaded with a second phosphate on the number-one carbon. There are now four phosphates in play, and in sequential steps, these are unloaded onto ADP to make four molecules of ATP. Net energy: 4 ATP – 2 ATP = 2 ATP. In addition, two molecules of NAD are reduced to NADH. These steps all occur without the need for oxygen. Pyruvate can be used anaerobically in fermentation; when this happens, the NADH is used to convert it to lactate. A much better use is the conversion into acetate and then entry into the Krebs cycle and ultimately, oxidation through the electron transport system. A single molecule of glucose can generate somewhere between 32 and 36 molecules of ATP if the latter pathway is pursued.

Krebs (tricarboxylic acid) cycle

Entry onto the Krebs (citric acid, tricarboxylic acid) wheel is accomplished by the two-carbon entity, acetyl-CoA (or acetyl-S-Co, to emphasize the importance of the sulfur atom). This molecule combines with the four-carbon oxaloacetate molecule to make a new six-carbon moiety, citric acid. In a series of enzymatic steps, two CO_2 molecules bleed off the cycle, three molecules of NAD are reduced to NADH, one molecule of GTP is created, and coenzyme Q is reduced to $CoQH_2$. It is critical to remember that it is the hydrogen ion gradient that ultimately drives ATP production in the mitochondria. (Electrons follow hydrogen. e^- follows H^+ to maintain electrical neutrality.)

Electron transport system

Electron transport occurs in an orderly sequence along the inner mitochondrial membranes, and hydrogen ions pass from the mitochondrial matrix into the intermembranous space as this occurs. It is the hydrogen gradient that drives ATP synthesis. Think of the membranes as factory table surfaces, where an array of receptor machinery processes electrons sequentially, ultimately delivering them to oxygen, the final "acceptor." The electron is passed toward receptors with increasing electronegativity. An electron moves through four protein complexes as it travels toward oxygen. A complex of cytochrome a and a3 facilitates the final transfer to oxygen. Electrons follow hydrogen ions to maintain electrical neutrality. Oxygen is reduced to water as the hydrogen ions ultimately pass from the intermembranous space back into the matrix through the ATP synthase molecule. Three ATP molecules are generated for each two electrons handled by the system. Cyanide ions bind to hemoglobin and compete for oxygen sites, but the most damaging problem they create is when they form a ligand with the cytochrome a and a3 system, preventing electrons from reaching their final receptor. The system backs up, and energy production ceases almost immediately.

Steroid synthesis

Steroids all have four attached rings – specifically, three six-carbon rings and a fourth ring with five carbons. The amazing array of steroid effects depends on attachments such as hydroxyl groups, the location of double bonds, and on the addition of side chains to the C-17 atom. The steroids include cholesterol, cortisol, estrogens, and androgens. Beginning with acetyl-CoA, and progressing through mevalonic acid in steps of conjugation, dehydration, and phosphorylation, the intermediate 22 carbon compound squalene is formed. This molecule is then folded into the familiar steroid ring arrangement. Statin drugs that are targeted at lowering cholesterol interfere with the synthesis of mevalonic acid. Cells in certain organs such as the adrenal gland can further modify the rings by simple steps such as dehydroxylation.

Gluconeogenesis

This process occurs mostly in hepatocytes, and it is not usually important until carbohydrate starvation occurs. The conversion of pyruvate to glucose occurs in a series of steps that exactly mirror those of glucose degradation. Almost all amino acids can undergo deamination and enter a cycle to produce carbohydrates in some manner, but some are ketogenic rather than glucogenic. (The brain can use ketone bodies as an alternate energy source.) This somewhat explains why diabetics are ketotic – their cells are deprived of all the glucose that is backed up in the bloodstream. The process requires considerable sacrifice of protein to produce the amounts of glucose needed for survival. Usually, protein degradation for gluconeogenesis begins as body fat stores are becoming exhausted, but the processes may occur simultaneously. It would be a mistake to believe that an obese, very ill patient is not consuming proteins just because they have not exhausted body lipid energy sources.

Adaptive cellular responses to varied external conditions

Temperature is a substantive problem for cells because enzyme systems function optimally at narrow ranges. In fact, if the body cannot cool cells (as, for example, in heat stroke), then irreversible denaturation of proteins may occur. Most of the time, this results in diminished activity in many pathways, so that there is less liberation of heat from high-energy bond cleavage. Sometimes, the cell cannot slow down, however, as in thyrotoxic crisis. Probably the most consistent challenge to cellular integrity is the onslaught of chemical attacks. Toxins can be detoxified or sometimes bound into inactive forms. Attempts to attach to or penetrate a cell can be thwarted by biochemicals that extend beyond the plasma membrane and either inactivate or entangle interlopers, whether they are macromolecules, viruses, or bacteria. Finally, sometimes cells execute entrapment maneuvers, opsonizing and phagocytosing invaders before extinguishing them in the comforts of the deep cellular bastions. Major hyposmolar challenges presented in the fluid surrounding cells is a very difficult for animal cells and one that is often fatal.

Homeostasis at the cellular level

Think of single-celled organisms swimming in the ocean. For them, there is only the world inside their plasma membrane and the universe beyond. It is not so different for man. Each cell must maintain a *milieu intérieur* against an external fluid compartment that may change dramatically in a short time. Most cells are electronegative (around 50 to 70 millivolts) inside compared to the outside. The electrical gradient occurs in nonliving systems in the form of concentration cells. Because cells like a high-potassium, low-sodium interior, the Nernst equation dictates that a transmembrane voltage will be present. Cells must deal with the issues presented by the tendency of positive ions to enter and be retained by the electrically negative cell contents; negative ions tend to be expelled. Aquaporin channels permit water to enter cells, and cellular chemicals with high hygroscopicity (proteins and complex carbohydrates) tend to retain it. Thus, cells have a volume control problem. Plants meet this challenge by using the cell wall to combat osmotic pressure with hydrostatic pressure. Animal cells do not have this luxury, so animals must maintain an extracellular set of fluid that is close to isotonic to the interior. Some cells face unusual problems, such as the change in cell shape that occurs during contraction of skeletal muscle. All cells face the challenges of temporary suspension of ordinary operations during division.

Intracellular inclusions

Cellular inclusions include foreign materials, infectious agents, and many forms of ordinary biochemicals that are present in excessive amounts. Certain inclusions are also a result of faulty cell development or injury, or else represent degenerative changes in the cell. The first question to be answered is whether the inclusion is nuclear or cytoplasmic, or both (which is unusual), and the second question regards its staining characteristics. A partial listing includes the following:
- crystals – silicon, asbestos – cytoplasmic
- infectious – intracellular bacteria or virus clumps such as Negri bodies in rabies (cytoplasmic) or cytomegalovirus (CMV) (intranuclear) or measles (both); merozoites of malaria (cytoplasmic)
- pigments – lipofuscin, iron (Hallervorden–Spatz neurodegenerative disease, or simple siderosis after a hemorrhage), copper (Wilson's disease) – all are cytoplasmic
- proteins – amyloid and neurofibrillary tangles of Alzheimer's – cytoplasmic
- cellular debris – many hemoglobinopathies or other red cell formation disorder – cytoplasmic
- storage products – glycogen, mucopolysaccharides, etc. – cytoplasmic.

Ischemic cellular changes and anoxic injury

A classic example of a hypoxic injury in which blood flow is preserved is that of carbon monoxide poisoning. In this situation, glucose is still delivered to tissues but it can only undergo the glycolytic and fermentative processes because the electron transport system and Krebs cycle are backed up. Cells rapidly accumulate lactic acid and can no longer control intracellular pH. A collateral example occurs when climbers get trapped on the upper reaches of Mount Everest in the "killing zone." They may have adequate calories and water, but they succumb to lactic acidosis because the FiO_2 at the summit is only about 44 torr. In ischemic injury, both nutrients and oxygen are delivered in lower amounts, so there is a better "match." Cells enter lowered or "idle" metabolic states, and they can often recover well if blood flow is restored. If the process continues, infarction will occur. Neurointerventionalists try to exploit this window of opportunity by restoring blood flow to ischemic areas of the brain as rapidly as possible to limit infarct size. Nerve cells in the penumbra (shadow) of an infarct may resume normal functioning. The microscopic pathology is what one would expect: leaky cellular and organelle membranes, dissociation of ribosomes from ER, and, ultimately, clumping of DNA. In both ischemia and hypoxic injury, waste metabolites cannot be removed as rapidly as they are produced (but for different reasons).

Cytotoxic insults to the cell

Any substance that interferes with the metabolism of a cell is cytotoxic. Divalent lead, for example, may compete with zinc as an enzyme cofactor. Cyanide ions bind to cytochrome oxidase and disturb the ability of the electron chain to function properly. The 2-deoxyglucose enters cells readily, but it cannot undergo glycolysis because of its altered chemical structure. If it is administered in large amounts, it will become toxic, in a sense, by depriving the cells of energy. It has been investigated as an antineoplastic agent for this very reason. In general, cells that are poisoned become more permeable and are unable to exclude marker dyes. The injury is dose dependent and somewhat reversible. Cytotoxic insults are different conceptually from other chemical damage to cells. For example, benzene is carcinogenic, but it is not usually described as directly cytotoxic.

Changes that occur in a cell due to freezing or thermal injury

The cooling of tissues is usually well tolerated, but freezing kills cells rapidly. Ice crystals basically pierce or lacerate the cell membranes (including those of organelles), so that when rewarming takes place, there is gross disruption of cell machinery. Often the cells lyse due to imbibition of water. Cellular defense mechanisms include the production of "antifreezes" (often unusual carbohydrates) in some species, brought on by chilling. This may allow survival a few degrees below 0°C and explains how some insects such as mosquitoes can survive winter. Heating gradually denatures proteins up to an irreversible level, ultimately resulting in coagulation necrosis. Such cells appear uniformly pink on hematoxylin and eosin (H&E) stained microscopic sections.

Apoptosis

Apoptosis refers to the biologically planned or programmed death of certain cells. The p53 gene is intimately related to the ability of an organism to regulate cell division, repair DNA, and regulate the involution of tissues. Defects in this gene lead to Li–Fraumeni syndrome, in which multiple unusual malignancies arise at a young age. Apoptosis involves an orderly process of loss of cell contacts, increased membrane permeability, and the formation of blebs on the cytoplasmic membrane. Failed apoptosis is evident in the rare persistence of a human tail, the failure of fingers to separate fully during embryogenesis, and as noted, in the occurrence of some forms of cancer.

Cell cycle

Cells that are not in line to divide – for example, hepatocytes, rhabdomyocytes, and neurons – are in the G_0 (gap zero) phase. Some are permanently in this pool, incapable of dividing ever again, and some can be recruited back into active division. As an example, an osteocyte can be stimulated by a bone fracture. This is sometimes called the "resting phase" of a cell's life, but the cell is indeed metabolically active, carrying out its primary functions. Cells in the G_1 (gap one) portion of the cycle have completed mitosis. They use this period to store nutrients, make organelles, and grow in physical size. Cyclin-dependent kinases (which are phosphorylases) govern entry into the S, or synthetic, phase. Unless certain intracellular "go" signals are detected, DNA replication will not be initiated. All chromosomal replication is complete by the end of the S phase. The cell then pauses, readying itself for the mitotic process during the G_2 period. At the next interface with the M, or mitotic, phase, there is a second signal-recognition mechanism that prevents mitosis from occurring if certain conditions are not met. Finally, mitosis proceeds through the familiar prophase-metaphase-anaphase-telophase steps until cytokinesis is completed. Cells then reenter the G_1 phase or pass out into G_0 life. The G_1/S checkpoint ultimately governs the rate of cell division.

Malignancy

Cells in a given tissue may become hypertrophic (larger), such as skeletal muscle cells that have been exercised; hyperplastic (more numerous), as is the case of residual liver cells after a partial donor hepatectomy; dysplastic, in which case they lose some of their normal features; or frankly anaplastic, at which point they have crossed over into malignancy. Dysplastic tissues show mild derangements of shape, size, and patterns of arrangement. In anaplastic neoplasia, one of the most consistent findings is a shift toward a 1:1 nuclear-to-cytoplasmic ratio. Nuclear chromatin may be unusually lacy or clumped when compared to the normal parent tissue. As malignancy of epithelia progresses, basement membranes are breached. Sometimes, sheets of almost-identical cells arise and in other cases, such as monstrocellular glioblastoma, in which bizarre, multinucleate syncytia dominate fields of much smaller cells. Prominent mitoses can be seen in many cases, and proliferation of blood vessels is common as the degree of malignancy and invasiveness progress.

Genetic factors, aging (ineffective DNA repair, loss of telomeres), infectious agents (especially viruses), and cumulative toxic insults to a cell may all play a role in the transformation of histologically benign processes into frank malignancies. Then, too, one must consider autostimulatory (autocrine) effects and possible paracrine effects of normally behaving cells upon cells that have already undergone subtle transformations. A variant on this question relates to how malignancy develops in burn scars. Finally, it is important to consider the effects of treatment on a histologically benign process. Biopsy, diagnostic X-rays, modification of the hormonal milieu—all of these have the potential to make a benign lump change in adverse ways.

A good example of an oncogene is myc, a gene identified on chromosome 8 because there are frequent translocations of this chromosome in Burkitt's lymphoma. Myc expression produces a protein that in turn is involved in the regulation of many other genes. Oncogenes include several families that regulate cytoplasmic or receptor-bound amino acid kinases, GTPase (particularly the ras gene), and growth factors. The expression of an oncogene is balanced by counterexpression of tumor-suppressor factors. Factors such as viral infections and exposure to carcinogenic compounds may initiate or perpetuate the expression of oncogenes.

Simple enlargement of a neoplasm is not synonymous with invasion. Breach of the basement membrane of an epithelium is the *sine qua non* step of invasion. This process is facilitated by dysfunction of epithelial cadherin and interference with integrin function. Lysis of the underlying stroma and pseudopodial intrusion of cancer cells into the resulting low-resistance space lead to further local spread. Attempts by the body to control the breakout of tumor cells include the response of immune cells and heavy deposition of collagen. As an example, heavy infiltration of lymphocytes around melanoma is considered to be an important positive prognostic factor.

Once a tumor has invaded locally, it possesses most if not all of the machinery necessary to spread further by invasion of the lymphatics or even the blood vessels. Germane to this level of aggressiveness is the ability to recruit vascular supply to sustain the metabolic demands of a rapidly growing tissue. Vascular endothelial growth factor (VEGF) and similar trophic substances cause tumor angiogenesis. Access to the lymph capillaries is easy for tumor cells that have breached a basement membrane. Nonetheless, loss of cell-cell contacts and the migration to new environments where the tumor cells will doubtless undergo attack once the unusual nature of surface proteins has been sensed by the immune system mean that only the most capable, robust tumor cells will be able to survive the trip and implant successfully. Migration into very hostile, low-nutrient environments such as the cerebrospinal fluid is usually unsuccessful. The progeny of cells that serve as the clones for metastatic lesions are very aggressive.

TNM cancer staging system

The letters stand for tumor, nodes, and metastases. This is different than a histologic grading system (which can be applied to the specimen on a single microscopic slide). Each letter is followed by subscripts: x means "cannot evaluate," is means "*in situ*," and the numbers 0 through 4 relate to degree, except for metastasis, where 0 means no and 1 means yes. For a small breast cancer presenting as a seizure due to a brain metastasis: T1N1M1 means small local tumor size, but with spread to a regional lymph node and a distant metastasis. With the advent of advanced imaging techniques, more micrometastases are being discovered, rendering comparison of contemporary and historical TNM classifications difficult. There are many other modifiers implicit to the system, and it is revised with some regularity. Special situations (leukemia, brain tumors) are not readily conformed to this staging system.

Golgi apparatus

The Golgi apparatus looks like a slightly concavo-convex stack of folded linen in electron micrographs. It is a perfect example of the structure–function theme of cellular biology. The convex, or trans, face is usually directed toward the plasmalemma. The organelle serves essentially as a packaging and reformatting center. The Golgi complex receives materials from the cisternae of the smooth and rough endoplasmic reticulum on its cis, or deeply oriented side, processes them, and then buds off secretory vesicles containing the finished product. Cells in which exocytosis is prominent, such as those surrounding the thyroid follicle, have a resplendent Golgi apparatus.

Microfilament and microtubule

Microfilaments are thin structural elements of the cytoskeleton composed of actin. They give cells a basic shape and orientation, and they may be seen as robust bundles or as a lacy background array. They are involved in the movement of cells and, of course, in muscular contraction. Microtubules are composed of tubulin; like actin microfilaments, microtubules undergo directed self-assembly, which requires the expenditure of energy. Microtubules are also important elements of the cytoskeleton and they are central to the function of cilia and flagella. Their most notable expression is during mitosis, when they act to draw chromosomes apart during anaphase.

Nucleolus

The nucleolus is a dark region of chromatin noted within the nuclei of many higher organisms. Nucleoli have a role (how much is not yet known) in the binding and inactivation of certain proteins within the nucleus. Their main importance, however, is in the transcription of ribosomal RNA. RNA polymerases I and III work in this region to create the ribosome structure, which is then exported through nuclear membrane pores into the endoplasmic reticulum. The nucleus communicates with the nucleolar depth via a series of channels. The nucleolus is NOT a membrane-bound structure.

Plasmalemma and the nuclear membrane

The cell membrane is a dynamic barrier whose core structure consists of a double layer of phospholipids. The hydrophilic phosphate heads face the two surfaces and the long lipid tails, with interspersed cholesterol molecules, overlap in the interior of what essentially amounts to a bilaminar entity. Floating in or attached to these layers are all manner of protein molecules, ion channels, glycoproteins, glycolipids, and receptors. The inner surfaces of the membrane are intimately associated with microfilaments and other cytoskeletal elements. Membrane-bound vesicles from inside arrive at the membrane and coalesce with it, discharging their contents to the exterior. Such a model is known as the fluid-mosaic membrane.

The nuclear membrane is similar, but it is associated with fewer complicated receptor chemicals and it is punctuated by many pores through which m-RNA must pass to get to the ribosomes. Additionally, the outer nuclear membrane is continuous with that of the endoplasmic reticulum. The nuclear membrane is similarly associated with microfilaments on its inner surface.

Sarcoplasmic reticulum and the T-tubule system

The sarcoplasmic reticulum is a modified endoplasmic reticulum unique to muscle cells. It serves as the principal reservoir of calcium, the ion that is released to initiate muscle contraction in response to nervous stimulation. Nerve action potentials cause release of acetylcholine into the specially modified synaptic cleft at the neuromuscular junction. A muscle action potential arises, and this wave of electrical depolarization invades deeply into muscle fibers via the transverse tube (T-tube) system. Each T-tube is associated with sarcoplasmic reticulum on two sides – a triad. The electrical signal invades the membrane of the sarcoplasmic reticulum, permitting calcium release into the sarcoplasm. Contraction ensues.

Microvilli

Microvilli are membrane-bound cytoplasmic extensions, which vastly increase the surface area of cuboidal or columnar cells; they are particularly prominent in absorptive surfaces such as the intestinal mucosa. They have an actin filament framework, but they otherwise are histologically rather unremarkable internally. In absorptive mucosae, they have a broad assortment of enzymes on their brush, or outermost, surfaces. Saccharidases and peptidases on the luminal surface are physiologically linked to transporter proteins on the abluminal surface of these cells. In other tissues, the microvilli use their extensive surface area as chemical receptors.

Cilia in the respiratory tract and the spermatic flagellum

Cilia and flagella are cytoplasm-contiguous, membrane-bound extensions of a cell. Flagella and motile cilia both have the same cross-sectional structure – nine pairs of microtubules with dynein extensions that surround a pair of central microtubules: this is called the "9+2" arrangement. Cilia beat in a coordinate fashion much like the oars of a crew boat; the process is ATP dependent and relates to the sliding of the microtubules along the dynein connectors (reminiscent of muscle contraction). Flagella have an identical appearance, but they are typically much longer and fewer in number. Some sensory functions have been attributed to flagellar surfaces (the ability to swim with or against chemical gradients, for example). Cilia and flagella in man are anchored to a basal body. In bacteria, flagella are anchored to a stator-rotor mechanism that spins the flagellum around a central axis; through the mechanism of a bend in the anchor, a whiplike undulant motion results.

Centriole, centrosome, and centromere

In contrast to the appearance of cilia, centrioles are composed of nine *triplets* of microtubules arranged in two cylindrical arrays situated at right angles to each other. Such arrays with appended microtubular components constitute the centrosome. They are important in creating and maintaining the spindle array necessary for cell division in eukaryotes. In contrast, centromeres are regions of heterochromatic DNA that assist in the attachment of homologous chromosomes to one another and that provide anchors for microtubules during cytokinesis. Centromere location is an important "gross anatomy" feature of individual chromosomes. They can be roughly in the middle of a chromosome (metacentric); asymmetrically disposed, creating short and long arms (submetacentric); near one end (acrocentric); or at the very end of a chromosome (telocentric).

Mitochondria

Mitochondria generate energy in the form of adenosine triphosphate (ATP). Not unlike the chloroplasts of plants, this organelle probably became incorporated into eukaryotic cells billions of years ago. The basic structure is that of an outer membrane, an extensively folded inner membrane (constituting the cristae), a matrix region in the center, and an intermembranous compartment between the inner and outer membranes. The exuberant surface area of the inner membrane allows the efficient physical arrangement of carriers in the electron transport system, like an assembly line in a factory. Further, the separation of aqueous compartments (matrix and intermembranous spaces) by the inner membrane allows for the development of a gradient in H$^+$ ions, and it is this gradient, ultimately, that drives the production of ATP.

Lysosomes

These acid-containing organelles are unique to animal tissues. Lytic enzymes are packaged inside rough endoplasmic reticulum and conveyed to the Golgi apparatus. A nascent lysosome receives a chemical designator that causes it to be extruded into the cytoplasm rather than being exocytosed. Lysosomes aid the chemical decomposition of a variety of materials, including foreign debris such as bacteria; aged, degenerating organelles or cytoplasmic castoffs; and some drugs. Peroxisomes, by contrast, are involved in fatty acid decomposition. Lysosomes are recognizable as medium-size organelles with a variety of inclusions; they of course stain well with basic stains.

Channelopathy

Cystic fibrosis is a classic example of a channel disorder. In this instance, chloride channels are genetically defective due to varied mutations in a single gene; the problems that arise include viscous pulmonary and pancreatic secretions, although the exact mechanism by which this occurs is not fully understood. Remember that genes code for protein and that proteins must have specific shapes to work properly. Even single amino acid substitutions may have disastrous consequences, depending on the protein involved. Another set of examples involves the multiple channel disorders that underlie various subsets of the prolonged QT syndrome.

Capillaries

Capillaries are of three main types:
- continuous, showing tight junctions between endothelial cells – the brain,
- discontinuous, with large open spaces between endothelial cells allowing very large molecules and even red cells to leave the circulatory system – the liver, and
- fenestrated, with membranous pores directly through the endothelial cell cytoplasm – the renal glomerulus and endocrine glands.

Gap junctions and tight junctions

Gap junctions are specially modified regions of two adjacent cells. The cell membranes are closely juxtaposed, and special channels between the two cells allow direct passage of large molecules between the cytoplasm of one cell to the cytoplasm of another. In effect, they create a syncytial arrangement. These are noted in electrically coupled tissues. Tight junctions (*zonulae occludentes*) are specially modified regions or bands between cells that close off the extracellular space. They are found in epithelia. Desmosomes are similar, but they occur in spots (*maculae adherentes*) rather than as strips or other completely occlusal connections.

Cell surface receptors and nuclear receptors

Cell surface receptors either project beyond the plasma membrane, loop through it or are suspended in it, or are on the interior surface of the plasmalemma. There are many classes of these signal-transducing molecules – glycoproteins, ion-specific channels (which might not be considered "receptors" in all classification schemes), and vital proteins such as tyrosine kinase and the G-receptor protein complexes that are involved with second messenger (cAMP) signaling. The surprising thing about nuclear receptors is that they actually bind with their ligand – such as a lipophilic steroid, a fat-soluble vitamin, or thyroxine – in the cytoplasm. They then pass through special pores into the nucleus, where the receptor-ligand complex directly binds to DNA and influences its transcription.

Negative feedback with enzyme systems and positive feedback in biological systems

Take as an example a hydrolytic enzyme that cleaves disaccharide XY. Suppose that X is normally rapidly consumed by some limb of the pathway, but Y is less useful metabolically. The enzyme might have an inhibitory, noncompetitive binding site for Y and hence be very sensitive to the concentration of Y, but this would lead to inadequate production of X. More likely, the enzyme has a noncompetitive, inhibitory binding site for X. If X does back up in the metabolic pathway, it is energetically conservative for the organism to stop producing so much of it. This is an example of negative feedback.

Positive feedback in biological systems occurs when there is an increased response to a stimulus over time. Examples include a cattle stampede or, in humans, mass hysteria due to an imagined odor or danger. A more common example is the uterus during late pregnancy. Braxton Hicks contractions begin in response to uterine distension by the fetus, and, ultimately, sustained smooth muscle contractions occur until parturition is complete.

Extracellular matrix

Two zones of chemicals must be considered as part of the extracellular matrix. First is a group of chemicals that extend far beyond the outer cell membrane, yet they are attached to it. These include receptor protein complexes and simpler molecules such as polysaccharides or sialic acid. They are technically components of the parent cell, most often functioning in signaling capacities. Far beyond this is the true extracellular matrix, which includes the "background stroma" of tissues. Here collagen, reticulin, elastin, and other fibers are laced against a number of other chemical moieties such as chondroitin and heparan. (The basement membrane of all epithelia is likewise a part of the extracellular matrix.) This compartment is most obvious in places such as loose areolar tissue.

Pedigree

Medical pedigrees depict the progression of heritable traits across generations. Squares universally represent males; circles typically represent females. Typically, those individuals expressing the phenotype of a certain trait are shown as black (filled-in) shapes, and those who do not carry the trait are white, or empty, shapes. Individuals who are carriers (heterozygotes who therefore do not express the trait) are usually indicated by an obliquely divided, half-black, half-white shape. The *propositus* or *proband*, indicated by an arrow, is usually an individual in the current generation who is known to have the trait. Generations are shown in vertical arrays, with the oldest at the top. Siblings are connected by short vertical lines attached to a common horizontal line emanating from the parents above them. Unions from (usually) different families are shown by horizontal lines connecting male and female members at the equator of each symbol. Multiple unions are arranged clocklike around the individual in question. Pedigrees usually indicate deceased members by a small cross next to their symbol. Age (present or age of death) is sometimes mentioned in a small font, often placed in parentheses. Family members of unknown status (for example, with premature death, adoption out of the family, etc.) are often shown as squares or circles with hatched edges rather than solid lines.

The propositus or immediate members of his/her family can usually identify most of the proximate members of a family, but rarely in a useful order without assistance. Careful interviewing is necessary. It is useful to sit alongside the family and construct the family tree with them. "Aunt Martha" might not truly be an aunt related by blood. The interviewer works backward through the siblings and parents of the propositus, then the siblings of each parent, then the parents of each parent, and so on. If possible, four generations should be included. Adopted children are sometimes noted on a pedigree, but they are not connected to the family tree. Once the pedigree has been established, it can be "read" forward or backward. The patterns that are particularly overt are those of traits inherited in a straight autosomal dominant-recessive manner or sex-linked conditions that skip generations. (Analysts must assume that all children arise from the stated union, and not from an undisclosed mating. The mother is always indisputable; not so for the father.) Some characteristics, such as dimples or a widow's peak in the hairline, may be seen in family photos, considerably amplifying the information in a pedigree.

Bearing in mind that pedigrees may be incomplete, it is still possible to determine the genotype of many individuals based on the phenotype of several of them. If condition A is autosomal dominant, it will appear in every member of the next generation if either parent is homozygous (AA). If both parents are heterozygous (Aa), then at least some of the following generation should be free of condition A, if there are enough of them to be reasonably certain. The problem, of course, is that couples have only a handful of offspring – rarely more than five or six in modern times. If, for example, two heterozygotes mate (Aa x Aa), then the chance of having a phenotypically affected child is 3/4; the chance of having two affected children is $(3/4)^2$, or about 56%; the chance of having three affected children is still $(3/4)^3$, or about 42%; the chance of having six affected offspring is still a whopping 18%! By scanning backward over generations, however, more information is acquired, and the geneticist can be increasingly sure whether or not an individual indeed is homozygous for A.

Hemophilia A, a condition in which blood clotting is abnormal either due to low levels of factor VIII or an inoperative form of the protein, is the classic example of an X-linked (sex-linked) recessive condition. The defective gene may arise due to spontaneous mutation, but typically it is conferred by the mother, who is XX^+ genotypically and therefore herself a carrier. Meiosis in the testis of the father produces sperm that are either X or Y. The maternal contribution of a normal X chromosome produces XX daughters who are normal or XX^+ female carriers who are not affected by the condition because their normal X chromosome allows reasonably normal production of factor VIII. Half their sons are normal, XY males, and half are afflicted X^+Y males who historically do not live to reproductive age. Note that the phenotypic pattern is different with dominant sex-linked characteristics.

Color blindness

Succinctly, a woman who is color blind must have both a color-blind father (X^+Y) and a mother who either a) herself is color blind (X^+X^+) or b) is a carrier (X^+X^0). Protanopia refers to the inability to detect red colors, and deuteranopia is the inability to discriminate green. The very unusual condition of tritanopia refers to the inability to see blue, and this may be inherited in an autosomal manner. Persons lacking normal color vision usually have better-than-normal scotopic vision, and they are able to see patterns better than normal people. During World War II, at least one member of each bomber crew was picked because of his color blindness. Normally, people see a blue and gold (gas and dust) tail on a small comet. Completely color-blind people see a comet as a huge luminosity in the sky.

Autosomal dominant

The man is either AA or Aa. If the condition is autosomal dominant, like Huntington's chorea, he will manifest the condition sooner or later, even if he is a heterozygote. The woman must be homozygous recessive, aa, because she is unaffected. (Assume for a moment that the age of presentation is not a factor.) If the man is AA, then each offspring will come to have the condition. If the man is Aa, then half of the children will develop the disease. Huntington's chorea is a particularly cruel neurodegenerative affliction because it usually does not declare itself until after people have ordinarily produced their offspring. Excessive copies of the CAG trinucleotide sequence are due to mutations in chromosome 4. Because CAG codes for glutamine, a defective protein results. Genetic testing is available, but if an individual is positive, his or her cognitive function, mobility, and longevity are doomed.

Conditions for a Hardy–Weinberg genetic equilibrium to exist

A stable (equilibrium) genetic state exists when the following five conditions are met:
- the population is large
- the gene itself is stable (very infrequent mutations)
- there is no migration into or out of the population
- mating is random
- there is no (natural) selection

In practice, these conditions are difficult to achieve in humans in the modern world. Nonetheless, for a rare condition such as cystic fibrosis, knowledge of the gene frequency in the population would allow fiscal planning relating to the number of anticipated lung transplants.

Example: In a certain population, the frequency of a homozygous, recessive condition is one in 10,000 persons. Assuming that Hardy–Weinberg principles obtain, what percentage of people are carriers for this disease?

In single-gene, dominant-recessive conditions, the number of normal (usually dominant) alleles of the gene is symbolized by p, and the opposite allele is represented by q. Obviously, the total must be 100%, or 1, so $p + q = 1$. In algebra, we can square both sides of an equation, and that is true here as well, so $(p + q)^2 = 1^2$ and therefore $p^2 + 2pq + q^2 = 1$. Here, p^2 represents the homozygous (dominant) state; $2pq$ is the number of heterozygotes, or carriers; and q^2 indicates the number of individuals with the (recessive) homozygous state. Substituting the numbers in the question, $q^2 = 10^{-4}$, so $q = 10^{-2} = 0.01$. Because $p + q = 1$, then p must equal 0.99. Now we evaluate for $2pq$ by substituting these numbers. The number of heterozygotes carriers is $2pq = 2(0.99)(0.01) = 0.0198$, or 1.98% of the total population.

Founder effect

Suppose that in certain birds, there is a gene A and an allele a. If 100,000 birds are blown by a storm onto an island with none of this species, it is quite likely that the resultant colony 100 years hence will have a gene distribution similar to the original pool, all other factors being equal. If, on the other hand, only 30, or just 10 birds were blown onto the island, then the resulting colony might, by dumb luck, eliminate one of the alleles entirely. (In other words, the gene frequency would be shifted because the gene pool was inadequately "sampled" by nature.) In humans, relatively small, (geographically, politically, socially) isolated groups of people may exhibit genetic conditions that arise in this manner.

Natural and artificial selection

Natural selection occurs in nature when mating is random between members of a species. This does not mean that there is no selection of mates. For example, the dominant bull elk mates with many elk cows, his "harem," which he guards from other competing males. The females naturally select the alpha male of their species. In humans, mating is not at all random because cultural, religious, and profound geographic barriers effectively limit the choice of partners. At best, it is semi-random. Artificial selection occurs when mates are specifically chosen for certain characteristics above all others – for example, in breeding racehorses, sheep, cows, or dogs. True natural selection is the underpinning of the theory of evolution.

Mutation-selection equilibrium

This concept addresses the issue of persistence of deleterious genes in a population. Of course, not every gene that creates disadvantages for its bearer is fatal. It would be expected, in fact, that the gene would "hang around" for many generations before disappearing entirely. Mutations may also create the harmful allele anew. It is important to recall that one of the criteria of a Hardy–Weinberg equilibrium is that there is a low spontaneous rate of mutation of a given gene. Additionally, the heterozygote state may actually be favored in some instances; it is almost always tolerated, and this indeed is the main reason for the persistence of "undesirable" genetic material.

Gene therapy

Gene therapy attempts to insert genes into a host that typically code for some vital product the host is not able to make. Viruses (especially neurotropic viruses or retroviruses) have been used to infect and transform human cells with some good initial results. There is also interest in other mechanical means of getting genetic information into cells, including the use of nanoparticles. The major problems with the technique are nonpersistence of the inserted DNA and immune reactions or other issues related to viral vectors.

Gene splicing

It is relatively easy to cut or to excise completely regions of the chromosome of bacteria using restriction enzymes that cleave the DNA at fixed recognition sites and then insert genes of one's choosing into the gap. Restriction scissors that make "sticky end" (irregular) cuts are generally preferred to those that make "clean" cuts straight across both DNA chains. It is also possible to insert genes into bacterial plasmids and then permit wild-type bacterium to take up these genetic elements from the environment. Either process results in a novel ability for the organism. In this way, bacteria can be modified to make biochemicals that are useful in human medical practice, such as human growth hormone. These techniques are now so routine that they are part of ordinary high school biology laboratory exercises!

Cloning

One oocyte from an adult sheep is taken, its nucleus is removed mechanically, and then the nucleus from a mature somatic cell of another adult sheep is swapped in, it is incubated in vitro for a bit, then it is placed into the uterus of yet a third sheep, and a cloned sheep is the result. The science is remarkable here in that mature DNA is able to direct the formation of an entire new mammal – all the embryological steps, all the apoptotic changes, etc. This shows that DNA that has been silenced or inactivated is still there to be expressed. However, the DNA that was used to make Dolly the cloned sheep in 1996 was old DNA with disappearing telomeres, and she died after just six years. So the clone was almost perfect; she had a young-appearing body that underwent premature aging and death.

Karyotype

Many cell types will suffice for karyotypes – chorionic villus cells harvested during amniocentesis, white blood cells, skin cells, cancer cells from biopsies, and so on. The cells are placed into tissue culture; colchicine, which disrupts spindles, is used to stop mitosis during the metaphase. Individual cells are then examined under the microscope after special staining of chromosomes. The size of each chromosome, the position of its centromere, and banding patterns are then compared to make a count and an analysis for deleted or transposed segments, etc. Spectral karyotyping is a newer technique in which the chromosomes are bathed in specific fluorescent molecular probes and then examined by digital optical techniques. In this way, the digital camera records small differences that cannot be detected by the eye. Chromosomes are assigned a color (for example, number three is hot pink) and paired in that manner.

Genetic counseling

Couples who are interested in becoming parenting or those who are pregnant with or have already borne a child afflicted with a genetic condition are naturally interested in a thorough explanation of the chances of a genetic disorder in future progeny. It is critical to advise them that not all chromosomal problems are *heritable*, but some are. The neurodegenerative condition known as Tay–Sachs disease is due to an autosomal recessive gene, and so the chances for occurrence or recurrence can be reasonably stated with a careful pedigree and demonstration to the parents of a simple Punnett square. Likewise, the inheritance of sex-linked traits – both dominant and recessive – is fairly predictable. Not all genetic disorders are due to gene problems, per se. For example, trisomy 21 (Down's syndrome) is due to nondisjunction of this autosomal chromosome, either in the mother (about 90% of cases) or in the father (the remaining 10%). Because the condition is very strongly linked to maternal age of 40+ years at conception, it has a reasonably high recurrence risk in older mothers. Likewise, schizophrenia and myelomeningocele, both complex disorders, have strong familial associations that must be articulated to the parents.

Amniocentesis

The tissues of the trophoblast are all fetal, as are amniotic membrane cells, and of course all the chemical products in the amniotic fluid. Thus, this is a reasonable way to biopsy the fetus, so to speak. The test is used for the determination of triploid states and to definitively prove the sex of the fetus. In addition, examination for alpha-fetoprotein is done to determine the likelihood of neural tube defects. (Note: fetal sex and myelomeningoceles are anatomic issues that are almost always clear on ultrasound, which is used to guide the amniocentesis needle.) Tests for chemicals found in pulmonary alveolar surfactant can also be done to assess the degree of fetal lung maturity. The risk of fetal death due to miscarriage is low – around 1/1,000–2,000, and infection is rare. The greatest problem is the ethical dilemma of what to do when a genetic abnormality is found.

Congenital condition and genetic condition

Congenital conditions are those you are born with – a ventricular septal defect, red hair, thalassemia, a myelomeningocele. Genetic problems are inherited and could be passed on to new generations. For example, you might be born with a defect in the p53 tumor suppressor gene and later develop the condition of multiple neoplasias known as Li–Fraumeni syndrome. There does not appear to be anything wrong at birth, but the problem is both congenital and heritable. If you die before you have offspring, the gene will die with you, but if you do have children, it will be passed as an autosomal dominant on chromosome 17.

Gene crossover

Crossover is key to genetic diversity. During meiosis (only), synaptonemal complexes form, in which homologous chromosomes lie adjacent to each other. Suppose that a given person has traits ABC on one chromosome and abc alleles on the other. Further assume that loci for A (or a) and B (or b) are fairly close together on the long arm, but both are far from locus C (or c). During meiosis, two ABC and two abc chromosomes are formed. One ABC chromosome will not be affected, and one abc will not be affected, so these will enter a germ cell unchanged. The remaining homologous ABC and abc lie alongside each other. They cross at multiple places, like two ropes lazily splayed over each other. DNA breaks and reforms without regard to the original order of chromosomes. A new pair of chromosomes is formed – perhaps ABc and abC, or possibly AbC and aBc, or it is possible that no change will occur at all. Because the loci for A (or a) and B (or b) are physically close together, they tend to travel together; that is, they show linkage. They are not as linked to C (or c), because it is remotely located.

Genetic mutation

Environmental factors such as ionizing radiation (tanning beds, gamma rays from the sun, medical x-rays, and radon gas) and chemicals (superoxides, chromium, aniline, benzene, nitrosoureas) can cause mutations, and some of these mutations are additionally carcinogenic. The carcinogenicity of viruses has been proven, but this is not exactly mutagenic in the usual sense of the word. Remember that genetic variation and hence evolution occur spontaneously. Genes may be more or less stable over time, or they may be more delicate and unstable. Probably the most important cause of mutation is intrinsic errors in copying, with base substitution, frame-shift reading errors, and the like. Chromosomal translocations or inversions may lead to faulty transcription, as well.

Trisomy

Trisomy occurs due to nondisjunction of autosomes or sex chromosomes during meiosis. The disorder can arises during meiosis stage I or II. Putative causes include faulty centromeres or improper attachment of microtubules to the centromere, adherence of sister chromatids, and microtubular dysfunction. Many malignant tumor cells demonstrate partial or complete aneuploidy – that is, they might have trisomy of just one autosome, or they might be 3n or 4n cells jammed with chromosomes.

Short arm deletion

Deletion of genetic material is usually a bad thing, but recall that there is evidence of a gradually shrinking Y chromosome. In autosomes, most deletions probably occur due to failure of a DNA crossover segment to attach to its new target strand. If a deletion is not fatal to the individual, then during the production of germ cells in this individual, homologous chromosomes will have to develop an unmatched loop to line up properly with the chromosomes that remain on its sister chromatic. Small losses can occur during translocation, as well.

Klinefelter's syndrome

Klinefelter's syndrome affects around 1 in 1,500 males. Patients demonstrate variable degrees of feminization. Due to nondisjunction of chromosomes during meiosis in either parent, the resulting offspring has a 47, XXY karyotype. Mosaic individuals (46, XY / 47, XXY) have been identified. The diagnosis is made by formal karyotyping or alternatively, by the demonstration of a Barr body in a phenotypic male. Diminished fertility is very common. The patients are described as weak, rather asthenic youngsters who later develop gynecomastia and endomorphic body habitus. Endocrine therapy and counseling may help these patients adapt to this genetic disorder.

Frame shift mutations

Frame shift mutations occur when one or two base pairs are deleted from the DNA chain. RNA polymerase just transcribes what is written, so it ends up coding for different amino acids from the error point all the way to the end of the protein. In fact, even the stop codons, UAA, UAG, and UGA might be "missed." The result might be acceptable (or not) if it was at the very end of a long polypeptide coding for an enzyme. If it was far removed from the active portion of the protein, then slight misfolding might not be disastrous. If the error is near the front end of m-RNA transcription, a meaningless protein will be constructed. If this is an important structural or enzymatic protein, death of the organism is likely.

Chromosomal inversion

There is nothing magic about having 46, XY genetics, nor is there anything special about having a gene for a given protein on chromosome 1 versus 4, for example. Chromosomal inversion refers to the upside-down reinsertion of a chromosome segment, and it is usually of limited consequence to the person bearing the altered arrangement, except that it makes meiosis more difficult and there may be faulty production of germ cells as a consequence. It arises when breakage repairs occur incorrectly. Although these are usually very small segments within one chromosome arm, they may also involve long segments including the centromere.

Chromosomal translocation

The Philadelphia chromosome is a reciprocal translocation (exchange) of genetic material between chromosome 22 and chromosome 9. Although the individual has the same amount of genetic information in the cells, the exact rearrangement creates a "fusion" of two genes with resultant overexpression of tyrosine kinase. This chromosome is a common marker in chronic myelogenous leukemia, and it occurs to a lesser extent in pediatric cases of acute lymphoblastic leukemia (ALL). (Balanced translocations are essentially exchanges of pieces of DNA between nonhomologous chromosomes.)

The Y chromosome

The Y chromosome is quite small. In humans, it is believed to bear fewer than 90 genes, and most of these do not directly code for proteins. In fact, microdeletion of the Y chromosome in men may have no discernible effect. The SRY gene, which directs testicular development in the fetus, is probably the most notable gene on the Y chromosome. There was a homology between X and Y chromosomes in antiquity when both were more autosomal in character. In view of the fact that the Y chromosome is unstable, that many high animals do not have a strict X-Y system relating to gender, and that the chromosome is growing smaller over time, it is no surprise that females do not need one. XYY males were once thought to be overly aggressive and more likely to commit crimes, but this idea has been refuted.

Trinucleotide expansion disease

Huntington's disease and certain spinocerebellar degenerations occur due to a so-called trinucleotide expansion. The CAG trinucleotide codes for glutamine, and in these disorders, useless sequences of 20 or more glutamines may be created. These polyglutamine tracts make the protein more subject to aggregation. From hundreds to thousands of CGG repetitions in the X chromosome underlie the fragile X syndrome. The concept of a stuttering allele implies that repetitions are progressively severe across generations.

DNA repair mechanisms

DNA undergoes different sorts of damage all the time, so there must be an array of repair strategies to deal with each. Damage to the bases is common. Radiation-induced pyrimidine dimerization is reversed by an enzyme that itself is activated by energetic radiation. Methylated guanine can be demethylated by a protein acceptor. Breaks in just one strand of DNA are fairly easy to fix by base or nucleotide excision repair enzymes. Double-strand breaks are corrected by end-joining techniques using DNA ligase type IV, or else by using a homologous template to scaffold a reconstruction.

Homeobox genes

Homeobox (Hox) genes are a set of genes coding for nuclear regulatory proteins that are key to the organization of the body during embryogenesis. The genes interact with each other in a complex, time-dependent mode to assure proper development of tissue layers, limb position, and anteroposterior orientation. Deletion or doubling of one Hox gene has the effect of shifting AP orientation of body parts. These genes are highly conserved in animals.

Single base substitution in DNA

This is a question about evolution. There are four possible effects:
- Nothing at all happens. Because there is some redundancy in the genetic code, it is possible that the same amino acid will be coded as the one originally intended.
- Something bad, but survivable, happens. A faulty structural or functional protein is created, but the individual is able to survive. The affected person may or may not be able to reproduce.
- Death. The resulting protein is so defective that the organism cannot live a normal lifespan, but reproduction might be possible.

- The organism improves. Slight changes in the protein confer evolutionary advantages as the environment changes. Over time, this new gene becomes more prevalent in a population. Somehow, Cro-Magnon man was able to dominate Neanderthal man.

Telomeres

TTAGGG. This sequence is repeated in man dozens if not hundreds of times at each end of each chromosome to constitute a telomere, or end segment. These should prevent inadvertent end-to-end attachment of one chromosome to another. Additionally, and most importantly, they allow genes near the end of chromosomes to be "read out" entirely. If they were not there, DNA polymerase would not be able to copy the terminal information in a chromosome, so information would be lost at each cell division. The enzyme telomerase is responsible for adding new telomeres as old ones are degraded. Loss of telomeres does occur with aging, and this has been investigated with regard to cancer and other conditions such as memory loss. Telomeres are also important in regulating the number of cell divisions that a given tissue may undergo.

Polygenetic trait

An example of a codominant trait due to two genes is ABO blood type. If a person has both A and B genes, then both are expressed on the surface of red cells, leading to an AB blood type. Histocompatibility locus antigens are a second, much more complex, example. In more pedestrian thinking, human eye colors go beyond brown and blue orhazel, green, and gray. All are manifestations of multiple genes controlling pigment production and distribution in the iris.

Cardinal (and anciently observed) signs of inflammation

The four cardinal signs of inflammation are as follows:
- rubor – redness due to increased blood flow to local tissues
- calor – warmth of the affected tissue, for the same reason
- dolor – pain in the affected region due to the release of cytokines
- tumor – swelling of tissues in an inflamed region due to increased vascular permeability

It is critical to recognize these signs of inflammation in the situation of acute infections, such as streptococcal cellulitis. Some of them may be masked if the inflammatory process occurs in deep tissues, and some of them may be more generalized. For example, there may be fever as well as localized warmth in a deep tissue. Only the febrile element is readily discernible.

Factors that mobilize neutrophils to a region of tissue injury

It is vital to mobilize polymorphonuclear cells to a region of injured tissue. Attraction of white blood cells (positive chemotaxis) is based on the recognition of signal molecules generated by bacteria or by the liberation of such markers from injured host cells. Demargination of white cells or detachment from anchorages in places such as the spleen, results in immediate increase in the white cell count far over what could occur by increased production. Once white cells are in a region of damaged tissue, they must adhere to capillary surfaces. The actual diapedesis of leucocytes may depend on activation of actin components in the cytoplasm of the white cells. One of the most important chemoattractants is the class of formylated peptides, which are generated by invading bacteria. Successful destruction of the bacteria results in diminished attraction of the pool leucocytes.

Opsonization

Opsonization refers to the binding of the fragment antigen-binding (Fab) portion of an antibody to an invasive pathogen, such as *Pneumococcus*. Obviously, both immunization and prior exposure lead to the development of antibodies that can recognize the bacterium. The effect of opsonization varies. In the classic sense, the Fc portion of the antibody binds to phagocyte receptors and facilitates the ingestion and then destruction of the bacterium. In some circumstance, the Fc component of the antibody binds with a natural killer cell, a monocyte, or a granulocyte to release lysins. Phagocytosis of the involved bacterium is then not necessary for killing it.

Cytokines

Cytokines are a diverse group of chemicals (mostly molecules such as polypeptides or glycoproteins) that are involved in cellular signaling. They include up to 36 interleukins and the interferons. Cytokine interaction with a target cell may stimulate or retard the expression of certain proteins, but the overall effect in the system is to coordinate cellular responses to perturbations such as oxidative stress, viral invasion, or the expression of novel proteins by host cells. In the latter capacity, they are important in autoimmune disease.

Platelet adherence to an area of injured vascular endothelium

Injured cells deep to the endothelium elaborate the membrane-bound glycoprotein thromboplastin into the interstitium. Some cells also produce a form that can be released into the bloodstream. Exposure of platelets to this "tissue factor" causes them to aggregate, which is the very first step in the control of hemorrhage. These platelet conglomerates plug holes in the endothelium and also attach to collagen fibers in exposed tissue. Aspirin irreversibly blocks the action of cyclooxygenase 1 (COX1), an enzyme in the chain responsible for making thromboxane. Adjacent platelets are not activated, and remote platelets are not attracted in this situation, so oozing occurs.

Thrombosis

Thrombosis, the formation of a clot, requires the participation of cellular elements along with a biochemical cascade. Working backward, the last thing that happens is the formation of fibrin from fibrinogen. Factor XIII shores up the fibrin by creating cross-linkages. The factor that converts fibrinogen to fibrin is the serine-protease enzyme thrombin. Thrombin itself arises from the conversion of prothrombin in the presence of activated factor X. Here, again going backward, the pathway diverges. Factor X can be activated either by a tissue factor-factor VII complex (the extrinsic system) or else by a cascade involving (going upstream) factors IX, XI, and XII (the intrinsic pathway). All of these steps are dependent upon the presence of calcium. Perhaps you noticed that factor VIII was missing from the discussion? This substance is used to treat hemophilia and it serves as a cofactor, along with calcium and a platelet membrane factor, to catalyze the conversion of factor X to factor X_a in the intrinsic pathway.

C-reactive protein (CRP)

This pentameric protein responds very nonspecifically to the presence of phosphocholine in the membranes of dying or dead cells. It works by activating the complement system, which signals for phagocytic cells to move toward an area of devitalized tissue. Levels of CRP are used as a general marker of inflammation, and it can be elevated due to gingivitis or a heart attack or in immune diseases. High random levels of CRP indicate chronic stimulation of the immune system, which has been linked to the occurrence of diabetes, cancer, and heart disease.

Complement system

"Complement" is actually a series of about 12 circulating proteins that serve as first-line defense agents in the immune system. Opsonization of bacteria is a function of (specific) IgG and (nonspecific) C3b. C3b can be activated by upstream members of the system (the classic pathway), but in an alternative schema, a fraction of it remains activated all the time. Other members of the system are involved in aggregating particles bearing antigens and in chemotaxis of polymorphonuclear cells (C5a). The most interesting function of complement is direct lysis of cells (C5b-C9), and this mechanism is involved in paroxysmal nocturnal hemoglobinuria. Members of this system are part of the innate defense mechanisms that do not undergo modification by "learning."

Allergens and the immune system

An allergy represents the reaction of the immune system to foreign chemicals (usually proteins). Persons who cannot blow up a natural rubber balloon because of lip swelling due to residual protein in the cheaply treated latex have no problem whatsoever with reactions to artificially produced medical grade silicone, which is a rubberlike polymer. The reaction to allergens such as pollen is usually limited to rhinitis and conjunctivitis because the IgE response that is elicited is local in character. Mast cells and basophils degranulate in response to the combination of the antigen with cell-surface fixed gamma globulin E, releasing histamine, which causes the local edema, erythema and pruritus. Small molecules, such as certain drugs, can act as haptens; these form a circulating protein-hapten complex and also trigger an immune response. Steroid treatment blunts the process.

Anaphylaxis

It is not only *that* large amounts of histamine are suddenly released in anaphylaxis, it is also a matter of *where*. Hymenoptera (sawflies, wasps, bees, and ants) stings, medications, and foods, particularly peanut products, can all trigger the mass release of histamine (and some serotonin) because unlike ragweed or a contact agent, they are injected or ingested. There are significant populations of mast cells in the vessels of the lungs and heart and in the digestive tract. A histamine dump causes dilation of venules and significant hypotension due to the activation of H1 receptors. Bronchoconstriction and edema are also effects of H1 receptor activation. H3 receptor activation interferes with neurotransmission in multiple systems. Prompt supportive care with oxygen, fluid administration, steroids, and general support of cardiac output may save some patients.

Interferon

The group of cytokine proteins known as interferons serves to inhibit the spread of (mostly viral) infections, but they also have antitumor activity. Antigens specific to the invader trigger the release of interferon by an infected host cell; this causes a variety of responses in cells adjacent to the organism. Upregulation of p53 is common, but another effect – downregulating host cell protein synthesis and actually destroying existing RNA with the RNAse-L enzyme – stops viral replication but also kills the host cell. Interferon preparations have been used to prevent the spread of respiratory viruses, and they are employed in oncology, but side effects, some of which are very serious, limit their effectiveness.

Natural killer (NK) cells

NK cells are members of the innate immune system, which means they do not need prior exposure to an antigen to do their job. They use "granulozymes" to induce apoptosis (or lysis) and death in the cells to which they bind. They establish contact by recognition of modified MHC type I cell surface markers. NK cells also have inhibitory receptors that recognize self-MHC, bind to it, and prevent the NK cell from destructive activity.

Chronic inflammation

At some point, acute inflammation progresses to a subacute and then to a chronic phase. Antibody responses wane, there are fewer granulocytes in a region of tissue injury, and tissue monocytes and macrophages move into the area. In some cases, the process resolves without substantive local tissue disruption; there may not even be much tissue scarring. In other cases, there is modification of host proteins sufficient to cause lingering, or autoimmune situations to evolve. Gamma interferon released from natural killer and T cells is believed to be important in sustaining this process. In fact, antigen processing of just this sort may explain the partial control of cancers by immune modulation.

Granuloma

Granulomas are characterized by the appearance of two types of cells – the Langhans type, in which an aggregation of multiple nuclei is located eccentrically in the cytoplasm, and the central type, in which the nuclei are more normal. These collections are composed of macrophages that have usually gone through an eosinophilic stage referred to as epithelioid formation. The appearance is somewhat that of a syncytium, with cell boundaries often being indistinct. Granulomas are classic in tuberculosis and fungal diseases such as histoplasmosis, but they also occur in autoimmune diseases and around foreign bodies. So-called caseating granulomas are those with central necrosis, and these are more common in infectious processes.

Abscess

Abscesses are collections of pus, which in turn is a localized accumulations of live and dead bacteria, dead host tissue, and a host of white blood cells. Initially, tissues respond to an infection with enlargement of regional microvasculature and capillary proliferation. As time goes on, say a week or more, the body attempts to wall off the infected area by surrounding it with exuberant deposits of fibrin. Over longer periods of time, these strands come to be replaced with robust layers of collagen. Abscesses develop considerable pressure within them, facilitating the transmural leakage of cytokines, which produces painful regional tissue inflammation. Antibiotics probably penetrate the abscess fairly well for the first few days, but as the blood supply becomes diminished with the fibrin/collagen deposition, the contents become increasingly acidotic and anoxic, and little antibiotic penetrates to the depths of the collection. Bacteria may not grow well in such a milieu, but neither are they effectively killed. Drainage of abscesses, either by open surgery or with a needle, irrigation with saline (good), irrigation with iodine or hydrogen peroxide (better), or all of the above with capstone instillation of antibiotics (where they will be in astronomical concentrations) (best) is effective in eliminating well-defined pus collections. The early stage of abscess formation is referred to classically as a phlegmon. This is an area of infected, soupy tissue without clear borders, and it is best treated with antibiotics alone.

Tumor angiogenesis

That some tumors are bloody far out of proportion to their size is no surprise to surgeons. About 40 years ago, it was suggested that they produced this effect through hormonal means, now known to include vascular endothelial growth factor (VEGF) and a group of similar vasogenic proteins. VEGF and its congeners cause endothelial cells to divide and migrate. A very interesting facet of tumor production of these hormones is their ability to induce vasodilation by the intermediate NO pathway. These hormones work through the familiar tyrosine kinase pathway. The VEGF3-type receptor may induce changes in the regional lymph capillaries that are supportive of metastasis. Part of this family of proteins participates in normal embryology.

Histologic findings in an autoimmune disorder

Failed self-tolerance due to immune system abnormalities underlies autoimmunity. These disorders can be systemwide, they can involve just a couple of organ systems (ulcerative colitis and spondylitis, for example), or they can be very tissue specific (autoimmune thyroiditis). Typical findings include antibody complex deposition, particularly on cell membranes (antiglomerular membrane basement disease). Special stains for lymphocyte populations may demonstrate mixed types or single varieties infiltrating a usually thickened, edematous, and hypervascularized tissue.

Rejection process in a transplanted solid organ

There are actually two forms of rejection – acute and chronic. (Hyperacute rejection is rarely observed, and it is usually due to gross MHC mismatch or even ABO blood group mismatch. Preformed antibodies to certain antigens may be involved as a result of previous transfusions or transplants.) Acute rejection (one to several weeks) is blunted by antilymphocyte globulin, steroids, and cyclosporine. This process is due to the infiltration of CD-8 lymphocytes (cytotoxic T cells). Chronic rejection is both antibody and T-cell mediated, and it is better suppressed by tacrolimus, which interferes with IL-2 secretion. This is an indirect way of diminishing the population of T cells, but it increases the risk of infection from Epstein–Barr virus and similar opportunistic organisms.

Graft-versus-host issues

Graft-versus-host issues are most prominent when bone marrow or stem cells are transplanted, and this falls in the subacute to chronic time period for rejection. Host antigens tease the graft T cells into responding by releasing a panoply of cytokines, and a slow standoff ensues. Skin rash and inflammation of mucosal surfaces occur and sometimes elevation of liver function tests. The process is blocked by corticosteroids and to some extent, methotrexate. The process can occur when severely immunocompromised patients are given transfusions of blood that has not been irradiated.

Monocytes

These cells, which ordinarily make up about 4%–5% of the leucocyte population on peripheral smears, live in the bloodstream for a few days before either taking up residence in the spleen or becoming tissue fixed at other locations throughout the body. They can express CD14, CD16, or both. The monocytes that enter the tissues morph into macrophages or into antigen-processing dendritic cells. Monocytes can phagocytose bacteria and deliver altered remnants to T cells for further information processing.

Serum sickness

Suppose that a person receives penicillin treatment for a serious infection. Because penicillin can act as a hapten, it has the potential to induce a type III hypersensitivity reaction in which antigen–antibody immune complexes form and are deposited upon membrane surfaces. These cause further inflammatory changes in the form of rashes, fever, and systemic complaints. This process can begin after just a few days, or it can take several weeks. Discontinuation of the causative agent and either nonsteroidal anti-inflammatory drugs (NSAIDs) or steroids usually blunt the progress of the condition, which usually resolves spontaneously thereafter.

Immunoglobulins

The five recognized classes are as follows:
- IgA: This is found in secretions such as tears. It does not fix complement. It attaches to bacteria and prevents them from adhering to cell surfaces.
- IgD: This is found in low levels in the blood, but it is also bound to B cells. Its exact function is unknown.
- IgE: This immunoglobulin is fixed to mast cells and basophils, where it triggers histamine and serotonin release. It is also involved in the reaction to helminth antigens.
- IgG: This immunoglobulin is produced in large amounts as a secondary response to immunizations or to bacterial antigen exposure. It crosses the placenta.
- IgM: This antibody is the first one formed in response to an antigen stimulus. It does not cross the placenta, but it does fix complement.

B cells and T cells

B cells are the category of lymphocytes responsible for making circulating and secreted antibody; that is, they underlie humoral immunity. Clones of B cells arise in the bone marrow. B cells that first encounter an antigen ("naïve B cells") may become activated in one of two ways. In one pathway, the B cell establishes a contact with a T helper cell after encountering an antigen that it has chemically processed and attached to a MHC type II molecule. This is then delivered to the T helper cell, which can become a memory cell in its own right. Signals passed back to the B cell direct it to focus subsequent antibody production to the antigen in question. B cells can also learn independently of T cells. T cells also arise in the bone marrow, but they mature in the thymus, differentiating into CD4 and CD8 varieties. In the lymph nodes, CD4 cells go on to become type 1 and type 2 T helper cells, whereas CD8 lymphocytes become cytotoxic cells.

Wound healing process in a surgical incision

Surgically incising tissue lacerates it in a controlled way, probably destroying only a few cell layers on either side of the incision and driving in from the skin follicles a small amount of bacteria. In addition to sealing and ultimately healing the wound, cell debris must be removed and bacteria must be mopped up by the system of opsonization and phagocytosis. This occurs in the background of the reparative process. First, small vessels must clot so that blood flow ceases at the wound margin. Granulocytes predominate in the hours after wounding, but shortly thereafter, monocytes leave the blood and become macrophages in the wound, where they are responsible for proteolytic activity. Driven by chemotaxic attractants and wound hypoxia, capillaries proliferate within a few days, leading to the appearance of slight reddening around a healing incision.

Large-dose, whole-body radiation

Without experienced, intensive medical care, large doses of ionizing radiation delivered at one time are fatal. Unusual forms of emissions, such as neutron beams, have been fatal in seconds, apparently by perforating cell membranes and creating cardiac arrhythmias. Ingestion or inhalation of alpha-emitting agents radiates hematopoietic tissues continuously and from the inside. These patients all die within a few weeks. As used in preparation for bone marrow or stem cell transplant, whole-body radiation is fractionated, but the dose is still massive. Any rapidly dividing tissue is affected the most – skin, GI mucosae from the lips to anus, and of course the entire hematopoietic line of cells. If the brain is included in radiation fields, cerebral edema and death may come on rapidly. A person can survive this near-lethal experience if stem or marrow cells implant and if there is not excessive damage to the basal layers of epithelia.

Bone fracture

Mature bone consists of hydroxyapatite crystals laid down on a protein osteoid matrix. In compact bone, idling osteocytes are found deep with the bone, and osteoblasts on the surface of compact bone and lying along the trabeculae of cancellous bone are driven by calcitonin; they are involved in laying down osteoid and facilitating mineralization. Osteoclasts lying in Howship's lacunae are dissolving bone minerals under the direction of parathormone. When a fracture occurs, the blood supply is interfered with and considerable bone remodeling begins almost immediately. Fibrous union occurs first. Micromovements of a stabilized fracture create piezoelectric effects that stimulate osteoblasts to produce more osteoid. Additionally, osteocytes may undergo dedifferentiation to osteoblasts. Osteoclasts also consume small bits of bone to free up the calcium and phosphate ions. Signaling molecules such as bone morphogenetic protein shepherd the process. The gradual coalition of fracture fragments usually tends to turn off the process, although overly exuberant bone healing is known to occur. Many of these processes are at work in the pedestrian remodeling of bone into a bone spur.

Keloids

The disorder underlying keloid formation is poorly understood, but it is known to have a genetic association. Most likely, there is a defect in cell-to-cell signaling that should tell wound fibroblasts to cease collagen deposition. The lesions are characterized by the presence of excess type 3 collagen; the same product is found in other spontaneously fibrosing conditions such as Dupuytren's contracture or Peyronie's disease. Over time, some or all of this is replaced by dense type 1 collagen. Radiation of wounds is effective in preventing recurrence after excision. This unusual disorder can probably inform us about processes such as the formation of adhesions after abdominal surgery.

Partial donor hepatectomy

Cells that do not normally divide can be stimulated to leave the G_0 pool and reenter the normal cell cycle. This means they are capable of dividing again. After the insults of ischemia and surgical manipulation, hepatocytes enter a stalled phase; markers of hepatic function, such as the production of clotting protein and the ability to conjugate bilirubin, are deranged. Following this, liver cells begin a period of hypertrophic enlargement, but a subpopulation also begins DNA synthesis and cell division. It is believed by transplant hepatologists that the hypertrophic phase is necessary to signal the mitotic phase.

Fibrinolysis

Even after repeated small hemorrhages into the subarachnoid space, the brain usually does not stick to the dura. Why? Spinal fluid contains fibrinolysins, and it is these very enzymes that make rehemorrhage from an aneurysm a problem – they dissolve the clot tamponading the artery. Plasminogen is a protein produced by the liver and converted to the active form, plasmin, by tissue plasminogen activator (tPA). Plasmin in turn acts to cleave fibrin into fibrin split products (FSPs). Measurement of the D-dimer of FSPs gives a good idea of the extent of fibrinolysins occurring. Ordinarily, this occurs very slowly near a site of wounding, allowing other tissue processes to seal the vascular leak from outside the vessel. Clinicians who wish to unblock a thrombosed vessel will give doses of tPA or urokinase (which has the same action) to hasten the conversion of plasminogen to plasmin. Here, the danger of course is precipitating a hemorrhagic problem. Finally, epsilon-aminocaproic acid is sometimes used to inhibit fibrinolysins.

Diabetics

General factors that impair wound healing are poor regional circulation, impaired sensation (leading to sustained pressure on a wound, etc.), and the propensity for diabetics to develop wound infections. A major factor not usually considered is the direct effect of high blood glucose on the tissues; it tends to make them edematous at the same time the cells are deprived of intracellular glucose. Also, it is known that hyperglycemia inhibits the function of granulocytes.

Neurological function at various stages of human development

Preterm infants are still undergoing maturation of many organs, but especially the brain. Even vital and primitive reflexes such as rooting and suckling may not be sufficiently developed for the infant to thrive. In contrast, term infants have an extensive repertoire of innate abilities. Infants rapidly gain antigravity function in the neck (at 2 to 3 months), then the trunk (4 to 6 months), and ultimately in the legs, permitting walking by about age 9 months or so. Speech is usually acquired by 12 to 15 months, and the typical 2-year-old has a spoken vocabulary of about 200 words; comprehension probably far outweighs this level. Motor speed and precision evolve in young children and progress through adolescence. Although brain mass is maximum by age 12 or so, adult behaviors are not fully developed until around age 25. Absent disease states, brain function is normal throughout adulthood, even though there is inexorable loss of brain mass (appreciable after the third decade of life). Loss of sensory input (presbycusis, presbyopia, peripheral neuropathies) adversely affects the function of cerebrally intact adults. At extreme ages, the effects of brain atrophy cannot be overcome by CNS redundancy, and forgetfulness, apathy, and frank dementia ensue.

Social and interpersonal development

Infants are instantly reactive to anything remotely unpleasant or simply at odds with their developing will. Small children are naturally somewhat reticent when it comes to strangers or nonfamiliar situations. Pediatricians are certainly skilled at eliciting the cooperation of children from about three years upward. Any parent knows that adolescence is a trying situation absent any medical issues and much more so if there are some. Friends become temporarily much more important than family until the high school years have passed. Young adults are just entering the discipline of a real job, and their behavior rapidly becomes more constrained than it was, for example, as a 20-year-old sophomore in college. It is fair to say that for any age below 30 or so, meeting the medical expectations of ostensibly healthy young adults is pretty easy. By middle age

(30 to 55), people tend to become more skeptical and demanding of the medical system. Also, these people are managing families, jobs, military assignments, and the stresses of caregiving for elderly parents. They are in positions of authority elsewhere in society. Appointment times are to be kept; laboratory results are to be available when stated. Yet, more experience in life teaches most individuals that doctors are people, that nothing is perfect, and that the medical system probably is doing its best most of the time; even people with substantial illnesses may show patience and understanding. These individuals begin to turn back to their family for various forms of assistance. Finally, during the senescent years, there is less involvement with the forms of care; some patients become passive and let their families and doctor make decisions for them.

Normal vital signs for a range of patients

The newborn will have a blood pressure in the 70/55 range, a pulse of 125 to 135, a respiratory rate around 30 to 35, and a temperature of 37°C, but these are all highly subject to the environment. The newborn vital signs are very sensitive to dehydration. A fifth and sixth vital sign might be added to newborns – the mass (3 to 4 kilos) and the head circumference (36 cm).

The 4-year-old has a higher blood pressure, say 80/50, a pulse around 90, a respiratory rate of 20, and a temperature of 37°C, virtually irrespective of the environment.

The adolescent has a blood pressure in the low-normal range of adults – about 110/60, a pulse of 70, a respiratory rate of about 12 to 14, and a temperature of 37°C.

The adult has a blood pressure of 120/80, a pulse of 70, a respiratory rate of 12, and a temperature of 37°C.

The elderly person has a blood pressure of 110/75, a pulse of 80, a respiratory rate of 10 to 12, and a temperature of 37°C, which is somewhat dependent upon the environment and body habitus.

Normal sexual development

There are two issues to consider – psychological development of sexuality and physical Tanner changes. Childhood is characterized by growing awareness that men and women are different anatomically and behaviorally. Preadolescents of age 11 to 12 or so have some understanding that sexual relations have societal taboos attached and that they involve genital contact. The physical development is not slaved to age. Male Tanner stages I–V demonstrate progressive enlargement of the testes and penis as well as the development of a male pubic hair pattern. Female Tanner stages contemplate the degree of breast tissue development (again staged I–V) as well as female pubic hair development. These are useful shorthand ways of describing the sexual maturation of children when considering endocrine disturbances. Coupled with bone age determination and dental eruption, they give a good estimate of the actual biological age of a normal child.

Physician–patient interview

Children who lack a substantive vocabulary must be interviewed through their parents. Even for 6 year olds, speech may remain infantilized – "boo-boo," "pee-pee," "owie," and so on. Children 6 to 10 years old with normal intelligence and social skills can usually be addressed directly as their parent sits nearby. Children entering puberty should certainly be able to describe symptoms to a physician and answer ordinary medical questions; at some point, it is important to ask both the patient and the parent(s) for permission to conduct this interview separate from the parent. Particularly sensitive areas relate to abdominal pain, low back pain, and any complaint whatsoever regarding the genitals or groin region. These may be coded statements related to sexual activity or sexual abuse. These are highly confusing and embarrassing matters for youngsters. Physicians examining older teenagers and college-age individuals must remember that these groups may fundamentally know nothing about how their bodies work and therefore do not know which symptoms might be important. It is a reasonable physician expectation that adults have some knowledge of why they have come to see the doctor, and they can usually direct the interview in productive ways. Very old adults may not be so clear about their complaints because they may have many coexisting problems, everything might hurt, and they may be depressed about their health.

Physician–patient relationship

Medicine is practiced in both a legal and a moral framework. In the former sense, the relationship is contractual in nature – both parties agree in advance to a mutual exchange of certain services for certain goods (remuneration). Because of the typically marked difference in knowledge of the parties in a medical transaction, coupled with the exotic nature of the services provided, and amplified by real dangers, misunderstandings and conflicts are certain to arise, sometimes leading to lawsuits. Then, too, medicine is so much more than a business. The physician must sometimes undertake the most diligent and demanding care of the most difficult patient with absolutely no expectation of being compensated because of the moral impositions freely entered into by recitation of the Hippocratic oath.

A passive-dependent patient is difficult to care for, because the entire burden of getting well is placed upon the provider. Indeed, it is sometimes almost a game to get information from these individuals that "normal" people would volunteer. The obsessive-compulsive family member will sit at the bedside of a sick relative and be able to account to the attending physician the next morning every nuance of ventilator setting, sputum production, and time of administration of antibiotics in a way that challenges and frustrates the health-care team. A cyclothymic patient will decide with enthusiasm to pursue a treatment plan, but when next seen in the office, it will be discovered that he has not complied with the plan at all because of having a "low" period. The sociopathic patient will do everything to manipulate the system to her advantage – frankly lying about facts, misrepresenting other issues, etc. Even when patients are clearly medically ill, they continue to be very difficult to manage.

Although medicine has been traditionally the bailiwick of males, females have come to represent the majority of medical students in many schools in the United States and in many other countries over the past three decades. Gender does play an important part of medical practice, particularly in obstetrics/gynecology and pediatrics, and also in urology. Adult patients may be more comfortable with physicians of the same gender, and women are frequently viewed as the more patient, kindly pediatricians. Certain cultures do not ordinarily view women as competent decision makers, however. Contrapuntally, certain groups may view male physicians as too authoritarian. Physicians of either gender must recognize that they will not be universally received well by certain patients or families strictly because of something beyond their control – their own gender.

By and large, socioeconomic status is directly correlated with education, although exceptions surely exist. A certain enlightened paternalism must underlie the discussion between certain underprivileged patients/families and their physician. There may be an unusually accepting attitude toward formidable procedures or treatments, or conversely there may be obstinate resistance to highly routine and rewarding interventions, such as an appendectomy. A good rule of thumb is for the physician to attempt to view things from the patient's vantage point. Wealthy patients may have arrived at that status by dint of hard work and strong intellect, and these patients are likely to understand the concepts of patience and uncertainty. Others may just be demanding – for instance, a "society mother" who demands antibiotics for her child with an obvious viral infection. Neither the wealth nor poverty of the patient should deter the physician from sound medical decision making.

Ethnicity and religion play important roles in all aspects of the physician–patient relationship, literally from cradle to grave. Certain cultures would discourage the attendance of males (physician, nurse, or husband) at births, for example. Autopsy is not welcome in certain religions because it is considered a defilement of the body. Matters as simple as dietary preferences and religious holidays impact the delivery of health care, often in unanticipated ways. Immigrants from rural portions of Southeast Asia originally encountered major difficulties with the pediatric community because of animist beliefs and the specific renunciation of surgical procedures; these problems lessened over time with acculturation of the older individuals in this society. It is important to recognize fundamentally patriarchal families from those that function under a matriarchal system. Mourning is quite protracted and public in some cultures and very private and subdued in others. It is a mistake to assume that ethnicity confers expected behaviors – not all Poles are Catholic; not all people from India are Hindu, refrain from eating beef, or bathe in the Ganges River; and some people from South America are Jewish or Muslim. Unfamiliar styles of clothes and foreign accents may accompany high degrees of sophistication and education.

Clinical interactions between doctors, patients, and families

Patients and their families may be wide-eyed novices to the medical experience, or they may be weary veterans with definite expectations. A single bad past experience (a frightening drug reaction, for example) may lead to increased wariness and questioning of what the physician considers routine decisions. On the other hand, a generally positive set of past experiences might dissuade patients from questioning the appropriateness of a major intervention, even when they should. Important negative experiences with the medical system (access issues, insurance or billing issues, negligent care, etc.) should be addressed by new caregivers at the onset of patient care. Likewise, a *laissez faire* or even flippant demeanor by patients should be discouraged. It is prudent to remind patients in either category that modern medical practice is fragmented and highly complex and that the best results will more likely be obtained if patient, family, and physician all work observantly and cooperatively, dealing with concerns before they become overt problems.

Adaptive responses to the stress of illness in a patient and her family

That which is adaptive for the patient and her family may seem odd or useless to the physician. Nonetheless, these coping mechanisms may help patients "hang on" in times of great stress. For example, it may aid a family to be informed of the smallest details of care, even though the nurses and physicians understand that these are medically inconsequential. Conversely, a spouse who stays away from the hospital may only be shielding himself from very unpleasant developments in the health of his wife, rather than being uncaring. A desire to "have everything possible done" to save a patient's life is partially intellectual and partially emotional: the patient and her family may not be able to confront a terrible situation immediately and head on. Behavioral health specialists may be able to help patients and families adopt better coping strategies over time.

Maladaptive behaviors that patients and families express in response to medical issues

Overly demanding patients or families are often acting out of fear – fear that treatments will not work, fear that the care providers will not be responsive to their needs, even fear of an overwhelming bill. Unpleasant confrontations are more common than frank belligerence. Requests for second opinions are reasonable, but requests for *n*th-order opinions are manipulative and counterproductive. Likewise, being very late for or entirely missing meetings with an assembled care team does nothing to help the medical or social situation. At times, a patient's relatives may present to the hospital drunk or drug intoxicated. Unwarranted threats to report the care team to administrators or licensing officials are further damaging to patient care, whether or not they are carried out. Medical social worker or psychiatric input to these situations is sometimes helpful. Transfer to other facilities usually results in repetition of the same behaviors elsewhere.

Americans presently spend approximately 18% of the GDP on "health" expenditures

Increasing longevity (females have a life span of approximately 82 years and males about 78 years) causes an increase in the number and severity of chronic diseases. Care for diabetes, obesity, hypertension, atherosclerosis and heart disease, osteoarthritis, and kidney disease in the last years of life dramatically impacts health-care expenditures. Advances in technology undoubtedly enhance the treatment of diseases, but at an immense cost. The demand for sophisticated technology further drives expenditures upward. Simultaneously, low-tech, commonsense measures such as diet, exercise, and immunization, all of which have easily demonstrable positive health outcomes, receive less attention and funding. It is always preferable to prevent a disease rather than to treat it.

Patient view of the health-care system

Patients view hospitals and the health-care team with a certain degree of naïveté; often, this attitude is quickly dispelled by an adverse occurrence. It is important to understand that most patients reasonably believe their physician is in charge of things and that she/he can circumvent almost any obstacle to bring about a desired result. Practitioners, of course, know that this is not the case in many situations. Patients and their families might believe, for instance, that physicians are in control of hospital-employed nurses – after all, they give orders, right? Many items on the social agenda – parking, driving, access to services for the disabled, school attendance, and athletic participation, to name a few – have been "medicalized" in the sense that a doctor's letter or other intervention may exert a permissive effect. As the most educated members of the health professions, it is incumbent upon physicians to serve as spirited advocates for their patients.

Patient compliance with medical instructions

Failure to understand the instructions regarding medications is a frequent cause for noncompliance, and no small amount is due to language barriers – meaning both English/non-English and noncomprehension of the unique language of medicalese. Common sense to the patient may not be the same as common sense to a doctor – witness the case of parents who placed an oral antibiotic for otitis in their baby's ear canal. Of course, cost highly influences whether or not patients take their medications as ordered; many elderly patients may skip doses or halve doses to stretch out their pill supply. The availability of dependable, cheap transportation often decides scheduled clinic attendance. Finally, perceived barriers to care – for example, long waiting times and the lack of privacy in crowded facilities –impact whether or not a patient sees a doctor and actually benefits from the interaction.

Impact of denial on patient adherence to treatment regimens

Denial is an extremely important defense mechanism that should not be immediately taken away from patients and their families by forcing them to "face facts." Sudden, catastrophic illnesses devastate and bewilder families. For instance, how can a family know, upon first meeting the neurosurgeon, that their matriarch's brain hemorrhage will indeed be fatal? It takes a physician time to build patient trust, and it takes the patient and family time to adjust to terrible news. Denial also comes in small, daily packets – the diabetic who fails to adhere to her diet; the person who ignores a sensitive tooth until he has a dental emergency; or the parent who, never imagining measles encephalitis, refuses to have her child immunized. Denial is an important short-term psychological defense mechanism, but it is a poor long-term approach to health.

Motivational interviewing

Motivational interviewing is a technique involving the use of open-ended questions that enlarge the range of possible patient responses. For example, in discussing blood pressure management, a patient might say, "The medicine the doctor gave me didn't work." The interviewer then steers the conversation so that the patient comes to a new and useful solution on his own. If the interviewer were to say, "Well, sometimes medications must be used in combination..." or "Did you try a different medicine?" then the discourse is fixed around pharmacologic management of the problem. If, on the other hand, the question is represented to the patient this way: "What do you think might work better?" then a new line of responses is possible. A patient might say, for instance, "Well, the job stress is causing my hypertension, so perhaps I need to change jobs..." or "Taking care of my sick mother is hurting my health, too, so maybe I need to address that issue with my doctor." The patient is allowed to use his unique knowledge of his own situation to formulate creative solutions to medical–social problems.

Approaches to patient education that might be offered in different settings

Some patients are great listeners, some only learn by doing, and some learn best by seeing a demonstration. More intelligent individuals might require only one pass to learn something, and slower learners may require repetition. Because the goal is to improve the patient's condition, education should be available in several forms to accommodate different learning styles. Pamphlets that describe stereotypic conditions and procedures are cheap and limit the information presented to palatable amounts. Reference to websites is highly effective for some computer-literate patients and families, but even with these individuals, there is the risk of distraction and of being overwhelmed by information that is sometimes at odds with prior learning. Nurse educators are very effective communicators; often, patients feel more comfortable with a patient nurse than a doctor whose time they (correctly) perceive as being very valuable. Patients are sometimes more willing to ask a nurse "stupid questions" that might be embarrassing or display a level of naïveté that they do not wish to show the physician. Short videos are a popular way to educate patients. Also, certain group-learning situations (for example, prenatal classes or instructions for diabetics on insulin administration) are also to be considered.

Communicating bad news to patients and their families

No one wants bad news, and patients and their families are likely to react with silence, tears, prayer, denial, anger, and other responses. If a physician already knows a patient and their family, the element of trust is (hopefully) established and the affected individuals are more likely to be receptive and meaningfully responsive to subsequent information. The emergency room staff doctor who does not know a patient or his family has a difficult task when she imparts news of a serious medical problem. In either situation, a kind and patient approach, with the delivery of bitter information in small aliquots, is almost always preferable to a hurried, blunt method. If critical decisions must be made very quickly – for example, in cases that warrant emergency surgery or the initiation of extracorporeal membrane oxygenation (ECMO) – it may be best for a colleague or a senior nurse to sit with the family and present the adverse information while another physician works to assist the patient. It is important, however, not to be so vague and open ended that families or patients fail to understand the gravity of dire events. The (sometimes ugly) truth must be fully conveyed in a manner that allows patient/family comprehension and ensuing cooperation in formulating a treatment strategy.

Difficult interview situations

Here are three reasonable scenarios:
- "It's time to put Mother in a nursing home" (in front of the mother). – Here, the family is most likely, though not necessarily, working in the best interest of the patient. Certainly the mother should be interviewed separately from her family. Additionally, it may be important to interview individual members of the family, as well as holding a joint patient–family conference later on.
- "We need to talk about the factors underlying your daughter's suicide attempt." In this situation, the parents and/or step- and grandparents may have very different views of what is going on in the life of this adolescent, and all inputs should be considered in managing the patient.
- My nurse tells me you think the other doctor committed malpractice." This patient or family already has an opinion of at least a part of the medical establishment. Here, without agreeing or disagreeing, the physician must elicit as fully as possible all the prior statements made to the patient/family, the treatments, the problems experienced, etc. The goal is to make subsequent interactions with the ill person as useful as possible.

Informed consent

A patient may *assent* to procedures they do not fully understand. Very limited discussion may have preceded procedures that are routine for the physician but exotic for the patient – for example, a lumbar puncture. Saying "Go ahead," does not constitute consent. To give legally effective consent, a patient and/or their relatives must be informed of the *reasonably foreseeable* expectations of gain from the procedure and the *reasonably foreseeable general spectrum of risks* associated with it, and all questions relevant to the procedure should be answered before having the patient execute a document indicating their consent. It is not necessary to obtain consent for procedures with no foreseeable risk (an electrocardiogram [EKG] or a blood draw, for example). Although verbal consent may be sufficient in extreme circumstances, written consent is always preferable, and certainly witnesses should be identified in writing either way. Parental consent is typically needed for minors (< 18 years), but there are exceptions for truly emergent conditions or sensitive areas relating to sexual health and diseases.

Disclosures that should be made to a patient who is asked to participate in medical research

In most medical research, a new drug or device is being compared for efficacy against a gold-standard treatment. Patients who are asked to risk being assigned to the experimental pool should know that the "best" treatment was most often established in just such a trial. If the disease is very serious and the available treatments are themselves often ineffective or intrinsically dangerous, it may be that the patient has little to lose. Nonetheless, it must be made clear that there may be a *deviation from best (to-date) established therapy*. The patient must be given the option to withdraw from the trial if he/she so desires. The patient must understand that an election not to enter the trial will not adversely affect their care. Finally, any confounding financial interests of the investigator should be made clear to an institutional review board (IRB) and then disclosed to the patient. In fact, IRBs offer patients substantial protections against unwarranted risks in experimental situations, all the more so when a multi-institutional trial is undertaken.

Boundary issues between physicians and patients

Patients and their families are vulnerable because illness has disrupted their lives. They may seek fellowship, friendship, or sexual fulfillment from a physician in these circumstances that try their lives. Dating and sexual relationships with patients are always forbidden, and physicians contemplating such matters must first distance themselves completely from the care of the patient by helping that individual find another treating doctor, preferably from a different practice. A "cooling-off" period of many months to a year is recommended, as well. Even so, romantic involvement with a former patient is dangerous and usually to be discouraged. Certain instances of emotional attachment between physicians – who are, after all is said and done, people – are permissible; an example might be a friendship that naturally develops between the parents of a child with leukemia and that child's oncologist. Even such innocent interactions have their problems, however. A slightly reserved, professional, emotionally detached demeanor allows the best medical decision making for the patient and avoids legal troubles for the doctor.

Management of the impaired physician

Physicians may become impaired because of alcoholism, the use of other drugs, age, mental illnesses, physical ailments, disturbances in their practices, or emotional problems arising from stresses at home (divorce, financial woes, spousal abuse, severe illness of a family member, etc.) Because society has invested so much capital and time in the education of a physician, efforts are usually directed at identifying the cause(s) of erratic behavior and attempts to rehabilitate the physician rather than at punishment of him or her. On the other hand, patients must be protected from harm while such attempts are being made on behalf of the physician. Larger hospitals have advisory systems in place to assist with management of physicians who are not practicing medicine safely, and it is the duty of all doctors to report instances of apparent impairment at once. Physicians who are helped to recognize their problem and report themselves to the state medical board usually are managed in a much more lenient fashion than physicians who minimize and try to conceal their issues.

Medical records

The medical record is a legal writing that is used for the purpose of caring for the patient. It is the property of the entity generating it, typically a hospital or doctor's office. Patients are entitled to the contents of the record, but never the original, and not to portions of it that could be damaging to their health (such as psychiatric diagnoses, etc.). If the record is lengthy, a reasonable abstract of it is usually sufficient for patient treatment needs. Doctors usually provide copies of pertinent records free of charge, but reasonable photocopying expenses may be billed to a patient for extensive record duplication. Notes provided to the doctor by other physicians, therapists, or psychologists should probably not be given to a patient, although the content may dictate differently in certain circumstances. The record should never be altered to conceal an error, but amplification or simple factual correction is allowed if the correction is noted as such and dated. Military time is preferred, along with very clear dating such as 05 June 2013, instead of 05/06/2013, which could be read as the fifth of June or the sixth of May. Laboratory or other reports that are physician reviewed (and they all should be) should be initialed. Medical records are subject to subpoena and also to governmental inspection.

Brain death and the organ donation procedure

Brain death refers to the *total* and *irreversible* cessation of all brain function. There must be loss of consciousness accompanied by complete loss of brainstem reflexes (to pupillary, corneal, caloric middle ear, and gag stimulation). It must be demonstrated that the patient still does not breathe when the blood gases have reached serious levels of hypoxia and hypercapnia. It must be irreversible and not due to toxins or hypothermia. Pronouncement of brain death is equivalent to the pronouncement of "ordinary" (or cardiac) death: the patient has died. Families understand brain death better if there is some obvious cause – a traffic accident, a gunshot wound, a fatal case of meningitis – and they accept the diagnosis more readily in older people. In the very young, even skilled pediatric intensivists may have lingering uncertainties about whether or not all brain function has indeed ceased. Organ donation cannot proceed without the pronouncement of brain death, typically by a neurosurgeon or a neurologist (although in principle, any physician can make the determination), and many situations call for reassessment in 12 to 24 hours, "to make sure." Those making the pronouncement should not be involved in organ procurement or transplantation, to avoid any taint of impropriety.

HIPAA

The Health Insurance Portability and Accountability Act of 1996 (HIPAA) specifies, among other things, certain patient privacy rights. These rights are not new, but confusion has arisen over many issues. Common sense may not suffice to avoid trouble. For example, a husband telephones a doctor's office, indicating that he needs to know what time to pick up his wife after a procedure. Even saying "Five o'clock." may be problematic, as it tells some party (is he really the husband?) where a given patient is at a certain time. It is probably illegal to disclose the procedure or any other details to the husband without specific consent of the patient-wife (who is sedated, and therefore cannot give consent). Therefore, saying, "Well, she was sedated for her needle breast biopsy, so...." is actionable by the patient, and it may incur a governmental sanction (a fine). One area of disclosure that raises many questions in pediatric practice is the ability of a noncustodial parent to learn about their child's illness. Generally speaking, both parents are always entitled to information, although only one of them may be making critical medical decisions.

EMTALA

Because certain hospitals and doctors' offices refused to see patients with acute medical situations due to their inability to pay, Congress enacted the Emergency Medical Treatment and Active Labor Act (EMTALA) about two decades ago. Any person presenting to a medical facility with an acute condition *must* be seen and medically stabilized before they are transported to another institution for the indigent. Problems of interpretation are fairly frequent, and genuine issues of delay of care or inappropriate venue of care can arise. For example, if a small child had a mild asthma attack, but came to an adult facility that cannot care for her, is there a risk of liability by referring them to the nearby children's hospital? Yes. The Inspector General of the United States enforces this rule strictly. There is always a presumption that transfer occurred for the wrong reasons. It is incumbent upon hospital systems and practitioners to make a full showing of good faith by doing everything possible to facilitate care of any ill persons who happen to be on medical property.

Medical malpractice

An attorney will identify four elements to this form of negligence. First, there must be a *duty* to the patient. A physician who is on call for her practice has a duty to act responsibly for all patients in that practice. She has no duty to patients of other practices, unless they present to a hospital where she is on call, in which case she must respond to requests to see any patients entering the system. She also has a general duty to be knowledgeable and competent. Second, the duty must be *breached.* She does not answer repeated pages, she refuses to see a disagreeable patient, she misdiagnoses a condition, she botches an ordinary operation: all of these are breaches of her duty to the patient. Third, the breach of an established duty must be the *proximate cause* of an injury to the patient. If a dermatologist refuses to come late in the evening to see an unusual skin rash afflicting a patient in the coronary care unit, and that patient dies during the night of a papillary muscle rupture, there is no proximate causation. Fourth, there must be *damages.* A completely bald actor who underwent a craniotomy could potentially sue his neurosurgeon for a very ugly, unusual scar, but he could not sue under the assertion that the craniotomy made him ineligible to be hired in a role demanding a robust head of hair.

Medicare patients

Medicare is a federally funded and administered program designed to compensate providers for medical services to the elderly (> 65 years old), the disabled, and those with end-stage renal disease. Although Medicare historically paid at rates far below those of private insurers, there is no longer such a great disparity in reimbursement. Hospitals, as recipients of federal dollars, typically require physicians on staff to care for those Medicare patients who enter the system. Physicians owe the same duties of diligence to Medicare-funded patients as they would to any other ill individual. The government is extraordinarily sensitive to any perceived discrimination against Medicare patients and to any fraudulent billing for services that are not actually provided, unnecessary, or even mistakenly improperly coded. Physicians must therefore be extremely diligent when submitting charges for these patients.

Medicaid

Medicaid is a program jointly funded by the United States government and that of each state. It is designed to provide some minimal reimbursement for services provided to the indigent, typically defined as those at or below a certain income level – typically some multiplier (often around 125%) of the local federally established poverty line. The program serves impoverished children, the working poor, and those with no employment or income whatsoever. Reimbursement for services is often below the actual administrative costs of patient billing, supplies, etc. The duties owed to these patients are, nonetheless, identical to those duties owed to the most fortunate members of society. Because coverage is linked to income level, a family might drop off Medicaid coverage at one time (when employed), and then return to this protected status at a later time.

Abortion

Probably no other medicolegal issue engenders as much emotion as the issue of who should be able to obtain an abortion and under what circumstances. State laws are highly variable. Third-trimester abortions are, for all intents and purposes, illegal everywhere. Neonatologists are usually able to save the lives of fetuses entering the seventh month of gestation, so really the issue becomes one of premature, controlled delivery. Midtrimester abortions are sometimes permissible in some places, but there is extreme controversy in this area and all physicians should consult competent legal authorities before deciding to proceed. Most jurisdictions allow first-trimester abortions on demand (at least for adult-age patients), although there is sometimes a requirement for a waiting or "cool-down" period of a few days. The treatment of pregnant minors raises special liability issues for the physician in the issue of consent.

Laws governing reproductive health

Many public schools have condoms freely available in the nurse's office, often to the consternation of parents in the school district. The availability of contraceptive pills depends on visits to the physician and also upon the ability to pay for the drugs. Recently, Food and Drug Administration (FDA) approval for over-the-counter sale of several "morning-after" medications (estrogens, progestins, or a combination of the two) to minors over 15 has received blessings from the court system. This of course begs the issue of what to do with younger girls seeking postcoital pregnancy prevention. It is likely that informed consent must be obtained from both the girl and her parent(s) or guardian for nonemergent contraceptive therapy. Placement of an intrauterine device (IUD), for example, is ordinarily safe and fairly effective, but there is a rare chance for uterine perforation. The physician would surely wish to be protected from accusations of lack of consent in this situation.

Relationship of a physician to her/his cognate specialty board and to the state medical board

Most physicians choose to pursue residencies leading to board certification by one of the 24 specialty boards recognized by the American Board of Medical Specialists. Many specialties have secondary certifying boards in the subspecialties. For example, there is a Board of Pediatric Cardiology affiliated with the American Board of Pediatrics. Certification by these organizations indicates that the diplomate has passed a qualifying examination after a certain period of residency instruction. Each board has normative standards for its members, and at least some limited sanctioning of diplomates is legally recognized. Recertification at (usually) 10-year intervals is now common, if not universal. Such certification is NOT a license to practice medicine within that specialty anywhere. In the United States, each and every state has its own appointed board of medical examiners, serving in an executive capacity to regulate the activity of medical practitioners. Physicians have a strongly vested property interest in their licenses, and adverse actions by a state board are usually vigorously defended with the help of legal counsel. State boards have considerable power to subpoena records, hold hearings, and issue disciplinary sanctions, but always within a legal framework that preserves the rights of physicians accused of wrongdoing.

Relationship of a physician to other health-care providers

The physician is the leader of the health-care team, and he/she has unique moral and ethical obligations to the patient. Although the legal system holds accountable all parties who interact with patients, there is an unspoken presumption that the physician will function as the captain of the ship in all situations. Physicians certainly must demonstrate respect for other doctors, even when they disagree or when doctors have markedly disparate levels of experience with a given condition or a certain patient. Resident physicians are, by definition, physicians who are still learning, and they should never be subject to ridicule, harassment of any sort, or battery (pushing them aside, striking their hand in the operating room, etc.). Likewise, all doctors must respect the professionalism of nurses, psychologists, pharmacists, social workers, therapists, and hospital administrators. Disputes between professions arising in the course of hospital practice can usually be handled through a chain of supervisors. Rarely, it may be additionally legally required directly to report a professional to a state licensing board. For example, if a physician becomes aware that a

- 43 -

pharmacist is intoxicated on duty, or that a psychologist is sexually abusing a patient, most states mandate that other licensed professionals submit this information to the authorities in a timely manner.

Birth and death certificates

The birth certificate is always filled out when a fetus is born alive, and in most jurisdictions it is also completed with stillborn fetuses older than a certain estimated gestational age. Legally this serves as the state's registration of a new citizen. Problems may arise in the delivery room if one observer believes they saw a baby move or take a breath but other observers disagree. When in doubt, immediately consult the hospital attorney. Death certificates are a little less contentious. Brain death declared in advance of organ donation usually mandates a note in the patient's chart written some hours before organ harvest. (Often, the organ harvest service assumes hospital charges after this point in time.) The official death certificate should reflect the time of official declaration of brain death. The most important problem with death certificates is the statement of the cause of death. For example, if a severe diabetic dies due to cellulites after an amputation, how should the primary cause of death be listed – cellulitis, postoperative wound infection, or diabetes? Most death certificates use a format that allows for a primary and up to three contributory causes of death. Because these are used for official record keeping by many government (funding) agencies, their accuracy is quite important.

Outcomes-based reimbursement

This method of payment is already being explored in many locales. Fundamentally, physicians are now compensated based on patient interactions. They are paid some for thinking (initial consultation, daily hospital visits, etc.) but they are paid much more for doing – lumbar puncture, thoracotomy, stress EKG, amniocentesis, C-section. An unlucky or unskilled neurosurgeon is presently reimbursed for the initial shunt and each subsequent revision, for example. Under outcomes-based reimbursement schemata, a given diagnostic code will be compensated at a fixed level (modified, perhaps, by confounding factors such as age and comorbidity). Some complications (a fracture from falling out of a hospital bed) will not be paid for (at least, not to the hospital) because they are considered preventable. The neurosurgeon who can effectively manage hydrocephalus with a single shunting procedure will be better compensated for her time than the less skilled or unlucky operator who has to do the same operation several times to achieve the same result. In theory, this practice will gradually identify and best compensate the most qualified, careful practitioners.

HMO and the role of the gatekeeper

A health maintenance organization (HMO) is a medical practice system that diligently strives for effective use of services and thereby, for cost containment. As a patient enters the practice, they are assigned to a primary care physician who is responsible for their routine care and for deciding when to consult, when to order non-routine testing, etc. Ordinarily, these group practices have established certain annualized fees for each patient enrolled from large employers such as the government, a manufacturer, etc. Suppose the annual fee per patient is $5,000. This means that the directing physician, the "gatekeeper" doctor, will have this much to allocate for medical care, administrative costs, and staff reimbursement per patient. Some patients may not use medical services at all, or use them far below the $5,000 level – a "profit" for the practice. A single morbidly ill or seriously injured patient would cost far in excess of this amount, a loss for the doctor group. The theory of cost control is thwarted, however, by overaggressive gatekeeping (sometimes leading to delay of care) as well as sloppy control of referrals and by the necessity to deal with other elements of patient care that are outside the control of the HMO – trauma systems, mental health facilities, the demand for referral "out of panel" to experts, and so on.

PPO

A preferred provider organization (PPO) has negotiated with insurers, or with an employer sponsor of a group of insured patients, to be (relatively) exclusive providers of a certain type of service for a defined group of patients. An orthopedic group that is big enough to staff several hospitals in a city might bid for exclusive services with, for example, government employees. Then, any such patient, no matter which hospital they go to, will be directed into the care of that orthopedic group. Likewise, elective orthopedic visits will be vectored toward this provider group. The orthopedists have likely negotiated rather low rates of reimbursement in return for a guaranteed stream of patients. Patients opting to see other orthopedists would usually pay 10%–20% more to leave the panel of providers, unless the group certifies that the needed services are beyond their abilities.

Cost containment

It is incumbent upon physicians not to bankrupt patients, and yet there is a duty to be comprehensive, complete, and certain in caring for them. (In fact, the most common cause of personal bankruptcy in the United States is medical bills.) Without a doubt, the advent of modern technology, including the revolution in radiological services, has vastly added to the national medical bill. Sometimes it is the doctor who orders unnecessary or redundant examinations, and sometimes it is the patient or family who demands more testing. A measured approach to the provision of medical services, ordering consultation when it is necessary, and using conservative approaches to common problems (think "diet and exercise" before "weight loss surgery") will help control medical costs.

Consultant

Physicians have a duty to consult other competent physicians when a matter falls outside their specialty, or outside their abilities, even if it is within the same specialty. For example, every obstetrician should be able to deliver twins. An obstetrician has an absolute duty to consult relevant experts at a major medical center when conjoined twins are diagnosed; however, ordinarily, care should be transferred, or at least shared, with physicians who have unique knowledge and experience with this unusual matter. The role of consultant is difficult, and the margins are indistinct. A doctor sometimes finds a consultant suddenly ordering all manner of tests and even other consults on a patient for whom she was just asked to render an opinion. Perhaps all this information is needed to form an opinion, but no one has informed the attending physician of what is going on. On the other hand, a consultant may sometimes find that a patient has more or less been transferred to their care without their acquiescence or even their knowledge. Then, too, there is the question of whether or not the recommendations of a consultant should be followed. And there is the very difficult legal problem of when a consultant owes a duty (and how much duty?) to a patient: when first informed of their existence, when the patient is actually first seen, or when care has been officially transferred to the consultant. Plaintiffs' attorneys thoroughly explore this gray zone in malpractice actions.

Basal metabolic rate (BMR)

Measuring BMR is actually quite difficult, and it is rarely done except in research applications. It reflects an awake but resting state without sympathetic nervous system stimulation. Age and muscle mass influence the results, but there are intrinsic and important differences between individuals. Around 70% of daily caloric intake is expended in the maintenance of homeostasis, and 10% is spent to digest food. Around 20% of the daily calories go to movements within and of the organism. Of course, athletic training or severe stresses such as burns, illnesses, and childbearing dramatically increase the requirements for food and redirect the expenditure of these energies.

Essential nutrients

There are nine essential amino acids – histidine, isoleucine, leucine, lysine, methionine, phenylalanine, threonine, tryptophan, and valine. All fat-soluble vitamins (A, D [the body can synthesize some D with adequate UV light exposure of the skin], E, and K) are required, as well as the water solubles – choline, thiamin (B_1), riboflavin (B_2), niacin (B_3), pantothenic acid (B_5), pyridoxine (B_6), biotin (B_7), folic acid (B_9), cobalamin (B_{12}), and vitamin C. In addition to the obvious metals – Na, K, Mg, Ca, Fe, Zn – and anions Cl, I – and phosphorous – there are also requirements for small amounts of selenium, chromium, molybdenum, manganese, copper, cobalt, and chromium. Two unsaturated fatty acids are also required – linoleic acid (18 carbons) and alpha-linoleic acid (also 18 carbons). Notice that there are no obligate carbohydrates.

Ordinary protein–calorie malnutrition, marasmus and kwashiorkor

Protein–calorie malnutrition could be called undernutrition. Probably all readers have had a viral illness leading to poor oral intake for just a few days with attendant weight loss and weakness in spite of adequate hydration. Even in such simple situations, the body is deficient several thousand kilocalories, and hence has shifted into a catabolic or consumptive state. In a great many hospitalized patients, protein–calorie malnutrition occurs as a result of being restricted to intravenous fluids for a period of days. This condition severely impacts the ability of the body to fight infections and to heal. Marasmus is an unusual state in which protein use seems adequate, but there are insufficient carbohydrates. This is also called "dry" starvation, because children so afflicted appear withered. Kwashiorkor, with its signature reddish hair discoloration, is caused by the opposite problem – seemingly adequate calories, but inadequate proteins. It is characterized as "wet" because there is edema. Both conditions may relate to the cessation of breast-feeding. Poverty, civil wars and similar problems underlie a great many instances of infant malnutrition.

Calorie count and caloric intake

It is important to recognize that a dietitian's calorie is actually a chemist's kilocalorie. A calorie is that degree of heat required to raise one gram of water 1°C. Thus, a single calorie would heat an entire kilogram (liter) of water 1°C. This is a considerable amount of heat. Nutritionists use the "4-9-4 rule," which is a very general but nonetheless useful estimate of caloric intake. Each gram of carbohydrate is multiplied by 4 cal/g, each gram of fat by 9 cal/g, and each gram of protein by 4 cal/g. Thus, a sandwich with two 15 g slices of bread, 10 g of mayo, and 25 g of meat has (2x15x4) + (10x9) + (25x4) = 310 cal. Sedentary, smaller adults might only need 1,600 cal per day, but very active, large athletes might need 4,000 cal or more! An overlooked "nutrient" with zero caloric value is water; most adults need around 2 liters per day, depending on climate conditions and altitude. Adults require somewhere around 1,800 to 2,500 calories per day, depending on their size and activity levels. Older adults may require less because of inactivity. A newborn needs around

100 calories per kilo per day, and adolescents require somewhere around 50 cal/kg/day, depending less on gender than activity level.

Parenteral nutrition and intravenous hyperalimentation

Parenteral "nutrition" usually isn't. In other words, most administration of IV fluids just supplements or complements the daily need for fluid and electrolytes and provides very little in the way of nutrients. A typical replacement regimen contemplates around 2 to 2.5 liters per day of IV fluids; 5% dextrose in normal saline given at 100 ml/hr can be used as an example. The arithmetic shows this to be only 120 grams of dextrose (D-glucose) per day – about 480 calories – hardly anything for a sick person. If the patient can begin alimentation within two or three days, nothing is lost. But a week at this level of caloric intake would mean that the patient is between 10,000 and 11,000 calories in arrears. It is no surprise that very ill patients would quickly enter a seriously catabolic state under these circumstances. As a consequence, "hyper"alimentation (total parenteral nutrition) by vein was described in the 1970s and is in common use today. Although it is always best to use the gut when possible, central venous administration of recipes tailored to the patient's individual needs are now available. Using a combination of dextrose, amino acids, and fats, basic calorie needs are met. Usually vitamins are added daily and trace elements at least weekly. The main complications occur with infection of the central lines or metabolic derangements associated with improper choice of ingredients or faulty patient monitoring.

Unusual trace components of the diet

Most trace substances function in ways one might guess: enzyme cofactors, electron receptors, in metalloproteins, free-radical scavenging, and so on. For example, molybdenum atoms are a cofactor for xanthine oxidase. Capers are loaded with quercetin, and although a number of salutary effects have been suggested, there is not clear evidence of its role in nutrition. Most of it is cleared as metabolites through the urine within a few days of ingestion. Unusual foods probably do contain useful biochemicals whose role in nutrition is not even suspected at this time. Overconsumption should be avoided, but there seems to be little harm of occasional consumption.

Cholesterol

Cholesterol is an important component of cell membranes, and it also serves as the starting point for synthesis of the steroids. Interestingly, although many foods have substantive amounts of cholesterol (steak and eggs, for example), it is poorly absorbed by the intestine. Therefore, almost all the cholesterol in the body is made, *de novo*, by liver, adrenal, and gonadal cells. Production and excretion are balanced at about one gram per day. Cholesterol is also critical to the production of vitamin D, and it is secreted into the bile, where it may form cholesterol crystal gallstones. Any cholesterol that is absorbed in the intestine (i.e., any that is not esterified by fatty acids) is taken up into chylomicrons. The latter are dynamic entities that exchange fats in the bloodstream and may help signal for low-density lipoprotein (LDL, known as "bad" cholesterol) and high-density lipoprotein (HDL, known as "good" cholesterol) production. Probably the most important factor of cholesterol in the diet is all the other fatty products that are consumed alongside it.

Vitamin B_{12} metabolism and deficiency states

Cyanocobalamin, vitamin B_{12}, cannot be produced by animals; humans acquire the vitamin by consumption of meat, eggs, fish, or other animal tissues. Parietal cells in the stomach make a protein, intrinsic factor, which is critical to B_{12} absorption in the distal ileum. Thus, mucosal atrophy in the fundal region of the stomach or Crohn's disease may impair the body's uptake of the vitamin. The liver converts ingested B_{12} to forms useful in human intermediary metabolism. The vitamin has generalized trophic effects on a great variety of tissues, but particularly the hematopoietic and nervous systems. Megaloblastic anemia with hypersegmented polymorphonuclear cells (six or more nuclear lobes) is almost pathognomonic of the deficiency state, pernicious anemia. Neurologic symptoms of deficiency vary from vague weakness and numbness to catastrophic and abrupt paralysis, blindness, and dementia. Recently, the recreational use of nitrous oxide (NO) as an inhalant has been linked to the abrupt onset of neurological deterioration; the gas causes valence changes in the cobalt atom, which is at the core of the vitamin molecule, rendering it useless.

Scurvy

Vitamin C, ascorbic acid, is water soluble. Although most animals can synthesize this vitamin, humans cannot. And while some tissues (especially central nervous system [CNS]) retain stores of the vitamin better than others, complete absence in the diet causes symptoms of scurvy to develop within a few months. Vitamin C is a cofactor in a number of enzymatic reactions, including those involved in the synthesis of collagen; it serves as a reducing agent, or antioxidant. The symptoms are initially manifest in the soft tissues – bleeding gums with loosening of the teeth, poor wound healing and skin eruptions. Gradually, lassitude and apathy ensue. The best dietary sources are fresh plants such as fruits. Cooking destroys much of the vitamin. In western societies, scurvy is almost never seen, except in alcoholics or street people.

Vitamin D metabolism and daily requirements

Vitamin D has two constituents – D_2 (ergocalciferol) and D_3 (cholecalciferol). The liver hydroxylates ingested vitamin D, and this metabolite is converted by the kidney to the useful form, calcitriol. Vitamin D acts through a D-carrier complex in the nuclei of cells, causing increased intestinal absorption of calcium and phosphorous. It works in the kidney to cause reabsorption of calcium across the tubules. Although it actually stimulates osteoclasts to dissolve the hydroxyapatite crystals in bone, it also makes this calcium available for remodeling and deposition under the direction of thyrocalcitonin. Low levels in adults lead to osteopenia and then osteoporosis; in children, the same condition is called rickets. The actual levels of vitamin D required in the diet are not known, because sunlight exposure varies so greatly across seasons and with lifestyles. The current recommendations hover around 1,000 to 2,000 international units (I.U.) per day for adults and 600 to 1,000 I.U. per day in children.

Vitamin intake in pregnant women

Folic acid supplementation in pregnancy is now known to lessen the chances of myelomeningocele and similar neural tube defects. (Very recently, there has also been a suggested association between excess intake and autism, however.) Most prenatal vitamins contain the recommended 400 micrograms in a pill intended to be taken once a day. Because there is a concern that vitamin A may be deleterious to the fetus in high doses, this is either eliminated or diminished from usual content levels in regular adult vitamins. Of course, the baby has to receive iron stores from the mother, so prenatal preparations contain variable amounts of this. The fetus derives its calcium from the mother, at the expense of her bone, so it is critical that pregnant women drink plenty of milk and eat broccoli or similar foods containing high calcium levels.

Metabolism of calcium and the effects of hyper- and hypocalcemia

The body maintains normal serum calcium levels by balancing absorption and excretion with deposition or leaching from bone. Normal blood levels of calcium are expressed one of three ways in hospital laboratory systems; normal ranges are about 9 to 10.5 mg/100 ml or 2.2 to 2.6 millimoles/liter, or around 3.5 to 5.5 milliequivalents per liter. The causes of increased calcium levels include hyperparathyroidism, malignancies, and some medications. Chronically high calcium levels cause renal stones, skeletal aching, abdominal pain and polyuria, and, sometimes, neuropsychiatric abnormalities. Acute elevations can cause flaccid paralysis and coma. The QT interval is shortened on the cardiogram. Treatment includes diuresis and redirection of calcium into bone by administration of calcitonin and pyrophosphates. Hypocalcemia is usually a symptom of parathormone deficiency, such as might occur after thyroid gland removal with inadvertent resection of all the parathyroid tissue. It can occur with severe pancreatitis. Neurologic symptoms are the opposite of those in hypercalcemia, to wit: irritability, seizures and contraction of muscles to light percussion. The QT interval is prolonged on electrocardiography (EKG). Treatment includes administration of calcium and treatment of the underlying problem.

Iron metabolism

Iron is a critical nutrient; among other functions, it is involved in electron transport and it is the metallic component of hemoglobin and myoglobin. On the other hand, ionic iron is toxic, so most of it is found either inside cells or in bound form. It is absorbed in the duodenum in its divalent (Fe^{+2}) form. It competes with calcium, zinc, and magnesium for transport across the brush border by the divalent *metal transporter I enzyme*. *Ferroportin* is an iron-binding protein that is used to regulate the amount of iron in intracellular versus plasma compartments of the body. The complex protein, *apoferritin*, when combined with iron ions, constitutes *ferritin*, which is involved both in transport and storage of iron. Iron deficiency occurs when the diet lacks sufficient supply or when there is excessive loss (blood loss, including menstrual loss and intestinal parasitism). Hemochromatosis is a condition associated with excessive iron storage in the body; fatal hepatic or cardiac damage may ensue. Acute iron poisoning is always associated with ingestion of large amounts of iron supplements. Chronic iron intoxication probably does not exist per se because the body is able to substantially, though incompletely, downregulate the amount of iron absorbed.

Normal sodium homeostasis, hyponatremia, and hypernatremia

Almost all Americans get plenty of dietary sodium – too much, most dietitians believe. Normal sodium ranges from a low of around 135 mEq/L to about 145 mEq/L. Because sodium is so vital to maintaining water balance, it is carefully conserved most of the time. Hypernatremia may come about when there is loss of low-electrolyte solutions (sweat or insensible loss through the lungs in hot, dry environments), inadequate water intake, or both. Watery diarrhea and ingestion of seawater (around 3.5%–4% salt, as opposed to normal body concentrations of 0.9%) are other causes. Symptoms include lethargy as well as irritability. The correction by mouth or by vein should be gradual, so as not to shift free water into brine-logged tissues, which would cause them to swell. Low sodium is seen in congestive heart failure, cirrhosis, and in glomerulonephritis. Because very low sodium levels can precipitate seizures, 3% sodium chloride can be cautiously given along with a diuretic until sodium levels are out of the danger range.

Disturbances of potassium homeostasis

Dyskalemia is a serious problem. Particularly because of the role of potassium in restoring excitability to nervous and cardiac tissues, careful attention to serum levels is warranted. Normal potassium levels are about 3.5 to 5.0 mEq/liter. Hyperkalemia occurs after accidental intake or administration, in acute renal failure, Addison's disease, use of potassium-sparing diuretics, and during any process that lyses cells. The symptoms are nonspecific, and the condition is most often recognized serendipitously by "routine" blood work or by tall, peaked T waves on EKG. It can be treated by changing patient management if it is mild, by potassium-eluting enemas, and most dramatically, by the administration of insulin, which drives potassium into cells along with glucose. Hypokalemia is often the result of diuretics, vomiting, or simple underconsumption in the diet. IV administration is commonplace to replace loses, but the agent can never be given quickly by vein because it may precipitate cardiac standstill.

Hypo- and hypermagnesemia

Normal magnesium levels are about 1.5 to 2.5 mg/100 ml. Dietary sources include green leafy vegetables, some nuts, and to a lesser extent, fish and meat. Alcoholism is probably the most common cause of hypomagnesemia in hospitalized patients, and this is the reason people with delirium tremens receive magnesium by vein. Diuretics and gut disease are other important causes of low magnesium levels. Seizures may come about, necessitating IV replacement with magnesium citrate; this is also administered in preeclampsia. Hypermagnesemia is usually iatrogenic because magnesium is divalent; sometimes the contents of a bottle are labeled as milligrams per unit volume, and sometimes as milliequivalents per unit volume. The difference is twofold: one milliequivalent of Mg^{+2} is equal to one-half of one milliformula weight of Mg^{+2}, so that 1 mEq of Mg^{+2} = 12.3 mg of Mg^{+2}.

Heavy metal poisoning

Recently, teenagers in many states have developed high mercury blood levels after finding large industrial stores in abandoned work sites. The Environmental Protection Agency (EPA) considers these vapor exposures to be very serious. Mercury can be accumulated as a result of eating too many large fish (who, as apex predators, accumulate the metal in their tissues). Without a doubt, exposure to organic mercury compounds is often fatal. The metal produces peripheral and central nervous system damage, principally by competition with selenium-dependent enzymes. Lead poisoning is fairly common; the metal can be inhaled or ingested, as with children who eat lead paint peelings (a behavior generally known as pica). Lead interferes with a number of enzymes because it competes for their divalent cofactors. Lead poisoning produces a microcytic, hypochromic anemia with classic basophilic stippling. Cadmium, thallium, bismuth, and even silver all have specific described intoxication states. Unusual presentations of systemic illnesses with vague or protean neurological components should trigger the measurement of heavy metal levels in the blood or urine. Treatment usually involves chelation therapy with ethylenediaminetetraacetic acid (EDTA), which may be quite prolonged.

Temperature homeostasis

The fact that nurses spend a not inconsequential amount of time cooling and warming patients attests to the fact that temperature homeostasis is not easy for sick people. Certainly, the thermal conservation problems of newborns are obvious. It is not until about the age of six months that children can reliably be left under a light cover at normal room temperatures. Small children are much more resistant to temperature change as long as they are well. Minor illness in youngsters mandates more careful attention to fevers, which can cause seizures, and to chilling, which occurs easily in normal rooms if the child is not fully clothed. Until old age sets in, adults are resistant to cooling. About half of heat loss in a clothed man occurs through the head. In patients in the operating room, body cavities are often irrigated with room-temperature solutions. Although slight cooling – to 35°C – may exert some neuroprotective effects, there are adverse consequences to shivering and tissue acidosis. Overall, more than a centigrade degree of body heating or cooling is not without physiological issues.

Oxyhemoglobin dissociation curve

The oxygen pressure in torr (a product of the percent of oxygen in air and the atmospheric pressure) is plotted on the abscissa against the percent of hemoglobin saturation on the ordinate. The curve has a sigmoidal shape, plateauing around 100 torr of oxygen pressure. Ambient air has about 20.5% oxygen at a pressure of 760 torr (at sea level), so that means that we are ordinarily breathing air with a partial oxygen pressure of $(0.205 \times 760) \sim 150$ torr. But reference to the curve shows that hemoglobin is completely saturated around 100 torr. Man can travel roughly 2,500 m up until the partial pressure of oxygen is only 100 torr. This is the reason commercial airliners are only pressurized to this extent. Moving along the curve, we see that even at an inspired pressure of 50 torr, hemoglobin is still around 80% saturated. Now, hemoglobin has to have extreme affinity for oxygen in the lung but not so much affinity in the tissues, where it has to unload the oxygen. Acidotic conditions shift the curve to the right (unload oxygen from its carrier) as do higher temperature and increased 2,3-diphosphoglycerate levels in red blood cells. The reverse conditions make oxygen have a greater affinity for hemoglobin. Different hemoglobins have altered affinities for oxygen, as well.

First- and second-degree sunburn

Intense insolation of the skin produces injury by action of ultraviolet light in 280 to 400 nanometer wavelengths. Capillaries dilate, leading to localized erythema, and painful cytokines are released, making even the least touching of skin quite painful. These inflammatory substances pass into the bloodstream, so generalized constitutional symptoms of mild fever and malaise may complicate the picture. Severely injured skin may form bullae and desquamate over the next week to 10 days. Very gentle management of damaged skin is important. Although cool compresses are often recommended, very little pressure can be borne by this injured tissue. Nonsteroidal anti-inflammatory drugs and even steroids may be needed. Intravenous rehydration improves the situation. Hospitalization for pain management is sometimes required, and if in doubt, consult the local burn unit.

Flash burn

Skin surface area is calculated using the rule of 9's – 9% for each arm and for the head, 18% for each leg and for the front of the torso and for the back of the torso, and 1% for the external genitalia/perineum. Here, a second-degree, or blistering, burn involves 9% of the body surface. Additional first-degree burns of the front half of the head (about 4.5%), half of the anterior torso (9%), and "most of" the left arm (another 8%–9%) are present, adding to around 22%–23% first-degree burns. Third-degree burns involve charring of soft tissues (and therefore, full-thickness skin loss), and the rare fourth-degree burn includes charring of muscle or bone. The latter condition is almost never seen, except with electrical burns.

> ➤ **Review Video:** <u>Rule of Nines</u>
> *Visit **mometrix.com/academy** and enter **Code: 846800***

Scuba diver during descent and ascent

People can develop symptoms of pressure problems in just 2 or 3 m of water. For example, complaints of ear pain due to Eustachian tube blockage can come about in some persons in an ordinary swimming pool. Each 10 m of water is equivalent to an additional atmosphere of pressure. During recreational diving, inspired gases are dissolved in the plasma of the bloodstream under the ambient pressure – 1 atmosphere (atm) at the surface, but 3 atm at a depth of only 20 m. Most people with normal cardiovascular physiology can tolerate diving to about 25 to 30 m, provided that they do not stay long on the bottom and given that they ascend slowly. This gives dissolved gases (mostly nitrogen) a chance to leave the liquid compartment of the circulation, cross over into the alveolus, and be expired. Sudden ascent (necessitated, for example by a shark or an impending medical crisis underwater) allows dissolved nitrogen to bubble out into tissues, a condition known as the bends because people double up with agonizing pain. Placing the patient back into a high-pressure chamber drives the gas back into solution, but then "surfacing" must be done over hours. Permanent neurological damage is possible even with the best of treatment. It is injudicious for pregnant women, persons with seizure disorders, patients with sickle cell anemia or other hemoglobinopathies, or anyone with serious medical conditions to subject themselves to the hostile conditions under the sea.

Organophosphate exposure

West Nile disease is a mosquito borne viral infection with an increasing United States seasonal presence. It produces substantial disability and even death. Urban regions have undertaken widespread spraying programs mostly at night because many organophosphates decompose in strong sunlight. This group of poisons acts by phosphorylating (and thereby inactivating) acetylcholinesterase. This causes buildup of acetylcholine in synaptic clefts, with resulting stimulation of the subsynaptic cell. Muscle cramps and fasciculations develop, with pallor, seizures, and general vascular collapse. The compounds can be inhaled, ingested, or absorbed percutaneously, so this worker needs to be undressed and bathed with soap and water, while taking precautions to ensure the safety of the doctors and nurses. Administration of atropine and pralidoxime is indicated, as well as general support of circulatory status. It is important to know that chronic low-level exposures can add up to such a sudden clinical presentation. Coworkers should be examined and tested for exposure.

Toxic gas exposures

Fire personnel are exposed, first and foremost, to carbon monoxide. Although firemen wear protective respirators, leakage is inevitable. Extremely active individuals will have more minute ventilation and thus take in more carbon monoxide than sedentary persons. It is typical to rest fire crews in areas close to the fire, where they will have removed their masks; even further intake is possible in such situations. Homes in America can be full of flammable synthetic building materials or household items that, when heated or burned, liberate cyanide. It is believed that many individuals who died in recent nightclub fires did so because of cyanide from burning ceiling tiles. Firefighters at the World Trade Center on 9/11 experienced very serious exposure to silicates and asbestos. It is possible that fire personnel will also be exposed to mustard gas, sarin, or other deadly agents in intentional bombings, not to mention the potential for weaponized bioagents or radioactive materials.

Chelation therapy

Compounds such as ethylenediaminetetraacetic acid (EDTA) can form coordination compounds with a variety of metals, including iron and lead. EDTA is usually given as calcium salt. As it circulates, the central calcium ion is replaced by the target ion, either already in solution or leaching from tissues. The complex is then cleared by the kidneys. Each treatment during chelation therapy removes only about 1% of the target metal in the case of lead. Nonetheless, over time, toxic levels of metals can be milked down in this manner.

Dehydration

Infant dehydration is most often due to severe diarrhea. Adult dehydration can occur from diarrheal illnesses such as cholera, but there are many other causes due to diminished intake, excessive fluid loss, or both. In infants, the pulse can best be used to guide fluid administration. For adults, a combination of vital signs including blood pressure are reliable indicators of dehydration. Lassitude in babies and confusion in adults are signs of impending circulatory collapse. Consider that the blood volume of an infant is about 80 to 85 cc per kilogram body mass and that of an adult is around 70 ml/kilogram. Thus, a newborn only has about 350 ml of circulating volume, and an adult has around 5 liters. A fluid bolus of 20 ml/kilogram in the infant and around 1 liter in an average adult (with a normal heart) will often restore vital signs rather well, and a repeat bolus (or half-volume bolus) can be considered shortly thereafter. Increased maintenance doses of relatively low concentration electrolyte solutions in the baby (5% dextrose in quarter normal saline with 10 milliequivalents of potassium added) and standard Ringer's lactate are required in adults. Constant bedside attention is required until hemodynamic stability is achieved.

Metabolic and respiratory acidosis

Metabolic acidosis occurs when the intake and production of acid compounds cannot be met by their excretion (almost exclusively in soluble form in the kidney). For example, one form of acidosis (renal tubular acidosis) occurs because the distal tubules do not secrete enough H^+ ions into the urine. Another form occurs with aspirin poisoning, when large amounts of acetylsalicylic acid are absorbed into the bloodstream. In these situations, two things will usually occur in an attempt to respond to the low blood pH: the respiratory rate will increase (and pCO_2 levels will fall) and/or there will be an attempt by the kidneys to increase bicarbonate ion reabsorption. In respiratory acidosis, there is underventilation. This might be due to CNS lesions (coma, drugs), obstruction of airways, or parenchymal lung disease (less common). Blood carbon dioxide levels will increase, and the compensatory mechanisms are to increase urinary hydrogen ion excretion and reabsorb more bicarbonate ions.

Starling's law

On the arteriolar side of the capillary beds of many tissues, fluids containing nutrients, electrolytes, hormones, and other small molecules are forced out of the capillary lumen by hydrostatic pressure. The blood remaining in the capillary thus loses some of its water and electrolytes, but it retains large proteins as well as the cellular contents of blood. The osmotic pressure (we can also loosely refer to it as "oncotic pressure," meaning protein derived) inside the capillary is then raised above the level of the blood when it first entered the most distal part of the circulatory bed. Some of the fluid that was driven out can now reenter the circulation on the venous side of the capillary bed, facilitated both by an oncotic gradient inward, and also a lower hydrostatic pressure than on the arteriolar side. Not all the fluid does reenter the capillary, however, leading to a third circulation of lymph. This fluid enters terminal lymph capillaries, proceeds to regional lymph nodes, and ultimately reenters the venous circulation. Around 1 to 2 liters of lymph is produced per day. It is a critical source of additional tissue drainage, however, as shown by the effect of its interruption – lymphedema.

Henderson–Hasselbalch equation

The Henderson–Hasselbalch equation relates to this relationship of an acid to water: $HA + H_2O \rightarrow A^- + H_3O^+$. The acid that is most important in medical practice is carbonic acid, composed of carbon dioxide and water. It can dissociate into bicarbonate and hydrogen ions (first dissociation) or fully back into CO_2 and water (second dissociation). It is roughly 100 times weaker than acetic acid, but it will dissolve dental enamel! The H-H equation itself states that blood pH $\sim pK_a + \log [HCO_3^-]/[H_2CO_3]$. The pK_a for the first dissociation is 6.37, so blood pH is this number plus the ratio, effectively, of the bicarbonate ion to the pCO_2. This sets the stage for understanding respiratory versus metabolic acidosis and alkalosis.

Pompe disease

Pompe disease is due to one of several gene mutations on chromosome 17 that result in disorders of the enzyme acid α-glucosidase. This normally cleaves glycogen into glucose units at both the 1,4 and 1,6 bonding positions. The effect is that normally acquired glycogen cannot be broken down in the cytoplasm or in lysosomes. Weakness, lassitude, and cardiac problems alert the clinician to the possibility of this disease. Once uniformly fatal, there is now a possibility of treating the condition with recombinant enzyme therapy, but it is exceedingly expensive.

Carnitine

Carnitine is a simple molecule – a quaternary ammonium derivative of hydroxybutanoic acid. It is often sold in bulk quantities in health stores for its alleged ability to enhance athletic performance or as an antioxidant. This molecule is synthesized in the body (principally in the liver) from methionine and lysine. It serves to transport long-chain fatty acid components across the mitochondrial membranes and into the matrix. Here, they are enzymatically converted to two-carbon groups and then acetyl-CoA so they can enter the Krebs cycle. Thus, carnitine is involved, indirectly, in energy metabolism. Deficiency states have been reported in man, and they chiefly involve weakness or myocardial dysfunction under stressful physiologic conditions. Absent congenital deficiencies involving the ability to synthesize carnitine or abnormalities of the mitochondrial enzymes leading to acetyl-CoA synthesis, there seems to be little rationale for dietary supplementation.

Renin-angiotensin-aldosterone system

This is a marvelously engineered blood pressure and volume control system involving the liver, kidney, and lung. The liver makes the protein angiotensinogen. If renal juxtaglomerular cells in the macula densa sense low blood pressure, they secrete renin, which converts angiotensinogen to angiotensin I. Mostly pulmonary endothelial cells use an angiotensin converting enzyme (ACE) to change angiotensin I into angiotensin II, the active form of the substance. This has four effects:
- it increases sympathetic tone (and it may also act directly to cause vasoconstriction),
- it causes renal tubular sodium reabsorption; water follows the salt to increase intravascular volume,
- it increases adrenal production of aldosterone, and
- it causes the neurohypophysis to secrete vasopressin.

Thus, this system adjusts intravascular volume and blood pressure by short-, medium-, and long-term means.

PKU

Phenylketonuria (PKU) is a disorder of metabolism of the amino acid phenylalanine (PHE). This autosomal (chromosome 12) recessive disorder results in defective phenylalanine hydroxylase activity, leading to elevated PHE blood levels and of the levels of other metabolites of this amino acid. Tyrosine production is blocked. Intellectual disability ensues because amino acid transport into the brain is stifled by the plasma phenylalanine. Early detection and severe dietary modifications have produced favorable results, so perinatal detection is critical. A variant of this enzyme deficiency exists where the cofactor tetrahydrobiopterin is deficient due to one of four inherited abnormalities.

Lesch–Nyhan syndrome

X-linked deficiency of the enzyme hypoxanthine-guanosine phosphoribosyl transferase (HGPRT) causes hypoxanthine and guanine to be converted to uric acid, rather than recycled to useful nucleotides. This further stimulates increased synthesis of purines. Afflicted children are floppy and intellectually disabled. Self-mutilation (chewing off lips and fingertips, for example) is a striking feature in youngsters, possibly due to sensory impairments. Gouty arthritis happens early in a foreshortened life. Similar but less severe disturbances of the function of this enzyme are present in ordinary gout.

Porphyria

Heme, the central component of the metalloprotein hemoglobin, consists of an iron atom loosely bonded to four porphyrin rings. Porphyrin is synthesized in a number of enzymatically mediated cytosolic and mitochondrial steps. A key early metabolite is delta-aminolevulinic acid. In the porphyrias, there is sufficient production of the compound to make normal amounts of hemoglobin, but there is accumulation of one or more of the intermediate metabolites, which are toxic. Elevated urine porphobilinogen levels are a clue to the possibility of such rare conditions. Hepatic, or acute, porphyrias have alarming presentations with abdominal pain, constipation, or diarrhea and mental aberrations including hallucinations. The cutaneous, or erythropoietic forms present with photosensitivity, chronic skin rashes, and sometimes hypertrichosis, leading to the familiar werewolf legend. Inheritance of some forms is autosomal dominant, but autosomal-recessive inheritance governs other forms. X-linked sideroblastic anemia affects the early stage of δ-ALA synthesis.

Mucopolysaccharidoses

The mucopolysaccharidosis (MPS) disorders are connective tissue diseases caused by deficiencies of one or more of the enzymes needed for lysosomal destruction of glycosaminoglycans. These stromal carbohydrates then accumulate in various tissues, protean in their manifestations, but most notably affecting the skeletal system (dwarfism and severe deformities), the nervous system (platybasia, hydrocephalus, retardation, and corneal clouding), and the liver. Nine different varieties are described, and the accumulated material is usually the sulfates of heparan, dermatan, or keratan. A ninth, milder form involving hyaluronidase deficiency and hyaluronic acid deposition has recently been described. Note that these are distinct from the mucolipidoses.

Pharmacokinetics

First to be considered is the separation of the drug from its delivery vehicle. For example, certain drugs are prepared for surgical implantation in the form of bioabsorbable wafers that leach the drug over time. In order for a drug to be effective (at least, beyond a distance of a few cell diameters), it must be absorbed into the bloodstream. Factors that affect absorption include tissue blood flow for parenterally administered drugs and bowel function for oral medications. Drugs are distributed to different compartments; some remain relatively free in the bloodstream, some are tightly bound to circulating carriers, and others rapidly sort themselves into specific tissues. Many compounds are metabolized in the liver, but others, such as insulin, are degraded by target tissues. Last to consider is the means of excretion of the drug.

For example, around three-quarters of a penicillin dose is secreted in the renal proximal tubule within four hours of administration. By competitively blocking this action with probenecid, plasma and tissue levels can be forced upward. The idea of pharmacokinetics, therefore, relates to the fate of the drug from the moment it is given until it is completely gone from the body.

Zero- and first-order drug elimination profiles

Zero-order kinetics means that a drug is eliminated at a constant rate, no matter how much or little of it there is. The notable example is alcohol: there is steady removal of the alcohol from the bloodstream. Because this plots as a straight line versus time, it is easy to calculate what the blood alcohol level would have been at some time prior to the acquisition of a sample. In first-order kinetics, which applies to most drugs, it is the logarithm of drug concentration that plots as a straight line against time. For example, if 10% is absorbed per hour, then for a 50 mg dose, at one hour the residual drug would amount to 45 mg, at two hours it would be 40.5 mg, and so on. In theory, the drug is never completely eliminated. The half-life of a drug is predicated on this concept, as well as "loading doses" of drugs such as phenytoin. For this anticonvulsant, initial elimination is closer to first-order kinetics, but it shifts toward zero-order kinetics at stable therapeutic levels when the receptors have been saturated.

Urine pH

To answer this question, one has to know the main structure of the drug in question. If it is an acid, such as aspirin, it will be best excreted in alkaline urine. If it is a base (typically they contain nitrogenous groups), then it will be best excreted in acidic urine. Recall that acid + base → salt + water. The goal is to get the drug into an aqueous (salt) form. Lipid-soluble forms of the drug get filtered out of the bloodstream in the glomerulus, but then they are reabsorbed across tubular membranes. The ionic forms tend to stay in the urine. Vitamin C is a cheap and easy way to acidify urine; oral bicarbonate, thiazide diuretics, and carbonic anhydrase inhibitors such as acetazolamide will all raise urine pH.

Drug half-life

Drugs with first-order excretion kinetics exhibit the phenomenon of half-life. An example is the inotropic drug digoxin. In individuals with normal kidneys, the half-life is about one and a half to two days. Suppose a patient is "dig. toxic" because of a plasma level of 3.0 ng/ml (therapeutic is 0.8 to 2.0 ng/ml). If the creatinine clearance is normal, then one would expect a level of 1.5 ng/ml in just 36 to 48 hours. If renal function is markedly impaired, then the half-life is extended accordingly.

Volume of distribution

This concept is a manifestation of the process of compartmentalization of drugs. Suppose that a given water-soluble drug is administered intravenously in a dose of 5 grams, or 5,000 mg. If it were uniformly distributed only in the blood plasma, which has a volume of about 2,500 ml, then we would expect a level of 2 mg/ml. Instead, we find that within a few minutes of administration, the level is 0.1 mg/ml. This means that the drug must have distributed itself uniformly to all aqueous compartments of the body – plasma, extracellular fluids, and intracellular fluids – about 50 liters, or a volume of distribution of 50,000 ml. Of course, drugs don't behave this strangely, but the point is made: the concentration helps pharmacologists to determine the compartments in which a drug is initially sequestered. The calculations for lipophilic drugs seem ridiculous, ten thousand or more liters of fluid, but, of course, the idea is that almost none of the drug remains in a fluid compartment of any sort – it all gets absorbed into body fats.

Effect of renal impairment on drug dosages

It is not usually necessary to adjust the loading dose of a drug in the situation of renal impairment because for practical purposes, the volume of distribution is approximately the same. A normal glomerular filtration rate (GFR) is about 125 ml/min, and it is convenient to adjust the doses of drugs that undergo renal clearance with this number in mind. Online calculators (and problems with oversimplification of the result) abound. For a patient with a creatinine of 1.0, GFR is about 100 ml/min; it is one-third this when the creatinine has risen to 2.0. Then, too, one must recognize that renal failure has protean effects on blood pH, protein binding of drugs, absorption from the gastrointestinal tract, and hepatic metabolism to ionic forms that can be renally excreted. Further, hemodialysis and peritoneal dialysis may markedly affect drug levels in an individual patient. Finally clouding the picture is the specter of narrow therapeutic index and the danger of toxicity.

Phase I and phase II metabolism of drugs

Phase I metabolism converts lipid-soluble drugs into water-soluble molecules by subjecting them to redox or hydrolytic reactions. Cytochrome p450 is involved in the redox parts of phase I conversions. The resulting metabolites often retain considerable activity. The next step in drug elimination is phase II modification by conjugation into compounds that are usually highly polar (and, therefore, water soluble = subject to renal elimination). Phase II conversions occur in several different tissues, but liver and kidney predominate over lung and others. A phase-I-modified drug could undergo the additional processes of sulfation, glucuronidation, methylation, or acetylation, or it could be coupled with the amino acid glycine or the tripeptide glutathione.

Bioavailability, potency, efficacy

Bioavailability refers to the percentage and rate at which an administered drug gets into the bloodstream. For example, atropine can be administered down an endotracheal tube during resuscitation because (theoretically) 100% can reach the bloodstream in seconds. Potency refers to the ability of a drug to create an effect at low doses. Thus, an investigator would look at blood levels of various anesthetic agents to determine that one of them was the most potent in producing surgical anesthesia at low doses. Efficacy relates to the ability of a drug to produce an effect through interaction with its receptor at *some* drug level. However, the effect may be limited even when the doses of the drug are increased. Another drug may require higher doses to act, but then its action is much more complete; in other words, it is more efficacious. We are not ordinarily too interested in the amount of a drug needed to achieve a therapeutic effect. Furosemide in low doses is not a great diuretic when the kidneys are failing (it has no potency), but in higher doses, it is fairly efficacious.

Therapeutic index (therapeutic margin)

Phenytoin is a very useful anticonvulsant. Clinicians usually try to achieve maintenance blood levels between 10 and 20 micrograms/ml. This seems simple enough, but this drug undergoes significant binding to plasma proteins. Very young children and elderly patients are often very sensitive to small dosage changes, probably because their plasma proteins are already saturated. Blood levels much above 22 to 25 μg/ml produce nystagmus and cerebellar signs, and cardiac arrhythmias can occur even this close to intended levels. Thus, the therapeutic margin is rather small – it may not be possible to control seizures with this drug at levels below 16 or 18 micrograms per ml in a given patient, but they may become overtly toxic at levels that are just slightly higher. Phenobarbital is another anticonvulsant that is somewhat safer because the early overdosage state is usually announced by the tolerable side effect of drowsiness.

Effects of competitive and noncompetitive antagonists on drug potency and drug efficacy

Consider a graph with the effect of drug A on the ordinate and the $\log_{10}$ drug dose A on the abscissa. The curve will be sigmoid in shape, with very low doses producing zero effect and very high doses producing only maximum effect. Concomitant use of a competitive antagonist will shift the drug A curve to the right, which is to say that more drug A will be needed to achieve the half-maximal effect (and for that matter, the 10%, 25%, and up to the 100% maximum effect). A noncompetitive antagonist, on the other hand, blunts the maximum effect of drug A at standard doses; it displaces the curve inferiorly. Intermediate curves are possible for competitors that function as weak agonists.

Structure-activity relationships in antineoplastic drugs

A good example of the structure-activity relationship is the agent Adriamycin, or doxorubicin. This is an antibiotic with a group of aromatic rings attached to an aminated sugar moiety. The flat rings are able to intercalate (fit between and around) base pairs, preventing DNA from forming a sealed double strand. This distorts the chain and interferes with histone binding. A second example is the modification of uracil into 5-fluorouracil. This compound blocks thymine synthesis during the S cycle by inhibition of the enzyme thymidylate synthase.

Level of an orally administered drug measured in a patient at one point in time

Compliance with dosing schedule and administration instructions is the first factor to consider; patients may forget or intentionally skip doses of a prescribed medication, take multiple doses ahead of schedule, or take the drug along with foods or alcohol that affect its bioavailability. Absorption of the drug by the bowel is additionally influenced by transit time and bowel disease. Once the drug is absorbed, it is principally metabolized by the liver or, alternatively, excreted by the kidney. Thus, hepatic or renal impairments tend to increase the level of drugs in the bloodstream. Additional factors affecting the measurement of drug levels are their binding to plasma proteins and the assay method itself, which may vary from one laboratory to another.

Individual factors that affect pharmacokinetics and pharmacodynamics

Pharmacokinetics deals with the amount of drug actually available to achieve an effect, and pharmacodynamics deals with factors influencing that effect other than just the amount available. Whether an individual takes a drug on an empty stomach or not may affect the amount liberated from the preparation and absorbed by the body. Idiosyncratic factors such as diabetic gastroparesis or gastrointestinal diseases affect absorption. Patient size affects drug distribution in terms of fluid and fat compartments available for redistribution. Liver, kidney, and lung disease all affect drug metabolism and excretion. Probably the most common individual pharmacodynamic factor is the presence of other drugs in the system. Deficiency of the enzyme pseudocholinesterase is notorious for producing sustained paralysis after standard doses of usually short-acting succinylcholine for surgical procedures.

Adverse drug reaction

Genetic sensitivity to certain anesthetic agents underlies the often fatal problem of malignant hyperthermia. Adverse drug effects due to interaction with other drugs are quite common in clinical practice. A patient may not consider oral contraceptives, aspirin, or sleeping medications to be "drugs" when interviewed for a health history, for example. Seizures due to rapid withdrawal from chronic barbiturate administration are not exactly an adverse effect of the drug, but rather, an adverse effect of suddenly not having it. Similarly, addiction is probably not the stated intent of the medical use of narcotics, but it is an adverse result. Some effects of a drug are unpredictable but good; consider the unexpected effects of amantadine, given for viral illnesses, on Parkinson's disease.

Stevens–Johnson syndrome

Patients experiencing this dramatic and sometimes life-threatening problem fall into two groups: those in whom it arises as an unusually severe drug allergy and those where it begins with a variety of commonplace infections. The disorder is characterized by a skin rash, conjunctivitis, and buccopharyngitis that rapidly progress to epidermolysis. Discontinuation of all drugs, initiation of high-dose corticosteroids, and administration of fluids according to burn protocols is indicated. Disfiguring scarring and blindness (from corneal ulceration) may occur. In the group where the syndrome is drug related, it is hypothesized that slow detoxification of certain drugs by failure promptly to acetylate them creates intermediate molecules that trigger the immune system as haptens. Activated lymphocytes then induce apoptosis in keratinocytes.

Toxic level of a drug

Some side effects due to excessive drug levels, such as mild nausea or drowsiness, might be tolerable if the drug is achieving its purpose and the treatment period is short. On the other hand, the literature might show that these very symptoms closely precede serious complications such as renal failure. The determination of a drug level gives the clinician a number and nothing more. The number is useful but cannot be used in isolation to manage a patient. For example, a blood alcohol level of 0.3% might be detected in an adult weekend drinker with chronic stimulation of his alcohol dehydrogenase enzyme system; such an individual might be drowsy and silly but talking. The same level in a teen novel to the experience of drinking might produce deep obtundation and clear signs of chemical poisoning. Sodium nitroprusside is quite useful in ICU settings for controlling blood pressure. Usage protocols encourage frequent changes of the rate of administration. Rather than rely on direct laboratory determinations (cyanide or methemoglobin levels) that may be unavailable for many hours, doctors will look at the emergence of cardiac arrhythmias or mental status changes as reliable indicators of an actual ill effect in the patient and adjust doses downward accordingly.

Drug overdosage

Patient factors, issues related to the prescriber, and drug peculiarities all contribute to unintentional overdosing. Particularly elderly patients, but also harried parents, might forget having already taken (or given) a dose of the drug and double up. Some patients may not understand the directions, and others may assume, that "if one works well, two will get me better faster." Patients waiting to hear about drug level testing may assume all is well and proceed to take more of a drug that is already near toxic levels. Physician failure to prescribe the correct loading or daily dose, or worse, somehow leaving in the orders loading doses *as* daily doses occasionally cause dangerous situations. Probably the most important physician-related cause is the failure to appreciate how hepatic, renal, and circulatory factors may necessitate decreasing dosages. Pregnancy should be an obvious red-flag situation for doctor and patient. Some of the most useful drugs in clinical medicine (e.g., phenytoin, digoxin, and Coumadin) are time and again the players in overdosage situations when scrupulous attention is not given to loading criteria and timely measurement of drug levels.

Mechanisms of drug interactions

It is not uncommon to admit elderly patients who are taking 15 to 20 different prescription medicines, a practice known as polypharmacy. Some of these might be eyedrops, some are only taken p.r.n., and others are vital medications that should be taken exactly as prescribed. It is small wonder that drug interactions are common. Drugs may act synergistically or antagonistically. Drug A, which competes for the same receptor as drug B, might be expected to block the effect of drug B, but drug A might be more potent than drug B, leading to the opposite therapeutic result. On the other hand, drug A might bind to the receptor and produce the exact opposite effect of drug B; this is a compounded unfavorable result, in that drug B is blocked and the effect of drug A worsens the clinical problem. Drugs may compete unevenly for the same plasma protein binding sites, leading to increased availability of the free form of one of them. Drugs can obviously compete for intracellular sites where they are modified into active forms or where they are detoxified. They compete for each other in the kidney at secretory sites; this is the mechanism by which probenecid blocks the loss of penicillin into the urine and enhances the loss of uric acid.

Nicotinic and muscarinic cholinergic receptors

These receptors bind acetylcholine. Nicotinic receptors are found in nerve and muscle (at synapses and neuromuscular junctions, respectively). Binding of acetylcholine (ACh) to the receptor induces increased membrane permeability to the sodium ion; an excitatory postsynaptic potential is produced in nerves, and a myoneural junctional potential is produced in muscle. Muscarinic receptors are found in glands, smooth muscle, autonomic ganglia, and the heart, and they rely on G-protein mechanisms to exert their effects, which are therefore usually somewhat slower in onset and last longer. It is debated whether the adrenal medullary (neuroendocrine) cells have nicotinic or muscarinic receptors.

α- and β-adrenergic-receptors

These are components of the adrenergic system of receptors, which respond to catecholamines (basically epinephrine and norepinephrine.) The exact response of a tissue will depend on the type of receptors present on its cells as well as the relative alpha- versus beta- stimulating effect of the specific drug. Alpha- and beta-receptors are further divided into alphanumeric subclasses. Alpha-1-receptors cause an increase in cellular permeability to calcium, whereas alpha-2- and beta-receptors work through cyclic AMP as a second messenger. Alpha-1-receptors are found throughout the body; vasoconstriction of arteries and veins occurs as well as stimulation of smooth muscle in the bowel and bladder. Alpha-2-receptors are found diffusely as well, with particular concentrations near alpha-1-receptors, where they exert an inhibitory effect. In general, they cause smooth-muscle relaxation. Beta-receptors exert positive chronoinotropic effects on the heart but relax smooth muscle.

Warfarin and vitamin K

Vitamin K, phytonadione, is obtained from leafy vegetables such as spinach. In humans, it is used to gamma-carboxylate glutamic acid residues in proteins that are involved in blood coagulation, including prothrombin and factors VII, IX, and X and proteins C, S, and Z. Modifications of these proteins induced by vitamin K_1 affect their ability to bind calcium. Oxidized vitamin K_1 is ordinarily conserved by reduction back to its active form by the enzyme vitamin K epoxide reductase. Warfarin (commonly called by the trade name Coumadin) exerts its action by inhibition of this enzyme. Thus, it is antagonistic to the actions of the vitamin, but only indirectly. Excessive Coumadin doses produce markedly elevated international normalized ratio (INR) results (the target dose achieves an INR of about 2, meaning that coagulation time is about doubled), sometimes as high as 8 or 10.

Heparin

Heparin is a glycoaminoglycan molecule that inhibits blood clotting by binding to and activating the enzyme, antithrombin III. This enzyme then inactivates thrombin, preventing blood clotting. Heparin is given only parenterally – intravenously in emergency situations and subcutaneously for some maintenance regimens. For example, in cases where there is life-threatening thrombosis, such as pulmonary thromboembolism, heparin is given IV in a loading dose of 10,000 units with follow-up IV doses averaging 1,000 units per hour. The target is an activated partial thromboplastin time (APTT) around 2 to 2.5 times the laboratory normal. Warfarin may be administered simultaneously because its effect is not manifested for a day or two. Heparin has the unusual effect of sometimes causing an immune-mediated thrombocytopenia, which can be severe and yet is often reversible. Many synthetic heparin analogs have been developed; these are generally somewhat safer and more convenient for longer term applications.

5-FU, vincristine, cis-platinum, and Adriamycin

5-fluorouracil is an antimetabolite that works during the S phase of the cell cycle in the same way as methotrexate – it complexes with folic acid, thereby inhibiting the thymidylate synthase enzyme. Cis-platinum works throughout much of the cell cycle, cross-linking DNA strands by binding to the base units. Vincristine and vinblastine disrupt spindle formation and action during the M phase. Like platinum drugs, Adriamycin works during much of the cell cycle, but by a different mechanism. Here, the antibiotic/antineoplastic agent intercalates (inserts itself) into the DNA strand between bases. This distorts the helix and makes transcription or duplication difficult. The idea of using combinations of antineoplastic drugs is identical to the notion of using multiple antibiotics for an infection – to assault the tumor at multiple points in the cell cycle, so that if it manages to escape control at one point, it will fail at another.

Estrogen receptor positivity

If a breast malignancy is "estrogen receptor positive," it means that estrogens (which are steroids) bind to nuclear receptors proteins, which then influence the expression of DNA. Such a complex can be stimulatory in certain tissues, such as the mammary gland, and inhibitory in others. The goal of establishing whether or not a given tumor expresses these receptors is to determine whether drugs such as tamoxifen (a competitive antagonist of estrogen) would be useful in the chemotherapy of a malignancy. Tissues are readily stained with estrogen receptor (ER) antibodies to make this determination microscopically. Expression is variable, so a given tumor might express much, some, little, or no estrogen effect. A second class of ERs is at the cell surface, members of the G-protein receptor family that is involved in signal transduction.

Glaucoma

Glaucoma is hydrocephalus of the eye. The problem is the inability to absorb into the canal of Schlemm (essentially an entry to the venous system) all the aqueous humor that is produced in the ciliary body. This is exactly analogous to production of cerebrospinal fluid (CSF) by the choroid plexus and its uptake by the arachnoid villi. For extremely acute cases, ophthalmologists use IV mannitol in exactly the same way and for the same reasons that neurosurgeons use this drug – to dehydrate the system and decrease pressures. Acetazolamide, a carbonic anhydrase inhibitor, can be used in the same way in both conditions. The parasympathomimetic drug pilocarpine works by stimulating the ciliary muscle, forcing mechanical opening of the ciliocorneal angle. Beta-agonist-adrenergic drugs diminish fluid production, and alpha-2-agonists both decrease production and dilate veins to facilitate drainage. Finally, there is interest in the use of certain prostaglandins to augment aqueous outflow.

Selective serotonin reuptake inhibitors in the treatment of depression

One biochemical model of depression and other mental illnesses relates to diminished effectiveness of serotonergic systems. Serotonin, or 5-hydoxytryptamine, exerts most of its effect on postsynaptic cells through the G-receptor protein system. Around 10% of released serotonin is taken up into the postsynaptic cell, and the remainder is taken back into the presynaptic neuron terminal for repackaging. Selective serotonin reuptake inhibitor (SSRI) drugs attempt to prevent the reuptake and have the chemical "linger" over the postsynaptic cell for an enhanced effect. Although there are many proposed uses, a withdrawal syndrome exists, and this class of agents has been linked to suicide in adolescents.

Federal regulatory system for controlled substances

The federal Drug Enforcement Agency (DEA) has classified drugs into five categories, or schedules, to govern their use. Doctors with a valid medical license may apply for a "narcotics license," which is a numbered certificate that the doctor can use to order or administer some, but never all, of the drugs in the five schedules. Category I drugs are either deemed to be extremely dangerous or they have no therapeutic purpose. Examples include gamma-hydroxybutyrate, peyote, heroin, and LSD. Schedule II drugs are those with a high abuse potential, which means this category includes many very useful substances, such as methylphenidate, morphine, and cocaine (which is used topically in ear, nose, and throat [ENT] practice). Schedule III preparations have less abuse potential and include such medications as paregoric and ketamine. Class IV drugs have even lower abuse potential and include such common medicines as diazepam and phenobarbital. Finally, schedule V drugs have almost no abuse potential, at least according to the DEA, and include codeine-laden cough syrup. Pharmacies and health-care systems attempt to monitor prescribing practices of individual physicians and use patterns by individual patients, but abuse of the system is unfortunately common by both. The penalties for illegal prescribing start at revocation of the drug license.

Role of the FDA in regulating drugs, devices, and nutritional supplements

The Food and Drug Administration (FDA) attempts to regulate drugs, medical devices, food production and food quality, vaccines, cosmetics, and veterinary products. Certain products, such as nutritional supplements and biotic preparations, strangely fall outside FDA review. The inexorable addition of new drugs to the pharmacopeia, as well as the expansion of indications for existing drugs makes the job formidable. When medical devices such as artificial joints, neurosurgical shunts, or pacemaker devices are added, the task is insurmountable. Reports of adverse drug reactions or of device failures are largely voluntary. Then, too, in the case of certain implants, the practitioners most likely to use them in high volumes are often the same (compensated) investigators involved in their genesis. Conflicts of interest are common. Certain drug problems, such as the notorious cases of mitral valve damage due to a combination weight-loss drug, do not materialize for a long period after treatment begins. Failure to identify complications for what they are, as well as underreporting, significantly hampers the effectiveness of this agency.

> ➤ **Review Video:** FDA Drug Categories
> Visit *mometrix.com/academy* and enter *Code:* **348438**

Signaling done by hormones

Hormones are chemical messengers. Usually we mean active agents, such as insulin or T3/T4, which are secreted into the bloodstream and work throughout the body. These might be termed "true" endocrine hormones, but there are other types. Some hormones act locally to stimulate the very cell or cells that produced them. This is called an autocrine effect, and it may be important in the conversion of idling, benign tumors into malignancies. A second type of local signal is paracrine, meaning that there is stimulation of a different, but juxtaposed, set of cells. Induction of nervous tissues by the primitive notochord is an example of such a paracrine effect. A modified form of this is the neuroendocrine response that occurs, for example, by sympathetic stimulation of adrenal medullary cells, leading to the release of catecholamines. In a sense, all synaptic activity (except electrical synapses) is paracrine in character.

Glucocorticoid activity

Glucocorticoids such as cortisol enter cells and then bind to cytosolic receptors, but without any initial result. These complexes must be translocated into the nucleus in order for the steroid molecule to have an effect through DNA binding. Both transactivation and transrepression occur; that is, the complex encourages expression of certain genes (glucose-6-phosphatase, for example) and downregulates the expression of others (those responsible for producing cytokines and interleukin). Thus, steroids have wanted and unwanted effects – they may decrease inflammation and pain, but they also cause hyperglycemia. Designer steroid adaptations can produce salutatory effects that outweigh the unwanted consequences of corticoid use.

Bacterium

Bacteria have been around for about 3.8 billion years. They have a single circular chromosome (although rare bacteria have two) and frequently have small extrachromosomal DNA fragments known as plastids. They multiply by simple mitosis, but they are capable of exchanging DNA information by plasmid transfer and through conjugation bridges. Bacteria lack organelles such as the mitochondrion, but they do have cytoskeletal elements lacing the cytoplasm. They have a conventional plasmalemma and they elaborate a variable amount of peptidoglycans to make a cell wall. Water dwellers have flagella. Some forms make a heavy capsule (*Haemophilus influenzae*), and others make a thick waxy coat (tuberculosis and leprosy).

Bacteria have natural enemies, including bacteriophages and fungi. *Penicillium* fungus inhibits the growth of certain bacteria by producing penicillin. Bacteria have been on the Earth approximately 3.8 billion years, so they have extensive experience in combating such problems. Plasmids (small pieces of extrachromosomal DNA) are routinely transferred between bacteria in the "soup" of the natural world. Some of these bits of information ("R" or resistance factor plasmids) contain plans for the elaboration of proteins such as the β-lactamase penicillinase. Bacteria were resistant to natural antibacterial agents in ancient times. When a new antibiotic is developed, most of the bacteria exposed to it are killed, but a few lucky ones persist because of their abilities to degrade the antibiotic more effectively and prohibit its entry into the bacterial cell. These become the new populace of the species. They may transfer their abilities to other species of bacteria through plasmids; hence, resistance to the new drug increases over time.

In routine clinical work, bacteria are described first by their staining characteristics and second by their shape. For example, a Gram-negative, comma-shaped bacterium is most likely *Vibrio cholerae*. The ability of a bacterium to retain the purple crystal violet stain after iodine exposure and alcohol washing relates to the amount of peptidoglycan in the cell wall of the organism. Gram-negative bacteria do not incorporate the dark purple stain and instead appear pink due to a safranin counterstain. Shapes are typically described as round (coccus), rodlike (bacillus), comma-shaped, or spiral, with some intermediate shapes possible. Pleomorphic (shape variable) forms may arise when the bacterium is growing in less-than-ideal conditions. Additional classification criteria include, for example, the presence or absence of flagellum or a capsule, whether the bacteria are visualized inside or outside of host immune cells, or colonial shapes (strands = strepto-, pairs = diplo-, or clusters). Bacteria are further classified by which sugars they are capable of metabolizing (and therefore, the special culture conditions they may require) and by their ability to grow in air (aerobic, facultatively aerobic [oxygen is not toxic to them], obligately anaerobic [oxygen exposure inhibits growth]). Other considerations are their ability to form spores under stressful conditions and their antibiotic sensitivity profiles.

Sporulation

Bacteria such as *Clostridium tetani* are able to form spores under adverse conditions of heat, starvation, or desiccation. Ordinarily residents of the intestine of animals such as horses, this organism is able to exist in spore form in the soil for decades. Because almost everyone has had a laceration or puncture wound while playing or working outside, routine vaccination of all children occurs in developed countries. Infants can develop tetanus from contamination of the umbilical stump when they are born in dirty conditions. The spore itself is a form of cryptobiote. It consists of the bacterial genome, a smidgeon of cytoplasm, and a very tough outer coat. It can resist extreme heat, radiation, extreme cold, and other conditions inhospitable to life. Under favorable conditions, the bacterium resumes normal functions and morphology. Anthrax is another agent that sporulates and is considered a potential tool for bioterrorism.

Penicillin

The mold *Penicillium* produces a class of agents collectively known as penicillin; these molecules inhibit bacterial growth nearby. Penicillin is a β-lactam compound, which means that it inhibits peptidoglycan cross-linkages in the bacterial cell wall. The result is a weakened or partially missing cell wall. The bacterium cannot resist the influx of water by cell wall counterpressure, and so it bursts. But bacteria have had millions of years to find a solution, and they have. The enzyme β-lactamase is able to hydrolyze the ring structure of penicillin, rendering it useless. Methylation of the penicillin molecule makes it resistant to beta-lactamases, and in effect creates a new, synthetic form of a natural antibiotic.

Aminoglycoside antibiotics

The naturally occurring aminoglycosides are bacterial products that serve to kill or at least inhibit the growth of competing bacteria. It was traditionally held that they operate as static or cidal agents based on their stable binding to ribosomes and the interference they exert at that level on protein synthesis. More recently, cell membrane effects have also been observed. They are named -mycin or -micin, or -kacin, and they are quite toxic. They are often administered only once or twice a day; blood levels should be monitored to avoid toxic complications, but they do not correlate very well with the therapeutic effect.

Lac operon

It would be quite wasteful for *Escherichia coli* to make the enzyme lactase if the substrate lactose was not actually available. On the other hand, if the bacterium could make the enzyme on demand, it would have an advantage when this sugar did become available as an energy source. This is precisely what happens. Three genes are encompassed in the model, but only lactose permease and beta-galactosidase will be discussed. The bacterium has used metabolic energy to create a repressor molecule that binds to the chromosome and prevents the transcription of *lac*-operon genes by RNA polymerase until lactose actually enters the cell. Lactose binds to the repressor, causing it to separate from the DNA (derepresses the gene) and allowing m-RNA to be created. This is then moved to ribosomal units for the translation into permease and galactosidase proteins. The former helps lactose enter the cell and the latter cleaves it hydrolytically to galactose and glucose. If lactose ceases to be available, the repressor molecule rebinds to the DNA and stops the transcription of this portion of the gene. Similar control mechanisms operate across all life forms.

Logarithmic growth

Under ideal conditions, bacteria can undergo mitotic replication every 20 to 30 minutes. Thus, from a single organism, there would be 2^n bacteria in a culture after $n + 1$ time periods. This pattern is logarithmic, or exponential, growth, and it does not occur commonly. Bacteria grow best in natural environments – ponds, mucosae, skin crypts, and so on. Putting bacteria on culture plates is about as organism-friendly as putting an astronaut on the surface of Mars. This reasoning underlies the fact that it is often difficult to culture bacteria in the laboratory, even when temperatures, ambient gas concentrations (either normal oxygen or completely anaerobic conditions, generally), and nutrients are ideal. Probably many bacteria die off during transportation to the clinical laboratory.

A common clinical experience is that the laboratory will report "scanty growth" after two or three days; colonial morphology cannot be stated under these conditions. Such factors lead to treatment delays.

Staphylococcal infections

Staphylococcus spp. commonly produces abscesses because of its limited repertoire of enzymes limits its invasive potential. Surgical drainage is often needed. One enzyme it can produce, however, is penicillinase, rendering ordinary penicillin G useless for treatment. Methicillin must be used instead. The emergence of strains resistant to methylpenicillin has emerged as a new problem in hospitals, nursing homes, schools, and other institutions over the past two decades. Streptococcal infections are characterized by opposite behaviors – highly invasive cellulitis, pharyngitis, and septicemias, but all are sensitive to penicillin. Streptococcus produces collagenase, hyaluronidase, and other similar digestive enzymes that allow it to spread rapidly through soft tissues. Streptococcus is famously unable to make penicillinase, rendering it exquisitely sensitive to penicillin. Thus, the enzymatic abilities of the two bacteria are almost perfectly inverse to one another.

L-forms

Some bacteria exist with fragile, incomplete, or absent cell walls – they are just a bag of cytoplasm waiting for a hyposmolar death. Because the cell wall is deficient, when they are placed in hypotonic, and possibly even isotonic, media, they swell, lyse, and die. Thus, they might be active in producing an infection, but they are very difficult to recover. Careful consultation with the hospital microbiologist, meticulous specimen collection, and rapid transfer to a hyperosmolar culture medium may allow recovery of these unusual organisms, particularly in the situation of an obvious infection that persistently cultures "negative" using ordinary techniques.

Baltimore classification system of viruses

This classification system is useful for understanding how viruses replicate themselves.

An example of a member of each class is listed below:
- Group I – double-stranded DNA – herpes viruses
- Group II – single-stranded DNA – parvovirus
- Group III – double-stranded RNA – rotavirus
- Group IV – single-stranded "sense" RNA – WEE
- Group V – single-stranded "antisense" RNA – Ebola virus
- Group VI – single-stranded RNA, reverse transcriptase – HIV
- Group VII – double-stranded DNA, reverse transcriptase – hepatitis B.

Virus structure

Viruses have protein coats (capsids) that more or less self-assemble to lower the energy state. These repeating units frequently assume geometric shapes such as icosahedrons. The protein coat can be varied, leading to the concept of a virus morphing over time and changing the "antigen package" that it presents to a host cell. Viruses contain DNA or RNA, but never both. Some viruses (bacteriophages) are modified with attachment. Filoviruses are rodlike or even curvilinear in shape. Some viruses are enveloped, meaning that they are surrounded by portions of the cell membrane or even the cell wall of the cell from which they budded off. Those with a lipid membrane are usually destroyed by exposure to diethyl ether.

Bacteriophage to combat bacterial disease

Scenario: fearing that production of antibiotics would be curtailed during World War III, cognizant of the fact that bacteria were developing polyresistant strains at a rapid rate, and further reasoning that Western governments would engineer new antibiotic resistance into probable biowarfare agents, the Soviet Union invests considerable resources in the middle portion of the twentieth century into the production of bacteriophages as alternative antibacterial agents. This idea is not at all far-fetched. There is some evidence that phages are effective in situations in which antibiotics cannot penetrate biofilms. This treatment idea is close to a century old, but it is used nowhere in the world (presently) except the Russian Federation and former Soviet block countries.

Lysogenic and lytic viral effects on a host cell

Viruses may invade a cell, capture its machinery, convert it to the production of many copies of the virus, and then rupture through the cell membrane, initiating new cycles in countless other cells. This is lytic behavior. Much more interesting is the ability of a virus to incorporate itself into the DNA of a host cell, take up residence there, and wait. In fact, a great many genes of higher organisms are very similar to viral genomes, so it is possible that the ability to "grow" and cope with a changing environment arose in just such a way. Varicella causes chickenpox, but then the virus enters a lysogenic phase where it is dormant in nerve cells for decades. Illnesses, cancer, or aging may unmask the virus, resulting in very painful, herpetiform eruptions of shingles. The lysogenic properties of some viruses are no doubt related to their ability to cause cancers.

Vaccines developed to prevent uterine cervical carcinoma due to human papilloma virus

The association of viruses with cancer is not a new idea. For example, the Rous sarcoma virus, which affects chickens, was discovered a century ago. The association of human papilloma virus (HPV) with cervical cancer was suspected because development of the malignancy was associated with early sexual activity, multiple partners, and of course the development of persisting genital warts. (Ironically, the types that are most commonly associated with cervical cancer are less associated with the development of obvious skin lesions.) These factors together suggest lingering infection – in other words, lysogeny. The virus causes slow proliferative changes in the squamous basal cell layer in the vagina and uterine cervix, but it has also been associated with malignancy of the buccopharyngeal tissues. Vaccination of both genders of adolescents is presently recommended.

Killed viral vaccine and live viral vaccine

The best way to assure immunity to a disease is to acquire it naturally, but that assumes one lives through the infection. The reason for this has to do with regional antigen processing by lymphatic tissues, as well as the "perfect" actual challenge of the organism. The more a virus is modified, either directly (chemically), or indirectly (by passing it through alternative hosts or tissue cultures), the more alterations occur in its capsid shell and the less faithful it is to the "real" virus. Hence, a killed viral vaccine might not be as effective as one that is merely attenuated by more modest modifications. Here, the opposite problem emerges – if not much is done to it, it might retain most of the virulence of the original pathogen, or even worse, it might mutate back to its original state. Killed vaccines may be safer in severely immunocompromised persons.

Retroviruses

HIV principally attacks cells in the immune system. There, it uses the enzyme reverse transcriptase to create host DNA that is complementary to its own RNA. Subsequent forward transcription of the host DNA leads to the production of many copies of the original viral RNA. Over time, cells in the immune system such as CD4 helper T cells and macrophages die off, leading to a loss of cellular immunity.

H7N9 influenza virus and "antigen packaging"

The protein capsids of some viruses that are tropic for the respiratory system contain hexosaminidase and neuraminidase. Each of these proteins functions as an enzyme, hydrolyzing chemical moieties on the host cell membrane, thereby facilitating attachment of the virus and subsequent infection of the cell. The capsid enzymes H and N are further categorized by assigning numbers for variants of the protein: 1, 2, etc. Thus, a virus might have H1N1 characteristics in a given year, but within a brief period of time, morph into, for example, a strain presenting modifications of one (H2N1) or both (H2N2) antigens. This is referred to as the "antigen package." Because vaccines against seasonal influenza are largely designed around the H and N antigens, public health officials must make educated guesses about the antigen package that will dominate in the following year. It takes around six months to create vaccines on a large scale, but smaller amounts can be generated in a few months to protect health-care workers.

Fungi reproduction

Fungi may reproduce by budding, and the classical example of this is simple baker's yeast. Fungi are regarded as monoploid, or "n," organisms – they have a single complement of DNA. Therefore, daughter buds are created by simple mitosis. Fungi that enter the mycelial phase may conjugate – that is, "plus" and "minus" mycelia with monoploid DNA may meet, fuse, and form a 2n form known as a sporangium. Ordinary meiosis then occurs, leading back to monoploid spores. The spores are disseminated and begin the life cycle anew. Although both forms may exist simultaneously in human infections, the elaboration of "fruiting bodies," as seen on laboratory plates, probably does not often occur in tissues.

Principal deep mycotic infections

Cryptococcal meningitis, due to *Cryptococcus neoformans*, is an important cause of central nervous system (CNS) infections in immunocompromised patients. Valley fever, or coccidioidomycosis, is a relatively frequent cause of pneumonia in the southwestern United States. Histoplasmosis and blastomycosis produce similar invasive disease, beginning in the lung and spreading hematogenously. In all cases, the fungus is inhaled. Certain occupations are at increased risk of developing fungal infections, especially agricultural workers and persons demolishing buildings (bird droppings contain fungal spores).

Amphotericin B

Amphotericin was derived from streptococci; it is a natural antifungal product that binds to the ergosterol component of fungus cell membranes. Unfortunately, mammals also have ergosterol in their cell membranes. The chemical interaction leads to the development of increased ionic permeability in affected cells, but it is not perfectly clear if this is the fungicidal element of its action. In man, orally administered amphotericin B is fairly well tolerated when it is used to treat candidiasis (thrush). Intravenous administration is accompanied by a panoply of systemic problems, including fever, chills, vascular collapse, organ system failure, and sometimes death.

Factors that make fungal infections notoriously difficult to identify and eradicate

Unlike garden fungi, which seem to spring up overnight, those causing human infection grow slowly in the body and even slower during attempts to culture them. Special culture media and extreme patience are required to identify certain pathogenic fungi. A little-known fact is that surface swabs often fail to capture the organism; submission of small tissue fragments is preferable. (Microscopic examination of tissue has to include fungal stains, typically silver methenamine, which shows black fungi against a green background.) Fungi exist in both yeast and mycelial forms. The yeast form is fairly nondescript, and during mycelial growth, the fungus sometimes does not conform strictly to a branched/nonbranched, septate, aseptate, or pseudoseptate pattern. Treatment requires even more patience and perseverance than does identification. Amphotericin B is a powerful antifungal medication, but it is so toxic that it must be administered in gradually increasing doses and over a long period of time. Radical surgical debridement is often thwarted by extensive fibrosis around the infectious mass.

Tuberculosis

Mycobacterium tuberculosis is an organism that should be regarded as intermediate between a normal bacterium and a fungus. It grows very slowly on culture media, commonly requiring six to eight weeks to develop an identifiable colony. Like many fungi, it makes an unusual biochemical product – in this case, a heavy, waxy, mycolic acid capsule that prevents Gram staining. Instead, acid-fast staining techniques are required. Because of its slow growth, prolonged treatment is needed; modern regimens include isonicotinoylhydrazine (INH), ethambutol, rifampin, and pyrazinamide. Reluctant, noncompliant, poorly educated, or itinerant patients constitute a special public health risk. Multidrug resistant (MDR) and extremely drug resistant (XDR) strains have emerged in immunocompromised populations.

Mycoplasma pneumoniae

Mycoplasma pneumoniae is one of the most frequent causes of primary atypical pneumonia. These bacteria are miniscule and therefore very difficult to identify under a light microscope. They have no cell wall and rely on obtaining sterols from their host environment to maintain their membranes. They are reminiscent of slime molds in that they can move along surfaces with a leading and a trailing edge. With a very limited biochemical repertoire, they are essentially saprophytic. Symptoms of low-grade fever, malaise, and productive cough may exist for several weeks prior to evaluation. Treatment with ordinary cell-wall-active antibiotics of course has no effect. Macrolides such as azithromycin, usually in combination with tetracycline, are effective treatments. Because DNA changes have been noted in tissue cultures contaminated with this organism, there is now research relating to its possible role in neoplasia.

"O and P" laboratory test for stool specimens

Enteric parasites (roundworms and segmented worms) shed their eggs into the intestinal lumen. (Entire segments of tapeworms are occasionally recovered.) A stool specimen is teased apart and a thin microscopic smear is examined for ova. An experienced parasitologist can easily differentiate the ova of common intestinal worms from each other. If symptoms are highly suggestive and the specimen is devoid of recognizable ova, repeat testing on different days may be needed. Modern serologic diagnosis of many parasitic species is now available, as well.

Malaria

Plasmodia have a complicated life cycle in which man is an intermediary host. *Anopheles* mosquitoes have sporozoite forms of the organism in their salivary glands. When they feed, they inoculate these into the bloodstream of the individual. The sporozoites are conveyed to the liver, where they divide to produce countless merozoites forms. These then infect (and cause lysis of) host erythrocytes in cycles that produce recurrent fever, chills, and hematuria due to the liberation of free hemoglobin into the bloodstream. Some merozoites differentiate into sexual gametocytes. When a second mosquito bites the human, these are transferred with the blood meal into the mosquito gut, where they produce sporozoites, perpetuating the cycle. Prevention of biting by destruction of adult and larval mosquitoes is the key to disease control. Five different *Plasmodium* species are capable of causing human disease. Mefloquine and doxycycline are fairly effective in prophylaxis. Because of the emergence of many resistant strains, an infectious disease or tropical medicine specialist should be consulted when initiating treatment of infected patients. Also, patients may be infected with more than one strain of *Plasmodium*.

Intestinal roundworms

Nematodes are ubiquitous in the environment. They vary in size from microscopic to roughly a meter in length. Perhaps three-quarters of puppies have roundworms by the time they are weaned.

Children become infected by the ingestion of eggs in dirt or animal feces. They develop anal itching and abdominal complaints; treatment is usually with single-dose mebendazole. Adults may become infected in the same way, although some roundworms may enter through skin fissures in agricultural workers or those exposed to contaminated waters. Large-scale infestations with large worms, such as *Ascaris*, are treated with the same drug regimen but are sometimes complicated by actual obstruction of the small bowel. A very important roundworm problem is heartworms in canine and feline pets; mosquitoes spread the disease, and rare human infections have been noted. Prophylaxis of pets is therefore crucial.

Amebas

Amebas are parasites that live in watery environments. Hence, they are mostly acquired through contaminated water, food, and drinks. However, certain forms can encyst and survive long periods in a dried state. These can be inhaled and become infectious. The most important amebic infection in man is dysentery due to *Entameba histolytica*. Diarrhea occurs in symptomatic cases, but many cases remain asymptomatic and the patient is effectively a carrier. Diagnosis is made based on examination of the stools and on the detection of specific blood antibodies. Treatment includes metronidazole; the organism may sometimes invade the liver and create abscesses. Consultation with an infectious disease specialist is needed in those circumstances. *Naegleria* species live in warm freshwater and invade the basifrontal lobes through the cribriform plate after inhalation of lake or river water. This infection is almost universally fatal.

Prion diseases

Creutzfeldt–Jakob spongiform encephalopathy is the most common example of a disease caused by a prion – a misfolded protein with the ability to replicate itself. Kuru, transmitted from human to human by cannibalism, is another classic example. Bovine spongiform encephalopathy (BSE, or mad cow disease) may occasionally jump to man if beef from affected cows is eaten. Chronic wasting disease of deer has afflicted a handful of people. It is controversial whether scrapie, the equivalent condition in sheep, can infect man. It is extremely difficult to kill prions by conventional sterilization techniques. Surgical instruments used for brain biopsy must be handled in an extraordinary manner. Spinal fluid markers proteins can also be used to establish the diagnosis.

Herd immunity

Infection with certain microbial agents (measles, for example) confers lasting and probably lifelong immunity. Similarly, proper vaccination with initial and booster doses "educates" the immune system to maintain immunoglobulin levels against the organism. It is not necessary to immunize each and every member of a population to prevent outbreaks of disease. Instead, vaccinating about two-thirds of a population is sufficient to prevent epidemics. Although sporadic outbreaks will continue to occur, they are self-limited because they are not spread through the immunized individuals. Levels of herd immunity substantially greater than 70% or so are nonetheless highly desirable, as they prevent individual cases of diseases that may be fatal, crippling, or merely annoying. All illnesses in man have economic and sociological costs.

Sterilization and disinfection

Disinfection refers to the log-kill of microorganisms on inanimate surfaces such as a kitchen counter or hospital wall. Numerous agents can be used, from isopropanol (which acts by denaturing protein) to quaternary ammonium salts such as benzalkonium chloride (which disrupts cell membranes). Probably the most important common agents are ordinary soap and water, with or without chlorine bleach. Some viruses and bacterial spores are highly resistant to surface disinfectants. Sterilization refers to the eradication of all life forms, including cryptobiotic spores. Autoclaving at high temperatures and for prolonged periods is necessary to kill sporulated bacteria; surgical instrument trays always include a "spore strip" to indicate that the autoclave has functioned properly in this regard. Prions, which are not life forms, are not eliminated by routine autoclaving. Exposure to extreme oxidizing agents and prolonged heating are required; the Centers for Disease Control and Prevention (CDC) has developed helpful protocols for this issue.

Pasteurization

Food can be sterilized by gamma-radiation, but this process has risks to those carrying it out and it is therefore rarely used. Prolonged boiling or other forms of cooking could sterilize many foods, but this alters the nutritional content and often makes them unpalatable. Pasteurization of (mostly liquid) foods involves sudden heating and then a quick return to normal temperatures. This eradicates or substantially eliminates many of the microbial agents that are likely to cause foodborne illness. In the case of milk, the main infectious problems (historically, at least) are tuberculosis, undulant fever, and listeriosis. Most Americans willingly embrace the texture and taste of pasteurized milk. The consumption of untreated milk is still associated with significant outbreaks of disease. The pasteurization of honey does not destroy *Clostridium botulinum* spores, of course – the temperature is inadequate; honey is therefore dangerous in infants and very young children.

Hospital-acquired infections

Nosocomial infection is a major problem in the contemporary setting of high-technology care. The use of indwelling central venous catheters is particularly associated with the development of bloodstream infections, or septicemias. Prolonged mechanical ventilation often leads to pneumonia. Scrupulous attention to preventive protocols is required. Lengthy operations with implantation of hardware are the recurrent theme of surgical wound infections; the sources of the bacteria include the patients themselves, the surgical environment, and improperly sterilized implants. The tendency to treat ever older, sicker, and immunocompromised patients undoubtedly increases the risk of infection. Although antibiotic resistance does not cause infection, it makes established infections persist longer and it makes routine prophylactic antibiotics less effective over time. The single best preventative measure is still frequent, careful handwashing and adherence to universal precautions when interacting with patients.

Outbreak of *Serratia spp.* wound infections occurs on a surgical ward

Serratia is a Gram-negative rod that prefers to grow in moist conditions. It is often resistant to multiple antibiotics. Individuals may present to the hospital with established *Serratia* infections, but more commonly, these develop after hospital admission. The organism is spread by health-care workers, so containment and eradication must focus on the conduct of hospital procedures. Affected patients must be isolated, and strict adherence to universal precautions (gown, mask, and gloves) must be observed. Careful disinfection of hospital room surfaces, followed by drying, will help control the pathogen. Doctors, nurses, therapists, food workers, and cleaning personnel – in short, anyone with patient contact – must adhere to these protocols. The hospital infectious disease service should be consulted, and their recommendations should be followed carefully. Persistence of the problem may necessitate consultation with state epidemiologists and occasionally requires closure of wards and even of entire operating suites.

Anamnestic responses that underlie permanent immunity

Anamnesis means "not forgetting," and it is a bit different conceptually from remembering. B-lymphocytes, and to a lesser extent, some T-4 memory cells exposed to an antigen such as the protein in a bacterial cell wall fragment differentiate into plasma cells. These cells persist for long periods of time. With a single exposure, IgM is produced in modest amounts for a few days until it is superseded by IgG. With multiple exposures (either naturally or in the form of booster immunizations), chronic low levels of IgG circulate in the bloodstream, effectively conferring long-term humoral immunity against the infectious agent. The reservoir lymphocyte/plasma cells are not exactly "thinking about" the antigen very much, but neither have they forgotten. Upon reexposure to the antigen, these immune cells generate an exuberant IgM and IgG response in a very brief period of time. Recent outbreaks of pertussis in correctly immunized, healthy individuals are probably due to shifts in the antigen surface profile of the microorganism, but whether or not immunity is truly lifelong has also been called into question.

Epidemic and endemic

Epidemics occur when there is a relatively sudden and somewhat sustained increase in the number of cases of a specified condition in a given timeframe. An epidemic need not be unexpected, such as the epidemic of influenza that typically occurs in winter months. Neither must it affect large numbers of people. As an example, 100 cases of whooping cough in a large state do constitute an epidemic, because so many people are immunized against it. Endemics exist when a disease is prevalent in a population over time. HIV/AIDS is endemic, with about 800,000 Americans afflicted by it presently.

Koch's postulates

Koch's time-honored postulates require certain proofs to link a microorganism to a disease state, to wit:
- the organism must be recovered from cases with the disease
- the organism must be grown in isolation in the laboratory
- inoculation of a sufficient number of the organisms into a healthy individual should lead to development of the disease

At times, these simple steps are difficult to achieve. Leprosy bacillus, for example, is notoriously difficult to grow in the laboratory; typically it is cultured in the footpad of an armadillo. Modern genetic techniques have rendered Koch's postulates somewhat dated. The linkage of *Helicobacter pylori* to enteric ulceration was established in exactly this classic manner, with the investigating gastroenterologists inoculating themselves to complete the cycle of proof.

Zoonotic conditions

The zoonoses are those diseases conveyed to man through (higher) animals. The broader concept includes transmission from one higher animal to man using an intermediate insect vector. West Nile encephalitis is an example of a bird virus that is transmitted to man by the bite of a mosquito. The disease is best controlled by elimination of the insect vector – capping, eliminating, or decontaminating bodies of water and insecticides are usually sufficient to stop an outbreak. Clearly, control of infected birds is beyond our reach. Another, now very rare, zoonosis is rabies. Mandatory canine vaccination has now virtually eliminated the disease from urban areas. Skunks, bats, raccoons, and other wild mammals constitute the only exposure risk for most people. Cysticercosis, due to ingestion of *Taenia solium* pork tapeworm eggs or larvae, can be considered a foodborne disease, but it is also a zoonosis. Direct fecal–oral ingestion is possible, although almost all cases come from eating improperly cooked meat. This disease is controlled by sanitary farming practices, proper food preparation, and occasionally joint pharmacologic treatment of pig herds and clusters of affected patients.

Blood test that has a sensitivity of 85% for detecting a condition

Sensitivity is the ability reliably to detect something. If 100 people have a disease and a test has a sensitivity of 85%, 15 patients will go undetected. If a second test was layered onto the first, even if it is not as sensitive--say it has a sensitivity of only 75%--it is still likely that it would detect some of the 15 patients missed by the first test.

Skin test has a specificity of 90% for detecting allergy to ragweed

If 100 patients had positive results from skin testing as described, only 90 of them would actually be allergic to ragweed. Others would have an allergy to something else, or perhaps they are just reacting to carriers in the allergen preparation, etc. Many tests are positive for multiple diseases and therefore are not solely diagnostic of any. An example of low specificity is rheumatoid factor, an autoantibody that is present in high levels in rheumatoid arthritis but is also elevated in related inflammatory conditions such as lupus or Sjögren's syndrome and in seemingly unrelated conditions such as hepatitis or infectious mononucleosis.

M-k-s system of measurement and its relationship to the *Système International*

All physical sciences use the metric system, and all units in that system are derived from the meter, kilogram, and second: measures of length, mass, and time, respectively. Scientific notation is used to avoid the clumsiness of zeros: the number of bacteria per milliliter in a sample is 10^7, rather than 10,000,000. In turn, prefixes of mega- (million) and kilo- (thousand) are commonly used, as well as deci- (tenth), centi- (hundredth), milli- (thousandth), and micro- or μ (millionth). Nano- describes 10^{-9} units, and pico- refers to 10^{-12}. Some measurements in medicine are not strictly derived from the metric system, however. Examples would include expressions of vitamins in international units, or the dosing of penicillin in units (of activity), and the bewildering expressions relating to radiation exposure – rads, roentgens, gray, etc. The persisting use of the English system of measurement in the United States is highly discouraged.

Scientific notation and its importance in medical practice

Expressions such as 5×10^5 platelets/mm^3 are just as straightforward as reporting 500,000 platelets per cubic mm or listing the count as 500, with the understanding that the latter expression is in thousands per cubic mm. On the other hand, expressing picogram (pg) amounts of a chemical is better handled as 5×10^{-12} grams or 5 pg, rather than the inordinately clumsy 0.000000000005 g. It is critical that laboratory reports are expressed in clear units.

Epidemiologic principles of incidence and prevalence

Incidence relates to acute conditions, such as appendicitis; it is the number of cases *occurring* within a group of subjects in a given time period. It is generally expressed as cases per 100,000 population per year. Prevalence relates more to chronic conditions, such as hypertension; it refers to the number of cases *existing* within a population at any given time. Asthma is a chronic condition, but it is punctuated with attacks leading to emergency room visits. Thus, there is a prevalence of asthma, but also an incidence of acute asthmatic attacks (often precipitated by environmental conditions such as air pollution, pollen, etc.).

Cured, impaired, alive, dead

Although the meaning of "cured" might seem obvious, it is not so simple. A patient who undergoes renal transplantation is cured of their renal failure but is certainly not healthy in the sense of a normal person who takes no medications. But neither is this patient necessarily impaired for any activity of daily life. Impairment exists in a range from mild and temporary (recovery from a fracture) to severe and completely disabling. Thus, many scales of impairment and disability have been created and many are disease specific. People may be alive but severely impaired and unable to participate in almost any normal activity. Death is fairly easy to demarcate, but here again, people die of causes completely unrelated to a disease that one might be studying. And how should the death be coded? If an epileptic patient has a seizure while driving and sustains deadly injuries, did this person die of epilepsy or trauma?

Disease association

Tuberculosis has a higher incidence in patients who live in poverty; there is a linkage between the two conditions. Smoking is associated with the development of lung cancer, but not every smoker gets cancer, and anyway, about one-third of lung cancers are believed to be due to radioactive radon gas. Perhaps the modern embodiment of a group of associations is the so-called metabolic syndrome, where there is a clear linkage between diabetes mellitus, obesity, coronary heart disease, and hypertension. Some "associations" are by default: only men develop prostate disease, and only those actually exposed to a toxin (as opposed to the greater population with potential exposure) can be injured by it.

QALY

Some conditions, such as appendicitis, are easily treated with outstanding results. Others, such as stroke, often have murky outcomes. Quality-adjusted life years (QALY) is the number of years a patient survives, multiplied by a scale denoting the medical quality of life experienced by the patient. For example, after a stroke, a patient remains hemiplegic until their death five years later of another stroke or a heart attack. If hemiplegia was assigned a scale of 0.4, then the patient has 5 x 0.4 = 2 QALY. A 10-year-old undergoing an appendectomy lives until age 85 without any medical trouble, and then dies in a fall. That individual would have 75 QALY as a result of a simple surgical procedure. When cost is added as a factor, the expression of QALY per dollar is generated, and this is a useful, if utilitarian, measure of the reasonableness of health-care expenditures.

Correlation value of 0.8 between hypertension and coronary heart disease

The correlation coefficient, r, has a range from –1 to +1. The value can be readily determined through available online calculators. A value of +1 means that there is perfect alignment between two variables. Here, it would mean that every single patient with hypertension also had coronary heart disease, and vice versa. Here, the value is 0.8, which indicates a strong association between the two conditions, but it is not invariant. Some people with hypertension will not have coronary disease, and vice versa. Values around –0.3 to +0.3 mean that there is no established or meaningful intersection of the two conditions. Strongly negative values such as –0.9 would mean that there is a negative correlation: having hypertension virtually excludes coronary heart disease as a comorbidity, and vice versa.

Hypothesis

Articulation of a hypothesis is a critical step in framing an experiment. The hypothesis is a statement, not a question, and it is written in such a way that the statement is either agreed to ("retained") or objected to ("rejected") after statistical analysis. Thus, the question, "Does antibiotic S cure streptococcal pharyngitis?" is not a hypothesis. The statement, "Antibiotic S, in doses of 10 mg/kg, given every 4 hours IV for a period of 5 days, cures streptococcal pharyngitis in children ages 6 to 18" is a hypothesis, and a very demanding one. It clearly frames the experimental subjects and the conditions of testing. If the resulting experimental paradigm is followed, and 37 of 42 patients are indeed cured after 5 days of treatment in the experimental group, but only 7 in the control group, then an X^2 test can be done to ascertain whether or not the hypothesis is a true or false statement. Here, the results are statistically significant at $p < 0.01$. Therefore, we retain the hypothesis – it's true that antibiotic S does work under the stated conditions. How sure are we of this? When we state that the hypothesis is retained with this statistical power, it means we will be wrong less than 1 time of every 100 such statements.

Null hypothesis

The null hypothesis is a statement of the hypothesis in negative terms; in the prior example, there will NOT be an effect of antibiotic S under the stated conditions. Here, the outcome is so obvious that the value of $p < 0.01$ clearly means that if you say there is no effect, you are (conversely) wrong more than 99 times out of 100. The problem with hypothesis and null hypothesis comes in the interpretation of data that are much closer to chance occurrences. In the prior example, if antibiotic S cured only a disappointing 14 of the 42, and the control group stayed the same, then the p value is about 0.08. This means you are wrong 8 times out of 100. Did the drug have an effect or not? Was the hypothesis stated positively or in "null" fashion? If written as a positive hypothesis, and you retain it, you are wrong 8 times in 100; in other words, there is some effect, but not to the magical 5% confidence limit. If, on the other hand, you accept the null statement that there is no effect, you are wrong 92 times of 100, but not to the mysterious 95/100 limit of being "significantly" wrong. With either statement, the results here are indeterminate.

Experimental control

Scientists sometimes just describe a phenomenon, but more often, they attempt to establish whether or not a certain manipulation or exposure has an effect. To do this, they must establish at least two groups of subjects – one or more groups ("controls") that are not subjected to the condition being tested, and one or more groups ("experimental") that are subject to the test condition. They must then eliminate all the confounding variables that might lead to a false result, so that the *only* difference between the control groups and the experimental groups is the condition that they seek to evaluate. Controls might include, for example, patients not receiving any drug or just a placebo (usually normal saline), but it also might include another group of patients who are already receiving drug A, a medication in common use. The experimental group might have subsets as well – for example, low-dose X and high-dose X. Such a paradigm would allow comparison of low- or high-dose X against no drug or placebo, but the study would discover the comparative outcome when drug A is a known and intentionally included confounding variable.

Variables

The independent variable is typically graphed on the abscissa (*x*-axis), and in the medical sciences, it is often time. The dependent variable is the condition being studied – for example, hemoglobin level, arterial diameter, or nerve conduction velocity. This variable, which is usually graphed on the ordinate or *y*-axis, is being examined against, or in the context of, the independent variable. Thus we would have hemoglobin level as a function of age, arterial diameter as a function of epinephrine concentration in a bath, or nerve conduction velocity as a function of limb temperature. It is easy to construct graphs showing multiple dependent variables against the same scale of a single independent variable – for example, multiple enzyme levels plotted over time. Confounding variables are many and often difficult to track down. Often, they constitute environmental problems, such as background sound level, room temperature, illumination, etc. A recently recognized confounding variable that seems to be much more important than previously recognized is gender as related to drug studies. Men and women have considerably different reactions to some commonly used pharmaceuticals. Identification of this item as a variable allows studies to be stratified into male and female compartments and may lead to clearer results in one or both groups.

Conditions for a double-blind, prospective study of the effects of an experimental drug

First, the principal investigators develop a study plan. They then consult with statisticians about the number of patients to enroll. If only a small positive effect is anticipated, it may be necessary to think of enrolling hundreds of patients, but if preliminary research has shown a dramatic effect, perhaps a biostatistics expert would only recommend an "*n*" of 120. Next, the patients will be randomized (e.g., by zip Code of residence, Social Security number, month of birth, etc.) to the control or experimental group. Typically, the control group receives either a placebo (intravenous injections of normal saline, for example) or a comparison gold-standard drug – digoxin in this case. The drug supplier will send to the hospital pharmacy envelopes marked in a manner that does not disclose which patient is receiving the control as opposed to the experimental drug. Once a patient signs the informed consent form, an investigator connected with the study will inform the pharmacy of the randomizing datum – say, zip Code. The pharmacists then send an "even" or "odd" envelope to the nursing station, and the patient receives that drug. Evaluators fill out forms relating to the severity of heart failure signs and symptoms before, during, and after treatment. No one except the coordinating study center knows whether the patient received the experimental drug until the study is completed and results are tallied.

Longitudinal observational study

Suppose that a researcher is interested in the long-term effects of estrogen use by postmenopausal women on the incidence of breast cancer. (For simplicity, let us assume that there is no genetic contribution to carcinoma in any of them.) A large number of women would be enrolled in the study and screened, probably by mammography, to ascertain that none of them had evidence of cancer at the inception of the study. No attempt would be made to influence their use or nonuse of estrogens. The results of the study might be clearer if routine rescreening was done at fixed intervals, but this is not a *sine qua non* for proceeding; one might just tally any woman who does have a cancer detected. At intervals of perhaps three to five years, the numbers of women with and without cancer would be determined and compared to their use of various estrogen preparations and doses. The key is that the study is purely observational – what happens, happens, and the research team is merely reporting observations.

Noninferiority

This relatively new expression is used in outcomes research when, for example, experimental drug B has about the same results in treating a disease as standard drug A. Even if drug B seems to work a little worse than drug A, the statistics show that it is the same, and hence, it is "noninferior" to standard drug A. This is very much like a rephrasing of the null hypothesis: there is no difference between A and B. If the p value for this statement is > 0.05, then the hypothesis is retained, and A and B have effects that cannot be described as different. Therefore, neither is superior to the other.

Drug study that found the control group and the experimental group are significantly different at a p value of 0.001

Science is, by its very nature, always open to new findings and to reinterpretation of prior understandings of a matter. In a pedantic sense, that is not comfortable to laypersons; scientists are never *absolutely* certain about anything. Nonetheless, they can be pretty sure about many things. The magic p value of 0.05 means, in the situation of this question, that there is only a 1 in 20 or 5% chance that the control group and experimental group are really the same (or not different from each other). This would happen by chance – dumb luck – due to the way the study was done, the manner in which individual patients reacted, and so on. If the p value fell to 0.01, this means that there is only a 1% chance that the two groups are not really different from each other. The 0.001 value means that there is a 1 in 1,000 chance that calling them the same (not different) is actually correct. In other words, it is very highly likely that they really are different.

Meta-analysis

Meta-analysis is the comparison and analysis of multiple reports relating to a substantially similar matter, usually generated over some period of time and at multiple institutions. Meta-analysis seeks to answer difficult therapeutic questions by increasing the "n" and therefore giving added statistical power to a conclusion. The difficulties are many. Case definitions may vary; for example, hypertension might be defined in terms of mean arterial pressure in one study, but diastolic pressures in another. Some studies might exclude persons over a certain age, say, 55, and other investigations include septuagenarians. Some publications are retrospective; others are prospective. One center might evaluate lung disease radiographically, whereas other investigators principally use pulmonary function testing.

T-test used to compare a control and experimental groups

Student's t-test is used to compare measurements in groups. For example, suppose that before the administration of a drug to 200 patients, the serum potassium is 4.5 ± 0.2 mEq/L. At some later date, the value is 3.9 ± 0.3 mEq/L. Is a value of 4.1 mEq/L in the before or after group? (Answer: it is impossible to say.) The t-test analyzes the partial overlap of the families of numbers to answer this question: "Are the groups different?" The null hypothesis states that they are the same. Taking into account the actual difference between means – here, 0.6 mEq/L, and dividing that number by the pooled standard deviations, a value is derived. This number is then sought in a t value table opposite the degrees of freedom, or absolute number of samples. The number residing at that intersection is the probability that the null hypothesis is wrong. Many variations of the simple test exist; online calculators are readily available.

Chi-square test used to evaluate the outcome of a study

The X^2, or chi-square test, is used when there is an expectation about the outcomes of an event. For example, in a mouse-breeding experiment, if Mendelian autosomal dominance pertains to black (dominant) and white (recessive) coat color, then breeding males and females who are both heterozygous for the condition should produce a 3:1 ratio of black to white offspring. Nature is not perfect, however: suppose in 948 offspring, there are 719 black mice and only 229 white mice. X^2 is calculated by determining observed minus the expected number for each category, squaring that number to get rid of the potential negative signs, then dividing that number for each category by the number of expected, and adding the two similarly treated categories together. Here, $(719 - 711)^2/711 + (229 - 237)^2/237 = 64/711 + 64/237 = 0.36$. The degrees of freedom (df) in the X^2 table is the number of possible outcomes (2, black or white) minus one; therefore, it is 1 in this case. Using standard tables, the observed results are not different from the expected results at about a 50% level of certainty; therefore, perhaps the predicted autosomal dominance pattern is working here, or perhaps not. The study must be repeated to get cleaner numbers to be "sure."

Example: In a study, the mean arterial pressure (MAP) of 500 control subjects was 78 ± 6 torr. Calculate the number with a MAP level greater than 90.

Assuming a normally distributed population (no skewness or kurtosis of the distribution curve), then about 68% will fall within the first standard deviation, or between 72 torr and 84 torr. Another 13.5% or so of the population will fall between 66 torr and 72 torr on the low end and 90 torr at the upper end (at the second standard deviation mark). So far, 95% of the population is accounted for. Only 2.5% will be less than 66 torr, and 2.5% will be greater than 90 torr. Therefore, 2.5% of 500 patients, or about 12 to 13 patients, will have MAP levels greater than 90 torr. Only 0.5% of patients (two or three) will have levels less than 78 – 3(6), or 60 torr, and a similar two or three will have levels greater than 78 + 3(6), or 96 torr.

Graph showing drug levels in a group of patients over time

At each point in time, a number of patients have undergone determination of the drug level. Suppose at the one-month point, only 47 of 54 enrolled study patients reported for their blood test. The results would be reported for those 47 as a mean ± standard deviation. This would appear as a dot (or equivalent symbol) with equal-length bars above and below the dot, showing the (first) standard deviation of the blood levels. A glance at such a figure gives the reader a sense of the "tightness" of the data (i.e., whether the blood levels were fairly consistent or all over the map). For each month, the numbers will be different. Next month, perhaps 52 individuals have their blood tested, and the results are more spread out. In this case, the standard deviation will be larger, so the error bars will be longer. Think of each point as a mean with a little bell curve superimposed upon it at a 90° orientation to the body of the graph.

Kaplan–Meier survival curve

Most patients with malignant brain tumors die within a year or two of diagnosis. A graph of the percentage surviving at various times after diagnosis would show gradual drop-off after a few months until the group of patients is almost, but not quite, extinguished altogether after perhaps four or five years. This is a standard K-M control curve, and it allows prediction of the lifespan remaining until, for example, 50% of the patients have expired. A treatment group undergoing radiation or immunotherapy can be compared to determine if overall survival is improved, worsened, or unaffected. If the curves are virtually superimposable, then there is no demonstrated treatment effect on time of death (although quality of life prior to that time might be the same, better, or worse). If the 50% survival time is meaningfully lengthened (say, from 9 months to 20 months), then the treatment might have some clinical utility. A special feature of K-M curves involving surgical treatment is that there is often about a 10% step-off of survival due to initial operative mortality.

Representative sample

A researcher who wants to know about a parameter in a population must decide how that population is to be sampled. If the population was all teachers at an elementary school, it might be possible to capture data from each and every one of them. On the other hand, if the researcher needs to learn the carbon monoxide levels of people living within 500 m of the Los Angeles freeway system, only a few of them can be counted, because of costs and other obvious limitations. But which ones? And on what day(s) of the week, and at what time of day? And during what meteorological conditions? Does the study contemplate including children? The researcher must think about the ultimate question that led to the research; in other words, what is to be done with the data once they are collected. This will help frame the scope of the research and define the sample population. Consultation with a statistician is generally needed to make sure that the sample size ("n") is large enough to have statistical power and that the sampling is done in carefully preplanned but numerically randomized manner.

Type I error

A type I (α) error occurs when a relationship is believed to exist when indeed it does not. As an example, suppose an investigator conducts an experiment to determine if a certain drug is toxic to mice at various doses. At a given dose, she finds that 75% of 200 experimental mice died abruptly, but only 2% of the 200 control mice. Doing an X^2 test, she determines that this is highly significant ($p < 0.01$)t and concludes that the drug is toxic. What she does not know is that a technician left a window open near the experimental cages, and most of the mice froze to death on a very cold night. The control group was near a radiator and mostly survived. Thus, the investigator makes a type I error because she is missing a critical piece of information.

Type II error

A type II (β) error occurs when a relationship *does* exist, but it is falsely believed not to. This might occur, for example, due to the "tyranny of small numbers" inherent in statistics. A multicenter drug study was conducted to determine whether or not a drug was useful for a condition that was extremely debilitating or fatal in most instances. Around 1,200 patients were enrolled, but only about 600 completed the study, roughly half in the placebo group and half in the experimental group. It was immediately apparent to all the practitioners at all centers that something new and positive was happening. As it turned out, there was only a weak statistical "proof" that the drug had any efficacy, irrespective of the observations of the clinicians. Had a single patient in the good-outcomes group been instead, by luck alone, in the bad-outcomes group, the drug would have failed statistical proof and been rejected – a type II error. Subsequent studies and broad clinical use of the drug were much more convincing for efficacy, and it is the gold-standard treatment today. A type II error was averted by the slimmest of margins – a single case.

Hematopoietic and Lymphoreticular Systems

Pre-embryonic development

During the pre-embryonic stage of development after fertilization, cellular multiplication and cellular differentiation occur. During cellular multiplication, the morula (a ball of 12 to 16 cells) forms. When the morula enters the uterus, the intracellular fluid increases, and a cavity forms within the morula. The inner mass of cells, the blastocyst, is surrounded by an outer layer that surrounds the cavity, the trophoblast. The trophoblast develops into the embryonic membrane called the chorion and the blastocyst develops into the embryonic disc (a double layer of cells), from which the embryo will develop, and into the amnion, another embryonic membrane. About 2 weeks after conception, the mass of blastocyst cells differentiate into germ layers—the ectoderm, the mesoderm, and the endoderm—from which all organs and organ systems develop. The hematopoietic and lymphoreticular system develop from the mesoderm.

Hematopoietic system

During embryonic development of the hematopoietic system, both blood cells and blood vessels, develops from the mesoderm. Blood vessels arise from vasculogenesis from blood islands as well as from angiogenesis with vessels sprouting from existing vessels. At about 2 to 3 weeks after conception, basic fibroblastic growth factor (FGF2) induces blood islands to begin to develop in the mesoderm in the wall of the yolk sac and a transitory population of blood cells arises from mesoderm cells that form hemangioblasts. The mesoderm cells secrete vascular endothelial growth factor (VEGF), which causes the hemangioblasts to develop the blood vessels and blood cells. From about the second week to the second month after conception, most erythropoiesis occurs in the wall of the yolk sac. This period of development is known as the mesoblastic period, during which primitive erythroblasts and embryonic hemoglobin are formed.

During fetal maturation of the hematopoietic system, while some primitive blood cells develop early from the wall of the yolk sac, the hematopoietic stem cells develop from mesoderm surrounding the aorta, the aorta-gonad-mesonephros (AGM) region. These blood cells colonize in the liver, where most red blood cells are formed from months 2 to 7 after conception. This is known as the hepatic period, during which (extramedullary) hematopoiesis occurs in the liver, which produces erythrocytes and fetal hemoglobin, as well as in the spleen, thymus, and lymph nodes, which produce some erythrocytes and lymphocytes. Leukocytes and megakaryocytes also begin to be produced in small numbers during this period. At about 7 months, the stem cells from the liver colonize the bone marrow (intramedullary hematopoiesis), which then takes over the primary role in hematopoiesis. At this time, adult hemoglobin A begins to form.

Perinatal period

Changes occur to the hematopoietic system in the perinatal period. During fetal maturation, fetal erythropoietin produced in the liver controls erythrocyte production as the mother's erythropoietin does not enter fetal circulation. Up to 90% of fetal erythrocytes contain fetal hemoglobin, which has a higher affinity to oxygen than adult hemoglobin. This fetal hemoglobin allows for increased oxygen transfer to the fetus; however, fetal hemoglobin less readily transfers oxygen to tissue cells, so this is not helpful after delivery. Thus, prior to delivery, the hemoglobin begins to shift from fetal to adult. After delivery, the production of erythropoietin shifts from the liver to the kidneys. The sudden increase in PaO_2 from about 30 mm Hg to at least 90 mm Hg after delivery causes erythropoietin levels to decrease, resulting in physiologic anemia because production of erythrocytes is depressed for up to 8 weeks.

Transport functions of the cardiovascular and lymphatic systems

The cardiovascular and lymphatic systems are the two organ systems involved in transport of substances throughout the body. The cardiovascular system includes the heart, arteries, veins, capillaries, and blood, while the lymphatic system includes lymphatic vessels, lymph nodes, lymphatic fluid, the thymus, and the spleen. Transport functions:
- Cardiovascular system/Blood: Carries gases (oxygen from the lungs to the cells and carbon dioxide from the cells to the lungs), hormones (from the endocrine organs to target cells), nutrients (from the GI system to the cells), and waste products (from the body cells to the kidneys and bladder).
- Lymphatic system: Carries excess fluids from the interstitial spaces back to the bloodstream and absorbs fatty acids from the intestines and transports them to the blood. The lymphatic system can also transport cancerous cells from one organ to another.

Thymus gland

The thymus gland, located anterior to the aortic arch and posterior to the upper body of the sternum, is positioned in front of the trachea and extends to the pericardium. At birth, the thymus is about 5 cm by 4 cm in size and 6 mm thick; it is largest during puberty and then shrinks during adulthood with adipose and connective tissue replacing thymus tissue in elderly persons. The thymus is bilobed and enclosed in fibrous connective tissue, which extends into the organ, creating lobules, which contain lymphocytes that migrated to the thymus from the bone marrow where they developed from progenitor cells. Some of these lymphocytes develop into T lymphocytes, which are part of the immune defense system. Each lobe comprises a cortex (superficial tissue that receives immature T lymphocytes and exposes them to antigens) and medulla (where T lymphocytes continue to mature). Protein hormones, thymosins, are secreted by epithelial cells in the thymus to stimulate maturation of the T lymphocytes after they leave the thymus.

Spleen

The spleen lies in the upper left abdominal cavity, inferior to the diaphragm and posterior and lateral to the stomach. It is similar to a lymph node but filters blood instead of lymph. The fist-shaped organ is 7 to 14 cm in length. The spleen is encased in connective tissue that extends inward, dividing the spleen into lobules. Nerves and blood vessels enter through a hilum on one surface. Tissue present in the lobules:
- White pulp: This is distributed throughout the lobules in tiny islands and comprises splenic nodules (similar to lymph nodes), which contain lymphocytes.
- Red pulp: This fills the spaces not filled by white pulp, surrounding the venous sinuses. The pulp contains primarily red blood cells as well as some lymphocytes and macrophages. The red pulp filters the blood. The blood capillaries are porous, allowing the red blood cells to enter the venous sinuses. Macrophages destroy foreign particles and cellular debris.
- Marginal zone: Stores white blood cells and platelets.

The spleen carries out four primary functions:
- Reservoir: About a third of the circulating platelets and granulocytes are stored in the spleen, posing a problem if the spleen is ruptured and large numbers of platelets abruptly enter peripheral circulation.
- Filtration: Red blood cells are filtered and those with abnormalities are culled from circulation by phagocytosis. Antibodies are removed, leaving smaller red blood cells called spherocytes. Inclusions are also removed.
- Immune response: The spleen promotes phagocytosis of encapsulated organisms and provides opsonizing antibodies to strip the capsules from bacteria, making the bacteria more susceptible to destruction by the phagocytic reticuloendothelial system (RES).
- Hematopoiesis: The spleen produces blood cells during fetal development and can assume production of blood cells if the bone marrow is not functioning properly (e.g., in leukemia).

Lymph nodes

The bean-shaped lymph nodes vary in size, 1 to 2 cm in length, and may occur singly or in groups. Each lymph node is enclosed in a fibrous connective tissue capsule, which extends into the node, forming trabeculae and partially dividing it into lymph nodules, the structural units. Afferent lymphatic vessels bring lymph flow into the lymph node at various points on the convex surface. The concave surface contains the hilum, where nerves and blood vessels join the lymph node, and efferent vessels, which carry lymph flow away from the node. The lymph node comprises an outer cortex, which contains packed follicles of leukocytes (primarily lymphocytes) and an inner medulla. Interior lymph sinuses contain the reticular network, chambers and channels, through which the lymph circulates and is filtered before draining into the medullary sinuses and then leaving through the efferent vessels. The primary functions of the lymph node are to filter harmful particles and to provide immune surveillance. Primary locations of lymph nodes include cervical, axillary, supratrochlear, thoracic, abdominal, pelvic, and inguinal areas.

Lymphatic pathway

The lymphatic pathway:
- Lymphatic capillaries: Extend into interstitial spaces, paralleling the network of blood capillaries. The thin walls allow fluid from interstitial spaces to enter the lymphatic capillaries as lymph. Lymphatic capillaries in the small intestine lining (lacteals) absorb digested fats.
- Lymphatic vessels (afferent): Drain capillaries and carry lymph to the lymph nodes.
- Lymph nodes: Filter the lymph.
- Lymphatic vessels (efferent): Carry filtered lymph away from the lymph nodes.
- Lymphatic trunk: Larger vessels formed from merging of efferent vessels and leading to collecting ducts. Trunks are named for the areas of the body that they serve: lumbar, intestinal, intercostal, bronchomediastinal, subclavian, and jugular.
- Collecting duct: Thoracic duct extends from the abdomen and empties into the left subclavian vein, draining all areas below the diaphragm and those on the left above the diaphragm. Right lymphatic duct extends from the right thorax and empties into the right subclavian vein, draining the right side above the diaphragm.
- Subclavian vein: Provides entry of lymph into venous system, incorporating it into the plasma.

Bone marrow

Bones are generally comprised of compact (cortical) bone overlying spongy (cancellous) bone, which contains branching bony plates (trabeculae). The ends of long bones are the epiphyses and the shafts the diaphyses. Compact bone in the diaphyses form medullary cavities, which are lined with bone-forming cells called endosteum and filled with marrow (soft connective tissue). Bone marrow is also found in spaces in spongy bone and in large central canals in other compact bone tissue. Two kinds of bone marrow include:

- Red: Contains erythroid (red) cells, myeloid (white) cells, and megakaryocytes (platelets) in different stages of maturation. Found in cavities of most bone in infants but recedes in adults and is replaced by yellow marrow. Red marrow in the adult is found primarily in spongy bone in the skull, ribs, sternum, clavicles, vertebra, and hips. Bone marrow sinuses allow mature cells to enter peripheral circulation.
- Yellow: Stores fat, but does not produce blood cells. Yellow marrow may convert back to red marrow if blood supply is inadequate.

Myeloid-erythroid ratio

The bone marrow produces both erythrocytes and leukocytes, and the proportion of each is used to determine the myeloid-erythroid ratio. Myeloid refers to the white cell elements and their precursors in the bone marrow and erythroid to the red cell elements and their precursors. Erythrocytes have a life span of approximately 120 days while leukocytes have much shorter life spans:

- Neutrophil: A few days in storage or 6 hours in circulation.
- Eosinophil: 8 to 12 days in storage and 4 to 5 hours in circulation.
- Basophil: A few hours to a few days.
- Lymphocyte: Weeks to years (depending on type).
- Monocyte: A few hours to a few days.

Because leukocytes generally have a very short life span compared with erythrocytes, many more leukocytes must be produced to provide a steady supply. Therefore, there are more myeloid elements and their precursors than erythroid. The normal myeloid to erythroid ratio is 3:1 or 4:1. This ratio may alter when hematological factors interfere with red cell production or life span, when overall production of blood cells is impaired, or when one particular cell markedly increases production.

Hemoglobin and transport proteins in oxygen and carbon dioxide transport

Gas exchange between oxygen and carbon dioxide occurs in the alveoli. Gas diffuses from an area of higher partial pressure to an area of lower partial pressure until a state of equilibrium is reached. Each erythrocyte contains about 280 million molecules of hemoglobin (Hgb) (comprising about a third of the cell). Hemoglobin is a transport protein because it carries oxygen and carbon dioxide. Hemoglobin (a tetramer) consists of heme, with each molecule of heme carrying one atom of iron (essential for hemoglobin synthesis), and globin, a protein chain consisting of four different globulins: $\alpha 1$, $\alpha 2$, $\beta 1$, and $\beta 2$. The alpha globulins contain 141 amino acids and the beta globulins 146. One molecule of heme and one protein chain of globin comprise one molecule of hemoglobin, and each molecule of hemoglobin can carry 4 molecules of oxygen (1.39 mL of oxygen per gram of Hgb). The two forms of hemoglobin include oxyhemoglobin (which is saturated with oxygen) and deoxyhemoglobin (which is saturated with carbon dioxide).

Arterial oxygen

Arterial oxygen is carried in the red blood cells by hemoglobin. Each hemoglobin molecule can carry 4 molecules of oxygen, with one gram of hemoglobin equal to 1.39 mL of oxygen (100 mL arterial blood carries 0.3 mL oxygen). When the hemoglobin is fully saturated (four O_2 molecules per molecule of hemoglobin), then arterial oxygen saturation is 100%. A small amount of oxygen remains dissolved in blood (PaO_2 x 0.0031), but this has little effect on arterial oxygen content. The formula to determine arterial oxygen (CaO_2) is as follows:

- CaO_2 = [hemoglobin x arterial oxygen saturation (SaO_2) x 1.39] + [arterial partial pressure of oxygen (PaO_2 x 0.003)]
- A simplified formula is sometimes used to evaluate oxygen delivery (O_2D):
- O_2D = [stroke volume (SV) x heart rate (HR)] x oxygen saturation (SpO_2).
- Perfusion pressure is estimated by the systolic blood pressure:
- Systolic blood pressure = cardiac output (CO) x systemic vascular resistance (SVR).

Because the oxygen in the blood is related to hemoglobin levels, correcting anemia more effectively increases PaO_2 than FiO_2.

Oxyhemoglobin dissociation curve

The oxyhemoglobin dissociation curve is a graph that plots the percentage of hemoglobin saturated with oxygen (Y-axis) different partial pressures of oxygen (PaO_2 levels) (X-axis). A curve shift to the right, as occurs with acidosis, represents conditions where hemoglobin has less affinity for oxygen and greater amounts of oxygen are released to the tissues. Low pH shifts the curve to the right, enabling increased off-loading of hemoglobin to tissues. A shift to the left, which occurs with hypothermia and alkalosis, has the opposite implications, increased binding of oxygen but less release to the tissues. Blood transfusions and elevated oxygen shift the curve to the left, causing increased affinity of hemoglobin for oxygen in the lungs. Normal PaO_2 is 80 to 100 mm Hg, equal to 95% to 98% oxygen saturation. Levels less than 40 mm Hg are dangerous.

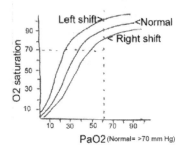

Erythrocytes

Erythrocytes (red blood cells) are biconcave discs about 7.5 µm in diameter. The shape increases surface area through which gases can diffuse for transport and also allows the cell to change shape to travel through narrow capillaries. Erythrocyte production takes place in myeloid tissue (bone marrow) in response to oxygen deficiency, which triggers release of erythropoietin by the kidneys and liver (to a lesser degree), which stimulates the bone marrow to produce red blood cells (RBCs). A nucleated precursor matures into a nonnucleated hemoglobin-filled cell. The nucleus is shed to allow space for hemoglobin, so the cell cannot synthesize messenger RNA or replicate. The cells contain no mitochondria and produce ATP by way of glycolysis and do not utilize the oxygen they

- 85 -

carry. The RBCs are released into the blood stream in an immature state called reticulocytes. They continue to mature over 24 to 36 hours and have a life span of about 120 days. About a third of an erythrocyte comprises hemoglobin. Normal values of RBC count vary by gender:

- Males older than 18 years: 4.5 to 5.5 million per mm³.
- Females older than 18 years: 4 to 5 million per mm³.

Plasma

Plasma is the straw-colored liquid portion of the blood, comprising about 55% of blood volume. It contains essential clotting factors. Constituents of plasma include:

- Water: 92% of volume.
- Proteins: 6% to 8% of volume. Over 500 proteins have been identified. The 3 main groups include albumin (60%), fibrinogen (4%), and globulins, including antibodies (36%). Plasma proteins help to maintain the colloid osmotic pressure of plasma, which tends to retain fluid in the capillaries because they are too large to diffuse through capillary walls. If the concentration of plasma proteins decreases, the osmotic pressure falls, resulting in edema as fluids shift to the interstitial spaces. Globulins (alpha, beta, and gamma) transport lipids and fat-soluble vitamins).
- Electrolytes: 0.8%.
- Lipids: 0.6%. Includes low-density lipoprotein (LDL), high-density lipoprotein (HDL), and triglycerides.
- Glucose: 0.1%. Plasma levels tend to be 10% to 15% higher than whole blood levels.

Platelets

Platelets (thrombocytes), produced from megakaryocytes in the bone marrow, are fragments of cytoplasm, lack a nucleus, and live about 10 days. Thrombopoietin (TPO), a hormone, is produced in the kidneys and liver and regulates production of both the megakaryocytes and platelets. The TPO stimulates production of megakaryocytes, which eventually break apart into platelets. A normal platelet count is 150,000 to 400,000/mm³. Platelets are disk-shaped at rest but change to a globular form with pseudopodia when activated, helping them to bind together. While some platelets circulate in the blood, others are held in reserve in the spleen until needed. At the end of their life cycle, platelets are destroyed by phagocytes in the spleen and liver. The primary role of platelets is in hemostasis. Once a vessel is damaged, it releases cytokines, adenosine diphosphate (ADP), thromboxane A1, and serotonin. Platelets respond by expressing glycoprotein IIb/IIA and platelet-endothelial cell adhesion molecule 1, which begin the process of clotting:

- Adhesion: Single platelets bind to wound site in response to release of tissue thromboplastin (factor III) from damaged blood vessels (extrinsic clotting mechanism).
- Activation: Tissue thromboplastin activates factor VII, which combines with and activates factor X, which combines with and activates factor V. These reactions require calcium ions (factor IV) and release prothrombin activator (factor II), which is converted into thrombin (factor IIa). Platelets change shape and release substances to activate other platelets and constrict vessels.
- Aggregation: Thrombin fragments soluble fibrinogen, forming insoluble fibrin, creating a mesh to stabilize the plug and stop bleeding.
- Clot: Bleeding contained.

The prothrombin time evaluates the time needed to form fibrin threads in blood plasma for the extrinsic clotting mechanism.

Age-associated changes in the hematopoietic system

There is some controversy regarding changes noted in the hematopoietic system with age, as it is not always clear if they are the result of aging or disease processes and hematopoietic stress. Some common changes:

- Decreased proliferative capacity of hematopoietic stem cells is believed to result from shortening of telomeres on chromosomes. When telomeres become too short, stem cell proliferation is impaired, so mature hematopoietic cells are reduced.
- Progenitor cells CD34+ begin to decrease in number in early stages of aging.
- Changes in cytokine production occur with age, interfering with the regulation of hematopoiesis. Peripheral blood produces less interleukin 3 and less granulocyte-macrophage colony-stimulating factor, resulting in decreased stimulation for production of hematopoietic cells, while interleukin 6 and tumor necrosis factor alpha have increased concentration, which may disrupt homeostatic regulation and may increase functional decline.
- Anemia related to decreased erythrocytes and hemoglobin is common in older adults, especially in men.

Intrinsic clotting mechanism

With the intrinsic clotting mechanism, all the factors necessary are already present in the blood. While the initial activation is different from that of the extrinsic clotting mechanism, the process is the same from the point where prothrombin activator is released. When blood is exposed to a foreign surface (collagen, glass), Hageman factor (factor XII) is activated, which in turns activates factor XI, which activates factor IX, which combines with factor VIII and platelet phospholipids to activate factor X. These activations also require factor IV (calcium ions) and result in release of prothrombin activator (factor II), which is converted into thrombin (factor IIa). Thrombin fragments soluble fibrinogen, forming insoluble fibrin, creating a mesh to stabilize the plug and form a clot. The partial thromboplastin test evaluates the time needed to form fibrin threads in blood plasma in intrinsic clotting.

Clotting factors I through XIII

Factor	Name	Synthesized	Active form	Clotting mechanism
I	Fibrinogen	Liver	Fibrin	Extrinsic/Intrinsic
II	Prothrombin	Liver with vit. K	Serine protease	Extrinsic/Intrinsic
III	Tissue thrombo-plastin	Damaged tissue	Receptor/cofactor	Extrinsic
IV	Calcium ions	Diet/bone		Extrinsic/Intrinsic
V	Proaccelerin	Liver, released by platelets	Cofactor	Extrinsic/Intrinsic
VII	Serum prothrombin conversion accelerator (Proconvertin)	Liver with vit. K	Serine protease	Extrinsic
VIII	Antihemophilic factor	Released by platelets and endothelial cells	Cofactor	Intrinsic
IX	Plasma thromboplastin component (Christmas factor)	Liver with vit. K	Serine protease	Intrinsic
X	Stuart-Prower factor	Liver with vit. K	Serine protease	Extrinsic/Intrinsic
XI	Plasma thromboplastin antecedent	Liver	Serine protease	Intrinsic
XII	Hageman factor	Liver	Serine protease	Intrinsic
XIII	Fibrin stabilizing factor Prekallikrein (Fletcher factor) HMWK (Fitzgerald factor)	Liver, released by platelets	Trans-gluta-minase Serine protease Cofactor	Extrinsic/Intrinsic

Age-associated changes in the immune system

Most studies of aging of the immune system have involved animal studies, but some common findings include:
- The innate immune system dysfunctions with fibroblasts and macrophages releasing increased levels of proinflammatory cytokines, leading to increased incidence of atherosclerosis and diseases, such as diabetes.
- Calcium deficiency, common in older adults, impairs cell signaling of the immune system and inhibits production of cytokines, necessary for adequate immune response.
- Decreased efficiency of phagocytosis results from inhibition caused by lower production of superoxide anion, necessary to destroy ingested foreign material.

- The thymus gland begins to atrophy (involution) during adolescence and continues so that by middle age serum activity related to thymic hormones is almost absent.
- IgM concentration decreases with age and IgA and IgG increase, so responses to vaccinations are less effective. Lower production of IgE results in decreased allergic and hypersensitivity reactions.

Age-related changes to the immune system include:
- T-cell activity declines with age and the thymus contains more immature T-cells. This T cell change can contribute to reactivation of viruses, such as herpes zoster, and other infections. The ratio of naïve to memory T cells changes with age with higher ratio of naïve to memory in the young and lower with age, so older adults have less effective response to new antigens. Replicative senescence occurs as B and T cells lose their ability to replicate.
- Cell signaling is impaired because CD28, which should be located on the surface of T cells so that they can respond to antigens, is often missing on T cells of older adults.
- Increased autoimmune responses are evident in older adults with increased numbers of T- and B-cell antibodies that attack the body's own cells, leading to autoimmune diseases, such as diabetes, rheumatoid arthritis, osteoporosis, and cardiovascular disorders.
- B-cell response to new antigens is decreased. B cells' changes develop slowly but increase more rapidly after age 60.

Bacteremia, septicemia, and systemic inflammatory response syndrome (SIRS)

A number of terms are used to refer to severe infections and they are often used interchangeably, but they are part of a continuum:
- Bacteremia is the presence of bacteria in the blood but without systemic infection.
- Septicemia is a systemic infection caused by pathogens (usually bacteria or fungi) present in the blood.
- Systemic inflammatory response syndrome (SIRS), a generalized inflammatory response affecting may organ systems, may be caused by infectious or non-infectious agents, such as trauma, burns, adrenal insufficiency, pulmonary embolism, and drug overdose. If an infectious agent is identified or suspected, SIRS is an aspect of sepsis. Infective agents include a wide range of bacteria and fungi, including *Streptococcus pneumoniae* and *Staphylococcus aureus.* SIRS includes 2 of the following:
  o Elevated (more than 38°C) or subnormal (less than 36°C) rectal temperature.
  o Tachypnea or $PaCO_2$ less than 32 mm Hg.
  o Tachycardia.
  o Leukocytosis (more than 12,000/mm³) or leukopenia (less than 4000/mm³).

Sepsis, severe sepsis, septic shock, and multi-organ dysfunction syndrome (MODS)

Infections can progress from bacteremia, septicemia, and SIRS to the following:
- Sepsis is presence of infection either locally or systemically in which there is a generalized life-threatening inflammatory response (SIRS). It includes all the indications for SIRS as well as one of the following:
  o Changes in mental status.
  o Hypoxemia (less than 72 mm Hg) without pulmonary disease.
  o Elevation in plasma lactate.
  o Decreased urinary output less than 5 mL/kg/wt for at least 1 hour.

- Severe sepsis includes both indications of SIRS and sepsis as well as indications of increasing organ dysfunction with inadequate perfusion and/or hypotension.
- Septic shock is a progression from severe sepsis in which refractory hypotension occurs despite treatment. There may be indications of lactic acidosis.
- Multi-organ dysfunction syndrome (MODS) is the most common cause of sepsis-related death. Cardiac function becomes depressed, acute respiratory distress syndrome (ARDS) may develop, and renal failure may follow acute tubular necrosis or cortical necrosis. Thrombocytopenia appears in about 30% of those affected and may result in disseminated intravascular coagulation (DIC). Liver damage and bowel necrosis may occur.

> ➤ **Review Video:** Multiple Organ Dysfunction System
> Visit **mometrix.com/academy** and enter **Code: 394302**

Cat scratch disease and tularemia

Cat scratch disease: Cats can develop a bacterial infection of the reticuloendothelial (phagocytic) system with the gram-negative bacillus, *Bartonella henselae*, when bitten by a tick or flea and pass it on to humans with a bite or scratch. Symptoms include a blister or sore at site of infection, regional lymphadenopathy, fever, malaise, and anorexia. Infections are usually mild and self-limiting, but rare complications may occur, including bacillary angiomatosis, Parinaud oculoglandular syndrome, encephalopathy, joint inflammation, atypical pneumonitis, neuroretinitis, osteomyelitis, and hepatitis/splenitis.

Tularemia: This acute febrile infectious disease is caused by the gram-negative bacterium *Francisella tularensis* and can be spread by ticks or fleas. There are 6 forms: ulceroglandular (spreads by proximal lymphatic system), glandular (gains access to the lymphatic system or bloodstream), oculoglandular (gains access through conjunctiva), oropharyngeal (from eating undercooked infected rabbit), pneumonic (inhaled), and typhoidal (mode of infection unknown). Tularemia is highly contagious. Symptoms include ulcerative lesions, fever, chills, headache, chest pain, sore throat, nausea and vomiting, rash, and diarrhea. Treatment is with streptomycin (drug of choice [DOC]) or other antibiotics.

Q fever

Q fever is an infection of the reticuloendothelial system by the gram-negative bacterium *Coxiella burnetii*, which in early stages can cause pneumonia and hepatitis, and in chronic stages endocarditis. Q fever is transmitted by inhalation of infected barnyard dust, ingestion of contaminated milk followed by regurgitation and inspiration of contaminated food, and tick bite. About 50% of those infected show no symptoms, but symptoms may be life-threatening in others:
- Acute stage: high fever, headache, malaise myalgia, confusion, sore throat, chills, sweats, cough (nonproductive) nausea and vomiting, diarrhea, hepatitis, and pneumonia (in 30% to 50%). Some may develop rash, neurologic syndrome, myocarditis, or pericarditis.
- Chronic stage (1 to 20 years after initial infection): endocarditis (usually of aortic valves), cirrhosis, interstitial pulmonary fibrosis, and death.

Treatment: DOC is doxycycline for 15 to 21 days (best if started within 3 days of onset). Endocarditis requires treatment with doxycycline and quinolones for at least 4 years and surgery may be required for damaged valves.

Brucellosis

Brucellosis is infection of the reticuloendothelial system by *Brucella* species, found in animals: *B. melitensis* (goats, sheep), *B. suis* (pigs), *B. abortus* (cattle), and *B. canis* (dog). *Brucella* are gram-negative aerobic bacteria that can invade both phagocytic cells and non-phagocytic and exist in the intracellular areas. The bacteria can replicate in virtually any organ. Transmission to humans occurs through ingesting undercooked meat or unpasteurized dairy products, inhaling bacteria, or contaminating open skin/mucous membranes. While rare, brucellosis can also be spread by sexual contact and through breastfeeding. People who work with the bacteria in laboratories or work with animals are most at risk. Diagnosis is per cultures and serology. Initial symptoms are flu-like (headache, myalgia, fatigue, fever, anorexia). Some symptoms may become chronic or recur: arthritis (pyogenic joint infusions), testicular/scrotal edema, endocarditis/valvular lesions, fatigue, depression, hepatomegaly/splenomegaly, fevers, and neurological abnormalities. Relapse rates are high (40%) with one antibiotic, so combinations (doxycycline and rifampin) are usually used. Surgical intervention may be needed to repair/replace heart valves and drain abscesses or effusions.

Ehrlichiosis

Ehrlichiosis, an infection of reticuloendothelial cells, results from several bacterial species in the genus *Ehrlichia*. *Ehrlichieae* are small, gram-negative rickettsial bacteria that primarily invade leukocytes, where they divide to form vacuole-bound colonies known as morulae (mulberry like clusters). Ehrlichiosis is spread by ticks. Initial symptoms occur in 5 to 10 days and include fever, lymphadenopathy, malaise, headache, and myalgia. Some may develop cough, nausea, vomiting, arthralgia, confusion, and fine petechial rash (60% of children). About half of patients develop severe symptoms, which can include renal failure, DIC, meningoencephalitis, adult respiratory distress syndrome, seizures, pancytopenia, coma, and death. Treatment is with immediate doxycycline (DOC) before laboratory confirmation because the condition is so life-threatening that waiting to give the medication may endanger the patient's life.

Bacillary angiomatosis

Bacillary angiomatosis is an infection of the endothelial cells resulting in vascular proliferation. BA is caused by *Bartonella henselae* (associated with cat scratch disease) and *Bartonella quintana* (associated with the human body louse). BA may also arise with immunosuppression, such as with HIV/AIDS. BA causes hemangioma-like lesions (red or black) of the skin and subcutaneous tissue, which may grow to 4 cm in size and bleed if traumatized. Lesions may also be nodular, friable pedunculated masses, or hyperkeratotic plaques. BA may also affect the mucous membranes and internal organs. Treatment includes appropriate antibiotics for the cultured organism. Erythromycin 500 mg four times daily for 2 to 3 months is DOC. Tetracycline is the second-line drug. A number of other antibiotics have been used successfully, but treatment failures with ciprofloxacin, trimethoprim-sulfamethoxazole, isoniazid, and rifampin have been reported.

Rocky Mountain spotted fever

Rocky Mountain spotted fever is an infection of endothelial cells caused by the bacterium *Rickettsia rickettsii,* spread by hard ticks. The classic triad of symptoms incudes fever, macular rash (day 6), and history of tick bite. The organism lives and multiplies primarily in the cells lining small- to medium-sized blood vessels. The organism multiplies and kills the cells, causing blood to leak through tiny holes in the vessel walls into adjacent tissues, resulting in the petechial rash and also causing damage to organs and tissue. Later symptoms can include abdominal pain, arthralgia, and diarrhea. Damage to the vessels may cause interstitial pneumonia or myocarditis, and perivascular glial nodules in the CNS, skin, muscles, GI tract, and organs. Thrombi may form, resulting in occlusion and vascular necrosis. Patients may develop CNS disorders, renal failure, hepatomegaly/splenomegaly, and death. Residual effects include partial paralysis (lower extremities), gangrene resulting in amputations, hearing loss, incontinence, and movement disorders. Doxycycline is DOC. Treatment should start with suspected disease rather than waiting for lab results.

Babesiosis

Babesiosis is a malaria-like infection of erythrocytes caused by hemo-protozoan *Babesia* parasites and spread by infected ticks. Most people are asymptomatic, but symptoms may be severe in immunocompromised and elderly patients. The incubation period may last from 1 week to 12 months. Moderate infection is characterized by flu-like symptoms and fatigue. Severe infection is characterized by capillary blockage or microvascular stasis occurring because of erythrocyte fragments, resulting in hypotension, hepatosplenomegaly, severe hemolytic anemia, hemophagocytic syndrome, kidney failure, and death. Treatment is with both antibiotics and antiparasitic drugs. DOC is clindamycin plus quinine sulfate (Formula Q). Exchange transfusions may be needed if patients have high rates of parasitemia (more than 10%), organ failure, or severe hemolysis. Intubation and mechanical ventilation may be needed.

Autoimmunity

Autoimmunity occurs when the body's immune system fails to recognize body cells from foreign cells and produces autoantibodies and cytotoxic T lymphocytes that attack the body cells, damaging tissue and organs. The causes of autoimmunity are not always clear but may relate to different processes, such as in response to a viral infection that uses host cell protein to replicate in a cell. In fighting the virus, the immune system may associate the protein with the invasive agent and begin to attack the protein in the body cells as well as the virus. Some T lymphocytes may be defective and unable to differentiate body cells for foreign agents. In some cases, a foreign antigen may closely resemble a body antigen. Autoimmune disorders include hemolytic anemia, pernicious anemia, and systemic lupus erythematosus.

Autoimmune hemolytic anemias (AIHAs)

With autoimmune hemolytic anemias, autoantibodies attack the person's erythrocytes, resulting in accelerated destruction. AIHA may be primary or associated with other autoimmune disorders, infections, malignancies, or medications. Typical findings include anemia with increased reticulocyte count, positive Coombs test, and peripheral blood smear that shows spherocytes or erythrocyte aggregates. Types include:
- Warm AIHA: Erythrocytes attacked by autoantibody immunoglobulin G (IgG). Patients may be asymptomatic or have fatigue or jaundice. Reactions may occur only in the laboratory or may cause life-threatening hemolysis. Severe anemia with changes in mental status is a medical emergency requiring immediate transfusion. Treatment is with glucocorticoids or rituximab.

- Cold agglutinin syndrome (CAS): Erythrocytes are coated with cold-activated immunoglobulin M (IgM) and C3d complement, triggering hemolysis. Acute CAS is associated with infections and most common in children and young adults, while chronic CAS is most common in adults older than 50 years and may be associated with lymphoma or chronic lymphocytic leukemia (CLL). Cold exposure may result in acrocyanosis and hematuria, nose and ear pain, and distal extremity pain. Treatment includes rituximab or avoiding cold.

Pernicious anemia

Pernicious anemia is an autoimmune megaloblastic anemia resulting from cobalamin (vitamin B12) deficiency because auto-antibodies attack vitamin B12 binding sites in the stomach. Intrinsic factor (IF) (normally produced by parietal cells of the gastric mucosa) is lacking because of atrophy or autoimmune destruction of parietal cells, decreasing hydrochloric acid secretion. Hydrochloric acid is necessary for secretion of IF, and IF is necessary for cobala-min absorption. Gastric surgery, removal of all or part of the ileum, Crohn disease, and long-term use of H_2-histmaine receptor blockers may also cause pernicious anemia. Diagnostic findings include decreased hemoglobin, hematocrit, reticulocytes, and cobalamin with increased mean cell volume (MCV) and mean cell hemoglobin ncentration (MCHC). RBCs are macrocytic, normochromic.

Signs and symptoms	Treatment
Sore tongue Anorexia Nausea and vomiting Weakness Peripheral paresthesia, reduced sense of position and vibration Ataxia Muscle weakness Confusion to dementia	Parenteral administration of cobalamin (B12). Typical dosage includes: Initially: 1000 mg IM daily for 14 days. Next: 1000 mg IM weekly until hematocrit is normal. Ongoing: 1000 mg IM monthly for life. Intranasal and sublingual medications are also available.

> ➤ **Review Video:** Pernicious Anemia (B12 Deficiency)
> *Visit **mometrix.com/academy** and enter **Code: 353419***

Anemia of chronic disease

Anemia of chronic disease is an inflammatory response that occurs secondary to autoimmune disorders (lupus erythematosus, rheumatoid arthritis, Crohn disease, and ulcerative colitis), cancer, liver disease, kidney disease, and long-standing infections (HIV/AIDS, endocarditis, osteomyelitis). Anemia of chronic disease is often mild and caused by an inflammatory response to disease that results in iron converted to unused ferritin, with decreased production of hemoglobin, common in patients with advanced malignancies. The cytotoxic effects of chemotherapy may worsen the anemia, which usually responds to erythropoietin rather than oral iron (which is usually ineffective). If the anemia is associated with inflammatory bowel disease, treatment with iron is usually all that is indicated; however, because of GI intolerance resulting from the disease, the iron may need to be administered parenterally. Patients with chronic infections, such as HIV, should not receive iron unless they have absolute iron deficiency because of concerns that the increased iron will also increase the risk of invasion of microorganisms. With chronic inflammation, such as rheumatoid arthritis, anemia is usually treated with erythropoietin.

- 93 -

Non-immunologically mediated transfusion complications

Transfusion-related complications include:
- Infection: Bacterial contamination of blood, especially platelets, can result in severe sepsis. A number of infective agents (viral, bacterial, and parasitic) can be transmitted. Infective agents include HIV, hepatitis C and B, human T-cell lymphotropic virus, cytomegalovirus, West Nile virus, malaria, Chagas disease, and variant Creutzfeldt-Jacob disease.
- Hypothermia: This may occur if blood products are not heated. Body temperature decrease of 0.5°C to 1°C increases oxygen consumption by 4 times.
- Circulatory overload: Patients present with cough, dyspnea, cyanosis, rales, headache, distended jugular veins, tachycardia, and orthopnea. Hypervolemia leads to pulmonary edema and cardiac failure.
- Mild allergic reaction: Release of histamine and other anaphylatoxins result in localized erythema, pruritus, flushing, and urticaria. If urticaria and pruritus are severe, this may indicate progression to anaphylaxis.
- Transient hypotension: This is associated with activation of bradykinin and use of bedside leukoreduction filters and apheresis. Risk also increases with use of ACE inhibitors.
- Hemosiderosis: Patients develop hepatomegaly, hepatic fibrosis, diabetes, cardiac failure, and bronzing of skin from accumulation of excess iron.

Transplant rejection

Transplant rejection, graft vs host disease (GVHD), may occur after bone marrow or stem cell transplant from a donor (30% to 40% incidence with related donor and 60% to 80% with unrelated). Two types include:
- Acute: Onset is within 90 days of transplant. Symptoms may include jaundice, pruritus, erythema, generalized rash, eye irritation, and GI upset (nausea, vomiting, pain, diarrhea).
- Chronic: Onset is more than 90 days after transplant. Symptoms may include eye irritation, vision changes, dry mouth and vaginal dryness, dyspnea, loss of weight, skin thickening, and raised rash. This condition may last for months or years.
- Both types are treated with anti-rejection drugs to suppress the immune system, such as corticosteroids. With both acute and chronic GVHD, some patients may develop more severe symptoms, including damage to major body organs and severe infection, because of immunocompromise related to preoperative radiation and/or chemotherapy. While GVHD may result in death, mild GVHD reactions can have a therapeutic effect because the transplanted cells may destroy remaining cancer cells.

Lymphocytes and granulocytes

Cell type	Radiation exposure	Traumatic injury
Lymphocytes	Count drops markedly within 24 hours and reaches lowest count at 48 hours. One type of T cell shows a slight increase after exposure.	Burns—B cells increase and helper T cells decrease. Trauma/Hemorrhage—immunosuppression related to shock. Increased rate of bone marrow apoptosis.
Granulocytes	Neutrophil count increases immediately after exposure and then pronounced neutropenia develops at 14 to 21 days.	Burns—Initially, granulocyte apoptosis decreases as well as functionality. Bone marrow progenitor cells and circulating granulocytes increase. If infection occurs with burns, the opposite effect is noted with decreased progenitor cells and circulating granulocytes. Wounds—Neutrophils and macrophages infiltrate the wound.

Thrombocytes and erythrocytes

Thrombocytes
Radiation exposure: Myeloid progenitor cells are lost and circulating platelets decrease. With moderate exposure, platelets may remain stable but drop 14 to 21 days after exposure. Traumatic injury: Burns—Mild decrease in thrombocytes within 1 hour and mild thrombocytosis between days 6 and 30. Megakaryocytes increase and life span of platelets is reduced for the first month.

Erythrocytes
Radiation exposure: Oxygen-carrying capacity of RBCs is impaired, although the cells are less sensitive to radiation than other blood cells.

Traumatic injury: Burns—Burn patients often exhibit anemia of critical illness, and studies suggest that in response to burns, the hematopoietic system shifts away from production of erythroid cells (with a marked fall in reticulocytes) to myeloid cells. Thus, the lower production of erythrocytes leads directly to anemia.

Trauma/Hemorrhagic shock—Production of hematopoietic cells is suppressed in the bone marrow but hematopoietic cells are released to travel to site of injury. Reticulocyte count is decreased.

Endothelial injury and hemorrhage

When endothelial injury and hemorrhage occur, collagen and clotting factors are released to bind thrombocytes to the injured area, and the coagulation process occurs, releasing byproducts that may increase permeability of the vascular system. If the hemorrhage is pronounced, then the thrombocyte count may not be sufficient to control bleeding, resulting in hypoperfusion, hypovolemic shock, and sometimes death. Trauma often leads to hemorrhage requiring resuscitative efforts, but this can cause hemodilution and hypothermia, which in turn can result in coagulopathy and more hemorrhage (dilutional coagulopathy). Hemorrhage can also lead to the "fatal triad" of shock, leading to acidosis and hypothermia, which also can cause coagulopathy.

Some degree of hypothermia is common in trauma patients because of exposed tissue and intravenous fluids, but mortality increases markedly when hypothermia is below 32°C (core temperature measurement) so temperature should be maintained at least at 33°C to 36°C.

Mechanical tissue trauma and coagulopathy

Mechanical tissue trauma may vary widely from simple lacerations to puncture wounds to extensive crush injuries, but tissue trauma is often associated with coagulopathy, which corresponds to the degree of injury. With trauma, damaged endothelial tissue exposes collagen (subendothelial, type 2) and tissue factor, which in turn bind von Willebrand factor, activated factor VII, and platelets, which activate plasma coagulation proteases. These effects then cause thrombin and fibrin formations. Hyperfibrinolysis is common after trauma because of release of tissue plasminogen activator (tPA) combined with inhibition of plasminogen activator inhibitor. Injuries associated with increased coagulopathy include severe traumatic brain injury, long bone fractures, and tissue damage. Other causes of coagulopathy include shock, hemodilution, hypothermia, acidemia, and inflammation.

Hodgkin disease

Hodgkin disease is a malignancy of the lymphatic system. It originates in a single node and then spreads contiguously along the lymphatic system. Common symptoms are swollen lymph nodes, night sweats, weight loss, red bruising associated with decreased platelet count, low-grade fever, pruritus, hepatomegaly, and splenomegaly. It is staged according to spread, with sub-stages (A and B) if specific symptoms (such as night sweats or weight loss) are present:

- Stage I A/B: Malignancy in one lymph node area (such as above the diaphragm on one side) or one area or organ (such as the stomach) outside of the lymph nodes.
- Stage II A/B: Malignancy in at least 2 lymph node areas on the same side of diaphragm OR malignancy is in only one area or organ outside of lymph nodes but the surrounding lymph nodes also have malignancy.
- Stage III A/B: Malignancy in lymph nodes on both sides of diaphragm and may spread to spleen or other organs near lymph nodes.
- Stage IV: Malignancy in organs outside of lymph nodes and may be in lymph nodes distant from organ involvement.

Treatment is chemotherapy and radiation or chemotherapy alone, depending on staging.

Non-Hodgkin lymphoma

Non-Hodgkin lymphoma (NHL) is a group of different lymphoid tumors rather than one cancer. Incidence has increased with a primary risk factor immune deficiency or dysfunction related to diseases, such as HIV, iatrogenic immune depression, congenital disorders, or autoimmune diseases. Other risk factors include infectious agents (herpesvirus, Epstein-Barr virus), human retroviruses, RNA viruses, and hepatitis C virus. Lymphomas are classified as B cell or T cell. NHL is classified with the Ann Arbor staging system (also used for Hodgkin). B-cell lymphomas have better prognosis than T-cell lymphoma. Symptoms and presentations vary widely but common symptoms include lymphadenopathy, fever, and weight loss. Lymphomas (usually B cell) may occur after bone marrow or stem cell transplantation.

Lymphomas include:
- B-cell: Burkitt lymphoma, chronic lymphocytic leukemia/small lymphocytic lymphoma (CLL/SLL), diffuse large B-cell lymphoma, follicular lymphoma, immunoblastic large cell lymphoma, precursor B-lymphoblastic lymphoma, and mantle cell lymphoma.
- T-cell: mycosis fungoides, anaplastic large cell lymphoma, and precursor T-lymphoblastic lymphoma.

Treatment involves chemotherapy, immunotherapy, and radiation therapy but depends on the type of lymphoma and whether it is indolent, relapsing, or aggressive.

> **Review Video:** Lymphoma
> Visit *mometrix.com/academy* and enter *Code:* **513277**

Acute lymphocytic leukemia (ALL)

Acute lymphocytic leukemia (ALL) is caused by a defect in the stem cells that differentiate into lymphocytes so that too many cells develop into lymphoblasts or lymphocytes, preventing development of other WBCs, RBCs, and platelets. ALL accounts for 15% of adult leukemia. Risk factors include male gender, Caucasian race, age (older than 70), history of chemotherapy or radiation exposure, and Down syndrome. Signs and symptoms:
- Weakness, lethargy.
- Increased bruising, petechiae.
- Abnormal bleeding, nosebleeds.
- Fever.
- Anorexia, weight loss.
- Anemia.
- Increased infection.
- Dyspnea.
- Bone or stomach pain.
- Painless lesions in neck, axillae, abdomen, and groin.
- Pain/fullness inferior to ribs.
- CNS manifestations including leukemic meningitis.

Treatment - Two-phase approach:
- Remission induction phase: Combination chemotherapy.
  CNS prophylaxis with intrathecal and/or systemic chemotherapy with/without radiation to the brain.
- Post-remission phase: Combination chemotherapy with/without tyrosine kinase inhibitors. Chemotherapy and stem cell transplant.
  CNS prophylaxis with intrathecal and/or systemic chemotherapy with/without radiation to the brain.
- Clinical trials (especially for recurrent ALL).

Acute myeloid leukemia (AML)

Acute myeloid/myelogenous leukemia (AML) is the most common adult leukemia (85%), often developing after 60 years of age (especially in males) and associated with a history of smoking, radiation, and/or chemotherapy (childhood treatment of ALL). AML is caused by a defect in the stem cells that differentiate into all mye-loid cells, causing immature white blood cells called myeloblasts (in-creasing risk of infection) and abnormal RBCs and platelets (increas-ing risk of anemia and bleeding). There are a number of subtypes.

Signs and symptoms	Treatment
Weakness, lethargy	Two-phase approach:
Increased bruising, petechiae	Remission induction phase.
Abnormal bleed-ing, nosebleeds	Post-remission phase.
Fever	Note: Treatment options (both phases) vary
Anorexia, weight loss	according to subtype, but may include:
Anemia	Combination chemotherapy.
Increased infection	High-dose chemotherapy with/without
Headache	radiation and stem cell transplant with own
Mouth sores	cells or donor cells.
	Anti-cancer drugs (arsenic trioxide and all-trans retinoic acid) for acute promyelocytic leukemia (one subtype).
	Clinical trials (especially for recurrent AML).

Chronic lymphocytic leukemia (CLL)

Chronic lymphocytic leukemia (CLL) develops primarily from a malignant clone of B lymphocytes. T-lymphocyte CLL is rare (1%). Chromosomal abnormalities include 13q deletion (in 50%) and trisomy 12 (in 15%). Most leukemic cells appear mature but do not function or die but accumulate in the bone marrow and blood. Most people survive 5 to 10 years, but thrombocytopenia and anemia indicate a more aggressive disease. CLL is classified in 2 ways: Rai classification (0 to IV) and Binet classification (A-C). CLL may progress to large cell lymphoma.

Signs and symptoms:
- Asymptomatic initially.
- Defects in humor and cell-mediated immune systems, increased risk of infections (herpes, *Pneumocystis jiroveci,* and *Candida albicans*).
- Fever, diaphoresis, weight loss, lymphadenopathy.
- Hepatomegaly/splenomegaly.
- Autoimmune diseases (hemolytic anemia, idiopathic thrombocytopenia purpura).

Treatment:
- Monitoring/Symptomatic support.
- Corticosteroids: autoimmune hemolytic anemia and thrombocytopenia.
- Fludarabine, alone or in combination with cyclophosphamide and/or rituximab (a monoclonal antibody).

- Alemtuzumab (a monoclonal antibody directed at CD52) is approved for use in CLL as both a first-line agent and for salvage in patients with fludarabine-refractory disease.
- Allogenic stem cell transplant (only curative Rx).

Chronic myeloid/myelogenous leukemia (CML)

Chronic myeloid/myelogenous leukemia (CML) is caused by mutation of the myeloid stem cells and proliferation of mature neoplastic granulocytes and blast forms in the bone marrow. The abnormal cells expand the bone marrow and spread to the peripheral circulation, infiltrating the liver and spleen, which form more cells (extramedullary hematopoiesis). About 95% of patients with CML have genetic markers in abnormal cells—the Philadelphia (Ph1) chromosome, a translocation between chromosomes 9 (ABL gene) and 22 (BCR gene).

Signs and symptoms	Treatment
PHASES: Chronic (2-5 years): WBCs increase but most cells mature and function appropriately. Fatigue, headache, splenomegaly. Accelerated (1-6 months with treatment and > 1 year without): Immature blasts increase and fewer mature cells. Immune system impaired. Fever, night sweats, weight loss, dyspnea, anemia. Blast crisis: Blast cells proliferate and other cells decrease. Bruising, bleeding, infections.	DOCs include imatinib mesylate (Gleevec): pro-motes apoptosis and inhibits tyrosine kinase activity in cells positive for BCR-ABL (Philadelphia). Remission rates higher with treatment during chronic phase (70%) than accelerat-ed (28%) or blast crisis (4%). Nilotinib and dasatinib have higher rates of remission but have more side effects.

Multiple myeloma

Multiple myeloma is proliferation and accumulation of mature B lymphocytes, the clonal plasma cells, which secrete antibodies necessary to fight infections. Malignant clones infiltrate the bone marrow, resulting in secretion of osteoclast-activating factors and cytokine as well as markedly increased levels of circulating immunoglobulin and/or free light chains and decreased immunity. Most patients present with back or neck pain. Normochromic-normocytic anemia causes weakness and fatigue. Renal insufficiency and hypercalcemia are common. Diagnosis requires at least one major and one minor or three minor criteria.

Major criteria	Minor criteria
Bone marrow plasmacytosis > 30% Plasmacytoma on biopsy. Monoclonal (M) protein in serum or urine	Bone marrow plasmacytosis 10%-30% M protein present but lesser concentration Lytic bone lesions Decreased normal immunoglobulin < 50%

Multiple myeloma is staged I to III according to beta-2 microglobulin and serum albumin levels. Patients at stage 1 may remain stable for years and not require treatment. Treatment regimens are varied and may include conventional chemotherapy, corticosteroids, dose-intensive chemotherapy with autologous hematopoietic cell rescue, allogenic stem cell transplantation, thalidomide, and bortezomib.

Dysproteinemia

Dysproteinemia is a condition in which there is excessive production of immunoglobulin (Ig) molecules because of cloning and proliferation of B lymphocytes or plasma cells. Dysproteinemias are associated with neoplastic disorders, such as multiple myeloma, thymoma, angioimmunoblastic lymphadenopathy (T-cell lymphoma), and other malignant tumors. The abnormal molecules (free light chains) circulate through the blood system to the kidneys, where they are deposited and form lesions or they form paraprotein lesions in other tissues, resulting in amyloidosis. Complications include hyperviscosity syndrome, characterized by changes in mental status, GI bleeding, retinopathy, and hypervolemia. Treatment includes therapeutic plasma exchange (TPE) to control hyperviscosity, and chemotherapy, which depends on the underlying cause, to control the malignancy.

Amyloidosis

Amyloidosis is a blood disorder that may occur with blood cancers, such as multiple myeloma. Primary amyloidosis is a clonal expansion of plasma cells with overproduction of monoclonal light chains. Amyloid is an abnormal protein that builds up in body tissues and organs. Types of amyloidosis include:
- AL (most common): kappa or lambda light chains accumulate in tissues, often linked with multiple myeloma.
- AA: AA protein accumulates in tissues and linked to chronic disease, such as diabetes RA, IBD, and TB.
- Hereditary (ATTR): transthyretin (TTR) protein made in liver accumulates in tissues, causes CNS problems, carpal tunnel syndrome, eye disorders.
- Beta-2 microglobulin: Can occur with chronic renal disease.

Diagnosis is per urine and blood tests for abnormal proteins and tissue biopsy. Symptoms depend on tissues and organs involved but can include peripheral edema, dyspnea, weight loss, skin changes, petechiae, ecchymosis, irregular heartbeat, dysphagia, and weakness. Treatment:
- Primary: Melphalan or cyclophosphamide and dexamethasone, peripheral blood stem cell transplantation.
- Secondary: Treatment aimed at underlying condition.
- Hereditary: Investigative drugs, liver transplantation.

Myelodysplastic syndromes

Myelodysplastic syndromes (MDS) are a group of clonal myeloid stem cell disorders in which hematopoiesis is impaired and there is increased risk of developing acute myelogenous leukemia. The bone marrow is typically hypercellular with abnormal stem cells. These disorders affect primarily adults older than 60. MDS results from progressive mutations of the hematopoietic stem cell. These mutations may result from previous chemotherapy or radiation and may be associated with aplastic anemia or Fanconi anemia. Symptoms usually present with anemia, mild at onset and progressing in severity to transfusion dependence. MDS is classified into the French-American-British (FAB) subtypes (5) according to bone marrow myeloblast count and risk of developing leukemia. Treatment includes platelet transfusion (single donor), aminocaproic acid, and growth factors. Specific treatment includes DNA methyltransferase inhibitors (azacytidine, daunorubicin, and decitabine), immunomodulatory agents (thalidomide, lenalidomide), immunosuppressive agents, histone deacetylase inhibitors, and chemotherapy. Allotransplant is curative, but prognosis is better in younger patients.

Iron deficiency anemia

A primary cause is iron deficiency anemia is GI blood loss, but melena only appears after loss of 50 to 75 mL of blood from the upper GI tract. Diagnostic findings include decreased Hgb, Hct, MCV, MCH, MCHC, and serum iron and increased total iron binding capacity (TIBC). Reticulocytes and bilirubin may be normal, or decreased, and platelets may be normal or increased. RBCs are microcytic, hypochromic. Iron deficiency anemia may also occur with bariatric surgery that bypasses the duodenum, blood loss (excessive menstruation), pregnancy, chronic renal failure, dialysis, and inadequate diet.

Signs and symptoms (Initial)	Signs and symptoms (Progressive)
Asymptomatic (initial). Pallor (most common). Glossitis and burning of the tongue. • Cheilitis Headache. Paresthesia. • Pica (unusual cravings, ice chewing)	General systemic symptoms resulting from hypoxia may occur as anemia worsens: Weakness, lethargy. Confusion. Ataxia. Cardiovascular abnormalities.

Treatment comprises diet high in iron, oral iron supplementation with vitamin C to increase absorption or parenteral (IV or IM) iron if patients don't respond to oral medications, and transfusion of packed RBCs with severe symptoms.

Folic acid deficiency anemia

Folic acid deficiency can result in megaloblastic anemia. Folic acid is necessary for DNA synthesis and formation and maturation of red blood cells. Causes of folic acid deficiency include inadequate diet, malabsorption syndromes (especially of the small intestine), medications that interfere with absorption (oral contraceptives, methotrexate, phenobarbital, and diphenylhydantoin), anorexia, alcoholism, and dialysis. Signs and symptoms are similar to those found in cobalamin (vitamin B12) deficiency except that folic acid deficiency does not cause neurological abnormalities. Diagnostic findings include decreased hemoglobin, hematocrit, and folate (normal value: 3 to 25 mg/mL), as well as increased MCV and MCHV. Cobalamin level is normal and gastric analysis is positive for hydrochloric acid. Other blood studies are usually within normal range. RBCs are macrocytic, normochromic.

Signs and symptoms	Treatment
• Asymptomatic (initial). • GI disturbances, such as indigestion, anorexia, and weight loss. • Red, beefy-appearing tongue. • Pallor. • Weakness, fatigue. • Forgetfulness, impaired concentration. • Pancytopenia.	Diet high in folic acid: green leafy vegetables, liver, citrus fruits, legumes, nuts, and grains. Oral supplementation: folic acid 1 to 5 mg/day (duration varies according to cause).

Polycythemia

Polycythemia is an increased volume of red blood cells (erythrocytes) greater than 50% in females:

- Polycythemia vera is a proliferative disease in which myeloid cells overproduce blood cells, primarily red blood cells, although other cells and platelets are also elevated. The hematocrit may be greater than 60%. Over time, the spleen enlarges and bone marrow becomes fibrotic, producing fewer cells. The disease may evolve into myeloid metaplasia with fibrosis or acute myelogenous leukemia. Patients are at increased risk of thrombosis because of increased viscosity of the blood. Treatment includes hydroxyurea to decrease production of RBCs, interferon to lower RBC counts, and scheduled phlebotomy to reduce RBC concentration. Hydration is especially important.
- Secondary polycythemia results from increased production of erythropoietin, which stimulates the bone marrow to produce more red blood cells. This may result from neoplasms (such as renal cell carcinoma), COPD, heart disease, or altitude sickness—conditions that cause hypoxia, which stimulates production of erythropoietin. Identifying the underlying cause is critical to treatment.

Disseminated intravascular coagulation (DIC)

Disseminated intravascular coagulation (DIC) (consumption coagulopathy) is a secondary disorder that is triggered by another, such as trauma, congenital heart disease, necrotizing enterocolitis, sepsis, and severe viral infections. DIC triggers both coagulation and hemorrhage through a complex series of events that includes trauma that causes tissue factor (transmembrane glycoprotein) to enter the circulation and bind with coagulation factors, triggering the coagulation cascade. This stimulates thrombin to convert fibrinogen to fibrin, causing aggregation and destruction of platelets and forming clots that can be disseminated throughout the intravascular system. These clots increase in size as platelets adhere to the clots, causing blockage of both the microvascular systems and larger vessels, and this can result in ischemia and necrosis. Clot formation triggers fibrinolysis and plasmin to break down fibrin and fibrinogen, causing destruction of clotting factors, resulting in hemorrhage. Both processes, clotting and hemorrhage, continue at the same time, placing the patient at high risk for death, even with treatment.

The onset of symptoms of DIC may be very rapid or a slower chronic progression from a disease. Those who develop the chronic manifestation of the disease usually have fewer acute symptoms and may slowly develop ecchymosis or bleeding wounds.

Symptoms	Treatment
<ul><li>Bleeding from surgical or venous puncture sites.</li><li>Evidence of GI bleeding with distention, bloody diarrhea.</li><li>Hypotension and acute symptoms of shock.</li><li>Petechiae and purpura with extensive bleeding into the tissues.</li><li>Laboratory abnormalities:<ul><li>Prolonged prothrombin and partial thromboplastin times.</li><li>Decreased platelet counts and fragmented RBCs.</li><li>Decreased fibrinogen.</li></ul></li></ul>	<ul><li>Identifying and treating underlying cause.</li><li>Replacement blood products, such as platelets and fresh frozen plasma.</li><li>Anticoagulation therapy (heparin) to increase clotting time.</li><li>Cryoprecipitate to increase fibrinogen levels.</li><li>Coagulation inhibitors and coagulation factors.</li></ul>

Von Willebrand disease

Von Willebrand disease is a group of autosomal congenital bleeding disorders (inherited from either parent) affecting 1% to 2% of the population, associated with deficiency or lack of von Willebrand factor (vWF), a glycoprotein that is synthesized, stored, and secreted by vascular endothelial cells. This protein interacts with thrombocytes to create a clot and prevent hemorrhage; however, with von Willebrand disease, this clotting mechanism is impaired. There are 3 types:
- Type I: low levels of vWF and also sometimes factor VIII (dominant inheritance).
- Type II: abnormal vWF (subtypes a, b) may increase or decrease clotting (dominant inheritance).
- Type III: absence of vWF and less than 10% factor VIII (recessive inheritance).

Symptoms vary in severity and include bruising, menorrhagia, recurrent epistaxis, and hemorrhage. Treatment includes:
- Desmopressin acetate parenterally or nasally to stimulate production of clotting factor (mild cases).
- Severe bleeding: factor VIII concentrate with vWF, such as Humate-P.

Thrombocytopenia

Inherited or acquired thrombocytopenia is a condition in which the platelet (thrombocyte) count is lower than normal because of increased consumption, reduced production, or increased sequestration of thrombocytes in the spleen (which usually holds about a third of the body's platelets). Thrombocytopenia is characterized by mucocutaneous bleeding, ecchymoses, petechiae, epistaxis, and gingival or conjunctival bleeding. When platelet count drops below 10,000 to 20,000/mcL, the risk of severe GI, GU, or CNS bleeding increases. Count alone does not predict bleeding; those with abnormal platelets may bleed at higher counts. If the platelet count is above 20,000 to 30,000/mcL, then the patient may be monitored but may not require immediate treatment. When risk of bleeding increases, treatment may include steroids, immunoglobulin/immunosuppressants, and blood/platelet transfusions. In some cases, splenectomy is indicated, usually for adults with immune thrombocytopenia.

Vascular disease

Vascular disease is associated with activation and dysfunction of endothelial cells in arteries. The cells secrete cytokines and chemokines, and adhesion molecules are expressed on the surface of the cells. These attract monocytes and lymphocytes, which begin to infiltrate the walls of the vessels, causing proliferation of smooth muscle cells and thickening of vessel walls and plaque formation. Treatment focuses on maximizing perfusion with antiplatelet agents, vasodilators, antilipemic agents, hemorheologic agents, and anticoagulants. Coronary artery disease is a common vascular disorder. Impairment of blood flow through the coronary arteries leads to ischemia of the cardiac muscle and angina pectoris. Stable angina episodes usually last for less than 5 minutes and are fairly predictable exercise-induced episodes caused by atherosclerotic lesions blocking more than 75% of the lumen of the affected coronary artery. Unstable angina is a progression of coronary artery disease and occurs when there is a change in the pattern of stable angina. The pain may increase, may not respond to a single nitroglycerine dose, and may persist for more than 5 minutes.

Peripheral vascular insufficiency (peripheral arterial disease)

Peripheral vascular insufficiency involves both arterial and venous disease; however, venous disease is a chronic condition that rarely causes acute care crises. Peripheral arterial disease involves the aorta, its branches, arteries, and arterioles. Peripheral arterial disease often involves occlusion of the arteries of the lower extremities, resulting in severe pain and ischemia. The arteries most often affected by peripheral arterial disease are the femoral, the popliteal, the distal aorta, and the iliac arteries. The most common cause of arterial occlusion is atherosclerosis. *Symptoms* of peripheral arterial disease include:

- Intermittent claudication, a cramping pain while walking.
- Rest pain, a progression of intermittent claudication that includes pain even at rest. This requires catheter or surgical treatment to repair blockage.
- Tissue changes include thickening of nails, hair loss, and dry skin. Ulcerations may occur.
- Acute occlusion, with pain, lack of pulses, decreased skin temperature, pallor, and loss of sensation and function. This requires immediate surgical intervention.

Antiphospholipid antibody syndrome (APS)

Antiphospholipid antibody syndrome is an autoimmune disease in which the immune system targets phospholipid (a fat found in all of the body cells). While patients may be essentially asymptomatic, in some cases the condition may result in thrombosis. Indications of APS include venous or arterial thrombosis, autoimmune thrombocytopenia purpura, endocarditis, and history of multiple spontaneous abortions (before week 10 of gestation). Thrombosis may be generalized, affecting multiple vessels and resulting in stroke and DVT. Risk factors include smoking and oral estrogen contraceptives. Treatment includes avoiding risk factors. Mild cases often require no treatment, but more serious cases may require treatment with steroids (prednisone) or other immunosuppressive agents (mycophenolate). After thrombosis, systemic anticoagulation (usually warfarin) is indicated for a prolonged period to prevent recurrence.

Systemic lupus erythematosus

Systemic lupus erythematosus is a systemic reaction to collagen or connective tissue in the body, believed triggered by an antibody-antigen immune response to an environmental agent, resulting in widespread damage of vessels and organs, primarily in females. Onset is usually 9 to 15 years of age and is more common in African American, Hispanic, and Asian females than Caucasian.

Symptoms (vary widely)	**Treatment** (varies with severity)
"Butterfly" rash (scaly erythematous maculopapular patches) on face, chest, and arms. Arthritic-type pain, stiffness, and swelling of joints. CNS involvement with seizures, headache, and psychosis. Heart/vessels (pericarditis, vasculitis) and lung (pleurisy) inflammation. Kidney failure. Anemia (erythrocytopenia and pancytopenia, hemolytic). Spleen, liver, and lymph nodes enlarged. • GI symptoms: nausea, vomiting, pain, and hepatitis.	NSAIDs for pain and inflammation. Steroids for organ inflammation, hemolytic anemia. Antimalarial drugs for skin involvement. Immunosuppressant agents if steroids not adequate.

Idiopathic thrombocytopenic purpura (ITP)

The autoimmune disorder idiopathic thrombocytopenic purpura (ITP) causes an immune response to platelets, resulting in decreased platelet counts. It may be triggered by viral infections. ITP affects primarily children and young women although it can occur at any age. The acute form primarily occurs in children, but the chronic form primarily affects adults. Platelet counts are usually 150,000 to 400,000/microL. With ITP, they may be as low as 0 or as high as 100,000/microL in less severe cases. A count of about 30,000/microL is necessary to prevent intracranial hemorrhage, the primary concern. The cause of ITP is unclear and may be precipitated by viral infection, sulfa drugs, and conditions, such as lupus erythematosus. ITP is usually not life-threatening and can be controlled. *Symptoms* include:

- Bruising and petechiae with hematoma in some cases
- Epistaxis
- Increased menstrual flow in females postpuberty

Treatment includes:

- Corticosteroids depress immune response and increase platelet count
- Splenectomy may be indicated for chronic conditions
- Platelet transfusions
- Avoiding aspirin or ibuprofen

Chronic idiopathic neutropenia

Chronic idiopathic neutropenia (absolute neutrophil count of less than 1800/mcL for Caucasians and 1500/mcL for African Americans) usually presents with mild symptoms, although some patients may develop more severe disease with lower absolute neutrophil counts and recurrent fevers, oropharyngeal infections, or systemic infections. Patients exhibit low serum immunoglobulin IgG3 levels, but these do not seem to increase risk of infection. Chronic idiopathic neutropenia is most common in middle-aged females. The risk of infection depends on a combination of factors: absolute neutrophil count, neutrophil reserve (bone marrow), and the duration of neutropenia. Risk increases as the absolute neutrophil count drops below 1000/mcL and is most severe with count below 500/mcL. Treatment focuses on controlling infections with antibiotics and relieving symptoms. With severe symptoms, patients are administered G-CSF. Common secondary complications include osteopenia (44%) and osteoporosis (15.6%). Rarely does chronic idiopathic neutropenia progress to acute myeloid leukemia.

Aplastic anemia

Aplastic anemia is a bone marrow failure syndrome that results in pancytopenia with hypocellular bone marrow. Myeloblasts and megakaryocytes are essentially absent. Aplastic anemia may be constitutional or acquired. Acquired aplastic anemia is currently most associated with NSAIDs, antithyroid drugs, penicillamine, allopurinol, and gold. Because stem cells are unable to produce mature cells, patients experience symptoms related to each cell line:

- Erythrocytopenia: anemia with fatigue, malaise, headaches, dyspnea, chest pain.
- Thrombocytopenia: mucosal bleeding and petechiae, GI bleeding, epistaxis, intracranial bleeding.
- Leukopenia/Neutropenia: infection.

The primary treatments are allogeneic hematopoietic stem cell transplantation (HSCT) or immunosuppression with anti-thymocyte globulin (ATG) and cyclosporine. HSCT is curative, but donor matches are not always available. About 66% of those undergoing immunosuppression achieve remission and are independent of transfusions. HSCT is recommended for those younger than 20 years and those who have failed immunosuppression.

Fanconi anemia

Fanconi anemia is a genetic disorder in which abnormal genes damage DNA and interfere with repair. Patients exhibit short stature, abnormal thumbs, small heads and eyes, abnormal ears and deafness, abnormal kidneys, abnormal or missing bones in forearms, underdeveloped testicles, and male infertility. Bone marrow failure is not present in all but is common, and patients usually develop aplastic anemia involving all cell lines with both decreased production and production of abnormal cells. Erythrocytopenia leads to anemia, thrombocytopenia to bleeding, and leukocytopenia to increased risk of infection. Patients are at increased risk over time of leukemia (10%), hepatic tumors, and solid organ tumors of the head and neck, female genitalia, and brain. Progression of the disease and prognosis are not always predictable. Treatment includes symptomatic support and bone marrow or hematopoietic stem cell transplantation (HSCT).

Heparin-induced thrombosis-thrombocytopenia syndrome (HITTS)

Heparin-induced thrombosis-thrombocytopenia syndrome (HITTS) occurs in patients receiving heparin for anticoagulation. There are two types:
- Type I is a transient condition occurring within a few days and causing depletion of platelets (less than $100,000/mm^3$), but heparin may be continued as the condition usually resolves without intervention.
- Type II is an autoimmune reaction to heparin that occurs in 3% to 5% of those receiving unfractionated heparin and also occurs with low-molecular-weight heparin. It is characterized by low platelets (less than $150,000/mm^3$) that are at least 50% below baseline. Onset is 5 to 14 days but can occur within hours of heparin rebound. Death rates are 30% or less. Heparin-antibody complexes form and release platelet factor 4 (PF4), which attracts heparin molecules and adheres to platelets and endothelial lining, stimulating thrombin and platelet clumping. This puts the patient at risk for thrombosis and vessel occlusion rather than hemorrhage, causing stroke, myocardial infarction, and limb ischemia with symptoms associated with the site of thrombosis. Treatment includes:
  o Discontinuation of heparin.
  o Direct thrombin inhibitors (lepirudin, argatroban).

ReoPro-induced coagulopathy

ReoPro (abciximab) is used to prevent cardiac ischemia for those undergoing percutaneous coronary intervention (PCI). It inhibits the aggregation of platelets. It is used with aspirin and/or weight-adjusted low-dose heparin and potentiates the action of anticoagulants. However, its use with non-weight-adjusted longer-acting heparin can cause thrombocytopenia with increased risk of hemorrhage, especially with readministration of the drug, which can induce the formation of antibodies and an allergic reaction that is characterized by anaphylaxis and thrombocytopenia, referred to as Reo-Pro-induced coagulopathy. Because of the danger of hemorrhage, ReoPro is contraindicated if there is active bleeding or a history of bleeding or cerebrovascular accident (CVA) within the 2 years prior, history of a CVA, platelet count less than $100,000/mm^3$, or recent history of oral anticoagulation. Careful monitoring of platelet counts prior to administration and the use of weight-adjusted low-dose heparin is important to prevent bleeding. Heparin should be discontinued after the PCI.

Sickle cell disease

Sickle cell disease is a recessive genetic disorder of chromosome 11, causing hemoglobin to be defective so that red blood cells (RBCs) are sickle-shaped and inflexible, resulting in their accumulation in small blood vessels and causing painful blockage. While normal RBCs survive 120 days, sickled cells may survive only 10-20 days, stressing the bone marrow that cannot produce fast enough and resulting in anemia. Different types of crises occur (aplastic, hemolytic, vaso-occlusive, and sequestrating), which cause infarctions in organs, severe pain, damage to organs, and rapid enlargement of liver and spleen. Sickle cell disease and crisis treatments include:
- Intravenous fluids to prevent dehydration.
- Analgesics (morphine) during painful crises.
- Folic acid for anemia.
- Hydroxyurea to decrease vaso-occlusive crises by stimulating production of fetal hemoglobin.
- Oxygen for congestive heart failure or pulmonary disease.
- Blood transfusions with chelation therapy to remove excess iron OR erythropheresis, in which red cells are removed and replaced with healthy cells, either autologous or from a donor.
- Hematopoietic stem cell transplantation (the only curative treatment).

Hemophilia

Hemophilia is an inherited disorder in which the child lacks adequate clotting factors. There are 3 types:
- Type A: lack of clotting factor VII (90% of cases)
- Type B: lack of clotting factor IX
- Type C: lack of clotting factor XI (affects both sexes, rarely occurs in the United States).

Both type A and B are usually X-linked disorders, affecting only males. The severity of the disease depends on the amount of clotting factor in the blood. Babies often show symptoms when more active, crawling or walking, with frequent bruises.

Symptoms	Treatment
<ul><li>Bleeding with severe trauma or stress (mild cases).</li><li>Unexplained bruises, bleeding, swelling, joint pain.</li><li>Spontaneous hemorrhage (severe cases), often in the joints but can be anywhere in the body.</li><li>Epistaxis.</li></ul>	<ul><li>Desmopressin parenterally or nasally to stimulate production of clotting factor (mild cases).</li><li>Infusions of clotting factor from donated blood or recombinant clotting factors (genetically engineered).</li><li>Infusions of plasma (type C).</li></ul>

Vascular Ehlers-Danlos syndrome type IV

Vascular Ehlers-Danlos syndrome type IV is an autosomal dominant genetic disorder of connective tissue with mutations in the COL3A1 gene coding for type III procollagen. The disease results in

- 107 -

marked fragility of connective tissue and vessels, predisposing the patient to rupture of vessels and gastrointestinal structures. The condition in children is frequently misdiagnosed as a coagulopathy. Typical findings in adults include unusual facial appearance (thin nose and lips, protruding eyes, unusually small chin), ecchymosis, visible veins in friable translucent skin (especially prevalent on the chest and abdomen), and ruptured vessels. Joints of hands and feet are hypermobile and infants may exhibit congenital talipes equinovarus or hip dislocations. About a quarter of patients experience rupture of the intestines, and women may experience tearing of the uterus during pregnancy. Arterial or organ rupture may be life-threatening. Treatment includes the beta-blocker celiprolol and elective surgical repair of vessels that area at risk of rupture.

Packed red blood cells (PRBCs)

Packed red blood cells may be refrigerated for up to 42 days and frozen for up to 10 years. PRBCs are indicated for chronic anemia, acute blood loss, low hemoglobin and hematocrit, and sickle cell disease. Some nonfunctioning platelets, plasma, and WBCs may remain in the PRBCs, and the WBCs may cause an adverse reaction, but this risk reduces with leukoreduction. Washed blood cells must be administered within 24 hours from the onset of the washing procedure, but these RBCs should not be considered leukocyte-reduced. Irradiation of the PRBCs reduces the risk of transfusion-associated graft vs host disease. PRBCs must be ABO/Rh compatible with recipient. One unit of PRBCs should increase hematocrit 3% and hemoglobin by 1 g/dL for a 155 lb adult. One unit of PRBCs usually comprises about 350 mL with 150 to 210 mL of RBCs, 100 mL of crystalloid solution, and 30 mL plasma. Pediatric/Divided units contain 45 to 50 mL of RBCs and 15 mL of plasma but no crystalloid solution.

Platelets

Platelets may be stored at room temperature for up to 5 days but must be agitated to prevent clumping. Platelets are administered for leukemia and other malignancies and to prevent and control bleeding from thrombocytopenia (less than 5000 to 10,000/microL). The number of red blood cells in platelets is usually too low to cause a reaction, but ABO/Rh compatibility is desired. Some nonfunctioning red and white blood cells remain. Single-donor platelets are preferred for patients requiring repeated administration of platelets as alloimmunization decreases if single donor is used instead of random donors. One unit of single-donor platelets is equivalent to 6 to 8 units of random platelets. Platelets should be tested with rapid culturing prior to administration because of their increased risk of infection. Platelet concentrate usually contains about 50 mL in volume and also contains 50 mL of plasma while platelet pheresis donation contains about 300 mL.

Whole blood and autotransfusion

Whole blood is rarely administered but is separated into components before administration. Storage varies depending on intended use. Whole blood may be administered for severe hemorrhage with loss of more than 25% of total blood volume. Blood is normally ordered in units, and a unit of whole blood generally contains about 450 mL of blood, but anticoagulant is added to the blood, bringing the total volume to about 500 to 520 mL. Autotransfusion of whole blood may be utilized with severe bleeding or trauma. Blood is usually collected from a body cavity, such as the pleural or peritoneal space, collected in a sterile container and reinfused. Commercial collection devices are available. The blood is filtered and citrate phosphate dextrose often added to prevent clotting (25 to 75 mL per 500 mL blood).

Cryoprecipitate and plasma

Cryoprecipitate (fibrinogen, AHF, von Willebrand factor, fibronectin) may be stored frozen for 1 year. Use of cryoprecipitate has generally been supplanted by pure factor VII or factor IX but may be used for bleeding associated with hemophilia A and von Willebrand disease if other clotting factors are unavailable. It may also be used for hypofibrinogenemia. ABO/Rh compatibility is not required. Cryoprecipitate is about 15 mL and contains 150 mg of fibrinogen and at least 80 units of other factors. Plasma is usually fractionated and administered as specific components. Plasma may be stored as fresh frozen plasma for up to 7 years but must be administered within 24 hours after thawing. Indications for use of plasma include control of bleeding associated with low levels of clotting factors, plasma replacement for blood loss, and plasmapheresis. Plasma must be ABO/Rh compatible. A standard dose of random plasma is equal to 4 units of pooled plasma, and a large dose of random plasma is equal to 6 units of pooled plasma. Fresh frozen plasma is about 225 mL.

Granulocytes (neutrophils) and lymphocytes (buffy coat)

The use of granulocytes for neutropenia is controversial, but when used, granulocytes (neutrophils) should be administered as soon as possible but may be stored for up to 24 hours at 20°C to 24°C without agitation and must be irradiated prior to administration to prevent transfusion-associated graft versus host disease. Because some lymphocytes, red blood cells, and platelets remain in the granulocytes, they must be ABO/Rh compatible. Granulocytes may cause febrile transfusion reactions and may transmit infectious diseases, such as cytomegalovirus. Generally, colony-stimulating factors are used to stimulate the body to produce neutrophils rather than transfusing patients with granulocytes. Lymphocytes (buffy coat) may be used fresh immediately or frozen for later use. Lymphocytes may be collected from a stem cell donor and stored. Lymphocytes are used to stimulate graft versus host disease effect after ablative and nonablative stem cell transplantation for treatment of leukemia with apheresis of lymphocytes from the original stem cell donor to prevent treatment failure.

Antihemophilic factor (AHF [factor VIII], factor IX concentrate, and factor IX complex [factors II, VII, IX and S])

Antihemophilic factor (AHF) (factor VIII) may be frozen for 1 year at 18°C or less, or 4 hours at 20°C to 24°C. It is used for treatment of hemophilia A, and ABO-Rh compatibility is not required. Factor IX concentrate may be refrigerated at 2°C to 8°C but not frozen. It must be stored away from light and moisture. It is used for hemophilia B, and ABO/Rh compatibility is not required. Factor IX complex (factors II, VII, IX, and S) requires that both the dry medication and the diluent be refrigerated at 2°C to 8°C and used within 3 hours of preparation. It is administered for factor VII, IX, and X deficiencies and hemophilia A with factor VII inhibitors. ABO/Rh compatibility is not required.

Albumin (5% and 25%), gamma globulin, and antithrombin III concentrate

Albumin (5% and 25%) may be stored at room temperature at 20°C to 25°C with short periods ranging from 15°C to 30°C. Albumin is used to treat hypoproteinemia and burns. It is used for volume expansion by 5% to increase volume of blood and by 25% to decrease hematocrit. ABO/Rh compatibility is not required. Gamma globulin (IV) must be refrigerated at 2°C to 8°C but must not be frozen. It is used to treated hypogammaglobulinemia related to CLL, ITP, and primary immunodeficiency. ABO/Rh compatibility is not required. Antithrombin III concentrate must be refrigerated at 2°C to 8°C but must not be frozen. It is used for antithrombin III deficiency with thrombosis or with increased risk of thrombosis. ABO/Rh compatibility is not required.

Leukoreduction, irradiation, and washing of red blood cells

Leukoreduction: Centrifugation or filtration is used to remove remaining white blood cells from whole blood, RBCs, or platelets to reduce post-transfusion infections and transmission of viruses. The process results in loss of about 10% of RBCs and adds to cost but is indicated for immunocompromised patients.

Irradiation: Gamma radiation (2500 rads) is used to destroy the T lymphocyte's ability to divide in whole blood RBCs, and granulocytes to prevent transfusion-associated graft versus host disease. Some RBCs are lost but platelet function is not impaired.

Washing of RBCs: Washing RBCs with 0.9% saline in a centrifuge or blood cell processor removes plasma, plasma proteins, micro-aggregates, cytokines, and antibodies. The process decreases the risk of allergic and anaphylactic reactions. Washed RBCs must be used within 24 hours of beginning the washing procedure and may be stored during that time at 1°C to 6°C, or for 4 hours at 20°C to 24°C.

Apheresis

Apheresis is a form of extracorporeal treatment in which the blood is removed and introduced into a centrifuge for removal of a specific component and then the treated blood is returned to the patient. The effect is temporary but may be used to give time for suppressive medications to work.
- Plasmapheresis: Removes plasma proteins for hyperviscosity syndromes and treatment of some renal and neurological diseases (Guillain-Barré, myasthenia gravis) to remove disease-producing autoantibodies. In some cases, all of a patient's plasma may be removed and replaced with donor fresh frozen plasma.
- Plateletpheresis: Removes platelets for severe thrombocytosis, essential thrombocytopenia, and single donor or random donor platelet transfusions.
- Leukapheresis: Removes white blood cells and can be specific to neutrophils or lymphocytes for extreme leukocytosis associated with acute or chronic leukemia (AML, CML) and to separate WBCs for transfusion.
- Erythropheresis: Removes red blood cells for RBC dyscrasias (such as sickle cell disease) and for replacement of RBCs.

Erythropoietin-stimulating agents (ESAs)

Erythropoietin-stimulating agents (ESAs), such as epoetin alfa (Procrit/Epogen), epoetin beta (NeoRecormon), darbepoetin alfa (Aranesp), and methoxy polyethylene glycol-epoetin beta (Mircera) are synthetically produced derivatives of the hormone erythropoietin. These agents stimulate erythrocyte progenitor cells in the bone marrow to produce erythrocytes. Epoetin alfa was approved in 1989 for treatment of anemia associated with chronic renal failure and was later used for chemotherapy-induced anemia. ESAs are administered to increase hemoglobin and prevent need for transfusions. However, a number of clinical trials have shown increased mortality rates and cardiovascular events as well as the potential for tumor progression related to the use of ESAs, so use has narrowed to avoid these adverse effects. ESAs should not be used with breast, head and neck, and non-small cell lung cancers, and the target hemoglobin should not exceed 12 g/dL. It is also recommended that ESAs be discontinued when chemotherapy is completed.

Granulocyte colony-stimulating factor (G-CSF) and granulocyte-macrophage colony-stimulating factor (GM-CSF)

Granulocyte colony-stimulating factor (G-CSF), such as filgrastim (Neupogen) and pegfilgrastim (Neulasta), is produced through recombinant DNA technology to stimulate progenitor cells for leukocytes, specifically the granulocytes (basophils, neutrophils, and eosinophils). G-CSF is used to treat chemotherapy-associated neutropenia and to stimulate production of neutrophils for those donating hematopoietic stem cells. G-CSFs oppose adverse effects of chemotherapeutic agents and enhance the immune system, so patients may tolerate higher doses of chemotherapy. A newer drug, sargramostim (Leukine), stimulates precursor cells that produce both granulocytes and monocytes (macrophages), so it is referred to as a granulocyte-macrophage colony-stimulating factor (GM-CSF). Sargramostim is used after bone marrow and peripheral blood stem cell transplantation to increase the number of leukocytes, and prevent infection, for bone marrow transplantation failure, and after induction chemotherapy for patients with AML. WBC counts must be monitored carefully during administration. Adverse effects of CSFs include fever, infection, edema, shortness of breath, splenomegaly or ruptured spleen, thrombocytopenia (increased risk of bleeding), hepatic injury, vasculitis, and allergic reactions.

Warfarin (Coumadin/Jantoven)

Warfarin (Coumadin/Jantoven) is an anticoagulant that inhibits bacterial synthesis of vitamin K in the gastrointestinal tract, thus inhibiting vitamin K–dependent activation of clotting factors II, VII, IX, and X, which are formed in the liver. Warfarin is derived from a natural plant anticoagulant, coumarin, and is the most commonly prescribed oral anticoagulant. The prothrombin time/international normalized ratio (PT/INR) must be carefully monitored during administration. The normal INR is 1, but with warfarin, the INR should range from 2 to 3.5, depending on use. Warfarin is indicated for pulmonary embolism, DVT, myocardial infarction (MI), rheumatic heart disease with damage to heart valves, prosthetic heart valves, and chronic atrial fibrillation. Adults older than 65 years may bleed more easily and have a lower threshold for INR. Warfarin may interact with numerous drugs, including acetaminophen. Cranberry juice and excessive alcohol intake may increase risk of bleeding, and high intake of vitamin K may impair anticoagulation. Adverse effects include hemorrhage, allergic reaction, hepatitis, fever, hematuria, dermatitis, angina, and GI disturbance. Vitamin K is the reversal drug for warfarin.

Heparin sodium (unfractionated heparin)

Heparin sodium (unfractionated heparin) is a naturally occurring heparin derived from the intestinal mucosa of pigs, sheep, or cows. Heparins prevent formation of clots by binding to antithrombin III (AT III), inhibiting clotting factors IIa (thrombin), Xa, and IXa, with thrombin (factor IIa) the most sensitive to the drug. Heparin sodium may be administered intravenously or subcutaneously and is used in lesser doses (10 units/mL or 100 units/mL) for heparin sodium flushes. Therapeutic doses often begin with 5000 to 10,000 units initially and then 10,000 units to 40,000 units daily, depending on the purpose. Heparin sodium is indicated for thrombosis/embolism, coagulopathies (such as DIC), DVT, and pulmonary prophylaxis, and for clotting prevention for open heart and brain surgery. Heparin sodium is incompatible with numerous drugs, including ampicillin, diazepam, dobutamine, morphine sulfate, and penicillin G, and may interact with other drugs and herbs. Frequent monitoring with activated partial thromboplastin time (aPTT) is required. Adverse effects include bleeding, hematoma, nausea, anemia, thrombocytopenia, fever, and edema. Protamine sulfate is the reversal drug for heparins.

> **Review Video:** Heparin - An Injectable Anti-Coagulant
> Visit *mometrix.com/academy* and enter *Code:* **127426**

Low-molecular-weight heparins, human antithrombin III, lepirudin, and bivalirudin

Low-molecular-weight heparins (LMWHs) are synthetic, obtained by cleaving large unfractionated heparin molecules into smaller fragments with enzymes. They work similarly to heparin sodium, although they are more specific for Xa than IIa, so they provide a more predictable anticoagulant response and do not require the frequent monitoring with aPTTs that unfractionated heparin requires. LMWHs include enoxaparin (Lovenox), dalteparin (Fragmin), and tinzaparin (Innohep). Adverse effects are similar to those of heparin sodium and include bleeding, hematoma, nausea, anemia, thrombocytopenia, fever, and edema. Antithrombin III (Thrombate III) is derived from human plasma so it may carry a slight risk of transmission of viruses or CJD (although it is pasteurized) and is indicated primarily for treatment of hereditary antithrombin III deficiency when patients require surgical procedures or obstetric procedures or have a thromboembolism. Common adverse effects include chest pain, dizziness, nausea, and impaired sense of taste. Lepirudin (Refludan) and bivalirudin (Angiomax) are direct thrombin inhibitors used for unstable angina and PCI, and for prophylaxis and treatment for thrombosis in heparin-induced thrombocytopenia.

Acetylsalicylic acid

Acetylsalicylic acid (ASA), generally referred to as aspirin, is commonly used as a prophylactic therapy for adults to reduce the risk of developing coronary artery disease or stroke. ASA irreversibly inhibits cyclooxygenase (COX), which activates thromboxane A2, necessary for platelets to aggregate and form a clot, with the effects lasting the life of the platelets (7 days). While both 81 mg and 325 mg are effective, 81 mg is usually recommended for those with increased risk of bleeding or gastrointestinal irritation. Current recommendations from the US Preventive Services Task Force advise daily aspirin for males 45 to 79 when potential benefit of reducing risk of MI outweighs risk of increased risk of GI bleeding and for women 55 to 79 when potential benefit of reducing risk of stroke outweighs increased risk of GI bleeding. However, recent studies have indicated that daily ASA does not decrease the risk of an initial MI or stroke; however, when taken after these events have occurred, ASA reduces the risk of a subsequent MI or stroke.

Dabigatran, rivaroxaban, apixaban, and edoxaban

Dabigatran (Pradaxa), a monovalent direct thrombin inhibitor that reduces the blood's ability to clot, is an alternative to warfarin to prevent stroke in those with atrial fibrillation not associated with heart valve disorders and does not require routine blood testing or dietary restriction. It is available in only two different dosages and is taken orally twice daily. Adverse effects include bleeding, allergic responses, indigestion, and gastric pain. Medication should not be stopped abruptly.

Rivaroxaban (Xarelto), apixaban (Eliquis), and edoxaban (pending FDA approval) are factor Xa inhibitors and are indicated to reduce risk of stroke in nonvalvular atrial fibrillation and to treat DVT and pulmonary embolism. They may be given as a prophylaxis for patients undergoing knee or hip replacement surgery to decrease risk of DVT and pulmonary edema. The most common adverse reaction is bleeding. Rivaroxaban and apixaban do not require routine blood monitoring or dietary restrictions.

Pentoxifylline (Trental) and cilostazol (Pletal)

Antiplatelet drugs interfere with the normal functions of platelets. When trauma to vessels occurs, the exposed collagen and fibronectin stimulate platelet adhesion; once the platelets become activated, they release stimulators that cause the platelets to aggregate: adenosine diphosphate (ADP), thrombin thromboxane A2 (TXA2), and prostaglandin H2. As the platelets change shape, they release ADP, serotonin and platelet factor 4 (PF4), which cause vasoconstriction and attract additional platelets. At this point, the intrinsic or extrinsic clotting cascade is initiated to create a more stable fibrin blood clot. Pentoxifylline (Trental) is an early anti-platelet drug that is a methylxanthine derivative and is referred to as a hemorheologic drug because it changes the fluid dynamics of the blood. Pentoxifylline inhibits ADP, serotonin, and PF4, and reduces the viscosity of the blood, increasing RBC flexibility and capillary blood flow and reducing platelet aggregation. It is indicated for intermittent claudication from chronic occlusive vascular disease. Adverse reactions include dizziness, headaches, indigestion, nausea, and vomiting.

Clopidogrel (Plavix)

Clopidogrel bisulfate (Plavix) is an adenosine phosphate (ADP) inhibitor, which alters the membrane of the platelet so it cannot receive the signal from fibrinogen molecules to aggregate and form a clot. Clopidogrel is used to reduce the risk of thrombosis in those with atherosclerosis and recent stroke, MI or peripheral arterial disease, those with acute coronary syndrome (unstable angina and non–Q-wave MI), including those receiving medications or PCI or coronary artery bypass graft, as well as those with ST-segment elevation acute MI and as a loading dose for patients undergoing placement of coronary stent. Clopidogrel should not be given with salicylates, NSAIDs, or red clover (herb) as the interactions may result in increased risk of bleeding. Overdose of clopidogrel can result in prolonged bleeding time and bleeding. Adverse reactions include intracranial bleeding, confusion, rhinitis, taste disorder, epistaxis, GI hemorrhage, indigestion, gastritis, ulcers, constipation, diarrhea, purpura, arthralgia, myalgia, pneumonitis, rash, pruritis, angioedema, and anaphylaxis.

Eptifibatide (Integrilin)

Eptifibatide (Integrilin) is an antiplatelet drug that reversibly binds to the GP IIb/IIIa receptor on platelets and inhibits platelet aggregation. Eptifibatide is available only for intravenous use and is used primarily in intensive care or cardiac catheterization labs where patients are closely monitored. It is indicated for acute coronary syndrome (unstable angina or non–ST-segment elevation MI) for those receiving drug therapy or having a PCI. The drug must be protected from light before administration and discarded if particles are evident in solution. Eptifibatide is incompatible with furosemide. Adverse reactions include hypotension, hematuria, bleeding, and thrombocytopenia. Eptifibatide is contraindicated in patients with creatinine levels at least 4 mg/dL or those receiving renal dialysis. Eptifibatide is intended for use with heparin and aspirin. Eptifibatide should be discontinued prior to CABG and if platelet count drops below 100,000/mm³.

Cilostazol (Pletal)

Cilostazol (Pletal) is an antiplatelet drug believed to inhibit the enzyme phosphodiesterase III, resulting in vasodilation and inhibiting platelet aggregation; however, this action decreases the chance of survival for those with class III and class IV heart failure. Cilostazol is indicated for treatment of intermittent claudication and is taken orally twice daily at least 30 minutes before meals or 2 hours after meals. Grapefruit juice may increase drug level, gingko biloba may prolong bleeding time, and smoking may decrease drug exposure. Benefits of the drug may not be evident for up to 12 weeks. Adverse reactions include dizziness, headache, tachycardia, peripheral edema, pharyngitis, rhinitis, indigestion, abdominal discomfort, flatus, nausea, abnormal stools, back pain, myalgia, increased cough, and infection. Drug-drug reactions may occur with diltiazem, erythromycin and other macrolides, omeprazole, and drugs that inhibit CYP3A4 (fluconazole, miconazole, sertraline).

Immunosuppressant drugs

Drugs	Actions	Side effects
Antibodies (Monoclonal)	Act to depress particular antigens, such a CD3, and lowers T-cell count. Used to treat acute rejection responses.	Marked cell-mediated immune depression increases risk of infection and development of cancer.
Antibodies (Polyclonal)	(Obtained from animal serum.) Inhibit T-cell production and promote destruction of T cells. Used with other immun-osuppressant drugs to reduce dosage. Depress cell-mediated immune response and used to prevent GVHD response.	Allergic/anaphylactic reactions to serum, including serum sickness, fever, arthralgia, urticaria, erythema.
Corticosteroids	Depress cell-mediated immune response, humoral immune response, and inflammation, reducing proliferation of T cells and B cells. Used with transplantations and to prevent GVHD disease.	Weight gain, edema, Cushing syndrome, bruising, and osteoporosis. Abruptly stopping drugs may trigger Addisonian crisis.
Ciclosporin	Inhibit activation of T cells. Used to prevent transplantation rejection and to treat autoimmune diseases and nephrotic syndrome.	Tremor, excessive facial hair, gingivitis, bone marrow suppression with increased risk of infection and cancer, especially skin cancer.
Methotrexate	Inhibits folic acid, which interferes with RNA/DNA synthesis and cell division. Used for many different cancers and many autoimmune diseases. Also used for elective abortions.	Nausea, vomiting, loss of hair, bone marrow suppression with leukopenia, stomatitis, Teratogenic.
Tacrolimus	Used after surgery to prevent rejection of heart, kidney and liver transplants (usually in combination with azathioprine or mycophenolate mofetil). Taken with adrenal corticosteroids.	(May interact with grapefruit juice.) Anaphylaxis, especially with IV infusion, tremor, headache, nausea, diarrhea, hypertension, and kidney dysfunction. Bone marrow suppression may result in increased risk of infection, bleeding, and cancer, especially skin cancer. Increases risk of developing diabetes.
Azathioprine	Inhibits cell reproduction, especially those that rep-licate quickly, such as B and T cells. Used with transplant-ations and autoimmune diseases, such as MS, Crohn disease, and restrictive lung disease.	Bone marrow suppres-sion, increasing risk of infection. Nausea, loss of hair, malaise, and rash. Increased risk of cancer, especially skin tumors, with long-term use.
Intravenous immuno-globulin (IVIG)	Used to combat immunosuppression by increasing antibodies to prevent infection or treat acute infection, such as Guillain-Barré. Used off-label for many different disorders and infections.	Dermatitis, headache, renal failure, venous thrombosis. Infections can occur because IVIG is extracted from pooled plasma.

Antibiotic classification

Antibiotics may be classified according to their chemical nature, origin, action, or range of effectiveness. There are hundreds of antibiotics. Broad-spectrum antibiotics are useful against both gram-positive and gram-negative bacteria. Medium-spectrum antibiotics are usually effective against gram-positive bacteria, although some may be effective against gram-negative as well. Narrow-spectrum antibiotics are effective against a small range of bacteria. Antibiotics function by killing the bacteria by interfering with their biological functions (bacteriocidal) or by preventing reproduction (bacteriostatic). The main classes of antibiotics include:

- Macrolides: Medium-spectrum antibiotics that prevent protein production by bacteria and are primarily bacteriostatic but may be bactericidal at high doses. They may be irritating to the gastric mucosa, but are less likely to cause allergic responses than penicillins or cephalosporins. Macrolides include erythromycin (E-Mycin), clarithromycin (Biaxin), and azithromycin (Zithromax).
- Fluoroquinolones: Broad-spectrum antibiotics that inhibit bacterial reproduction and repair of genetic material in the bacterial DNA. Drugs include ciprofloxacin (Cipro), levofloxacin (Levaquin), and ofloxacin (Floxin). Adverse effects include CNS and cardiac toxicity and may increase risk of MRSA and C. difficile infections.
- Sulfonamides: Sulfonamides are medium spectrum with action against gram-positive and many gram-negative organisms as well as Plasmodium and Toxoplasma. Some people are sensitive and may develop an allergic response. Resistance to sulfa drugs is widespread. Sulfa drugs interfere with folate synthesis and prevent cell division, so they are bacteriostatic. Sulfonamides include co-trimoxazole (Bactrim) and trimethoprim (Proloprim).
- Tetracyclines: Broad-spectrum antibiotics. They are also used for rickettsias- and psittacosis-producing agents. Tetracyclines include tetracycline, doxycycline (Vibramycin), and minocycline. Adverse effects include phototoxicity, nausea, vomiting, diarrhea, and fever.
- Aminoglycosides: Effective against gram-negative bacteria. They interfere with protein production in the bacteria and are bacteriocidal. Aminoglycosides cannot be taken orally. They are often given in conjunction with other classes of antibiotics, such as penicillin. Aminoglycosides include gentamicin (Garamycin) and tobramycin (Tobrex), neomycin, and streptomycin. Side effects include nausea, vomiting, dizziness, seizures, anorexia, and rash.
- Penicillins: Medium-spectrum antibiotics may be combined with β-lactamase inhibitors. They are bacteriocidal and cause breakdown of the bacterial cell wall. Penicillins may cause severe allergic reactions in sensitive individuals. Penicillins include penicillin, ampicillin, and amoxicillin.
- Cephalosporins: Medium-spectrum antibiotics effective against gram-negative organisms. They are bacteriocidal and inhibit cell wall synthesis. They are divided into different "generations" according to antimicrobial properties with succeeding generations having more powerful effect against resistant strains. First generation includes cephazolin (Kefzol), cephalexin (Keflex), and cephradine (Velosef). Second generation includes cefaclor (Ceclor), cefuroxime (Zinacef), and loracarbef (Lorabid). Third generation includes cefotaxime (Claforan), cefixime (Suprax), cefpodoxime (Vantin), ceftazidime (Fortaz), and cefdinir (Omnicef). Fourth generation includes cefepime (Maxipime).
- Polymyxins: Narrow-spectrum antibiotics effective against gram-negative organisms. They interfere with the cell membrane of bacteria and are bactericidal. Polymyxins have both neurotoxic and nephrotoxic properties and are not used unless other antibiotics are ineffective. They must be given intravenously. Polymyxins include polymyxin B Sulfate.

Antiviral agents

Antiviral agents target viral proteins at different stages in the replication process:
- Entry: Drugs to block viral entry into cells bind to the cellular receptor of the virus-associated protein (VAP) to prevent the virus from binding and entering. Other drugs bind to the VAP directly, preventing it from binding to cells. Entry blockers include amantadine (Symmetrel), an antiviral that has been used to prevent and treat influenza, although there is increasing resistance by current viruses. Additionally, amantadine has dopaminergic and adrenergic properties that can cause central nervous system side effects. In 1969, it was discovered to have anti-Parkinson properties and is routinely used for treatment of Parkinson disease. Rimantadine (Flumadine) is a closely related drug that is used to treat influenza A virus. It has fewer side effects than amantadine but can also be used to treat Parkinson disease. Fusion inhibitors (Fuzeon) are also entry blockers.

Antiviral agents target viral proteins at different stages in the replication process:
- Synthesis: Many current antiviral (and antiretroviral) drugs target viruses during synthesis, after they enter the host cells, disrupting processes essential to replication. These include the nucleoside analogues, such as acyclovir (Zovirax), which is used to treat herpes simplex and herpes zoster. Another nucleoside analogue is zidovudine (AZT), the first drug approved to treat HIV/AIDS. Nonnucleoside reverse transcriptase inhibitors and nucleoside reverse transcriptase inhibitors also target the virus during synthesis. Lamivudine (3TC) has been approved for the treatment of hepatitis B virus. Protease inhibitors prevent protease from cutting apart viral protein chains.
- Release: The two most common antiviral drugs used to combat influenza, zanamivir (Relenza) and oseltamivir (Tamiflu), block release of viral particles from the host cell by blocking neuraminidase (molecule on surface of viruses).

Thrombolytics

Thrombolytics	
Alteplase tissue-type plasminogen activator (t-PA) (Activase)	An enzyme that converts plasminogen to plasmin, which is a fibrinolytic enzyme. t-PA is used for ischemic stroke, MI, and pulmonary embolism, and must be given IV within 3 hours or by catheter directly to the site of occlusion within 6 hours.
Anistreplase (Eminase)	Used for treatment of acute MI and given intravenously in a 30-unit dose over 2-5 minutes.
Reteplase (Retavase)	A plasminogen activator used after MI to prevent CHF in 2 doses, a 10-unit bolus over 2 minutes and then repeated in 30 minutes.
Strepto-kinase (Streptase)	Used for pulmonary emboli, acute MI, intracoronary thrombi, DVT, and arterial thromboembolism. It should be given within 4 hours but can be given up to 24 hours
Tenecteplase (TNKase)	Used to treat acute MI with large ST-segment elevation. Administered in a one-time bolus over 5 seconds and should be administered within 30 minutes of event.
Urokinase (Abbokinase)	Used for DVT and pulmonary embolism. Dose is calculated according to patient's weight. Urokinase is given in an initial loading dose of 15 mL over 10 minutes and then with an infusion pump, 15 mL/h over 12 hours.

Antineoplastic chemotherapeutic agents

There are numerous antineoplastic chemotherapeutic agents and many clinical trials in progress. Protocols are established for different types of cancers and doses are titrated for the individual patient. Many agents target particular phases of cell division and must be given in repeating cycles at those specific phases of the cell cycle (time required for a tissue cell to divide into two daughter cells). Cells are most susceptible to drugs during proliferation, while non-dividing cells are least responsive:
- G1 phase: Synthesis of RNA and proteins takes place.
- S phase: Synthesis of DNA takes place.
- G2 (premitotic) phase: Synthesis of DNA is complete and mitotic spindle forms.
- M (mitotic) phase: Cell divides to produce daughter cells.
- G0 phase: This is a resting phase that can occur after M phase or during G1.

Each treatment may destroy from 20% to 99% of malignant cells, depending on many variables. It is almost impossible to destroy all malignant cells; the goal is to reduce the number so that the body's immune system can destroy those remaining.

Antineoplastic chemotherapeutic agents

Antineoplastic chemotherapeutic agents include:
- Alkylating agents (busulfan, carboplatin, chlorambucil, cisplatin, cyclophosphamide, dacarbazine, hexamethyl melamine, ifosfamide, melphalan, nitrogen mustard, thiotepa) alter the structure of DNA and may be given at any point in the cell cycle. Some may cause suppression of bone marrow, vomiting, cystitis, stomatitis, hair loss, gonadal suppression, and kidney damage.
- Nitrosoureas (carmustine, lomustine, semustine, streptozocin) are similar to alkylating agents but cross the blood brain barrier. They may be given at any point in the cell cycle. Adverse effects include myelosuppression, especially causing thrombocytopenia, nausea, and vomiting.
- Topoisomerase I inhibitors (irinotecan, topotecan) bind to the topoisomerase I enzyme, causing the DNA to break and preventing cell division. They must be given at a specific point in the cell cycle and may cause bone marrow suppression, liver toxicity, and gastrointestinal disorders.
- Antimetabolites (5-fluoroucil, 5-azacytadine, methotrexate, hydroxyurea, FUDR, edatrexate, fludarabine, gemcitabine, 6-mercaptopurine, pentostatin, 6-thioguanine cladribine) target the S phase of cell division and interfere with RNA and DNA synthesis. Adverse effects include gastrointestinal disorders, bone marrow suppression, stomatitis, kidney and liver toxicity.
- Antitumor antibiotics, such as bleomycin, dactinomycin, daunorubicin, doxorubicin (Adriamycin), idarubicin, mitomycin, mitoxantrone, and plicamycin, are not cell cycle specific but prevent RNA synthesis and interfere with synthesis of DNA by binding to the DNA. Adverse effects include bone marrow suppression, gastrointestinal disorders, alopecia, anorexic, and cardiac toxicity.
- Mitotic spindle poisons, such as plant alkaloids (etoposide, teniposide, vinblastine, vincristine, vindesine, and vinorelbine) and taxanes (paclitaxel, docetaxel), target the M phase of cell division and arrest the metaphase by inhibiting tubular formation and tubulin

depolymerization as well as inhibiting DNA and synthesis of proteins. Adverse effects include bone marrow suppression, neuropathy, and stomatitis.

- Hormones, such as androgens, anti-androgens, estrogens, anti-estrogens, progestins, anti-progestins, aromatase inhibitors, luteinizing hormone-releasing hormones, and steroids (prednisone), are not cell cycle specific but bind to hormone receptor sites that affect cell growth. Adverse effects include bone marrow suppression, anorexia, gastrointestinal disorders, anaphylaxis, hypertension, impaired glucose metabolism, and hepatotoxicity.
- Corticosteroids (prednisone, cortisone, dexamethasone) are cell cycle nonspecific and disrupt cell membrane, decrease circulating lymphocytes, and depress the immune system. Adverse effects include increased appetite, acne, mood changes, and rapid mood swings, GI irritation, tachycardia, nausea, insomnia, metallic taste in mouth, muscle weakness, bruising, osteoporosis, Cushing syndrome, cataracts, glaucoma, and hypertension.
- Varied targeted therapy includes signal transduction inhibitors (imatinib mesylate, gefitinib, cetuximab, and lapatinib), biologic response modifier agents (denileukin, diftitox), and proteasome inhibitor (bortezomib). Small molecules enter cancer cells and disrupt cell function, resulting in death of the cell.
- Angiogenesis inhibitors (bevacizumab, sunitinib, everolimus, sorafenib) target blood vessels that supply nutrients to the cells to starve the cells of nutrients. Some monoclonal antibodies have antiangiogenic activity.

Some drugs used for chemotherapy do not fit into the other classes of drugs and are usually used in conjunction with other chemotherapeutic agents:

- Asparaginase (Elspar), an enzyme, is used for the treatment of leukemia. It interferes with the ability of leukemic cells to obtain nutrition necessary for life. Adverse effects include impairment of liver function, decreased clotting time, allergic reactions, and rash.
- Procarbazine (Matulane), a hydrazine derivative, is used for some brain tumors (glioblastoma multiforme) and stage III and IV Hodgkin lymphoma with nitrogen mustard, vincristine, and prednisone (MOPP). It interferes with DNA, breaking the strands, but the mechanism is not clear. Adverse effects include leukopenia, thrombocytopenia, and anemia, as well as gastrointestinal disorders.
- Trastuzumab (Herceptin) is and HER_2-neu receptor antagonist used for HER_2-positive breast tumors, often with other drugs initially and then after completion of other therapy. Adverse effects include cardiomyopathy, pulmonary toxicity, and exacerbation of neutropenia. Cardiac status must be monitored during treatment.

Antiparasitic agents

Parasite	Drugs
Nematodes (pin-, hook-, whip- and roundworms.	Albendazole (Albenza), mebendazole (Vermox), pyrantel pamoate (Pin-Rid), and ivermectin.
Cestodes (tapeworms)	Praziquantel (Biltricide), nitazoxanide, and niclosamide.
Trematodes (flukes)	Praziquantel and albendazole.
Giardia intestinalis	Metronidazole (Flagyl), nitazoxanide, and tinidazole.
Dientamoeba fragilis	Iodoquinol, paromomycin, tetracycline, and metronidazole.
Entamoeba histolytica	Asymptomatic infections: iodoquinol, paromomycin, and diloxanide furoate. Mild to severe disease: metronidazole and tinidazole.
Balantidium coli	Metronidazole, tetracycline, and iodoquinol.
Cryptosporidium parvum/hominis	Nitazoxanide
Isospora belli	Trimethoprim-sulfamethoxazole-no alternative
Cyclospora cayetanensis	Trimethoprim-sulfamethoxazole or nitazoxanide
Microsporidia	E. intestinalis: albendazole 400 mg twice daily for 14 days. E. bieneusi: fumagillin 60 mg daily for 14 days

Hematopoietic stem cell transplantation

Hematopoietic stem cell transplantation (HSCT) from stem cells harvested from bone marrow, peripheral blood, or cord blood may be done for leukemia, some solid tumors, aplastic anemia, genetic, or immune deficiency disorders. HSCT offers long-term remission, but the risks are high. Graft versus host disease (GVHD) is a common complication.

- Allogenic transplants use donor stem cells from family members or an unrelated donor.
- Syngenic transplants are from identical twins.
- Autologous transplants, using the patient's stem cells, has a lower risk than allogenic transplants, but if used for leukemia, cancer cells may inadvertently be transplanted with the cells.

Transplants from related donors have lower rates of GVHD and lower mortality rates. Transplantation is done through intravenous transfusion. If used for cancers that affect the bone marrow, such as leukemia, the patient must undergo either ablative doses of chemotherapy or total body irradiation to destroy the bone marrow and disease that exists prior to transplantation, leaving the patient susceptible to infection and disease.

Emotional and behavioral factors that affect disease, treatment, and prevention

Emotional responses, especially negative ones such as depression and anxiety, put patients at increased risk for disease, although the exact mechanism by which this happens is not always clear.

For example, researchers believe that biochemical changes related to depression may increase plaque buildup in the arteries, leading to cardiovascular disease. Patients with emotional problems may not seek medical help when needed or may be resistive to following through with medications and treatments. Patients with depression or undergoing emotional stress may attempt to self-medicate by resorting to substance abuse, such as drinking, smoking, using illicit drugs, and withdrawing from social contact. All of these may have negative effects on disease, treatment, and prevention, and counteract many preventive efforts, which often begin with basics, such as smoking cessation, limited alcohol consumption, and increased exercise.

Influence of person, family, and society on disease treatment and prevention

The healthcare provider must always consider the influence of person, family, and society on disease treatment and prevention:
- Person: The individual's emotional stability and maturity as well as cognitive and knowledge levels and religious/spiritual beliefs can influence the response to treatment, cooperation, and compliance, and willingness to carry out preventive strategies.
- Family: Support of the family, emotional and financial, is often critical to treatment and preventive methods. Family members' reactions to treatment and prevention may be influenced by their ethnicity and cultural and religious/spiritual beliefs. Different ethnic groups view the family and individual autonomy differently, so decisions about treatment may be made by someone other than the patient, such as by the eldest male in the family.
- Society: The society the patient operates within has established norms for behavior and often applies value and judgment to diseases, treatment, and preventive methods that influence the patient's attitudes. Social pressure to conform may influence the patient's behavior.

Alcohol abuse

Alcohol abuse can have a number of negative effects on the hematopoietic and lymphoreticular systems:
- Alcohol-associated GI bleeding may lead to inadequate stores of iron. On the other hand, iron absorption from the intestines may be increased, resulting in excess iron and hemochromatosis.
- The bone marrow precursors of both erythrocytes and granulocytes (to a lesser degree) develop vacuoles.
- Blood cell production is decreased overall and blood cell precursors may be abnormal, producing abnormal cells.
- Erythrocyte production decreases and alcohol-associated hypersplenism increases the rate of erythrocyte destruction.
- Alcohol interferes with hemoglobin synthesis, resulting in sideroblastic anemia.
- Increased mean corpuscular volume may indicate macrocytosis.
- Stomatocyte, spur-cell, and hypophosphatemic hemolysis may develop.
- Decreased production of leukocytes and abnormal production interfere with the immune system, increasing risk of infection.
- The monocyte-macrophage system is impaired.
- Thrombocytopenia and thrombocytopathy may occur, impairing blood clotting.

Jehovah's Witnesses and administration of blood products

Jehovah's Witnesses have traditionally shunned transfusions and blood products as part of their religious belief. In 2004, *The Watchtower,* a Jehovah's Witness publication, presented a guide for members. When medical care indicates the need for blood transfusion or blood products and the patient and/or family members are practicing Jehovah's Witnesses, this may present a conflict. It's important to approach the patient/family with full information and reasons for the transfusion or blood components without being judgmental, and to allow them to express their feelings. In fact, studies show that while adults often refuse transfusions for themselves, they frequently allow their children to receive blood products, so one should never assume that an individual would refuse blood products based on the religion alone. Jehovah's Witnesses can receive fractionated blood cells, thus allowing hemoglobin-based blood substitutes. The following guidelines are provided to church members:

Basic blood standards for Jehovah's Witnesses	
Not acceptable	Whole blood: red cells, white cells, platelets, plasma
Acceptable	Fractions from red cells, white cells, platelets, and plasma

Effects of occupations and exposure to chemicals on the blood and vascular system

Agent	Occupations/Industries	Negative effects
Arsenic	Pharmaceuticals, smelting workers, farm workers.	Increases coronary artery disease.
Benzene	Oil/Gasoline workers, chemical plant workers, shoe manufacturing	Increases risk of developing acute myeloid leukemia.
Carbon disulfide	Dry cleaning, various types of manufacturing	Increases atherosclerosis and coronary artery disease.
Carbon monoxide	Oil refinery workers, paper industry workers, firefighters, workers in operations with combustion	Binds more readily to hemoglobin than oxygen, displacing the oxygen and leading to hypoxia.
Cyanide	Jewelers (utilizing electroplating), steel workers, workers exposed to pesticides, plastic manufacturing	Decreases the ability of hemoglobin to uptake oxygen and inhibits tissue metabolism.
Tobacco	Smokers and those exposed to secondary smoke, such as waitresses and bartenders.	Increases risk of acute myeloid leukemia.

Environmental agents and drugs that can impair the hematopoietic system

Environmental agents can inhibit synthesis of hemoglobin, inhibit cell production, inhibit cell function, and increase the rate of red cell destruction. Methemoglobinemia is a condition that may be inherited or acquired by contact with environmental agents. With methemoglobinemia, abnormal hemoglobin is unable to release oxygen to the cells. Environmental agents and drugs that may cause methemoglobinemia include:
- Benzocaine and similar anesthetics
- Some antibiotics (dapsone, chloroquine)
- Nitrous gases utilized in welding

- 122 -

- Aniline dyes
- Nitrates and nitrites found in food
- Naphthalene (an ingredient in moth balls)
- Potassium chlorate
- Benzenes

Symptoms include bluish tinge to skin, dyspnea, fatigue, and headache. Treatments include methylene blue (may not be used with G6PD deficiency), ascorbic acid, hyperbaric oxygen treatment, and exchange transfusions. Patients usually recover after treatment once the environmental agent is identified and exposure reduced or eliminated.

Race and ethnicity

Race and ethnicity can be a factor in disorders of the blood and blood types. Anemia occurs in African Americans more than 3 times the rate of anemia in Caucasians. African Americans tend to have lower hemoglobins and higher rates of microcytosis. Additionally, those with anemia tend to have more comorbid conditions, such as diabetes, hypertension, and vascular disease. Sickle cell disease is most common in persons of African, Indian, Mediterranean, and Middle Eastern background, while thalassemia is most common among those of Mediterranean ancestry (such as Greek). Hereditary hemochromatosis is most common among Caucasians of Northern European ancestry (especially Celtic). Another factor is that rare blood types are often found only in specific racial or ethnic groups (the reason that blood is labeled by the donor's race). Rare blood types specific to ethnic groups include:
- RzRz: Native Americans
- Jk (a-b-): Asians or Pacific Islanders
- Di(b-): Hispanics
- U- : African descent
- Vel-: Caucasians
- Dr(a-): Russian Jews/East European

Gender differences

Gender differences can be an important factor. Females often metabolize medications differently from males, and since most dosages were initially determined for male subjects, the dosages may be inaccurate for females and may alter the course of treatment. After puberty and before menopause, females usually have lower red blood cell, hemoglobin, and ferritin levels, probably associated with iron loss during menstruation. Estrogen has a vasodilatory effect through binding with endothelial receptors and stimulating nitric oxide release, and this can have a protective effect on the cardiovascular system. Recent studies also indicate that estrogen causes hematopoietic stem cells to divide more quickly in females than males, as evidenced by increased production during pregnancy when estrogen levels increase. Estrogen affects release of growth hormones so that they maintain a consistent level in the plasma, and this in turn results in increased lymphoid proliferation, affecting the immune response.

Central and Peripheral Nervous Systems

Neural tube derivatives

The neural tube derivatives differentiate into the central nervous system. The central nervous system consists of the brain and spinal cord. Between days 18 and 25 postfertilization, the neural tube is formed from ectoderm, indenting into a neural groove and then forming a neural tube. The surrounding mesoderm forms the notochord and somites. Signaling from the notochord stimulates the neural induction process, which forms the neural tube. The expression of different genes, including bone morphogenic protein and hedgehog, influences further differentiation of the notochord. The closure of the spinal cord is dependent on folic acid and cholesterol levels. The neural tube eventually forms the neural pituitary, motor neurons, and retina in addition to the spinal cord and brain.

Cerebral ventricles

The cavity of the neural tube is what eventually leads to the development of the cerebral ventricles. Around day 21–28 postfertilization, the forebrain has formed three vesicles: the forebrain or prosencephalon, the midbrain or mesencephalon, and the hindbrain or rhombencephalon. By about day 35, the prosencephalon has differentiated into the telencephalon and diencephalon. The rhombencephalon has differentiated into the metencephalon and myelencephalon. The telencephalon becomes the lateral ventricle, and the diencephalon becomes the third ventricle. The mesencephalon becomes the cerebral aqueduct. The metencephalon becomes the fourth ventricle, pons, and cerebellum, while the mesencephalon becomes the medulla. The ventricles are lined by choroid plexus cells, which produce cerebrospinal fluid. The fourth ventricle has openings through which cerebrospinal fluid (CSF) can circulate. If there is a blockage of the circulatory system of CSF at any point during fetal or perinatal development, hydrocephalus will result, which can lead to brain damage or death.

Neural crest derivatives

After formation of the neural tube, the neural crest cells differentiate into the peripheral nervous system and the autonomic nervous system. Neural crest cells migrate along the neural tube, and these multipotent cells are influenced by different genetic expression to form different cells. The development of the neural crest cells can be divided by region: cranial, cardiac, trunk, and vagal/sacral. The cranial part forms the structures of the head and neck; the cardiac part forms the heart outflow tract; the trunk part forms the melanocytes, adrenal medulla, and sympathetic ganglia; and the vagal/sacral part forms the nerves of the gastrointestinal tract. The neural crest cells eventually form the adrenal medulla (chromaffin cells), melanocytes, facial cartilage, and dentine of teeth in addition to the peripheral nervous system. Within the peripheral nervous system, the neural crest cells form Schwann cells, neuroglial cells, and the sympathetic and parasympathetic nervous systems.

Spinal cord

The spinal cord is part of the central nervous system and is enclosed within the spinal column. It begins at the foramen magnum and ends in the filum terminale in the sacral area. The spinal cord in surrounded by three layers: the dura mater (outer layer), arachnoid mater (middle layer), and pia mater (inner layer). The spinal cord is made up of inner gray matter and outer white matter. The white matter contains sensory and motor neurons, and the gray matter contains nerve cell bodies. The spinal cord is surrounded by three parallel arteries that run the length: the anterior, the right posterior, and the left posterior spinal arteries. The radicular arteries, which do not run the length of the spinal cord, are important contributors to blood supply. Spinal reflexes are neural responses that bypass the brain to occur in fractions of a second. They involve monosynaptic activation of muscles and pass only through the spinal cord.

Brain

The human brain is what is known as the cerebrum, part of the central nervous system, and is made up of many gyri or folds, which increase the surface area. The cerebrum is divided into two hemispheres, which are connected by the corpus callosum. The internal carotid and vertebral arteries, which are both paired, provide blood supply to the cerebrum. The cerebrum is divided into lobes, including the frontal lobes, parietal lobes, temporal lobes, and occipital lobes. Cognition is not limited to one lobe, but the mind–brain connection has been established through the study of various diseases. Language is lateralized in most people to the left hemisphere. Two key areas for language within this hemisphere are Broca's and Wernicke's areas. The search for how the brain makes and stores memory has eluded scientists though it is known to involve the hippocampus and the frontal lobe.

Brain stem

The brain stem is the posterior part of the brain before the spinal cord starts. It includes the medulla oblongata, the pons, and the midbrain. The cranial nerves, which provide motor and sensory innervation to the face, are contained within the brain stem. All neural tracts must pass through the brain stem on their way to and from the cerebrum and cerebellum. These tracts include tracts for pain, temperature, proprioception, and touch. The brain stem is responsible for physical processes that occur without the need to think about them, or autonomic functions of the peripheral nervous system. These include the sleep–wake cycle; cardiac and respiratory functions, such as breathing, heart rate, and blood pressure; and regulation of the central nervous system. The brain stem is responsible for consciousness, and traumatic injury to it can lead to coma and death.

Brain hypothalamic function, limbic system, and emotional behavior

The hypothalamus is a small region of the cerebrum located right above the sphenoid sinuses at the skull base. It connects the nervous system to the endocrine system via the pituitary gland. The hypothalamus is responsible for body temperature, hunger, thirst, fatigue, attachment behaviors, and circadian cycles. The hypothalamus is responsible for homeostasis, including regulation of blood pressure, heart rate, and temperature. It releases the following hormones: thyrotropin-releasing hormone, gonadotropin-releasing hormone, growth hormone–releasing hormone, corticotropin-releasing hormone, somatostatin, dopamine, vasopressin, and oxytocin. The limbic system is primarily responsible for emotional behavior. It is composed of the hippocampus, amygdalae, anterior thalamic nuclei, septum, limbic cortex, and fornix. Like the hypothalamus, it works by influencing the endocrine system. It supports a variety of functions, including emotion, behavior, motivation, long-term memory, and olfaction.

Brain circadian rhythms, sleep, and control of eye movement

Circadian rhythms are biological processes that are governed by an internal clock of approximately 24 hours. These rhythms can be reset by zeitgebers, or external cues, like daylight. In the absence of external cues, the human body demonstrates a circadian rhythm to sleep patterns with an increase and decrease in sleepiness every 24 hours. This rhythm is controlled by the suprachiasmatic nucleus in the hypothalamus. The sleep cycle is composed of four stages, which are followed by rapid eye movement sleep (REM). During this stage, intense dreaming occurs along with paralysis of voluntary muscles. The eyes move back and forth rapidly under the eyelids, and a distinctive pattern on a polysomnogram is present. Heart rate and respiration speed up, and the level of brain activity increases. Circadian rhythm leads to an average of 16 hours awake and 8 hours asleep. During sleep, each REM stage increases in length.

Sensory systems

Sensory systems consist of sensory receptors, a neural pathway, and a corresponding part of the brain to process the information. Proprioception and pain are processed using somatosensory area 1, which is then processed in Brodmann areas 1–4. Vision is processed through vision area 1 and processed in the specialized visual cortex located in the occipital lobe. Hearing travels through auditory area 1 and is processed in the auditory cortex, corresponding with Brodmann area 41 and 42 in the temporal lobe. Balance is a form of proprioception but is handled by the cerebellum, not the cerebrum, for processing. Taste is processed in gustatory area 1 and does not reflect the flavor of food, which is related to olfaction. The five qualities of taste include sourness, bitterness, sweetness, saltiness, and a recently discovered protein taste quality called umami. Olfaction is processed by olfactory area 1, and the olfactory bulbs do not cross hemispheres. The olfactory cranial nerve is the only nerve whose ganglia are present outside the central nervous system.

Motor systems

The motor systems responsible for voluntary movement are innervated by motor neurons in the spinal cord and hindbrain. The motor systems are controlled by both spinal reflexes for basic movements and reflexes and by higher connections from the brain, which allow for more sophisticated movements. The prefrontal cortex in the brain controls executive functions, while the premotor cortex groups muscle movements into coordinated functions. The supplementary motor area of the frontal lobe puts movements into temporal sequence, and the motor cortex of the frontal lobe directly activates spinal motor circuits. The basal ganglia are located in the forebrain and are responsible for action selection on the basis of motivation. The cerebellum in the hindbrain controls the precision and timing of movements. The oculomotor nuclei in the hindbrain are responsible for neurons that directly control eye movements. The ventral horn in the spinal cord contains motor neurons that directly activate muscles.

Autonomic nervous system

The autonomic nervous system is part of the peripheral nervous system. It controls functions that are not at the conscious level. This includes heart rate, digestion, respiratory rate, salivation, perspiration, pupillary dilation, micturition (urination), and sexual arousal. The medulla oblongata contains the autonomic nervous system, and this area primarily focuses on respiration, cardiac functions, and reflexes. The autonomic nervous system is composed of both the parasympathetic and sympathetic nervous systems. The sympathetic component has outflow tracts in the thoracic and lumbar regions of the spinal cord. The parasympathetic component has outflow tracts in the cervical and sacral regions of the spinal cord. The sympathetic nervous system has been thought to act in opposition to the parasympathetic nervous system, but this is too simplified. They work together in functions, such as heart rate and blood pressure. The sympathetic nervous system is thought to produce the fight or flight responses, and the parasympathetic nervous system is thought to produce the rest and digest responses.

Peripheral nerve structure

The peripheral nervous system consists of nerves outside of the brain and spinal cord. The structure of the peripheral nerves allows transmission of nerve impulses from the spinal cord out to distant effector muscles. The cell body is located in the ganglia or ventral horn of the spinal cord, while the axon must extend all the way to the intended target or terminal. Axons are surrounded by three layers that protect the nerve impulse transmission. The inner layer is the endoneurium; the middle layer is the perineurium; and the outer layer is the epineurium. The epineurium contains multiple fascicles, which are bundles of axons, Schwann cells, and perineurium. Schwann cells are supporting cells that produce the myelin to protect the axon. The main neurotransmitters of the peripheral nervous system are acetylcholine and noradrenaline. These neurotransmitters are used to transmit the nerve impulse across synapses, or spaces between nerves and from the nerve to the target.

Axonal transport

Axonal transport refers to the transport of organelles to and from the cell body through its cytoplasm along the axon. Movement toward the cell body is called retrograde transport, and movement toward the synapse is called anterograde transport. Microtubules, which are made of tubulin, run the length of the axon and serve as tracts on which transported items can travel. Motor proteins help to move the items: dynein is used for retrograde transport, and kinesin is used for anterograde transport. The items that can be transported by axonal transport include mitochondria; lipids; synaptic vesicles, which contain neurotransmitters; proteins; and other cell parts. Axonal transport can be divided into fast and slow transport, but this must be clarified as the transit speed is the same in both types. The slow transport of proteins, however, involves many more stops along the way.

Excitable properties of neurons, axons, and dendrites

Neurons transmit information via chemical and electrical signals. Neurons are electrically excitable via voltage gradients maintained across their cell membranes. Ion pumps maintain these gradients by pumping ion, such as sodium, potassium, chloride, and calcium across the cell membrane. The voltage-dependent ion channels can be altered when the voltage differential becomes high enough and an action potential can be generated. This action potential will then travel the length of the axon and be dispersed via the axon terminal to spread to adjacent neurons or targets across a synapse. The traveling action potential is also known as a wave of depolarization, referring to its electrical component. Dendrites extending off the cell bodies at adjacent neurons receive the signal, and a voltage gradient is created, which helps to transmit the signal to the next neuron.

Neurotransmitters and neuromodulators

Neurotransmitters and neuromodulators are endogenous chemicals that are used to transmit signals from a neuron to a target cell or other neuron across the synapse. The neurotransmitters are carried in vesicles that form at the cell body or dendrites from the cell membrane when the

- 127 -

signal is received. These synaptic vesicles are carried down the length of the axon, fuse with the cell membrane, and release their contents across the synapse to propagate the signal. The presynaptic neuron forms vesicles of the excess neurotransmitters that remain in the synapse and uses enzymes to degrade these neurotransmitters. Neuromodulation involves the use of multiple neurotransmitters to modulate or influence the signals being transmitted. Neuromodulation is used in the central nervous system and allows a few neurons to influence many neurons via the diffusion neurotransmitters through large areas. Examples of neuromodulators include dopamine, serotonin, acetylcholine, and histamine.

Pre- and postsynaptic receptors

Presynaptic receptors are located on the axon terminal of the proximal neuron, while postsynaptic receptors are located on the cell body or dendrites of the distal neuron. Presynaptic receptors can function as autoreceptors, which feed information back to the nerve cell about the presence of neurotransmitter in the synapse. This functions as a negative feedback, preventing the further release of that particular neurotransmitter. Postsynaptic receptors bind to neurotransmitters and help facilitate the formation of vesicles to transport the neurotransmitters. Trophic factors are signals that tell a cell to maintain its existence. In the absence of such factors, the cell commits suicide, usually by apoptosis. Growth factors are substances that stimulate cellular growth, such as cytokines or hormones. They are often involved in cellular differentiation and maturation.

Brain metabolism

The brain, unlike muscle or other components, cannot store energy, for example, as glycogen. The brain primarily uses glucose for energy metabolism and in times of unavailability, it can use ketone bodies or lactate. Other forms of energy, such as fatty acids, are unable to cross the blood–brain barrier. The brain is responsible for up to 20% of the total body energy consumption. Though the human brain represents only 2% of the human body weight, it receives 15% of the cardiac output, 20% of total body oxygen consumption, and 25% percent of total body glucose utilization. Active areas of the brain demonstrate increased glucose utilization, and this can be visualized, using positron emission tomography. These active areas have increased rates of glycolysis versus oxidative phosphorylation.

Glia and myelin

Glial cells or neuroglial cells provide support and protection for nerve cells in the central and peripheral nervous systems. There are four main functions attributed to glial cells: to surround neurons and hold them in place, to supply nutrients and oxygen to neurons, to insulate one neuron from another, and to destroy pathogens and remove dead neurons. Glial cells are capable of mitosis and can assist the neuron in releasing and reuptaking neurotransmitter. However, glial cells are not capable of action potentials. Myelin is the covering that surrounds axons. It serves as insulation to prevent dissipation of the nerve impulse and also functions to increase the speed of impulses along the neuron. Schwann cells supply the myelin for peripheral neurons, whereas oligodendrocytes myelinate the axons of the central nervous system. Myelin of the peripheral nervous system is capable of regeneration.

Brain homeostasis

The blood–brain barrier is a strict separation of the circulating blood from the brain extracellular fluid. Tight junctions along capillaries prevent the passage of microscopic and large hydrophobic objects into the cerebrospinal fluid (CSF). Astrocytic feet also contribute to its integrity. The CSF is also protected by a barrier from the circulating blood. The choroidal cells of the choroid plexus function as this barrier. The choroid plexus produces CSF, which is a clear bodily fluid that surrounds the central nervous system. It is secreted into the subarachnoid space between the arachnoid mater and the pia mater. The CSF serves as buoyancy, protection, and chemical stability, and assists in preventing brain ischemia. The weight of the brain without the buoyancy provided by CSF would compress the vascular supply to the brain, resulting in necrosis. The CSF also prevents injury that may result from the brain hitting the skull during trauma. It also helps to remove metabolic waste from the brain, and brain ischemia is prevented by the regulation of the production of CSF, which can decrease intracranial pressure.

Central and peripheral nervous systems

The central nervous system is unable to repair itself after serious injury, which often leads to paralysis or even death. The peripheral nervous system is capable of repair if the nerve has not been transected completely. The degree of injury to a peripheral nerve can be classified as neurapraxia (class I), axonotmesis (class II), and neurotmesis (class III). In neurapraxia, the epineurium, perineurium, and endoneurium are intact. In axonotmesis, the epineurium and perineurium are intact. Axonotmesis is total disruption of the entire nerve fiber, which requires surgical repair. After injury, Wallerian degradation takes place in the part of the axon that is separated from the neuron's cell body, which degenerates distal to the injury. However, errors can still be made in peripheral nerve repair.

The central nervous system is incapable of regeneration. Although this incapacity has been studied, it is poorly understood. Research has pointed to the role of astrocytes in blocking this regeneration. Upon nerve injury, astrocytes secrete glial fibrillary acidic protein (GFAP) and vimentin, which isolate the damaged neuron to prevent interference with the operation of the central nervous system. This is protective in the short term; however, over the long term, it leads to the development of scar tissue, which prevents regeneration and axonal transmission. The peripheral nervous system is capable of regeneration after injury as long as the nerve has not been completely transected. Distal to the injury, Wallerian degeneration removes the damaged part at which point chemotactic factors secreted by Schwann cells promote regeneration of the axon within the endoneurial tube.

Some common infections of the central nervous system include brain abscesses, meningitis, neurosyphilis, and rabies. Brain abscesses occur when a bacterial infection spreads to the brain and becomes walled off into a cavity. This makes antibiotic penetration difficult. These infections can spread from adjacent areas, such as the sinuses and the mastoid (related to ear infections). Brain abscesses can present with fever and increased white blood cell counts but may also present with seizures. Meningitis can be either bacterial or viral, and the presentations are different. Bacterial meningitis is an infection of the cerebrospinal fluid (CSF) and can present with high fever, high white cell count, stiff neck, and seizures. Viral meningitis is more insidious in its presentation but still involves infection of the CSF. It can present with a dull headache, light sensitivity, and a sore neck. A lumbar puncture examines the cellular composition and can help differentiate between viral and bacterial causes.

Some common infections of the peripheral nervous system include Guillain-Barré, shingles, HIV, and Lyme disease. Peripheral neuropathy is the most common presentation for infections of the peripheral nervous system. Shingles is a herpetic (varicella-zoster virus) infection of a peripheral nerve and usually presents with blistering and pain along a skin dermatome. HIV and Lyme disease

- 129 -

can present with weakness or pain associated with a peripheral nerve. Guillain-Barré is an acute polyneuropathy, which presents with ascending paralysis. It is most commonly triggered by an infection. Untreated, it can lead to paralysis of the diaphragm and respiratory failure. It can also affect the autonomic nervous system, leading to cardiac issues. Guillain-Barré is treated with intravenous immunoglobulins or plasmapheresis, in addition to supportive care, such as ventilatory support. Six subtypes exist and are differentiated by the parts of the peripheral nervous system that are involved.

Inflammation of the central nervous system is known as encephalitis if it involves the brain. It is known as meningitis if it involves inflammation of the meninges surrounding the central nervous system. These inflammatory conditions can be caused by bacterial or viral infections. Foreign substances can also be responsible. Inflammatory conditions of the peripheral nervous system can lead to peripheral neuropathy. Neuritis is the general term for inflammation of a nerve or nerves in the peripheral nervous system. The neuritis can cause compression of the nerve, which can block the transmission of action potentials along the axon. Symptoms of neuritis may include pain, paresthesia (pins and needles), paresis (weakness), hypoesthesia (numbness), anesthesia, paralysis, wasting, and disappearance of the reflexes. This may be caused by physical injury, infection, radiation, chemical injury, or underlying medical conditions, such as vitamin deficiencies.

As patients age, the central and peripheral nervous systems undergo changes. Nerve cells in the central nervous system begin to atrophy and lose weight. They may transmit signals more slowly, leading to reduced or absent reflexes or sensation. Waste products begin to accumulate, leading to plaques and tangles. Brain death is the irreversible cessation of all brain activity necessary to sustain life. It is due to complete necrosis of the cerebral neurons due to lack of oxygenation. Brain death is the legal definition of death in many jurisdictions. Patients who are brain dead can have their organs removed for transplant as circulatory functions will continue. The medical criteria for brain death include no response to pain and no cranial nerve reflexes. These reflexes include pupillary response (fixed pupils), oculocephalic reflex, corneal reflex, no response to the caloric reflex test, and no spontaneous respirations.

Immunologic disorders

Multiple sclerosis is an immunologic disorder of the central nervous system. In this disease, the myelin surrounding the nerves of the brain and spinal cord become inflamed, leading to demyelination and scarring. This inflammation is triggered by the patient's own immune system, although the stimulus for this reaction has not yet been elucidated. Systemic lupus erythematosus (SLE) is an autoimmune disease, which can affect many parts of the body. When SLE affects the brain and nervous system, it can lead to headaches, numbness, tingling, seizures, vision problems, and personality changes. SLE is frequently treated with nonsteroidal anti-inflammatory medications, but there is no cure. Sarcoidosis is a disease process that leads to inflammation in many different tissues of the body. The cause is postulated to be an overexuberant immune reaction to an infection, leading to the formation of granulomas in the body. When these granulomas form in the nervous system, they can lead to headaches, seizures and Bell's palsy (i.e., temporary paralysis on one side of the face).

Demyelinating disorders

Demyelinating disorders can target the central or peripheral nervous systems. These disorders lead to destruction of the myelin sheath that covers and protects the axon of nerves. This leads to impairment in nerve conduction, which can cause deficits in sensation, movement, cognition, or other functions, depending on which nerves are involved. These disorders can be caused by genetics, infectious agents, and autoimmune conditions; some causes are unknown. Some chemical agents, such as organophosphates, and medications, such as neuroleptics, can also lead to demyelination. Treatment involves improving a patient's quality of life. This may involve medication, lifestyle changes, relaxation, exercise, or counseling. Long-term progression of these diseases cannot be prevented, only slowed, and complications are related to which nerves are affected. Some diseases, such as transverse myelitis, can resolve in 2–12 weeks.

Myasthenia gravis and muscle channelopathies

Myasthenia gravis is a neuromuscular disorder that is classified as an autoimmune disorder. In this disease, the body makes antibodies that block the nerve from transmitting the nerve signal to the muscle. It is most common in young women and older men and can be related to disorders of the thymus. Myasthenia gravis typically presents with breathing or swallowing difficulties or difficulty climbing stairs, lifting objects, and rising from a seated position. It can also present with headaches, double vision, hoarseness of the voice, and eyelid drooping. Nerve conduction studies are done to aid in the diagnosis, but there is no cure. Treatment can lead to periods of remission. Lifestyle changes, such as rest periods, an eye patch, and avoidance of stress and heat, can help to minimize episodes. Medications, such as neostigmine and prednisone, are used to reduce the symptoms by improving communication between nerves and muscles or reducing the immune response, respectively. Muscle channelopathies are dysfunctions of the ion-gated voltage channels necessary for nerve transmission. This can lead to periodic paralysis, hypotonia, or susceptibility to malignant hyperthermia.

Nervous system disorders

Traumatic
Trauma to the central nervous system can result in death, paralysis, and coma. Trauma can be penetrating, resulting in an open injury, or blunt, resulting in a closed injury. Traumatic brain injury results in damage to the brain via anoxic injury. The damage causes bleeding to occur inside a closed space (i.e., the skull), which cuts off vital oxygen and blood supplies to the brain. This can present with a brief loss of consciousness, which resolves, or can be permanent, depending on the severity of the injury. Trauma to the spinal cord can result in bleeding, scar tissue formation, or transection, which, in turn, can result in paresis, paralysis, and neuropathies. If the spinal cord is transected, permanent paralysis will result for all nerves below the injury. If blunt trauma occurs, a hematoma or blood clot can develop that can cut off oxygen, resulting in temporary or permanent paralysis, depending on the length of anoxia. Scar tissue can result chronically from any injury, and this can impede nerve transmission.

Traumatic disorders of the peripheral nervous system can lead to peripheral neuropathy and paresthesias. The most common area for injury is the brachial plexus with the most commonly involved nerves being the radial, peroneal, and ulnar. Motor vehicle accidents are a frequent cause for peripheral nerve injuries. Neuropathic pain is a common complaint and can lead to disability. Unlike in the central nervous system, regeneration is possible in the peripheral nervous system, but errors can occur. Scar tissue can form while the healing or regeneration process takes place, leading to the formation of neuromas (i.e., localized areas of scar tissue). Neuromas of this type are known as traumatic neuromas, which can be very painful and can impair the transmission of nerve impulses. Acutely, peripheral nerve trauma can present with pain, numbness, and paresthesias.

Mechanical

The central nervous system, especially the spine, is vulnerable to mechanical disorders. The normal wear and tear associated with the aging process can lead to the breakdown of normal protective measures that surround the spine. The spinal vertebrae are separated by a cushioning layer called intervertebral discs that are made of cartilage. The effects of gravity combined with the fact that humans walk upright puts compressive pressure on the intervertebral bodies. The erosion of the intervertebral bodies can compress the spinal nerves as they exit from the vertebrae. This can lead to compression neuropathy, paresthesias, or paralysis. Pain, numbness and tingling can be felt along the course of the compressed spinal nerve. If a disc tears, leaks, protrudes, or slips forward, the nerves send a message to the brain, which translates the signal as pain.

Mechanical disorders of the peripheral nervous system most commonly result from laceration, compression, or entrapment. Trauma can lead to laceration of the nerves, often seen with bone fractures. Without immediate repair, the nerve may regrow improperly or not at all. This can lead to decreased motor or sensory function of the area innervated by that nerve. Carpal tunnel syndrome is a common complaint of patients who must type for their job. The median nerve can become compressed in the carpal tunnel of the wrist, leading to entrapment. The ulnar nerve can also become compressed and entrapped at the medial epicondyle of the humerus. This leads to inflammation and prevents the nerve signals from being properly transmitted, which can present with numbness and paresthesias of the hand. The common peroneal nerve can become compressed and entrapped at the neck of the fibula, leading to numbness and paresthesias of the foot.

Primary neoplastic

Central nervous system neoplasms are quite difficult to treat and have dire consequences due to their location in a vital area of the human body. Brain tumors include all solid neoplasms within the brain or central spinal canal. Primary brain tumors are commonly located in the posterior cranial fossa in children and in the anterior two-thirds of the cerebrum in adults. The cells from which the neoplasm is derived can originate from lymphatic tissue, blood vessels, cranial nerves, the meninges, skull, pituitary gland, or pineal gland. The cells may also be neurons or glial cells, which include astrocytes, oligodendrocytes, and ependymal cells. These neoplasms can present with seizures, focal deficits (i.e., vision, speech, hearing), and headaches. The most commonly seen peripheral nervous system neoplasms include neurofibromas and schwannomas. Neurofibromas are seen in patients with neurofibromatosis in which benign neoplasms are formed along the nerve sheath. These can cause compression symptoms and are cosmetically disfiguring. Schwannomas are benign nerve tumors of the Schwann cells, which produce myelin and can also cause compressive symptoms.

Metastatic neoplastic

The central nervous system, specifically the brain is a common location for metastases from other types of cancers. Metastatic brain lesions are far more common than primary brain tumors and can occur months to years after treatment for the primary cancer. Patients can present with nausea, vomiting, headaches, vision disturbances, memory loss, ataxia, or seizures. The most common primary cancers that metastasize to the brain are: lung, breast, genitourinary, and osteosarcoma. Treatment centers around palliative care as the lesions are usually multiple and poorly responsive to chemotherapy and radiation. Metastases to the peripheral nervous system tend to affect cranial nerves, nerve roots, and plexi. These tumors can cause compressive and entrapment symptoms, such as numbness and paresthesias. Surgical treatment can be used if the lesions are solitary, and chemotherapy and radiation are useful for multiple lesions.

Metabolic

Metabolic disorders can affect the nervous system. Disorders of pyruvate metabolism can impact the nervous system. Pyruvate dehydrogenase is a mitochondrial enzyme, which when not functioning can lead to the buildup of lactic acid. Symptoms can include episodic dystonia, hypotonia, weakness, areflexia, or hemiplegia. Dietary changes can modulate the effects of this disease. Phenylketonuria is a metabolic disorder in which the body is unable to metabolize phenylalanine. Untreated, this disease can lead to severe intellectual disability, microcephaly, and epilepsy. It is completely treatable with dietary restrictions. Glycosylation disorders can lead to storage disorders of metabolism, such as Gaucher, Niemann-Pick, and Tay-Sachs diseases. These disorders can lead to intellectual disability and death. Galactosemia disorders involve deficits in the metabolic pathway for galactose conversion to glucose. Dietary restrictions can help, but if untreated intellectual deficits, and cerebellar and cortical tract signs can develop, even resulting in death.

Regulatory

Regulatory disorders of the central and peripheral nervous systems can interfere with many vital functions. Regulatory disorders of the autonomic nervous system can lead to problems with regulation of cardiac functions. The heart rate and blood pressure in the human body are regulated by the autonomic nervous system. The autonomic nervous system depends on the interplay between the sympathetic and parasympathetic divisions. If one of these divisions is under- or over-regulating, the brain may receive not enough or too much oxygen and blood supply. This can lead to stroke, loss of consciousness, and death. Digestion is also controlled by the autonomic nervous system, and impairment can lead to diarrhea, constipation, bowel obstruction and abdominal pain. Temperature regulation is controlled by the autonomic nervous system, and problems such as hypo- or hyperthermia and sweating can result from dysregulation.

Vascular

Vascular disease can affect any vessels in the human body, but when it targets the central nervous system, the consequences can be severe. The carotid arteries are the predominant supply of arterial blood and oxygen to the brain. Carotid artery vascular disease can result in stenosis of the artery, thereby restricting the blood flow available for the brain. This can lead to vision disturbances, loss of consciousness, and permanent brain damage if severe. The plaques that can form on the carotid artery can also break loose and travel into the central nervous system, resulting in stroke. If the obstruction or stenosis affects vessels that supply the spinal cord, such as the vertebral arteries, then problems with motor function can develop. If the blood supply is cut off acutely or chronically for a long period of time, then the spinal cord may not receive enough oxygen or nutrients, and neural death may occur, which leads to paralysis.

Vascular disorders can affect the peripheral nervous system as can a decrease in the supply of oxygen and nutrients to peripheral nerves. Plaques can also form and travel, resulting in acute loss of blood supply. Depending on which nerves are affected, one can suffer from motor or sensory deficits. These deficits can be temporary or permanent, depending on the length of time that the nerve lacks oxygen and nutrients. Vascular disorders can also affect the autonomic nerves, leading to problems with regulating cardiac function, digestion, and temperature. Ischemic vascular disease can also lead to peripheral neuropathy. Without a proper supply of nutrients, the nerves are unable to transmit signals appropriately between the brain and the body. They may transmit signals of damage that the brain interprets as pain.

Systemic

Many systemic disorders can affect the brain and spinal cord. Systemic lupus erythematosus can affect the brain in what is known as neuropsychiatric lupus. In this condition, there is inflammation around the brain commonly leading to headaches. It can also lead to mood disorders, seizures, problems thinking clearly or performing mental tasks, anxiety disorders, acute confusional states, and nerve inflammation. Vasculitis is a systemic disorder that can cause serious dysfunction in the brain. In systemic vasculitis, targeting small- to medium-sized vessels, central nervous system involvement is a predictor of poor prognosis and is one of the factors considered to recommend aggressive treatment with cyclophosphamide in addition to high-dose steroids. Vascular intervention procedures or anticoagulation therapy may be used in large-vessel disease. Rheumatoid arthritis may affect the brain and spinal cord, leading to cerebral vasculitis and cervical myelopathy.

Many systemic disorders can affect the peripheral nervous system. Sjögren's syndrome can result in neuropathy. The neuropathy may be either sensory or motor and can be diagnosed by nerve conduction studies. Trigeminal and other cranial nerve neuropathies, autonomic neuropathies, and demyelinating polyradiculoneuropathies may also develop. Rheumatoid arthritis can lead to peripheral neuropathy due to nodules of chronic inflammatory cells in the peripheral nerves. The development of peripheral neuropathy has prognostic value in the disease course as these patients have decreased survival rates. Synovitis of the wrist is a common symptom and can lead to carpal tunnel syndrome and median nerve entrapment. Peripheral neuropathy can also be due to vasculitis as rheumatoid arthritis affects the blood vessels supplying oxygen and nutrients to the nerve.

Idiopathic

Diffuse idiopathic skeletal hyperostosis affects the spine, leading to calcification and ossification of spinal ligaments and the regions where tendons and ligaments attach to bone. This can affect the entire spine and is usually diagnosed radiographically. It most commonly occurs on the right side with the descending aorta offering some protection to the left side. It usually affects patients in their sixties, and complications include paralysis, dysphagia, and pulmonary infections. Lung involvement is only secondary to this disease affecting the ribs. The most frequent complaint is thoracic spine pain. Physiotherapy and manipulative therapy show beneficial results for decreasing pain and increasing spinal range of motion. There is no cure, but acute episodes can be relieved by the use of nonsteroidal anti-inflammatory drugs, such as ibuprofen. It is hoped that minimizing the inflammation in these areas will lead to a reduction in the growth rate of these hyperostotic areas.

Idiopathic disorders affect the peripheral nervous system and can cause many problems, including peripheral neuropathies. Idiopathic inflammatory demyelinating diseases are diseases in which, for unknown reasons, the body's immune system begins to attack its own nerve cells and cellular components. These diseases include multiple sclerosis, acute disseminated encephalitis, and Devic's disease. Multiple sclerosis is when inflammatory conditions occur, leading to demyelination and scarring of the myelin sheaths in the brain and spinal cord. The axons become damaged and are unable to transmit nerve signals properly. Acute disseminated encephalitis is triggered by a virus or vaccine and results in autoimmunity against myelin. Devic's disease is an autoimmune disorder that affects the optic nerve and spinal cord. The lesions that develop can lead to weakness or paralysis in the legs or arms, loss of sensation, blindness, and bladder and bowel dysfunction.

Congenital

Many congenital disorders can affect the central nervous system. Agenesis of the corpus callosum is a congenital defect in which the connection between the cerebral hemispheres, the corpus callosum, is missing. This leads to vision impairments; low muscle tone (hypotonia); poor motor coordination; a delay in motor milestones, such as sitting and walking; low perception of pain; delayed toilet training; and chewing and swallowing difficulties. Cognitive difficulties arise because of the inability to pass information across hemispheres. There is no cure, but developmental therapies may benefit patients. Spina bifida is a congenital defect in which the neural tube fails to close completely during development. The most common areas are the lumbar and sacral regions of the spinal cord. This leads to an outpouching of the spinal cord contents as the vertebral bodies are not fully closed. These patients suffer from leg weakness or paralysis, and dysfunction of the bowel and bladder.

Congenital myasthenia is a disorder of the peripheral nervous system that resembles myasthenia gravis but is not autoimmune in origin. It is caused by several types of defects at neuromuscular junctions. Presynaptic symptoms include brief stops in breathing and weakness of the eye, mouth, and throat muscles. This can result in double vision and difficulty chewing and swallowing. Postsynaptic symptoms in infants include severe muscle weakness, feeding and respiratory problems, and delays in the ability to sit, crawl, and walk. Ephedrine sulfate and salbutamol can help in some forms of the disease. Congenital hypomyelinating neuropathy is a congenital disorder that involves abnormal myelination of peripheral nerves. It is a motor and sensory neuropathy that presents soon after birth and can lead to respiratory failure. It presents at birth with hypotonia and limb weakness, neuropathy, and arthrogryposis (i.e., multiple joint contractures). It may initially be confused with spinal muscular atrophy.

Genetic
Genetic disorders can affect the central nervous system, including metabolic disorders. Canavan disease is part of a group of disorders called leukodystrophies. It causes degradation of the myelin covering of nerve axons. The course of the disease is variable but can include delays in motor skills, such as turning over, controlling head movement, and sitting without support. It can also lead to intellectual difficulties and macrocephaly. Krabbe disease, also known as globoid-cell leukodystrophy, is an inherited metabolic storage disorder that affects the muscles, vision, and mental abilities. It is also in the class of leukodystrophies and can be fatal if untreated. Lack of the galactocerebrosidase enzyme leads to buildup of a product toxic to myelin. There is both an early-onset and late-onset form. Both share presentations of weakness, stiffness, and a loss of developmental and mental abilities. The only treatment thus far is a bone marrow transplant, which will introduce healthy cells with the ability to make the galactocerebrosidase enzyme.

Genetic disorders of the peripheral nervous system can lead to peripheral neuropathy and other problems. Charcot-Marie-Tooth (CMT) is an inherited set of disorders in which the neurons and myelin sheath are not made properly. CMT diseases involve dysfunctional proteins. These proteins are used to form the nerve axon or myelin, and their dysfunction impairs the transmission of nerve signals. Patients can present with extreme weakening and wasting of the muscles in the lower legs and feet, gait abnormalities, loss of tendon reflexes, and numbness in the lower limbs. This disease can affect both motor and sensory nerves and usually presents with motor difficulties in the feet and lower legs (i.e., foot drop, a high-stepped gait). The onset is gradual, and supportive care, including braces and pain medications, can be helpful. Sufferers can have a normal life expectancy.

Degenerative
Alzheimer's disease is a degenerative disorder of the brain that results in dementia. It also affects memory, thinking, and behavior. The disease can progress slowly or rapidly, and in the later stages can be characterized by the inability to understand language, recognize family members, perform activities of daily living as well as incontinence and swallowing problems (i.e., dysphagia,

- 135 -

aspiration). There is no cure for Alzheimer's disease, and there may be a familial tendency toward its development. Autopsies have shown the accumulation of beta-amyloid plaques and tangles in the cerebrum. These plaques and tangles interfere with the transmission of nerve signals and can lead to the death of nerve cells. Medications, such as donepezil (Aricept) and memantine (Namenda), may help symptoms. Amyotrophic lateral sclerosis is a degenerative disorder of the nerves in the brain and spinal cord. It targets the nerves that supply the voluntary muscles, leading to weakness, trouble walking, problems with speech, and writing difficulties. There is no cure, and the disease is fatal due to respiratory failure.

Degenerative disorders of the peripheral nervous system include Friedreich's ataxia in which the nerves that control muscle movement in the arms and legs become nonfunctional. It is an inherited disorder in which foot problems, hearing loss, scoliosis, speech, vision problems, muscle weakness, and loss of reflexes can develop. It is a progressive disorder that can lead to premature death. Complications can include heart failure and diabetes. Treatment centers around counseling, physical and speech therapies, and the need for wheelchairs, which usually occurs 10–15 years post-diagnosis. Peripheral nerve degeneration can also be linked to chronic intoxication, metabolic and inflammatory disorders, nutritional disorders, and infectious diseases. This can lead to pain and loss of motor function. The presenting symptoms include flaccid paralysis, wasting, loss of reflexes, pain of varying intensity, loss of ability to perceive vibratory sensations, numbness, tingling, increased sensitivity to pain or touch, or anesthesia in the hands and feet. Deep-tendon reflexes can be diminished or absent, and atrophied muscles can be tender or hypersensitive to pressure or palpation.

Paroxysmal
Paroxysmal disorders of the nervous system, disorders in which the nervous system functions normally between attacks of symptoms, appear to be due primarily to abnormalities of ion channel function. It has also been linked to demyelination of the nerves. Paroxysmal disorders are characterized by their transient symptoms, their brevity (usually no more than 2 minutes), frequency (a few to hundreds of times per day), stereotyped fashion, and excellent response to drugs. Carbamazepine (Tegretol) is the drug of choice. Withdrawal of symptoms without any residual neurological finding is another key feature in their recognition. When this occurs in the brain, it can lead to a seizure. When it occurs in peripheral muscles due to disorders in the spinal column or peripheral nervous system, it can lead to spasms. It can be seen in conjunction with multiple sclerosis, pertussis, encephalitis, stroke, head trauma, epilepsy, and malaria.

Eye
Leber's hereditary optic neuropathy (LHON) is a genetic disorder that leads to dysfunction of the nerves related to the eye. It is a mitochondrially inherited condition that leads to degeneration of retinal ganglion cells and their axons, which, in turn, leads to an acute or subacute loss of central vision. Because of the inheritance pattern, it affects predominantly males. Presentation involves acute loss of vision in one eye, followed weeks to months later in the other eye. It typically presents in young adulthood. The pathophysiology involves degeneration along the axonal pathways from the retinal ganglion cell bodies to the lateral geniculate nuclei. This is mediated by impaired glutamate transport and increased reactive oxygen species, causing apoptosis of retinal ganglion cells. Genetic counseling is available for those affected, and regular corrected visual acuity and perimetry checks are advised for follow up of affected individuals. Fundal examinations can show the progression of disease via swelling of the optic nerve fiber layer.

Sight

Nervous system disorders that affect sight often involve the optic nerve, which is responsible for transmitting images to the brain for interpretation. Optic neuritis is an inflammatory condition of the optic nerve. It can lead to sudden vision loss over hours to days. This can be temporary or permanent, depending on how quickly treatment is administered and the severity of the disease. It can be seen with bacterial and viral infections, autoimmune diseases, cryptococcal infection, multiple sclerosis, and some respiratory infections. Treatment involves corticosteroids, which can hasten recovery. Prognosis is good for isolated cases with no underlying systemic conditions. Friedreich's ataxia is an inherited disorder in which areas of the brain and spinal cord degenerate. It is characterized by visual problems, commonly a loss of color vision. There is no cure, merely supportive treatments.

Ear

Vestibular neuritis is an inflammatory disorders of the nerves related to the ear. The ear is supplied by cranial nerves seven and eight; cranial nerve seven is related to auditory function, and cranial nerve eight is related to balance. When cranial nerve eight is inflamed this leads to problems with balance. This inflammation disrupts the transmission of sensory information from the ear to the brain. Vertigo and dizziness may result. Vertigo is a violent feeling that the room is spinning around oneself. It can be accompanied by nausea, vomiting, difficulty with vision, and impaired concentration. This inflammation can be due to infectious causes, mostly commonly viral. The acute phase may lead to a visit to the emergency room due to the severity of symptoms, but the disease can progress to a chronic phase that impairs activities of daily living.

Hearing

Nervous system disorders that affect hearing often involve cranial nerve VIII, which is the vestibulocochlear nerve. Friedreich's ataxia is an inherited disorder in which 10% of patients can suffer from hearing loss. This disease is characterized by degeneration of tracts in the brain and spine for which there is no cure. Sensorineural hearing loss is the most common form of hearing loss and can be linked to chronic noise exposure. Central hearing impairment occurs when the nerve and areas of the brain that process sound become damaged over time and their function decreases. Certain conditions, such as meningitis and head trauma, that affect the temporal bone can cause damage to the nerve, leading to hearing loss. Vestibular neuritis is an inflammatory condition along cranial nerve eight that can lead to hearing loss. It usually linked to viral infections.

Touch

Nervous system disorders that can affect the sense of touch are usually linked to damage to the peripheral nerves responsible for transmitting the sensation of touch. This is a form of peripheral neuropathy. Patients with diabetes can suffer from diabetic neuropathy, a form of peripheral neuropathy. Uncontrolled or poorly controlled blood glucose levels lead to glycosylation of the peripheral nerves. Over time, symptoms will develop and worsen. It may present with tingling or burning sensations in the peripheral extremities. These patients are also highly prone to wound infections and injuries because they become insensate to pain and temperature extremes. The primary treatment involves tight blood glucose control, but medications such as gabapentin (Neurontin) and carbamazepine (Tegretol) can help with the neuropathic pain. Peripheral vascular disease refers to the accumulation of atherosclerotic plaques in the arteries of the peripheral areas of the body. These plaques can disrupt and reduce blood flow, thereby cutting off oxygen and nutrients to the peripheral nerves. This can lead to peripheral neuropathy and is best treated by managing the underlying condition and smoking cessation.

Taste and smell

The sense of taste is a complex sense and is intimately affected by the sense of smell. Diseases that damage these nerves can affect the sense of taste. Alzheimer's disease is a type of dementia in which neurofibrillary tangles and plaques form in the brain. It is a progressive disease and can lead to changes in taste or loss of taste in patients. This can lead to malnutrition and dehydration in older adults. Due to the dementia, patients may not remember what certain tastes are like or what they enjoyed as a flavor. In addition, with age the sensation of taste is weakened and changes. Disorders related to smell can be characterized by complete loss (anosmia), a decrease (hyposmia), or a change in smell (dysosmia). Disorders of smell are often related to damage to cranial nerve I, the olfactory nerve. This can be due to mechanical trauma or due to an infection, commonly viral, which can affect the nerve transmissions.

Early onset

Some disorders of the nervous system can be characterized by their early onset. Many diseases that are differentiated into early- and late-onset are inherited disorders, which are characterized by defective proteins. The temporality of onset can be related to the number of these defective proteins. Huntington's disease is a neurodegenerative genetic disorder that affects muscle coordination and leads to cognitive decline and psychiatric problems. The defective gene codes for a protein huntingtin, and the number of copies of the defective gene is proportional to how much huntingtin is made. Friedreich's ataxia is a neurodegenerative disease caused by a genetic coding repeat. The more copies of this repeat that a patient has, the earlier in life the disease starts and the faster it progresses. This disease impacts the muscles and the heart, leading to muscle weakness, loss of coordination and balance, heart disease, and heart failure.

Mood

Mood disorders are often involved in changes in the central nervous system. Major depression is a mood disorder in which feelings of sadness, loss, anger, or frustration interfere with everyday life. This disorder may be due to an imbalance of neurotransmitter levels in the brain, specifically serotonin, norepinephrine, and dopamine. Antidepressant medications work by increasing the amount of certain neurotransmitters in the brain synapses. However, neurotransmitter imbalance alone does not precipitate depression. Imaging studies of depressed patients showed increased volume of the lateral ventricles and adrenal glands and smaller volumes of the basal ganglia, thalamus, hippocampus, and frontal lobe (including the orbitofrontal cortex and gyrus rectus). Bipolar disorder is a mood disorder that involves episodes of mania and depression. Imaging has shown an increase in the volume of the lateral ventricles and globus pallidus and an increase in the rates of deep white matter hyperintensities in the brain. The prefrontal region and amygdala regulation are also likely involved.

Anxiety

Anxiety disorders can impact the nervous system and the underlying causes can be tied to central nervous system characteristics. Generalized anxiety disorder involves excessive, exaggerated anxiety about everyday life events. This disorder is thought to involve depressed amounts of serotonin and norepinephrine in the brain synapses. This is the basis for treatment with reuptake inhibitor drugs that target serotonin and norepinephrine. There is thought to be a disruption of the functional processing of the amygdala. The adjacent central nucleus of the amygdala shows increased gray matter and less distinct connections to the brain, cerebellum, and hypothalamus. Anxiety interferes with daily life and is constant. Obsessive-compulsive disorder is another mood disorder linked to low levels of synaptic serotonin. Different patterns of brain activity are seen in patients with obsessive-compulsive disorder, including dopaminergic hyperfunction in the prefrontal cortex and serotonergic hypofunction in the basal ganglia.

Somatoform

Somatoform disorders are those psychiatric disorders that suggest injury or trauma, but there is no physical cause for these feelings or any drug to which it could be attributed. The etiology is thought to involve the misfiring of neural signals from the autonomic system to the body instead of to the brain for processing. Testing does not reveal any source of the symptoms or physical malfunctioning. Somatoform disorders include hypochondriasis, conversion disorder, somatization disorder, body dysmorphic disorder, and pain disorder. One theory behind somatization disorder is that the catastrophic thinking causes the brain to interpret signals of discomfort. Imaging studies show changes in the dorsolateral prefrontal, insular, rostral, anterior cingulate, premotor, and parietal cortices that support this theory. Conversion disorder has long been differentiated by neuroimaging, but some of these have been questioned, such as more prominent symptoms on the nondominant side. However, studies have shown that conversion can be distinguished from feigning by frontal lobe activity.

Personality

Personality disorders are a set of personality characteristics that deviate from social expectations and are associated with distress or disability. Personality disorders can be divided into three clusters. Cluster 1 is eccentric and includes paranoid, schizoid, and schizotypal disorders. Cluster 2 is dramatic/erratic and includes borderline, antisocial, narcissistic, and histrionic disorders. Cluster 3 is anxious and includes avoidant, dependent, and obsessive-compulsive personality disorders. Borderline personality disorder involves the inability to regulate emotion. Imaging has shown that patients with borderline personality disorder are unable to activate the anterior cingulate cortex and intraparietal sulci areas of the brain that are active in healthy people under stressful conditions. Underperforming areas, such as the subgenual anterior cingulate cortex and the medial orbitofrontal cortex areas, on imaging were linked with behavioral control. High levels of activation are seen in the amygdala and limbic regions.

Cocaine

Cocaine can have negative effects on many parts of the body, but its effects on the brain and central nervous system can be devastating. Cocaine blocks the reuptake of dopamine in the brain's synapses, leading to an overall feeling of well-being. Over time, the body down-regulates the production of dopamine, and autopsies have shown lower numbers of dopamine neurons in chronic cocaine users. This makes it much more difficult to stop using the drug, as feelings of hopelessness and depression will be worse than before one began taking cocaine. In addition, cocaine also leads to vasoconstriction of the blood vessels, increases the heart rate and blood pressure, and increases body temperature. Over time, this increased blood pressure in the brain can lead to stroke, cerebral hemorrhage, and permanent brain damage. In addition, the user faces an increased risk of seizures, convulsions, heart attack, respiratory failure, and death.

Lysergic acid diethylamide

Lysergic acid diethylamide, or LSD, is a potent psychedelic drug with effects on the central and peripheral nervous systems. LSD is a hallucinogenic drug and is thought to interfere with the brain's serotonin receptors. Serotonin is a neurotransmitter responsible for regulating moods, appetite, muscle control, sexuality, sleep, and sensory perception. LSD also interferes with how the retina perceives images and how the brain interprets these images. It is thought that there are no lasting effects from LSD use. There have been reports of heart attacks and strokes, and death associated with LSD use. It is not an addictive drug, but the negative effects come from the hallucinations that accompany its use. Users can develop social problems, completely ruin their sleep cycles, and lose interest in eating and personal hygiene. They are also prone to bad decisions regarding their safety when under the influence of LSD.

Schizophrenia

Schizophrenia is a psychiatric disorder thought to be related to the levels of certain neurotransmitters in the brain. Common symptoms include auditory hallucinations, paranoid or bizarre delusions, disorganized speech and thought, and significant social or occupational dysfunction. Treatment centers on medications that suppress dopamine- and serotonin-receptor activity. However, long-term use of these medications predisposes patients to develop tardive dyskinesia, a form of involuntary, repetitive motor movements. Genetic and environmental factors are thought to play a role in the development of schizophrenia. There is also a high risk for drug and alcohol abuse as these can alleviate or change symptoms temporarily. Imaging has shown a reduction in size as compared to normal in the frontal and temporal lobes of the brain. Autopsies have also shown a reduction in the number of glutamate receptors in the brains of schizophrenics.

Physical and sexual abuse

Physical and sexual abuse can be linked to many changes in the central and peripheral nervous systems. Both forms of abuse can lead to post-traumatic stress disorder (PTSD), which involves intrusive recollections of a traumatic event. There are three areas of the brain that are different in patients with PTSD compared with those in control subjects: the hippocampus, the amygdala, and the medial frontal cortex. Characteristic symptoms of PTSD include an exaggerated startle reflex and flashbacks of the traumatic event. These may be linked to the failure of the hippocampus and the medial frontal cortex to modulate emotional processing from the amygdala. Shaken baby syndrome is another form of physical child abuse and occurs when a caregiver shakes a baby too hard. This shaking can lead to whiplash and can prevent the brain cells from getting enough oxygen, leading to brain damage or death.

Torture

Torture can be both physical and mental and can result in changes in the nervous system. Both forms of torture, especially when conducted over a long period of time, can lead to post-traumatic stress disorder (PTSD). Patients suffering from PTSD show differences on neuroimaging from control subjects. These differences are in the hippocampus, the amygdala, and the medial frontal cortex. The amygdala may send out information about the emotional state that is not properly regulated by the hippocampus and medial frontal cortex. Torture also is an extreme form of stress and leads to the release of cortisol. Cortisol can impair cognitive function, including that of the prefrontal cortex and hippocampus. Torture also leads to the release of norepinephrine, which can enlarge the amygdala, making it more difficult to distinguish a true from a false memory. Torture triggers abnormal patterns of activation in the frontal and temporal lobes, impairing the ability to recall memories.

Prednisone

Prednisone is a corticosteroid used to treat inflammatory conditions. The side effects seen with this medication are directly proportional to the dosage and length of time the medication is taken. Unfortunately, chronic use can impact the nervous system negatively. Prednisone has been shown to do permanent damage to the hippocampus in rats, the area of the brain responsible for short-

and long-term memory storage and retrieval. This is due to neuron cell death in these areas. The prefrontal cortex is also affected by neuron cell death, leading to an inability to concentrate and make decisions. In the short term, prednisone can lead to mood changes, such as agitation, palpitations and inability to sleep. At high doses, it can lead to psychotic behavior. Additional side effects include headache, dizziness, extreme fatigue, decreased libido, and increased sweating.

Anticancer drugs

Chemotherapy drugs target rapidly dividing cells and cause cellular apoptosis. Antineoplastic drugs can lead to central nervous system toxicity. Patients receiving these drugs may develop encephalopathy, extrapyramidal reactions, seizures, cerebellar dysfunction, retinopathy, cerebral venous thrombosis, myelopathy, cognitive impairment, and psychiatric symptoms. Taxanes are a class of antitubulin chemotherapeutic drugs, which can have a toxic effect on the peripheral nervous system, leading to peripheral neurotoxicity. Microtubules are used for transport within the axon and as structural support for the neuron. This toxicity is dependent on the dose administered, the duration of the infusion, and the schedule of administration. Peripheral sensory neuropathy is the most common complaint. Risk factors that may predispose patients to develop severe peripheral neurotoxicity include significant prior exposure to neurotoxic agents and concomitant medical disorders that are associated with peripheral neurotoxicity, such as diabetes mellitus.

Ethambutol

Ethambutol (Myambutol) is a common first-line drug in the treatment of tuberculosis and other atypical mycobacterial infections. Ethambutol may bind zinc, thereby decreasing its concentration and ability to be used as a cofactor for many biological enzymes. Ethambutol has been shown to lead to optic neuritis and peripheral neuropathy. The most common complaints are numbness and tingling of the extremities. Both symptoms of optic neuritis and peripheral neuropathy appear around 6–9 months after starting treatment and are usually reversible once treatment has been discontinued. Ethambutol leads to inflammation of the optic nerve, and this inflammation may progress to the optic chiasm, resulting in bitemporal hemianopia. Early signs of optic nerve involvement may be red–green color blindness. Factors that may increase the risk for developing ethambutol complications include underlying kidney disease and the concomitant use of isoniazid. It is important that patients be followed closely for the development of these side effects so that the medication can be stopped.

Neuropathy

Peripheral neuropathy can result from many medical conditions and medications. Peripheral neuropathy symptoms depend on the nerve involved. Some people may experience temporary numbness, tingling, and paresthesias, sensitivity to touch, or muscle weakness. Others may suffer more extreme symptoms, including burning pain, muscle wasting, paralysis, and organ or gland dysfunction. Patients may become unable to digest food easily, maintain safe levels of blood pressure, sweat normally, or experience normal sexual function. The neuropathy may be acute as in Guillain-Barré or chronic as in diabetes mellitus. Many peripheral neuropathies start in the distal lower extremities and progress superiorly. There are many causes of peripheral neuropathy including trauma, systemic diseases, inherited conditions, infections, and autoimmune disorders. There are no cures for peripheral neuropathy, but there are medications that can help to alleviate the symptoms. Control of systemic diseases and smoking cessation can also lessen symptoms.

Neuralgia

There are different causes for neuralgias, and the symptoms usually include sharp, stabbing pain. This pain is due to irritation or damage to the nerve. Some examples include trigeminal neuralgia and shingles. This irritation can also be due to chemical irritation, chronic renal insufficiency, diabetes, infections, medications, porphyria, pressure, and trauma. Symptoms can also include increased sensitivity, numbness, and paralysis of the area supplied by the nerve. Trigeminal neuralgia is specific neuropathic pain along the trigeminal nerve, which supplies sensation to the head and neck. Shingles is pain due to a herpetic reactivation in a specific dorsal root ganglion, the symptoms of which appear along a dermatome or area of skin supplied by that nerve. There are no cures, but medications, such as lidocaine patches, antiseizure drugs, antidepressant drugs, and narcotics can help with symptoms.

Central pain syndrome

Central pain syndrome is a neurologic condition caused by damage to the central nervous system. Neuropathic pain can be a symptom with the sensation of pins and needles or burning pain. Damage to the central nervous system from trauma, spinal cord injury, tumors, stroke, multiple sclerosis, Parkinson's disease, and epilepsy can lead to the development of central pain syndrome though the pain lasts much longer than the initial insult. This damage is commonly located in the thalamus. It can be chronically debilitating, and patients can try to avoid clothing or objects touching the painful area or cold temperatures. Treatment centers on the use of neurologic drugs, such as antidepressants and antiepileptics. Drugs, such as amitriptyline (Elavil), gabapentin (Neurontin), and pregabalin (Lyrica) can be used. There is no cure, and diagnosis is difficult, so patients may suffer from pain for a long time before being properly diagnosed.

Anesthetics

Anesthetic agents can act either locally or generally and block the transmission of pain signals from the body to the central nervous system. Anesthetics do not change the injury to the body, but they block the information of the pain receptors, known as nociceptors from the central nervous system. Local anesthetics work only at the site of injury. They block the sodium–potassium channel, preventing the transmission of impulses. Local nerve blocks can be used to treat specific areas of pain. Spinal anesthetics are used to block sensation below a certain level of the spinal column, the area superior remains sensate. The anesthetic travels down the spinal column, blocking impulse transmission. It is commonly called an epidural and is used for procedures in which the patient can be conscious but will not feel pain in the lower body. General anesthetics to suppress pain information and induce sleep may be delivered intravenously or via inhalation to render a patient unconscious for major surgical procedures.

Hypnotic sedatives

Sedative hypnotics are medications that limit excitement and induce drowsiness or sleep via central nervous system depression. Many function by targeting the gamma-aminobutyric acid (GABA) receptor. Many drugs enhance the chloride channel at the GABA receptor, mediating inhibition of the central nervous system. Benzodiazepines are a class of drugs that have sedative-hypnotic properties and work by targeting the GABA receptors. These medications work to promote sleep and reduce anxiety; they are also used as anticonvulsants and muscle relaxants. They can also interact with serotonergic receptors. They can be classified as short-, intermediate-, or long-acting based on the length of time the effects are seen. They are useful in treating anxiety, insomnia, agitation, seizures, muscle spasms, and alcohol withdrawal and can be used as a premedication for medical or dental procedures. Overdoses can lead to stupor or coma and can lead in some cases to respiratory depression and death, especially when combined with alcohol.

Psychopharmacologic agents

Psychopharmacologic agents are used to treat psychological disorders. They may act as a precursor to neurotransmitter synthesis; inhibit neurotransmitter synthesis; and prevent the storage or release of neurotransmitters, stimulating or blocking receptors or inhibiting neurotransmitter breakdown in the synapse or reuptake. Antidepressants include tricyclics, monoamine oxidase inhibitors (MAOIs), and selective serotonin reuptake inhibitors (SSRIs). As depression is sometimes linked to low levels of these neurotransmitters in the synapse, these medications increase their availability. Tricyclics block reuptake of norepinephrine and serotonin. The MAOIs inhibit the enzyme that breaks down serotonin, dopamine, and norepinephrine. The SSRIs block the reuptake of serotonin. Antipsychotic medications are dopamine antagonists acting as postsynaptic dopamine receptor blockers. Benzodiazepines act on GABA receptors and are used as anxiolytic, sedative, and anticonvulsants medications.

Anticonvulsants

Anticonvulsant medications are used in the treatment of epileptic seizures. They are also used to treat mood disorders, such as bipolar disorder, and for neuropathic pain relief. In epilepsy, the cortex is highly irritable, and these medications suppress the rapid and excessive firing of neurons that start a seizure and prevent the spread of the seizure. These drugs work by targeting sodium channels and blocking them or enhancing gamma-aminobutyric acid (GABA) activity. Benzodiazepines are a class of anticonvulsants that work by enhancing GABA activity and act as a central nervous system depressant. Barbiturates, such as phenobarbital, are also central nervous system depressants that enhance the activity of GABA. They can also be used as anxiolytics and hypnotics but have a high potential for lethal overdose. Hydantoins, such as phenytoin, are anticonvulsants that act by stabilizing the inactive state of voltage-gated sodium channels.

Analgesics

Analgesics can be used to treat various pain syndromes and work by blocking or reducing the pain signals that are transmitted to the central nervous system. Common analgesics include ibuprofen and acetaminophen, which are available over the counter. Ibuprofen is a nonsteroidal anti-inflammatory drug, which blocks the COX-2 enzyme responsible for pain and inflammation. These drugs also suppress platelet clotting. Acetaminophen is used to relieve minor pain, but it does not relieve inflammation or have antiplatelet properties. Its mechanism of action is not well understood. Ibuprofen and acetaminophen are non-narcotic medications, but acetaminophen can be combined with narcotic medications. Caution must be exercised as acetaminophen overdoses can lead to liver failure. Narcotic medications work in the central nervous system at mu pain receptors by increasing the availability of serotonin and norepinephrine, leading to a decrease in the perception of pain. Overdose can lead to respiratory depression, and tolerance develops, leading to a need for higher doses.

Stimulants and amphetamines

Amphetamines are psychostimulant drugs that stimulate the central nervous system. They enhance wakefulness and focus and act as appetite suppressants. These drugs are commonly used to treat attention deficit hyperactivity disorder, to treat weight problems, and to increase wakefulness in people who work night shifts and long hours. Amphetamines enhance the synaptic activity of three neurotransmitters: dopamine, serotonin, and norepinephrine. It has been postulated that the norepinephrine release correlates to the potency of the drug. Amphetamines bind to and block the presynaptic transporters used for reuptake of these neurotransmitters. They act in a similar fashion to cocaine and can raise blood pressure and heart rate. Long-term use can lead to psychosis, tremors, hallucinations, restlessness, insomnia, and anxiety. Tolerance to these drugs may develop, leading to withdrawal symptoms if abruptly discontinued.

Antiparkinsonian drugs

Antiparkinsonian drugs can be classified into two types, one that slows the loss of dopamine in the brain and the other that improves the symptoms of Parkinson's disease. Levodopa–carbidopa (Sinemet) attempts to replace lost dopamine in the central nervous system. It can have long-term side effects, such as tardive dyskinesia, restlessness, and confusion. Dopamine agonists, such as ropinirole (Requip), are better tolerated and have fewer long-term side effects as compared to levodopa–carbidopa. These drugs also increase the effect of dopamine in the central nervous system. Amantadine (Symmetrel) also increases the amount of dopamine available in the central nervous system. Anticholinergics reduce the amount of acetylcholine and can reduce tremor and muscle stiffness. Selegiline (Eldepryl, Deprenyl) conserve the amount of dopamine available by preventing the dopamine from being destroyed.

Dementia (Alzheimer type)

Alzheimer's disease targets the brain and destroys the synaptic connections between neurons, leading to nerve cell death. There are two classes of Alzheimer medications that can slow the progress of the disease. Cholinesterase inhibitors slow down the disease activity that breaks down a key neurotransmitter. Donepezil (Aricept), galantamine (Razadyne), rivastigmine (Exelon), and tacrine (Cognex) are cholinesterase inhibitors. The second class includes memantine (Namenda), which is an N-methyl-D-aspartate (NMDA) receptor antagonist that regulates the activity of glutamate, a chemical messenger involved in learning and memory. Glutamate is released in large quantities by nerve cells damaged by Alzheimer's disease, and this medication helps to protect the brain from the excess glutamate. Glutamate binds to the NMDA receptors, leading to an influx of calcium, which, if excessive, can damage the cell.

Multiple sclerosis

Multiple sclerosis is an autoimmune disorder of the central nervous system that leads to inflammation and damage to the myelin of the nerves. As in other autoimmune disorders, the use of corticosteroid medications can be helpful in decreasing the immune response and inflammation. Beta-interferons can slow the progress of multiple sclerosis, reduce the number of attacks, and lessen the severity of attacks. Glatiramer (Copaxone) can reduce the number of multiple sclerosis attacks by blocking the immune attacks on myelin. Fingolimod (Gilenya) can trap immune cells in lymph nodes, preventing them from attacking the myelin covering. Natalizumab (Tysabri) can interfere with the movement of potentially damaging immune cells from the bloodstream to the brain and spinal cord; it is a humanized monoclonal antibody that acts against the cell adhesion molecule α4-integrin, which may prevent the movement of immune cells through the intestine and blood–brain barrier.

Restless leg syndrome

Restless leg syndrome is a condition in which the legs become extremely uncomfortable, typically when one is sitting or lying down in the evenings. This can interfere with sleep and can worsen as one ages. It is common for symptoms to fluctuate in severity, and occasionally symptoms disappear for periods of time. This can also be associated with nighttime leg twitching. Many medications that are used to treat other conditions can be used to treat restless leg syndrome. Antiparkinsonian drugs, such as ropinirole (Requip) and pramipexole (Mirapex), which are dopamine agonists, and carbidopa–levodopa (Sinemet), which increases synaptic dopamine, can be used to reduce symptoms. Antiepileptic drugs, such as gabapentin (Neurontin), which is a gamma-aminobutyric acid analogue, can be used as treatment. Opioids, such as codeine and oxycodone (Oxycontin), can work as pain relievers by acting on muscle receptors in the central nervous system. Muscle relaxants, such as benzodiazepines, can aid in sleep but do not reduce the leg cramps.

Skeletal muscle relaxants

Skeletal muscle relaxants can lessen or eliminate the action of specific skeletal muscles and can be used to treat spastic disorders. There are two classes of skeletal muscle relaxants: neuromuscular blockers and spasmolytics. Neuromuscular blockers act at the motor end plate by blocking acetylcholine from binding to postsynaptic receptors, preventing depolarization, or by binding to these postsynaptic receptors, initiating so much depolarization that desensitization occurs, thereby preventing activation of the muscle. Spasmolytic agents work by either enhancing the level of inhibition or reducing the level of excitation. Generally, this involves action on gamma-aminobutyric acid. They are often used in conjunction with other pain-relieving medication as they have side effects of sedation and drowsiness and may cause dependence with long-term use. Botulinum toxin is a purified form of neurotoxin that can be injected into specific muscles, resulting in paralysis. This is especially useful in areas when a specific muscle is having spasms (i.e., blepharospasm). Botulinum toxin inhibits presynaptic release of acetylcholine, preventing depolarization.

Neuromuscular junction

The neuromuscular junction is the location when the neural signal is transmitted to the muscle, resulting in muscle action. Neuromuscular blocking agents act at the presynaptic nerve, interfering with acetylcholine release, or at the postsynaptic muscle, interfering with the binding of acetylcholine to the postsynaptic receptors. Neuromuscular blocking agents are used in surgery to paralyze the muscles to prevent interference with the surgery and to paralyze the vocal cords, allowing intubation. Mechanical ventilation is needed as the diaphragm is paralyzed. Quaternary ammonium muscle relaxants block the nicotinic acetylcholine receptor, preventing activation of the postsynaptic muscle. These are classified as nondepolarizing blocking agents. The other class is depolarizing blocking agents, which includes succinylcholine (Anectine). These agents can more persistently depolarize the muscle fibers as they are resistant to acetylcholinesterase, the enzyme responsible for degrading acetylcholine. This permits long-term muscle paralysis.

Antiglaucoma drugs

Glaucoma is the state of increased pressure within the eyeball (i.e., intraocular pressure). This can lead to vision loss, and therefore, medications are prescribed that lower this pressure. These are often in the form of eye drops and include: prostaglandins, beta-blockers, alpha-adrenergic agonists, carbonic anhydrase inhibitors, and cholinergic agents. Prostaglandins increase the outflow of fluid from the eye by binding to receptors and stimulating the relaxation of smooth muscle. Beta-blockers block the beta receptor and prevent the binding of stress hormones to receptors on the smooth muscle. Alpha-adrenergic agonists bind to alpha receptors and inhibit the enzyme adenylate cyclase. This leads to the inactivation of the secondary messenger cyclic adenosine monophosphate and smooth muscle and blood vessel constriction. Carbonic anhydrase inhibitors can also be delivered orally. These medications work by slowing the formation of bicarbonate ions with subsequent reduction in sodium and fluid transport. Cholinergic agents work by stimulating the parasympathetic system, leading to muscle relaxation.

Drugs used to decrease intracranial pressure

Increased intracranial pressure can cause serious adverse effects on the brain. The brain exists in a fixed cavity, and increased pressure in that cavity decreases the blood supply, the delivery of oxygen, and the delivery of nutrients to the brain. Many drugs can be used to reduce this pressure, including mannitol and pentobarbital sodium. Mannitol is an osmotic diuretic agent and a weak renal vasodilator. It is delivered intravenously and filtered through the kidney where it is incapable of being reabsorbed from the renal tubule, resulting in decreased water and sodium reabsorption via its osmotic effect. Therefore, mannitol increases water and sodium excretion and decreases extracellular fluid volume. It is a sugar alcohol formed by the reduction of mannose or fructose. Pentobarbital sodium is a short-acting barbiturate, which is thought to down-regulate cellular metabolism in the brain. This results in a decreased need for oxygen and nutrients, leading to less cellular damage and consequent edema, which can further increase intracranial pressure.

Pain-relieving antimigraine agents

Migraine headaches are headaches characterized by photosensitivity, nausea, and vomiting. The medications used to treat these headaches can be classified as pain-relieving or preventative. Pain-relieving medications include ibuprofen, acetaminophen, triptans, ergots, opioids, antinausea medications, and dexamethasone. Ibuprofen is a nonsteroidal anti-inflammatory, and acetaminophen is an analgesic, both of which inhibit the inflammatory enzyme cyclooxygenase. Triptans have agonist effects on serotonin receptors in cranial blood vessels, causing their constriction. They also inhibit proinflammatory neuropeptide release. Ergots contribute to vasoconstriction in the brain but also interact with a variety of receptors. Opioids act at mu pain receptors to decrease pain, while antinausea medications help with side effects from the migraine headache. Dexamethasone is a glucocorticoid and has anti-inflammatory properties. It is used as an adjunct to other medications and can help to reduce short-term headache recurrence.

Preventative antimigraine agents

There are two classes of medications designed to treat migraine headaches: pain-relieving and preventative. Migraine headaches are characterized by photosensitivity, nausea, and vomiting and can be quite debilitating. Preventive medications can reduce the frequency, severity, and length of migraines and may increase the effectiveness of symptom-relieving medicines used during migraine attacks. Preventative medications include cardiovascular drugs, antiseizures medications, antidepressants, cyproheptadine, and botulinum toxin. Cardiovascular drugs, such as beta-blockers and calcium channel blockers, can reduce the severity and length of a migraine by preventing vasoconstriction, thought to be a cause of migraine headaches. Antiseizure medications, such as valproic acid (Valproate), topiramate (Topamax), and gabapentin (Neurontin), can reduce the frequency of migraines. These medications reduce the excitability of the nerves in the brain. Antidepressant drugs, such as tricyclics and some selective serotonin reuptake inhibitors, can prevent migraines by increasing the synaptic concentration of serotonin. Cyproheptadine (Periactin) is an antihistamine that can increase serotonin activity. Botulinum toxin inhibits the presynaptic release of acetylcholine, which paralyzes the muscles. When injected into trigger sites along the cranium, it can prevent the muscle constriction that may trigger migraines.

Drugs affecting the autonomic nervous system

Drugs that can affect the autonomic nervous system include adrenergic drugs, adrenergic-blocking drugs, cholinergic agonists, ganglionic blockers, and diuretic drugs. Adrenergic drugs include albuterol (Ventolin) and amphetamine. Albuterol acts at beta receptors to cause smooth muscle relaxation. Amphetamines stimulate the brain and are used to treat attention deficit hyperactivity disorder through the release of dopamine, norepinephrine, and serotonin. Adrenergic-blocking drugs, such as atenolol (Tenormin), block the beta receptor, thereby blocking the sympathetic nervous system. Cholinergic agonists, such as pilocarpine (Carpine), mimic the effects of acetylcholine and can be used to stimulate salivation and tear production. Ganglionic blockers, such as mecamylamine (Inversine), are used to treat hypertension by acting as a noncompetitive antagonist of nicotinic acetylcholine receptors. Diuretic drugs, such as furosemide (Lasix), facilitate the excretion of water, thereby lowering the total blood volume and blood pressure. In the kidney glomerulus, furosemide acts on the luminal sodium–potassium–chloride transporters in the thick ascending limb of the loop of Henle.

Antineoplastic drugs

Antineoplastic drugs are used to treat cancers of different parts of the body. Patients receiving anticancer treatment may develop encephalopathy, extrapyramidal reactions, seizures, cerebellar dysfunction, retinopathy, cerebral venous thrombosis, myelopathy, cognitive impairment, and psychiatric symptoms. Peripheral neuropathy is also a common side effect with tingling, burning, weakness, or numbness in the hands and feet. Tamoxifen, which is used in the treatment of breast cancer, competitively inhibits estrogen receptors. A reduction in cognition and memory can be seen with patients on this drug. Methotrexate inhibits the metabolism of folic acid. Myelopathies and leukoencephalopathies have been seen with the use of this drug, especially if delivered intrathecally. Cisplatin acts to crosslink DNA in cells, which leads to apoptosis. It can lead to neurotoxicity and peripheral neuropathy. Fluorouracil works through irreversible inhibition of thymidylate synthase. It causes damage to the oligodendrocytes that produce the insulating myelin sheaths, leading to delayed degeneration of the central nervous system.

Antimicrobials

Antimicrobial drugs can work in many different ways, but all are designed to combat bacterial infections. The blood brain–barrier provides an obstacle to the delivery of drugs to the central nervous system. Ceftriaxone is a third-generation cephalosporin antibiotic that has broad-spectrum activity against gram-positive and gram-negative bacteria. It is used in the treatment of bacterial meningitis and has good penetration into the central nervous system. Vancomycin is a glycopeptide antibiotic used in the prophylaxis and treatment of infections caused by gram-positive bacteria by inhibiting cell-wall synthesis. It must be given intravenously and can have nephrotoxicity and ototoxicity but has good penetration into the central nervous system. Acyclovir is a guanosine analogue antiviral drug used in the treatment of herpes simplex virus, varicella zoster (chickenpox), and herpes zoster (shingles) infections. After phosphorylation, acyclo-guanosine triphosphate is incorporated into the viral DNA, resulting in termination of replication. It is inactive against latent viruses in dorsal root nerve ganglia.

- 147 -

Antiparasitics

Antiparasitic drugs are used to treat parasitic infections and can be classified as antinematodes, anticestodes, antitrematodes, antiamoebics, and antiprotozoals. Ivermectin (Stromectol) is an antinematode used to treat river blindness or onchocerciasis. The drug binds and activates glutamate-gated chloride channels. It has potent central nervous system toxicity, including central nervous system depression and consequent ataxia. Praziquantel (Biltricide) is an anticestode with central nervous system side effects. It is thought to act by increasing the cellular permeability to calcium ions or interfere with adenosine uptake. Side effects in humans result from the death of the parasites, and include dizziness, headache, and malaise, drowsiness, somnolence, fatigue, and vertigo. Cerebral parasitic infection known as cerebral cysticercosis can result in seizures, meningitis and encephalitis. Corticosteroids are used during treatment to minimize these side effects.

Cerebrovascular disorders

Cerebrovascular disorders encompass brain dysfunctions related to disease of the blood vessels supplying the brain. They can be classified as transient ischemic attacks, strokes, embolisms, and aneurysms. Major risk factors for cerebrovascular disease include hypertension, smoking, obesity, and diabetes. Aspirin and other antiplatelet drugs are frequently used in treatment. These drugs inhibit the clotting activities of platelets, thereby preventing the formation of blood clots, which can obstruct blood vessels or break off and travel to the brain, leading to a stroke. Aspirin inhibits the production of thromboxane, which binds platelet molecules together. Clopidogrel (Plavix) is also used to prevent clotting. It irreversibly inhibits an adenosine diphosphate chemoreceptor on the platelet cell membrane. While the risks of these medications include hemorrhage, they can be used to prevent the serious complications of cerebrovascular disorders. Treatment of the underlying conditions should also be included in any treatment regimen.

Substance abuse disorders

Patients with substance abuse disorders are a serious problem for those in the medical field. The tolerance and addiction seen with many medications, especially pain medications, make treatment difficult. Methadone is a synthetic opioid used in the treatment of narcotic addiction. It is an acyclic analog of morphine and binds to the same mu pain receptors. Methadone lasts much longer than other opioids and can reduce or eliminate the withdrawal symptoms associated with substance abuse disorders. It also can block the pleasurable effects of opioids when given at high doses. Naltrexone is an opioid antagonist used in the treatment of alcohol dependence. This medication blocks the receptors eliminating the pleasure that users achieve when consuming alcohol. It can help to reduce the frequency and severity of relapses. Ceftriaxone has been investigated in the prevention of cocaine addiction relapse.

Emotions

Emotions can play a large role in the disease process. Stress can lead to the activation of the sympathetic nervous system with the resultant release of cortisol, adrenaline, serotonin, and norepinephrine. The hypothalamus, amygdala, and hippocampus are involved in the central nervous system response to stress. The spinal cord is responsible for transmitting the signals of stress to the organs and muscles that respond to it. The release of cortisol weakens the immune system, putting it at risk for disease or infection and slowing wound healing. Chronic stress can raise blood pressure, increase the risk of heart attack and stroke, increase the likelihood of anxiety and depression, contribute to infertility, and hasten the aging process. It can also slow the pituitary's release of growth hormone, leading to growth deficiencies in children. Cortisol can directly affect the parts of the brain where memories are stored, impairing the formation of memories.

Behaviors

Many behaviors can have a negative impact on the nervous system, both in the short term and the long term. The diet that a patient follows can negatively impact the nervous system. High-fat, high-cholesterol diets can lead to atherosclerosis, which diminishes the blood supply to the brain and spinal cord. The atherosclerotic plaques can break off and travel through the blood vessels to the brain, obstructing blood flow acutely and leading to stroke. Smoking can also lead to the development of atherosclerotic disease and increase the risk of stroke and damage to the brain. Drug abuse, especially with cocaine, can lead to hemorrhagic stroke, paralysis, or death. Cocaine can also lead to damage and death of dopamine neurons, which can lead to depression and mental health issues. Exposure to lead, especially during early childhood and development can lead to permanent learning and behavior disorders. Symptoms include abdominal pain, confusion, headache, anemia, irritability, and in severe cases, seizures, coma, and death.

Family and society

The views of one's family and society can influence behaviors, which, in turn, have an impact on disease. Smoking in the home exposes family members to second-hand smoke and creates an atmosphere of acceptance and encouragement of tobacco use. This also holds true for a diet high in fat and cholesterol or a propensity to exercise. Smoking, poor diet, and lack of exercise increase a patient's risk of developing atherosclerotic disease. The development of atherosclerotic plaques can chronically decrease the blood supply of oxygen and nutrients to the brain. These plaques can migrate and cut off the blood supply to the brain, resulting in a stroke. If one's family or society does not hold Western medicine or the use of drugs in high regard, the patient may be less likely to visit a physician for proper diagnosis and treatment. If that treatment involves drugs, the patient may refuse to take them because of family or societal values.

Over the last century, societal perceptions and scientific knowledge have changed and advanced, leading to a shift in disease treatment and prevention. In the past, for example, physicians attributed many psychological disorders to the mother. Current research has elucidated the presence and role of neurotransmitters in the brain. Mental diseases that were thought to be untreatable or due to psychological issues can now be linked to insufficient levels of specific neurotransmitters, and drugs have been developed to treat these abnormal levels. Drugs, such as selective serotonin reuptake inhibitors, can be used to treat depression and other mood disorders. Drugs have been developed such as levodopa–carbidopa (Sinemet) to help to raise the dopamine levels in the brain in patients suffering from movement disorders, such as Parkinson's disease. Treatments for Alzheimer's disease can now focus on increasing the level of the neurotransmitter acetylcholine in the brain.

Occupational factors

Occupational exposure to harmful chemicals, such as antineoplastic drugs or radioactive substances, can lead to damage to the nervous system. The risk of central nervous system malignancies increases with exposure to electromagnetic fields, methylene chloride, insecticides, and fungicides. Exposure to lead also increases the risk of meningioma. Occupations that show an increased risk of central nervous system cancers are textile mills, paper mills, printing and publishing industries, petroleum refining, motor-vehicle manufacturing, telephone and electric utilities, department stores, health care services, elementary and secondary schools, and colleges and universities. Governmental agencies, such as the Occupational Safety and Health Administration, have been established to monitor occupational exposure to dangerous substances that have shown links to increased cancer risk. Prevention includes protective clothing, respirators, proper ventilation, thresholds for exposure, and mandatory time off.

Environmental factors

Environmental factors can also influence the nervous system. Exposure to electromagnetic fields, including cell phones and cordless phones has been postulated to increase the risk of central nervous system malignancies. Asbestos, arsenic, wood dust, benzene, mercury, lead, pesticides, and other chemicals can be found in buildings and houses, and chronic exposure may lead to health problems, including cancer of the brain. Industrial toxins, when they are not properly contained, may pollute the environment. They may leach into drinking water that may infect mammals that are then eaten by humans. In addition, children are at greater risk from environmental exposure as their nervous system is still developing. Exposure to pesticides, lead, and household chemicals can lead to intellectual disability and growth deficiencies.

Gender

The role that gender plays in disease occurrence, treatment, and prevention is only beginning to be fully understood. Many research studies on the toxicity and side effects of drugs, especially to the central nervous system, have only involved men who metabolize and store chemicals differently than women. Women also have a higher rate of autoimmune diseases, such as multiple sclerosis and myasthenia gravis. Male patients tend lack attention to medical appointments, diet, and exercise. This puts them at higher risk for more advanced diseases and their complications. Alcohol abuse and smoking are more prevalent in men, leading to a higher rate of atherosclerotic disease, which can lead to stroke, paralysis, or death. Prevention is harder in the men as they are more resistant to making changes that are beneficial in the long term, such as smoking and alcohol cessation.

Ethnic and cultural factors

Different ethnic groups and cultures value certain types of behaviors and appearances; for example, certain ethnicities and cultures have a higher prevalence of tobacco use because it is widely accepted. In addition, the excessive use of alcohol and drugs may be tolerated in certain cultures. These substances can lead to damage to the central nervous system over the short and long term. Each culture or ethnic group has a certain cuisine and diet that is prominent. If these cuisines are high in fat and cholesterol, they may lead to a high risk of atherosclerotic disease. Atherosclerotic disease increases the risk for brain damage, paralysis, stroke, and death. Certain ethnic groups and cultures place emphasis on non-Western medicine, eschewing interventions, such as medications, surgeries, or basic preventative care, in favor of their own religious or cultural interventions.

Skin and Related Connective Tissue

Embryonic/fetal development of the skin and connective tissue

At 4 weeks, the embryo consists of a layer of simple ectoderm epithelium covering the mesenchyme. Between 1–3 months, the ectoderm develops into the epidermis, while the mesoderm develops into the mesenchyme from which derive the dermis and connective tissue. At 4 months, neural crest cells develop into melanocytes. Basal cells proliferate, forming the basement membrane. Nails are formed from ectoderm epidermal thickening. Epithelial cords extend into the mesoderm, forming hair follicles and sebaceous glands. At 5 months, hair growth begins at the base of these cords. Mammary glands also begin to develop and elongate. The skin becomes less transparent as fat is stored under the skin in the third trimester.

Changes in the skin and connective tissue after birth

Newborn skin is much thinner than that of an infant. It can also look cracked, peeling, or blotchy, but this is not permanent. The fetal skin is covered with a fine layer of hair called lanugo. This is replaced by vellus hair by 33 weeks' gestation. The vernix caseosa is a fetal skin coating with high-water content, composed of sebum, fetal skin cells, and lanugo. This coating develops in conjunction with terminal differentiation of the epidermis and formation of the stratum corneum. The vernix caseosa is shed soon after birth. When these protective coverings are lost, the infant begins to lose heat, and skin receptors signal the body to burn stores of brown fat. Brown fat is a specialized type of fat found only in newborns; it is replaced by normal adipose tissue within a few months.

Adult and fetal skin

Adult and fetal skin is different as fetal skin does not contain elastin, but it contains higher amounts of hyaluronic acid, chondroitin sulfate, and glycosaminoglycans, making up the dermis and epidermis. Type 3 collagen is present in a higher ratio in fetal skin, as compared to type 1 collagen, than in adult skin. Fetal surgery has demonstrated that fetal skin can heal without the formation of scars. After injury, fetal skin is characterized by rapid re-epithelialization; lack of inflammation; and restoration of normal extracellular matrix architecture, strength, and function. In adult skin, there is slow regeneration with fibrosis and scar formation. It is believed that the dermal components of the fetal skin are responsible for these characteristics. Fetuses also contain pluripotent stem cells, which can differentiate into many different cells. Further research may enable the use of fetal skin cells to allow adult wounds and injuries to heal without scars.

Errors in fetal development

Any errors in the formation of the skin barrier result in skin that is unable to protect the body properly from infection and injury. For example, harlequin ichthyosis, which can be fatal, develops from abnormal keratinization of the fetal skin. The keratin layer, the top layer of the epidermis, is abnormally thickened, resulting in an appearance of large scales, which can be red in color and diamond shaped. These large scales are not as flexible as normal skin, resulting in cracks, which provide entry for bacteria. Xeroderma pigmentosum is a genetic disorder that results in the inability of skin cells to repair DNA damage caused by ultraviolet radiation. Children with this disorder are forced to avoid the sun completely as exposure will lead to severe blistering. They also have an increased risk of skin cancers.

Layers of the skin

From the surface downward, the layers of the skin include the stratum corneum, stratum lucidum, stratum granulosum, stratum spinosum, and stratum basale. The stratum corneum acts as a barrier, preventing molecules from entering the lower layers of the skin. The stratum lucidum contains eleidin, which forms keratin. The stratum granulosum contains lipids and desmosomal connections, creating a waterproof barrier. The stratum spinosum protects against foreign material and produces lipids. The stratum basale is responsible for generating new cells, which slowly migrate superficially to replenish all the other layers of the skin. The dermis is made of dense connective tissue and can be divided into two layers: the papillary and reticular layers; these layers give the skin its strength, elasticity, and firmness.

Microscopic appearance of skin layers

Under the microscope, the five layers of the epidermis can be seen, as each stains differently. From the surface downward, these include the stratum corneum, stratum lucidum, stratum granulosum, stratum spinosum, and stratum basale. The stratum basale contains the tightly packed cells in a line, which stain darker than the dermis. The stratum lucidum is a thin, wispy layer that lets in much light on microscopy, hence the name. The stratum granulosum is a darker layer with keratohyalin granules, which promote hydration crosslinking of keratin. The dermis is made of dense connective tissue and can be divided into two layers: the papillary and reticular layer. The dermis stains lighter than the epidermis, and the dermal layer contains more tightly packed cells than the reticular layer.

Cellular components of the skin

The epidermis contains three specialized cells: melanocytes, Langerhans' cells, and Merkel cells. Melanocytes are found in the stratum basale. Langerhans' cells are most prominent in the stratum spinosum. As epidermal cells are produced in the stratum basale, they are pushed upward and are shed eventually by the stratum corneum. These cells flatten out as they move close to the surface. The dermis contains the small arrectores pileum muscles attached to hair follicles, sebaceous and apocrine glands, eccrine glands, blood vessels, and nerves. Specialized nerve cells are also present in the dermis of certain areas of the body that are sensitive to touch and pressure (e.g., extremities). These cells are called Meissner's cells for touch sensation and Pacini's corpuscles for pressure sensation.

In the epidermis, melanocytes are responsible for pigment production. This pigment, known as melanin, protects the hypodermis from damage from ultraviolet-B (UV-B) light by absorbing the UV-B light. Langerhans' cells are immune cells, which can take up, process, and present microbial antigens. They contain Birbeck granules, which are tennis-racket shaped. Merkel cells are thought to be involved with light touch sensation, but this has been difficult to prove definitively. They contain dense core granules, suggesting a neuroendocrine function. In the dermis, Meissner's cells are responsible for touch sensation, and Pacini's corpuscles are responsible for pressure sensation; these tend to be concentrated in the extremities.

Cellular components and function of connective tissue

Connective tissue is made up of areolar/loose connective tissue, fibrous/dense connective tissue, elastic connective tissue, reticular connective tissue, and adipose tissue. Areolar connective tissue contains collagen and elastin and holds organs and epithelium in place. Fibrous connective tissue forms ligaments and tendons, which attach muscles and bones. Elastic connective tissue allows the stretching of organs, including the lungs, arteries, and vocal cords. Reticular connective tissue is composed of collagen type 3 and supports lymph nodes, bone marrow, and the spleen. Adipose tissue is made up of adipocytes, which are commonly referred to as fat cells. These are used for thermal insulation, lubrication, energy storage, and cushioning.

Skin as an organ

The skin is the largest organ of the body and serves multiple functions. These include barrier functions, thermal regulation, and eccrine functions. The skin contains and protects all of the internal components of the body, preventing the loss of moisture or the entrance of microorganisms and pathogens. The skin contains specialized nerve cells that sense temperature, touch, pressure, and vibration. The skin controls thermal regulation through the dilation and constriction of cutaneous blood vessels. Arrectores pileum muscles create a barrier of air between the skin and hair, which traps and preserves heat. The production of sweat acts as an evaporation device for cooling.

Sweat

The autonomic nervous system, especially the hypothalamus, controls the production of sweat. It is produced in response to heat, stress, and nausea. The hypothalamus activates the sweat glands, which are located in the epidermis to produce sweat. Myoepithelial cells surround the sweat gland and pump the sweat out toward the surface of the skin. Sweat is composed primarily of water, minerals, lactate, and urea. The minerals can include sodium, potassium, calcium, and magnesium. The trace metals that can be found in sweat include zinc, copper, iron, chromium, nickel, and lead.

Eccrine glands

The eccrine glands are responsible for the production of sweat and are present only in primates. They are different from apocrine glands, which are found only in the perianal and axilla areas and do not contribute much to thermal regulation in humans. Eccrine glands are coiled structures found in the epidermis that work in concert with adjacent myoepithelial cells to pump the sweat to the skin's surface. These glands and their resultant sweat cool the skin and reduce body temperature, are an excretion route for water and electrolytes, and protect the skin from bacteria and pathogens.

Wound healing

After injury or surgery, normal skin is replaced by scar tissue, which can have a lighter or darker appearance than surrounding skin. Within minutes after an injury to the skin, platelets begin to form a fibrin clot, known as hemostasis. The second phase of wound healing is inflammatory; this takes place over hours after injury. Bacteria and debris are phagocytosed by macrophages and white blood cells, and growth factors are released to attract more healing cells. The proliferative phase occurs days to weeks after injury and involves angiogenesis, collagen and granulation tissue formation, epithelialization, and wound contraction. New blood vessels are formed; fibroblasts deposit a new extracellular matrix; and epithelial cells migrate across the wound, creating a new layer of epidermis. Myofibroblasts then contract to lessen the size of the wound. Maturation and remodeling are the last phases of wound healing, and they continue for years to remodel collagen.

Skin regeneration

The stratum basale and the stratum spinosum are responsible for skin regeneration by producing new cells that migrate superficially through the epidermis. In young skin, the epidermal layer is regenerated every 2–3 weeks. Burns are classified according to the level of injury: First-degree burns involve the epidermis; second-degree burns extend into the dermis; third-degree burns involve the entire dermis; and fourth-degree burns extend into underlying muscle and bone. In first- and second-degree burns, the dermis is still present to aid in re-epithelialization. However, third- and fourth-degree burns lack the dermis; thus, the ability to regenerate in those areas is lost. Third- and fourth-degree injuries must be dealt with surgically, using skin grafts to promote re-epithelialization.

Skin and connective tissue aging

As skin ages, the ability to regenerate is adversely affected. Exposure to sunlight contributes to this process by decreasing the production of collagen and elastin and by increasing the evaporation of moisture. Loss of collagen and elastin makes the skin thinner and decreases its strength. Dehydration makes it more difficult for the skin to repair and regenerate. The subcutaneous fat and soft tissue also decrease, leading to a loss of volume that, combined with the pull of gravity, makes the skin droop with folds and wrinkles. Photoaging, due to exposure to the sun, accounts for many of the changes discussed above, but it can be prevented with the use of broad-spectrum sunscreen lotions.

Caucasian, African American, and Asian skin

The most obvious difference among Caucasians, African Americans, and Asians is skin color, which is due to the differences in melanin production by melanocytes. High levels of melanin, such as that found in African Americans, provide protection from photoaging. Asians have more collagen than Caucasians, which contributes to a low incidence of wrinkling and sagging skin among Asians. Caucasians have earlier wrinkling and sagging of the skin than either African Americans or Asians. Populations with dark pigmentation have a strong stratum corneum. Asian and Caucasian skin suffers from transepidermal water loss, but Asian skin has the weakest barrier function as compared to Caucasians and African Americans. Asians and African Americans have more problems with melasma and pigmentary issues than Caucasians. Asians also have a thin stratum corneum and high eccrine gland density. African Americans have increased pore size, sebum secretion, and skin surface microflora.

Bacterial composition

A normal epidermis is likely colonized by approximately 1000 different types of bacteria. These bacteria are more prevalent in moist areas and in intertriginous areas (i.e., where two areas of skin touch each other, such as under the arms). Healthy bacteria commonly found on the skin include species of *Staphylococcus*, *Streptococcus*, *Enterobacter*, and *Neisseria*. *Staphylococcus aureus* can be benign in some people and harmful in others. This is why it is important to identify *S. aureus* carriers, especially among hospital workers. Harmful bacteria include those species that have become drug-resistant, such as methicillin-resistant *S. aureus* and vancomycin-resistant *Enterococcus*. *Pseudomonas* and *Haemophilus influenzae* can also be harmful when spread to others through skin contact.

Cellular components of the skin that aid in defense

The eccrine glands produce sweat, which protects the skin and helps to flush away pathogens. Melanin protects the hypodermis from damage from ultraviolet-B (UV-B) light by absorbing the UV-B light. Langerhans' cells are immune cells that can take up, process, and present microbial antigens. The stratum basale contains tightly packed cells with desmosomes and tight junctions and acts as an impermeable layer separating the body from the outside environment. The stratum basale is continuously producing new cells that migrate superficially and are then shed at the stratum corneum. This helps to rid the skin of any bacteria or viruses that may have attached or colonized.

Skin infections

The skin acts as an impenetrable defense barrier, but when this barrier is compromised, infections can develop. Dehydration, genetic predisposition, congenital defects, systemic conditions, and medications can all lead to breaks in the skin barrier. Cracks in the epidermis allow the entry of bacteria and viruses, which can then penetrate into the bloodstream. This activates the immune system, and T lymphocytes are able to migrate to the epidermis and provide a defense mechanism along with Langerhans' and Merkel cells. Viruses, such as human papillomavirus, may take up residence in the keratinocytes, using the host mechanisms for reproduction. This leads to the overgrowth of cells, known as a wart. This usurpation of host replication can also lead to malignant growth.

Factors that impair skin defense

Any factors that impair the barrier function of the skin will lead to a lowered defense. Sun exposure leads to decreased collagen and elastin production as well as increased dehydration of the skin. This leaves the skin vulnerable to cracking and the entry of pathogens. Diseases, such as eczema and psoriasis, also create cracks in the epidermis, allowing the entry of bacteria and viruses. Xeroderma pigmentosum is a genetic condition that impairs the skin's ability to repair damage caused by sunlight; individuals affected by this disease are predisposed to skin malignancies at an early age. Diseases involving Langerhans' or Merkel cells decrease the skin's ability to defend itself against pathogens.

Bacterial infections

Bacterial infections of the skin occur when bacteria are able to penetrate the epidermal barrier. The most common skin bacterial infections involve *Streptococcus* and *Staphylococcus* bacteria, which are also found as normal flora on the skin. Bacterial infections typically present with erythema (redness), edema (swelling), and calor (warmness). These are indications of the defense cells working to fight the infection. A localized area of whiteness in the center of the red area can indicate the source of the infection as the white blood cells and debris congregate in the area. Many skin infections are associated with hair follicles, such as folliculitis, as they can provide entry for bacteria.

Bacterial skin infections can sometimes be fought by the host's defense mechanisms alone; warm compresses with peroxide or salt-water soaks can help. Often, however, antibiotics are needed to resolve skin infections. Broad-spectrum antibiotics, such as amoxicillin, cephalexin, or clindamycin, interfere with bacterial replication and fight infection. If skin infections go untreated, the bacteria continue to proliferate and spread either locally or through the bloodstream. When a bacterial infection develops a thick wall around it that prevents the entry of antibiotics or host immune cells, it is called an abscess. The treatment for an abscess is surgical drainage.

Herpesvirus infections

The most common herpesvirus skin infections belong to the genus *Simplexvirus* (e.g., herpes simplex) and the genus *Varicellovirus* (e.g., herpes zoster). Herpes simplex is classified into type 1, which appears most commonly in the oral region, and type 2, which appears most commonly in the genital region. Herpesviruses remain dormant in the dorsal ganglion (herpes simplex) and in the nerve cell bodies (herpes zoster) and are reactivated during periods of stress, such as injury, sun exposure, decreased sleep, changes in diet, and decreased immunity. Both herpes simplex infections (type 1 and 2) present as painful vesicles or blisters that contain actively replicating viruses; they are shed and spread easily to others. Once the infection has resolved, scabs cover the affected areas at which point there is no shedding of the virus. Herpes zoster, which causes chickenpox, most often in children, can become reactivated at a later time and cause shingles. Shingles is characterized by extremely painful vesicles or blisters usually along a single dermatome. There is now a vaccine to prevent shingles.

Viral infection treatments

Viral skin infections usually resolve without treatment but may require medications to control the pain. Other times, antiviral medications, such as acyclovir, are used to prevent further spread of the infection. Untreated infections or infections not successfully controlled with antiviral medications can result in scarring and pockmarks on the skin. Since these viruses of the skin are never totally eradicated from the body, they can become periodically reactivated. These viral infections also disrupt the skin barrier and can become secondarily infected with bacteria or other pathogens.

Fungal infections

Fungal infections of the skin are common and occur most commonly in areas of skin that are moist, such as intertriginous areas. Common fungal skin infections include: tinea pedis (athlete's foot), tinea cruris (jock itch), and tinea corporis (ringworm). Tinea pedis presents as itching, cracking, and redness of the skin. It is caused by a fungus that lives on the dead tissue of the feet and nails. Tinea cruris presents as a red itchy rash that is often ring-shaped. It is caused by a fungus that lives in warm, moist areas of the body; therefore, it is most often found around the thighs, genitals, and buttocks. Tinea corporis presents as a red circular flat sore that can be accompanied by scaling. It can appear anywhere on the body, but it favors warm, moist areas.

Fungal infections can be definitively diagnosed by performing a skin scraping and examining the tissue under the microscope. After treatment with potassium hydroxide, filamentous fungal hyphae will be apparent. Often, clinical suspicion will warrant treatment without microscopic examination if the patient has been exposed to other persons or animals with the fungus. The best prevention is to remove the favorable conditions for fungal growth by keeping the skin clean, dry, and cool. Also, the use of sandals in common shower areas will help prevent the spread of tinea pedis since it can thrive on the shower room floor. Cotton clothing, cotton socks, and powders, all of which can absorb moisture, help to prevent fungal infections on the skin.

Parasitic infections

The most common parasitic skin infections include creeping eruption, scabies, and lice. Characteristics of creeping eruption include itching, blisters, and a curving, snake-like rash. This rash is caused by the burrowing of the hookworm. Hookworm infections can be spread from skin contact with feces from cats and dogs. The infection is most commonly found on the legs, feet, buttocks, and back. Scabies is characterized by severe itching, a rash with small bumps, and scaly skin. Tiny mites are responsible for this infection, and it is highly contagious through skin contact. The mites burrow through the skin and lay eggs, which causes the itching and small bumps. Lice are typed, according to location: body lice, pubic lice, and head lice. Severe itching and the appearance of small white balls characterize this infestation. The small white balls are the egg sacs, also known as nits, and are visible to the naked eye.

Mycobacterial infections

The most common mycobacterial skin infections are *Mycobacterium leprae*, *Mycobacterium ulcerans*, and *Mycobacterium marinum*. *M. leprae* is the mycobacteria responsible for leprosy or Hansen's disease. Leprosy can have a long incubation period and then present as skin lesions with decreased sensation and a lighter color than surrounding skin. Muscle weakness and numbness are also characteristics of the disease. *M. ulcerans* is the cause of the Buruli ulcer. The Buruli ulcer presents as a nodule that leads to extensive destruction of the skin and soft tissue with accompanying ulcers. This can lead to restriction of joint movement and secondary infection. *M. marinum* is also known as fish tank infection and is the most common of the three types seen in the United States. Exposure occurs through broken skin contact with a fish tank and presents as a small granuloma or cluster of granulomas known as sporotrichotic lymphangitis.

Scleroderma

Scleroderma is an autoimmune disease that affects the skin and connective tissue. It can be seen as part of the CREST syndrome (i.e., calcinosis or calcium deposits under the skin; Raynaud's phenomenon or vasoconstrictive disease of the fingers and toes; esophageal dysfunction; sclerodactyly or thickening of skin around fingers and toes; telangiectasia or dilation of blood vessels, leading to red patches or systemic scleroderma). The skin in localized scleroderma presents as thick white patches. It is predominant among 30- to 50-year-old women. Treatment centers on suppressing the immune system with anti-inflammatory and immunosuppressive medications. The skin changes associated with Raynaud's phenomenon can be treated with calcium channel blockers. Research in drugs that target the excess collagen deposition underlying scleroderma has been disappointing.

Erythema multiforme

Erythema multiforme is an allergic reaction that commonly presents as skin lesions and affects children and young adults. Patients may be allergic to drugs or infections. It is also known as erythema multiforme because of the multiple red rings around a central core. These lesions may have associated vesicles and blisters. Symptoms also include fever, malaise, aches, and itching of the skin. Erythema multiforme minor is usually due to viral or mycoplasmal infections and is mild. Erythema multiforme major is severe and usually results from drug allergies. Patients may be positive for Nikolsky's sign where the top layers of the skin slip away from the lower layers when rubbed. A skin biopsy can be done to aid the clinical diagnosis. This will show an acute interface dermatitis with damage to basal keratinocytes, leading to clefting or detachment of the epidermis from the underlying dermis.

Thermal injury

Burns are classified according to the level of injury. First-degree burns involve the epidermis; second-degree burns extend into the dermis; third-degree burns involve the entire dermis; and fourth-degree burns extend into underlying muscle and bone. Second-degree burns can be further subdivided into superficial (papillary) and deep (reticular) dermal involvement. The coloration helps to classify a burn: first-degree burns appear red; second-degree burns appear red with blisters; third-degree burns appear white or brown, and fourth-degree burns appear black. Second-degree burns will blanch with pressure, indicating that the vascular supply remains intact. This is crucial for healing. Third- and fourth-degree burns have eliminated the ability of the skin to regenerate in those areas and must be dealt with surgically.

Decubitus ulcers

Decubitus or pressure ulcers form as a result of unrelenting pressure and a compromised vascular supply to the skin, leading to ischemia and possibly necrosis. They are classified by stage: stage 1 involves intact skin with redness; stage 2 involves partial thickness loss of the dermis; stage 3 involves full thickness tissue loss and may reveal underlying subcutaneous fat; and stage 4 involves full thickness tissue loss with exposure of underlying bone, muscle, or tendon. Healing time increases with the high stages of the ulcer. Prevention revolves around movement and rotation of the body or extremity so that prolonged periods of compromised vascular supply to the skin do not elapse. Treatment involves debriding the pressure ulcer so that healthy skin and tissue can regrow to cover the wound.

Ultraviolet light

Ultraviolet (UV) light comes from the sun and is classified as UV-A (longwave), UV-B (shortwave), or UV-C light. UV-A light is responsible for aging, and UV-B light is responsible for burns. Most UV-C light does not reach the earth. Short-term exposure to UV light causes damage to the epidermis, resulting in edema, erythema, and shedding of the stratum corneum as the inflammatory cells migrate and assist in cellular repair. Long-term exposure to UV light causes cellular and DNA damage, which adversely affects the cells' ability to repair damage; in addition, the DNA can become mutated, leading to uncontrolled cellular replication or malignancy.

Radiation

Radiation is frequently used as treatment for many malignancies of the body. However, to reach these targets, it must pass through the skin. Immediate reactions to radiation exposure are erythema, edema, and peeling at later stages; this is commonly known as a radiation burn. In addition, the hair cells in the epidermis, which are rapidly dividing, are also unintentionally targeted, resulting in hair loss. Repeated exposure leads to darkening and drying of the skin. Long-term exposure to radiation may lead to permanent darkening or redness of the skin along with the appearance of telangiectasias. Radiation can lead to changes in DNA structure and repair mechanisms, leading to malignant growth.

Squamous cell carcinoma

Squamous cells make up the outer layer of the epidermis and are, therefore, exposed directly to multiple insults. Risk factors include lighter skin coloring, especially with light-colored eyes or hair, severe sunburns in childhood, age, repeated exposure to radiation or chemicals, and repeated exposure over the long term to the sun. The earliest form of squamous cell carcinoma, in situ, is known as Bowen's disease. This skin cancer usually presents as an itchy, rough patch or bump on the skin that does not heal and may bleed. Sun-exposed areas are at high risk, including the scalp, ears, nose, lips, forehead, hands, and arms. The best prevention is to use aggressive sun-protection measures, such as avoid the sun during peak hours; use hats, long-sleeved shirts, and sunglasses; reapply sunscreen often; and have routine skin checks by a professional.

Basal cell carcinoma

Basal cell carcinoma is a slow-growing cancer of the basal cells of the epidermis and is the most common form of skin cancer in the United States. Risk factors include light-colored skin with light-colored hair and eyes, multiple exposures to radiation sources, multiple moles, severe sunburns in childhood, close relatives with skin cancer, and long-term exposure to the sun. A basal cell cancer presents as a raised, flesh-colored bump that appears pearly or waxy. It can also present as a sore that does not heal. Sun-exposed areas are at high risk, including the scalp, ears, nose, lips, forehead, hands, and arms. Prevention centers on sun avoidance, especially during peak hours, hats, long-sleeved shirts, sunglasses, and reapplication of sunscreen, as well as routine skin checks by a professional.

Neoplastic disorders of melanocytes

Melanoma is the malignant growth of melanocytes and can develop from normal skin or from preexisting moles. There are four types of melanoma: superficial spreading, the most common; nodular; lentigo maligna; and acral lentiginous, the least common form, which is most prevalent in African Americans. Melanomas most commonly present on the skin; however, they can also appear in the mouth, nose, back of the eye, inside the vagina, esophagus, anus, urinary tract, and small intestine. Melanomas can grow rapidly and are at high risk for metastasizing after they have penetrated the basement membrane and entered the blood and lymphatic system. Once melanoma has spread to other organs or the lymph nodes, surgical excision is less likely to result in a cure, and interferon is commonly used as treatment. However, the success with interferon is low.

Risk factors for melanoma include fair skin with light-colored hair and eyes; daily exposure to sun, especially high-intensity sunlight at high altitude or locations close to the equator; severe sunburns in childhood; the use of tanning beds; close family relative with a history of melanoma; a personal history of dysplastic nevi; and a weakened immune system. The acronym ABCDE can assist in identifying moles or lesions at high risk for melanoma: asymmetry where one half of the lesion is different from the other, border irregularity, color changes within one lesion or mole, a diameter of greater than 6 mm, and evolution in which the lesion has a progressive change in appearance. Any suspicious lesions should be evaluated immediately by a medical professional.

Hemangioma versus a hemangiopericytoma

A hemangioma is an abnormal collection of blood vessels. A capillary hemangioma appears in the top layers of skin, while a cavernous hemangioma appears deeper in the skin. A hemangioma appears at birth or soon after as a red or purple lesion that is raised; sometimes blood vessels can be seen in it. Most frequently these appear on the head and neck. Recently, lasers have been used to reduce the size of hemangiomas with or without oral steroid medications or injections directly into the lesion. A hemangiopericytoma is a soft tissue tumor that develops from pericytes, cells found primarily in the walls of capillaries in the central nervous system, especially in the brain. A hemangiopericytoma can be benign or malignant and, in infancy, presents as rapidly growing multiple nodules.

Congenital vascular neoplasms

Congenital vascular neoplasms, such as capillary and cavernous hemangiomas, can have negative effects on development though they usually regress on their own: about 50% regress by age 5, and 90%, by age 9. However, hemangiomas can cause problems with bleeding, depending on their location. They can also become secondarily infected. Hemangiomas on the head and neck and around the vocal cords can cause breathing and eating difficulties. The presence of upper eyelid hemangiomas can cause difficulty opening the eye, resulting in amblyopia, strabismus, or decreased vision in that eye. In these cases, when time is of the essence, laser treatments and steroids, either orally or injected into the lesion, are used to reduce the size and, therefore, the negative effects on development.

Neoplasm

A neoplasm is defined as the abnormal growth of tissue, which can be either malignant or benign. Risk factors for skin neoplasms are long-term sun exposure, radiation exposure, immune compromise, trauma, genetic problems, and viruses. Skin malignancies include squamous cell carcinoma, basal cell carcinoma, and melanoma. Benign skin neoplasms include common warts or papillomas, which are caused by the human papillomavirus. Neoplasms of connective tissue include sarcomas, which can be either malignant or benign. Risk factors for these include exposure to industrial chemicals, radiation exposure, viruses, and genetic disorders. Viruses, such as human herpesvirus 8 and HIV, are both linked to Kaposi's sarcoma, which presents with dark purple skin lesions.

Metastatic disease is defined as the spread of disease from one organ to another nonadjacent organ and is most commonly used to refer to malignancies. Malignant cells have lost the ability to stop cell mitosis and continue to grow, producing a tumor. Metastasis can occur through the blood, hematogenously, or through the lymphatic system. A tumor cell must penetrate the basement membrane to reach the underlying blood and lymph vessels to metastasize. Basal cell carcinoma is not prone to metastasize; it spreads locally. Squamous cell carcinoma tends to spread locally but can spread lymphatically. Melanomas, which can easily metastasize, spread both lymphatically and hematogenously after very little local growth.

Metabolic disorders

There are skin and connective tissue manifestations of many metabolic disorders, including gout, calcinosis, xanthomatosis, amyloidosis, myxedema, and porphyria. All of these metabolic disorders cause an excess of a chemical or component of the blood, which is then deposited in the skin. Gout results when uric acid salts are deposited in the skin around joints; these are known as tophi, which characteristically affect the big toe. Calcinosis cutis results in calcium salt deposits in the skin, resulting in nodules or plaques. Xanthomatosis results in yellow, fatty deposits under the skin; these are known as xanthomas. Amyloidosis results in the deposition of amyloid proteins and is classified by the amyloid protein that is deposited. Myxedema results in edema secondary to the deposition of hyaluronic acid, glycosaminoglycans, and other mucopolysaccharides in the subcutaneous tissue. Porphyria is an inherited disorder that involves the hepatic or erythropoietic system that produces heme. It results in photosensitivity, which can cause rashes and blisters.

Regulatory disorders

Regulatory disorders of the skin and connective tissue involve dysfunction in how the cells regulate growth and cell division. Many regulatory disorders concern dysregulation of an attack by the immune system. Rheumatoid arthritis, scleroderma, lupus, and dermatomyositis are some examples. Rheumatoid arthritis involves an attack by the immune system on the joints of the wrists, fingers, knees, feet, and ankles. It presents with morning stiffness, joint pain, and deformity. Systemic scleroderma can result in skin patches with thickening, sores, changes in pigmentation, and decreased elasticity. Systemic lupus erythematosus classically presents with a butterfly rash across the cheeks and nose. It can also present with light sensitivity, hair loss, fatigue, and malaise. With skin symptoms alone, it is known as discoid lupus. Dermatomyositis is characterized by inflammation of the skin and muscles. Gottron's papules are present across the metacarpal and interphalangeal joints, resulting in red patches.

Structural disorders

Structural disorders of the skin include epidermolysis bullosa and bullous pemphigoid. These diseases result from abnormalities in the dermoepidermal junction and basement membrane. When the attachments form incorrectly, the epidermis can slide over the dermis, resulting in blistering and shearing from minor trauma. These blisters can break open, forming open sores, and this can lead to secondary infections. Epidermolysis bullosa is an inherited disorder that can also cause blisters in the mouth and throat, leading to feeding difficulties. It is associated with nail loss, alopecia, and dental problems. Bullous pemphigoid has an unknown etiology but presents mostly in elderly people and can resolve on its own. Steroid medications can be used to treat both diseases with limited success.

Structural disorders of the connective tissue include Marfan's disease, Ehlers-Danlos, osteogenesis imperfecta, and fibrodysplasia ossificans progressiva. Marfan's disease results from a defect in the fibrillin protein, leading to aortic root aneurysms, long limbs and fingers, and dislocated lenses. This disease is an autosomal dominant genetic disease. Ehlers-Danlos syndrome is caused by a defect in the synthesis of collagen, leading to increased flexibility in joints, degenerative joint disease, osteoarthritis, weak muscle tone in infants, spinal deformities, and fragile skin with poor wound healing. There are six major types. Osteogenesis imperfecta, also known as brittle bone disease, concerns a deficiency of type 1 collagen. This results in blue sclera, hearing loss, loose joints, poor muscle tone, and multiple bone fractures. There are eight types with type 2 and 8 being lethal. Fibrodysplasia ossificans progressiva causes fibrous tissue to become ossified when injured as a result of a mutation of the cellular repair system.

Treatment options for metabolic, regulatory, and structural disorders

Metabolic disorders of the skin and connective tissue, including gout, amyloidosis, and porphyria, can be treated by dietary modification, including avoiding alcohol. Medications may also be used to treat the symptoms of the disease, such as propranolol to control the heart rate in porphyria. Sunlight must also be avoided in porphyria. Regulatory disorders, such as lupus and rheumatoid arthritis, can be treated with oral steroid medications and nonsteroidal anti-inflammatory drugs. Methotrexate, an antineoplastic drug, is also used to treat rheumatoid arthritis and psoriasis. There is no definitive treatment for structural disorders of the skin and connective tissue, such as epidermolysis bullosa, Marfan's syndrome, Ehlers-Danlos syndrome, and osteogenesis imperfecta; many of these conditions are lethal. Surgical interventions are used to treat the complications of these diseases.

Hypertension

Hypertension is defined as blood pressure above 140/90 mm Hg and can lead to complications that involve the skin and connective tissue. Hypertension when left untreated can lead to hardening of the arteries in the extremities, known as peripheral artery disease. This can present as decreased skin temperature and shiny brittle skin, especially on the legs. This condition leads to ischemia of the extremities and decreased wound healing, which can ultimately lead to skin necrosis, osteonecrosis, and amputation. Connective tissue disorders can be associated with pulmonary arterial hypertension, which leads to increased pulmonary vascular resistance as a result of proliferation and remodeling of the pulmonary vascular vessels. This can lead to right heart failure and death.

Rosacea

Rosacea is a chronic vascular skin condition that presents as redness and flushing. It can also result in telangiectasias around the nose and cheeks, leading to chronic enlargement of the tip of the nose. It is often mistaken for acne and occurs in middle-aged, fair-skinned women. It is exacerbated by alcohol, stress, sun exposure, and spicy foods. Treatment centers on avoiding these triggers and topical ointments, such as azelaic acid or metronidazole. Laser treatments help to reduce the visible vessels and red appearance of the skin. Rosacea does not negatively affect a person's health, but it often causes embarrassment and loss of self-esteem for sufferers.

> ➤ **Review Video:** L.A.S.E.R.
> *Visit* **mometrix.com/academy** *and enter* **Code: 703707**

Raynaud's phenomenon

Raynaud's phenomenon can appear alone (primary Raynaud's or Raynaud's disease) or with other diseases (secondary Raynaud's or Raynaud's syndrome) in the CREST syndrome (calcinosis, Raynaud's phenomenon, esophageal dysfunction, sclerodactyly, telangiectasia). It is present in about 10% of all women and a smaller proportion of men. The etiology of this disease is unknown, but the symptoms are caused by vasospasm often after exposure to the cold. It is most prominent in the fingers, which display a characteristic color change after exposure to cold of white to blue to red. This condition is also very painful during attacks. Attacks are precipitated by exposure to cold, emotional stress, smoking, and tools that vibrate the hands; treatment centers on prevention. Medications, such as calcium channel blockers, are also used to prevent vasospasm.

Buerger's disease

Buerger's disease, also known as thromboangiitis obliterans, is caused by blood vessel inflammation, leading to blockage of the vessels, especially of the hands and feet. This disease appears predominantly in men age 20–40 with a history of heavy exposure to tobacco. Color changes may resemble those of Raynaud's phenomenon, and symptoms include intermittent claudication and skin sores and ulcers in the peripheral extremities. Diagnosis is by Doppler ultrasonography or angiography to demonstrate blockage of the vessels in the extremities.

Treatment centers on avoiding triggers, such as cold temperatures and tight clothing, and discontinuing the use of tobacco. Complications can lead to nonhealing sores and ulcers, gangrene, and amputation of limbs.

Polyarteritis nodosa

Polyarteritis nodosa is a vascular skin condition that primarily affects the small- and medium-sized blood vessels. It is commonly seen in adults, and patients with hepatitis B and C are at high risk. The etiology is thought to be autoimmune, but this has not been proven definitively. Symptoms are caused by vascular insufficiency to affected organs, which often include the skin, heart, kidneys, and nerves. The skin of the extremities can show red nodules, which are painful. Ischemia of the tissue can lead to skin sores and ulcers as well as serious complications with the kidneys and gastrointestinal tract. Treatment centers on immune suppression with steroids and cyclophosphamide.

HIV/AIDS

HIV is the virus that causes AIDS, which leads to a compromised immune system and serious infections. HIV/AIDS can present with skin and connective tissue manifestations. The most well known is Kaposi's sarcoma, a purplish lesion on the skin, which is related to the herpesvirus. Thrush is also frequently seen as red or cracked lesions in the mouth, which can be covered by a white cheesy material that is easily scraped off. This is caused by the *Candida* fungus and is found in the mouth and throat. Oral hairy leukoplakia is an infection caused by the Epstein-Barr virus that appears in the mouth and on the tongue. Molluscum contagiosum is also caused by a virus and appears as white or flesh-colored bumps on the skin. Herpesvirus, both type 1 (oral) and type 2 (genital), can become reactivated in HIV/AIDS patients, leading to painful outbreaks of bumps filled with clear fluid. Shingles, caused by a reactivation of the chickenpox virus, is also seen among HIV/AIDS patients.

Autoimmune disorders

Addison's disease, dermatomyositis, rheumatoid arthritis, Sjögren syndrome, and systemic lupus erythematosus are all autoimmune disorders with skin manifestations. Addison's disease is a disorder where the adrenal glands do not produce enough hormones. This results in darkening of the skin in patches with overall paleness. Rheumatoid arthritis leads to inflammation of the joints, especially those of the wrist and fingers. In severe forms, nodules develop under the skin. Sjögren syndrome results from an autoimmune attack of the glands that produce saliva and tears. This results in dry mouth with mouth sores. It can be associated with Raynaud's phenomenon with color changes in the hands and feet. Systemic lupus erythematosus leads to chronic inflammation and is characteristically seen with a butterfly rash across the nose and cheeks. It can also be associated with hair loss, sun sensitivity, mouth sores, and Raynaud's phenomenon.

Diabetes mellitus

Some common skin manifestations of diabetes mellitus include skin thickening, frequent and severe skin infections, yellowing of the skin and nails, and peripheral neuropathy of the distal extremities, which increases the risk for trauma. More uncommon manifestations include diabetic bullae or skin blisters, usually on the extremities, necrobiosis lipoidica, disseminated granuloma annulare, and Kyrle disease. Necrobiosis lipoidica is frequently seen as a hard, raised area on the shin that may present as a bruise and then develop into a central red area surrounded by yellowish skin. This can develop into an open sore. Disseminated granuloma annulare is an inflammatory dermatitis that can present with papules and plaques. Kyrle disease presents as a large papule with a central keratin plug.

Hyperlipidemia

There are many manifestations of hyperlipidemia on the skin, including the following: tendinous xanthoma, tuberous xanthoma, planar xanthoma, and eruptive xanthoma. A xanthoma is a deposit of lipids or fat under the skin giving the skin a yellowish or tan color. Tendinous xanthomas result in xanthomas deposited along tendons, classically of the hands, feet, and Achilles tendon. This condition is seen with type 2 hyperlipidemia, chronic biliary tract obstruction, and primary biliary cirrhosis. Tuberous xanthomas present as flat or elevated yellow nodules on the skin over joints, typically the elbow and knee. It is associated with hyperlipoproteinemia types 2A and 3, less commonly with types 2B and 4. Planar xanthomas are characterized by macules and plaques sometimes with a central white area, spread over large parts of the body. This may be associated with hyperlipidemia and hypertriglyceridemia. Eruptive xanthomas present as small red-yellow papules most commonly over the buttocks, shoulders, arms, and legs. This is associated with hypertriglyceridemia, often found in patients with diabetes mellitus.

Dermatomyositis

Dermatomyositis is a type of inflammatory myopathy with an unknown cause. It occurs most commonly in children between the ages of 5 and 15, in adults between the ages of 40 and 60, and in more women than men. It is characterized by muscle weakness, difficulty swallowing, and a purple-red skin rash with purple upper eyelids. The rash occurs in the areas of the face, knuckles, neck, shoulders, upper chest, and back. Raising the arms over the head becomes difficult. It can be diagnosed through electromyography or a muscle biopsy. Treatment centers on reducing the inflammatory response through the use of steroid medications and immunosuppressive medications. Complications from the disease include acute renal failure, malignancy, pericarditis, joint pain, and lung disease. Some cases have been known to regress spontaneously.

Psoriasis

Psoriasis is a common condition with a genetic predisposition that leads to thick red skin with flaky white patches, which resemble scales. These commonly appear on the elbows, knees, and trunk of the body. Nail changes include thick nails, yellow-brown colored nails, and early separation of the nail from the nail bed. It usually presents between the ages of 15 and 35 and can be triggered by bacterial and viral infections, dryness, injury, stress, alcohol, sun exposure, and some medications. A more severe form can be seen in immunocompromised patients. A clinical diagnosis or skin biopsy can be done, and treatment centers on preventing infection and controlling the symptoms. Phototherapy can be used, as well as topical ointment and creams containing cortisone, tar, salicylic or lactic acid, and retinoids. Drugs that suppress the immune system can be used in severe cases.

Chronic urticaria

Chronic urticaria is defined as a skin reaction of hives and wheals, resulting from mast cell degranulation and the release of histamine that lasts for more than 6 weeks. There is intense pruritus associated with it. It is unknown what triggers the urticaria, but laboratory studies that evaluate the chronic urticarial index can differentiate an autoimmune from an idiopathic etiology. The autoimmune etiology has a positive functional test result for the autoantibody to the Fc receptor of immunoglobulin E. Treatment centers on blocking the histamine response with antihistamine medications, often up to four times the normal dosage, and avoiding triggers, including stress, alcohol, nonsteroidal anti-inflammatory drugs, and tight-fitting clothing. Anti-inflammatory medications, tricyclic antidepressants, and leukotriene-receptor antagonists can also be added to the treatment regimen.

Erythema multiforme

Erythema multiforme is a type of hypersensitivity reaction that results in damage to the blood vessels of the skin, resulting in damage to skin tissues. Certain medications or infections can trigger it, but the exact cause is unknown. Erythema multiforme presents as two types: minor (a mild, self-limited skin rash) and major (life-threatening inflammation). It presents with itching, joint aches, and multiple skin lesions that resemble hives or bulls eye lesions. These typically appear on the upper body, legs, arms, palms, hands, and feet and may involve the face and lips. The diagnosis is typically clinical, based on the skin lesions. Treatment involves preventing infection and treating the symptoms. Topical anesthetics, antihistamines, antibiotics, corticosteroids, and in severe cases, intravenous immunoglobulin can be used. The major form of erythema multiforme is often mistaken for the Stevens-Johnson syndrome, but they are not the same disease.

Ehlers-Danlos

Ehlers-Danlos syndrome, also known as cutis hyperelastica, is an inherited degenerative disorder characterized by problems with collagen, type 1 or 3. There are six major types. The syndrome presents with extremely loose joints; skin that is soft, thin, and hyperelastic; and easily damaged blood vessels, which can lead to bruising. This can also lead to easy scarring, poor wound healing, increased joint mobility with early arthritis and dislocation, and joint pain. Diagnosis can be made by skin biopsy or genetic testing. There is no specific treatment or cure for Ehlers-Danlos, and other symptoms must be treated individually. This disease also affects the digestive, excretory, and cardiovascular systems, which must be monitored.

Rheumatoid arthritis

Rheumatoid arthritis has an unknown etiology and leads to chronic inflammation of the joints and surrounding tissues. It commonly appears in middle-aged women. The body recognizes healthy tissue as foreign, and the immune system attacks it. Joint pain and stiffness, especially in the morning, affect the wrists, fingers, knees, feet, and ankles. Numbness, tingling, or burning can be felt in the extremities, and nodules may appear under the skin in more severe forms of the disease. Laboratory studies often show elevated rheumatoid factor and erythrocyte sedimentation rate. Treatment includes anti-inflammatory medications, such as nonsteroidal anti-inflammatory drugs, methotrexate, and antimalarial drugs, such as hydroxychloroquine. In severe cases, biologic drugs, such as white blood cell modulators, tumor necrosis factor inhibitors, and interleukin-6 inhibitors, are given.

Scleroderma

Scleroderma is an autoimmune disorder with an unknown etiology in which the body attacks healthy connective tissue, recognizing it as foreign. It usually affects women from age 30 to 50, and it can appear in both localized and systemic forms. Scleroderma presents as hair loss, skin hardness, thickening, stiffness, skin discoloration, and sores on the extremities. It can also present with joint pain, stiffness, and swelling of the fingers and joints. Laboratory studies may show elevated antinuclear antibody, erythrocyte sedimentation rate, or rheumatoid factor. Treatment attempts to control the symptoms and prevent complications. Corticosteroids, nonsteroidal anti-inflammatory drugs, and immunosuppressive medications, such as methotrexate, are used to reduce the inflammatory response. Phototherapy can also be used to treat skin symptoms.

Degenerative disorders

Degenerative disorders of the skin and connective tissue commonly result when the body's immune system recognizes healthy tissue as foreign. In the short term, this leads to inflammation and destruction of skin and connective tissue. This presents as skin lesions and rashes, joint inflammation, pain, stiffness, and overall myalgias. Laboratory studies show an inflammatory response with an elevated erythrocyte sedimentation rate and rheumatoid factor. Over time, chronic inflammation leads to early osteoarthritis, joint deformities with decreased flexibility, and a higher susceptibility to skin infections. Systemic forms of some of these diseases can lead to organ failure or rupture and inflammation, leading to fibrosis, especially of the lungs.

Cocaine

Cocaine is drug that has both medical and abuse potential. It acts as a serotonin, norepinephrine, and dopamine reuptake inhibitor and thus stimulates the nervous system and acts as topical anesthetic. After acute use, users can develop itching and hallucinations, especially one in which bugs are crawling on them, which, in turn, causes self-injury to the skin and subsequent bacterial infections. Cocaine also acts as a vasoconstrictor, which after long-term use can lead to tissue ischemia and necrosis. Cocaine raises the body temperature and blood pressure, leading to vasodilation. Chronic use raises the risk of developing Stevens-Johnson syndrome, lupus, and vasculitis. Recently, cocaine users have been identified with purple, discolored patches of skin and permanent ear disfigurement. This is due to an impurity, levamisole, a veterinary medicine used for deworming, which is often mixed with street cocaine and has many adverse effects on users. Levamisole was taken off the market for use in human patients because of these adverse effects.

Prednisone

Prednisone is a corticosteroid used to treat inflammatory conditions. The side effects seen with this medication are directly proportional to the dosage and length of time the medication is taken. Hirsutism, or excessive body hair growth, can be seen with even low doses. Redistribution of body fat can occur, specifically in the upper back, known as a buffalo hump. Increased susceptibility to infections, such as thrush, can occur as well as thin skin. Patients on moderate-to-high doses bruise easily and suffer cracks in the epidermis from only minor trauma, which increases the risk of skin infections. Abdominal striae appear as purplish lesions, which resemble stretch marks, in those taking prednisone for long periods of time. Even after short periods of time, acne breakouts increase.

Anti-cancer drugs

Chemotherapy drugs target rapidly dividing cells and, through different mechanisms, cause cellular apoptosis. Cells of the bone marrow, digestive tract, skin, and hair follicles are all composed of rapidly dividing cells and are targeted unintentionally by these drugs. Easy bruising and bleeding from trauma can be seen due to a decreased platelet population. Depression of the immune system makes bacterial and viral infections (e.g., shingles) more likely. Hair loss and brittle nails can result from chemotherapy; these effects, however, can be lessened with the use of cooling caps, hand wraps, and foot wraps, which cause local vasoconstriction, decreasing the amount of chemotherapeutic medication to which the skin is exposed.

Vancomycin

Vancomycin is an intravenous antibiotic used commonly to treat infections resistant to other antibiotics. It can cause a hypersensitivity reaction of the skin known as red man syndrome, caused by the release of histamine. This reaction is characterized by flushing, erythema (redness), and pruritus and usually affects the upper body. Corticosteroids, epinephrine, and antihistamines can help alleviate the symptoms. Vancomycin can also cause skin rashes, representing eosinophilia induced by a delayed hypersensitivity reaction. Local reactions include skin necrosis at the site of infusion if peripheral veins are used to gain access. The mechanism responsible for this reaction is thought to be phlebitis of the vein.

Marfan syndrome

Marfan syndrome is a genetic disorder that causes a defect in the connective tissue by affecting the protein fibrillin-1. It can also appear sporadically as a new gene mutation in about 30% of cases. This disease is characterized by overgrowth of the long bones; aortic root dilation and aneurysm; eye problems, such as lens dislocation; pectus excavatum; extremely flexible joints; scoliosis; nearsightedness; and learning disabilities. Treatment centers around preventing the complications associated with this disease. Patients must be followed regularly with eye exams to identify retinal detachment, lens dislocation, and cataracts. They must also be followed by a cardiologist who administers echocardiograms, as the leading cause of death is related to aortic root aneurysm.

Osteogenesis imperfecta

Osteogenesis imperfecta is a congenital disorder divided into four subtypes, which have variable severity. It is an autosomal dominant disorder. All subtypes have defects in type 1 collagen and present with blue sclera, progressive deafness, and susceptibility to bone fractures. Definitive diagnosis can be made by skin biopsy or in utero with chorionic villus sampling. Type 1 is the most common and is mild. Type 2 is severe and is usually fatal before 1-year-old. Type 3 is also severe with a shortened life expectancy. Type 4 is moderate, and patients have a normal life expectancy, although they may require assistance with walking. Treatment attempts to reduce the pain and complications associated with the disease. Bisphosphonate medications can help increase the strength and density of bone. Physical therapy and low-impact exercise help to build muscle tone and strength, although surgical rod placement and reconstructive surgery may be needed in some cases.

Epidermolysis bullosa

Epidermolysis bullosa is an inherited disorder in which the skin sloughs and blisters in response to minor trauma. It is classified under four main types: dystrophic epidermolysis bullosa, epidermolysis bullosa simplex, hemi desmosomal epidermolysis bullosa, and junctional epidermolysis bullosa. This disease is usually seen in adults over 50 who present with alopecia; multiple skin blisters, including in the mouth and throat; milia; deformed nails; dental problems; and breathing problems. Children can be born with blistering at birth. Diagnosis is confirmed with a skin biopsy. Treatment attempts to prevent complications from the disease. Ointments and antibiotics must be used to prevent infection, and trauma must be avoided. Proper nutrition can help with wound healing, and oral steroids may be used in severe cases. These patients are at high risk for skin cancer and may suffer joint contractures.

Gorlin syndrome

Gorlin syndrome, also known as basal cell nevus syndrome, is an autosomal dominant disorder. Patients with Gorlin syndrome have a distinct facial appearance with a protruding brow, broad nose, wide-set eyes, and cleft palate. In addition to the propensity to develop basal cell cancers starting around puberty, patients may also suffer blindness, deafness, intellectual disability, and seizures. Brain tumors and cysts in the jaw along with rib abnormalities are also seen. Clinical diagnosis is confirmed by genetic testing. Treatment centers on close dermatological follow-up to excise the basal cell cancers before they metastasize. Avoidance of the sun and radiation help to decrease the risk of skin cancers.

Anti-inflammatory agents

Prednisone is a corticosteroid that decreases the precursors (e.g., arachidonic acid) that are needed to produce inflammatory mediators. It helps to reduce redness, swelling, and the immune response. Prednisone can be used to treat rheumatoid arthritis, systemic lupus erythematosus, psoriasis, scleroderma, erythema multiforme, and other inflammatory skin and connective tissue disorders. Ibuprofen (e.g., Advil, Nuprin) is less potent than the corticosteroids but is also used to treat inflammation. Ibuprofen is a nonsteroidal anti-inflammatory drug, and this class also includes aspirin and naproxen, which are all available without a prescription. Nonsteroidal anti-inflammatory drugs are used to treat rheumatoid arthritis, psoriatic arthritis, gout, and any acute or chronic condition that presents with inflammatory properties.

Corticosteroids come in two classes, mineralocorticoids and glucocorticoids, and enter cells where they bind to steroid receptors in the cytoplasm; they enter the nucleus where they downregulate the synthesis of enzymes responsible for inflammation. Corticosteroids also inhibit the formation of phospholipase-A2, which, in turn, decreases the amount of arachidonic acid, which is needed for the formation of inflammatory mediators. These compounds also act on cell membranes to change ion permeability and alter the production of neurohormones. Nonsteroidal anti-inflammatory drugs oppose the action of the cyclooxygenase enzyme, which is responsible for the production of prostaglandin, which is, in turn, responsible for inflammation. Herbs, such as Arnica Montana, contain tumor necrosis factor-kB, which inhibits inflammation. Rest, ice, compression, and elevation, also known as RICE, diminish localized inflammation by decreasing blood flow to the area.

Emollients

Emollients are prescription drugs or over-the-counter medications that work to soothe the skin and protect it from dehydration. Moisturizers serve the same function but also contain humectants to hydrate the top layer of the epidermis. Both of these classes of drugs soften and moisturize the skin. The composition of these drugs often includes lipids, fats, and oils, such as lanolin and liquid paraffin. Skin diseases are often worsened by the breakdown of the epidermal barrier due to loss of water content and the subsequent development of cracks. These cracks can get infected and can also be bothersome and unattractive. Topical emollients are applied to the skin, creating a barrier that traps the moisture, keeping it in the epidermal layer.

Emollients like Vaseline and Aquaphor contain petroleum jelly and act a barrier against evaporation. These can be used for any skin condition, including dryness, such as eczema and psoriasis. Lac-Hydrin and AmLactin contain ammonium lactate, which is used to treat pruritus associated with any condition and ichthyosis vulgaris. Carmol and Keralac contain urea, which promotes the softening of hyperkeratotic areas (scaly skin). It is used to treat dermatitis, psoriasis, ichthyosis, eczema, keratosis, and calluses. It can also be used for nail bed debridement. Kerasal contains salicylic acid and urea and is used for the foot, specifically in diabetic foot care. It helps to repair dry, cracked skin and calluses. Aloe vera is a gel that comes from the aloe vera plant leaves and is used to soothe skin inflammation from sunburn, insect bites, cuts, rashes, and blisters. It helps promote healing while protecting the skin underneath.

Sunscreen

Sunscreen is also known as sunblock, although this is a misnomer because no lotion or cream can block the ultraviolet (UV) rays completely. Sunscreen is a topical product that blocks some of the ultraviolet rays, reducing the skin damage associated with UV radiation. Sunscreens contain chemical compounds, inorganic particulates, or organic particulates to absorb or reflect the UV rays. Sunscreens are classified as either physical sunscreens or chemical sunscreens based on whether they reflect or absorb the UV rays, respectively. Use of broad-spectrum sunscreen has been shown to reduce the risk of skin cancers, including melanoma. Broad-spectrum signifies that the sunscreen acts against UV-A and UV-B radiation. Sunscreen is currently measured, using a sun protection factor, which measures the amount of time required for a sunburn with the sunscreen as a multiple of the time without the sunscreen.

Sunscreens can be classified as chemical or physical sunscreens. Chemical sunscreens contain chemical compounds that absorb the ultraviolet (UV) radiation. Complexes such as Mexoryl, a chemical designed by L'Oreal to filter out UV-A rays and Helioplex, a chemical mixture of avobenzone and oxybenzone designed by Neutrogena to provide broad-spectrum UV protection. Titanium dioxide and zinc oxide are physical compounds that can be micronized to eliminate the white tinge, which acts as a reflector of the UV rays. Both of these compounds can act against UV-A and UV-B rays. The use of both physical and chemical sunscreens is indicated for everyone exposed to sunlight but especially those who have a light skin tone as this correlates with less melanin in the skin. Melanin can also act as a protective mechanism against the UV rays.

Retinoids

Retinoids are a class of compounds derived from vitamin A. All of these compounds are involved in regulating epithelial growth and turnover. Retinoids are used in the treatment of many skin disorders, including skin cancers, inflammatory skin conditions, psoriasis, photoaging, and acne. Retinoids increase skin cell turnover, reducing the number of dead skin cells in the top layer of the epidermis. The buildup of dead skin cells can block pores and cause acne. The oral form of retinoid fights the inflammation and bacteria that cause acne; it can also help to reduce the oil production in the skin. Topical retinoid can treat photoaging by stimulating new blood vessels, increasing the production of collagen, fading discoloration, and reducing actinic keratoses.

Accutane is the oral form of a retinoid known as isotretinoin. It is used in cases of severe cystic or nodular acne by reducing the amount of oil that is produced by the skin and increasing the cell turnover rate. Retinol, Retin-A, and Accutane belong to the first generation of retinoids. Retin-A is a topical form of retinol, which is used to combat acne, photoaging, and pigmentation changes in the skin, especially of the face. The second generation of retinoids includes etretinate, which was

- 169 -

developed to treat severe psoriasis. Because etretinate is stored in the adipose tissue and side effects are seen long after discontinuation of use, it has been removed from the market. The third generation of retinoids includes tazarotene, known as Tazorac. It is used to treat acne, photoaging, and psoriasis.

Sunscreen and sun avoidance during peak hours are crucial if one is using any form of retinoid. These medications increase the skin's sensitivity to the sun, and sun damage can occur in a much shorter period of time. Vitamin A, used as a supplement, should be avoided as this can lead to vitamin A toxicity when combined with the use of retinoids. Symptoms of vitamin A overdose include yellowish color to skin along with dry skin, hair, lips, and eyes. Glycolic acid, salicylic acid, and any other topical preparations with the word acid in them should be avoided, as these will increase skin cell turnover too. This may result in skin peeling and irritation. Laser treatments of any kind should also be avoided as they ablate the top layer of the epidermis, which is not as thick in patients using retinoids. Chemical peels of any strength should be avoided as these may burn off the top layer of the epidermis.

Antimicrobial agents

Antimicrobial substances kill or inhibit the growth of bacteria, fungi, or viruses. Antibiotics are used to treat bacterial infections and can be in topical or oral form. Beta-lactam antibiotics work by inhibiting the synthesis of the bacterial cell wall, leading to death. Protein synthesis inhibitors usually act at the ribosomal level by interfering with protein synthesis at the level of mRNA translation. Antivirals are used to fight viral infections and are in topical or oral form. These drugs work by inhibiting the entrance of the virus, preventing replication, or preventing the exit and spread of the virus. Antifungals work by disrupting the fungal cell membrane, resulting in the leakage of the contents of the cell. Essential oils found in plants have also been discovered to have bacteriostatic and antiviral properties and can be used as treatment.

Antibiotics, such as penicillin and sulfa, are used to treat bacterial infections, such as *Staphylococcus aureus*. For methicillin-resistant *S. aureus* infections, stronger antibiotics, such as vancomycin, are sometimes needed. Antivirals, such as acyclovir, protease inhibitors, and nucleoside/nucleotide reverse transcriptase inhibitors, are used to treat viral infections. These viral infections can include the herpesvirus and HIV. Antifungals, such as Lamisil and nystatin, are used to treat yeast infections and various tinea infections. Amphotericin B can be used in oral or intravenous forms as an antifungal agent to treat thrush and serious systemic infections, such as cryptococcal meningitis. Essential oils, such as oil of bay, cinnamon, clove, and thyme, can be used to treat both bacterial and viral infections. For example, cinnamon has anti-HIV properties.

Antiparasitic agents

Antiparasitic agents are used in parasitic infections and can work by inhibiting microtubule formation, glucose transport, and glycogen depletion. Parasitic infections are more common in third-world countries or in poor, rural areas where there is fecal contamination of water sources. Intestinal nematode infection, such as roundworm, pinworm, hookworm, whipworm, trichinosis, and neurocysticercosis, can be treated with antiparasitic medications. Antimalarial drugs can be used for the treatment or prevention of parasitic malarial infections. Many parasites can cross the blood-brain barrier and form cysts in the brain, causing seizures. Neurocysticercosis and toxoplasmosis are examples of this, and other parasites can cause serious disfigurements, such as elephantiasis. Once complications develop, the antiparasitic agents are not as effective as they would be earlier in the disease process.

Mebendazole is a benzimidazole drug that treats nematode infections, such as pinworms, roundworms, tapeworms, hookworms, and whipworms. Experimental studies show a potential oncologic treatment potential. Albendazole is also a benzimidazole compound used to treat tapeworms, roundworms, and flukes. Ivermectin is an avermectin medication used to treat onchocerciasis, river blindness, strongyloidiasis, ascariasis, filariasis, and enterobiasis. Niclosamide is a teniacide used specifically to treat tapeworms in humans. Chloroquine is a 4-aminoquinoline drug used to treat or prevent malaria. Malaria is caused by infection of heme cells with *Plasmodium vivax*, *Plasmodium falciparum*, *Plasmodium ovale*, and *Plasmodium malariae* parasites. Nitroimidazole is an imidazole derivative medication that is designed to treat amebic parasitic infections and anaerobic bacteria in the form metronidazole.

Cytotoxic agents

Cytotoxic drugs are those that are used to kill tumors or malignant cells. However, many have been found to also assist in relieving the inflammation associated with chronic rheumatological conditions as well as some skin conditions. Cytotoxic drugs work by interfering with cellular mitosis in rapidly dividing cells. Cytotoxic drugs can be divided into classes: alkylating agents; antimetabolites; plant alkaloids, including taxanes and vinca alkaloids; topoisomerase inhibitors; and cytotoxic antibiotics. Some drugs promote cell death or apoptosis. Cytotoxic drugs are used as chemotherapy for various cancers. They work better on more differentiated tumors that are still dividing. These same drugs can be used to suppress the immune system in such conditions as rheumatoid arthritis, psoriasis, and systemic lupus erythematosus.

Alkylating agents, such as cisplatin and cyclophosphamide, work by impairing cell function. Cisplatin is used to treat solid tumors, such as sarcoma and germ cell tumors. Cyclophosphamide is used to treat systemic lupus erythematosus (SLE) and rheumatoid arthritis. Antimetabolites, such as methotrexate, are used to treat cancers of the head and neck, breast, bladder, and lung; leukemia; lymphomas; and osteosarcoma. They are also used to treat autoimmune disorders, such as psoriasis, rheumatoid arthritis, and SLE. Azathioprine is also an antimetabolite, which can be used to treat eczema, atopic dermatitis, SLE, rheumatoid arthritis, and pemphigus. It is used in transplant patients to suppress organ rejection and is thought to lead to an increased risk of cancer, including skin cancers.

Immunologic agents

Immunologic agents are those that modify the immune system, either enhancing or suppressing it. They can be used as antineoplastic medications to treat inflammatory conditions and to prevent graft rejection. Immunoglobulins are antibodies normally produced by the body but which can be given intravenously to patients who are lacking or do not have sufficient quantities of the immunoglobulin. Antibodies bind to antigens and promote their removal and destruction. Immunoglobulins can be used to treat people with deficiencies, such as immunoglobulin G, or given Rhesus factor to prevent fetal destruction. Immunostimulants include interferons, interleukins, and colony-stimulating factors. These are used to stimulate the immune system to produce certain products that can be used to fight both bacterial and viral infections. Immunosuppressive agents, such as interleukin inhibitors, calcineurin inhibitors, and tumor necrosis factor–alpha inhibitors, can be used to suppress an immune response to avoid symptoms associated with chronic inflammation.

Immunoglobulins are given to supplement or replace a patient's own supply if a condition is present that necessitates it. These conditions include immunoglobulin G deficiency, X-linked agammaglobulinemia, immunoglobulin A deficiency, common variable immunodeficiency, and transient hypogammaglobulinemia of infancy. In these conditions, the lacking immunoglobulin must be given either for a short period of time or in regular intervals. Immunostimulants stimulate the immune system and include vaccines, colony-stimulating factors, interferons, and interleukins. Colony-stimulating factors promote the productions of white blood cells, which can fight infection. Vaccines stimulate the production of antibodies to specific antigens to prevent infection by viruses or bacteria. Immunosuppressive agents downregulate the immune response; these include calcineurin inhibitors, interleukin inhibitors, and tumor necrosis factor–alpha inhibitors. For example, calcineurin inhibitors are used to treat pemphigus, psoriatic arthritis, and rheumatoid arthritis.

Antineoplastic agents

Antineoplastic agents work by targeting rapidly dividing cells and preventing mitosis. They can be used against cancer cells but also to help the symptoms of psoriasis, psoriatic arthritis, rheumatoid arthritis, and scleroderma. Antineoplastic drugs can be divided into classes: alkylating agents; antimetabolites; plant alkaloids, including taxanes and vinca alkaloids; topoisomerase inhibitors; and cytotoxic antibiotics. Alkylating agents work by incorporating themselves during DNA replication and preventing the correct DNA synthesis. Antimetabolites work by forming covalent bonds with certain molecules preventing replication. Plant alkaloids include vinca alkaloids and taxanes, which interfere with microtubule construction. Topoisomerase inhibitors disrupt DNA transcription and replication. Cytotoxic antibiotics induce cell damage and prevent cellular replication.

Cyclophosphamide is an alkylating agent that is used to treat systemic lupus erythematosus (SLE) and rheumatoid arthritis. Methotrexate is an antimetabolite that is used to treat autoimmune disorders, such as psoriasis, rheumatoid arthritis, and SLE. Azathioprine is also an antimetabolite that can be used to treat eczema, atopic dermatitis, SLE, rheumatoid arthritis, and pemphigus. Vincristine and vinblastine bind to microtubule components, preventing their assembly. It is used to treat non-Hodgkin's lymphoma. Taxol inhibits mitosis by stabilizing microtubules and is used to treat tumors of the lung, ovary, breast, head, and neck, and Kaposi's sarcoma. Amsacrine can intercalate into tumor DNA and is used to treat acute lymphoblastic leukemia. Bleomycin acts through forming free radicals, which cause DNA damage.

Solar and light therapy

Solar therapy can be used to treat certain skin conditions, albeit in limited amounts with concern for the increased risk for skin cancers. Skin diseases, such as psoriasis, can have symptoms lessened by sun exposure, specifically to ultraviolet-B (UV-B) rays. Short, multiple exposures are ideal to avoid sunburn and sun damage. Tanning beds are discouraged because they primarily emit UV-A rays and can increase the risk of skin cancers. Lasers, such as intense pulsed light therapy or photorejuvenation, can be used to lessen the symptoms of rosacea and to treat broken capillaries/telangiectasias, vascular lesions, acne, and photoaging. The light targets pigment in the skin and vaporizes it, stimulating its removal by macrophages.

Psychological treatments

Psychological tension can be a contributing factor in many skin disorders, and treating the psychology may help improve the skin condition. Massage, meditation, and biofeedback have been shown to improve the symptoms exacerbated by stress and tension in inflammatory skin and joint disorders, such as rheumatic arthritis, psoriatic arthritis, eczema, acne, and systemic lupus erythematosus. Cognitive-behavioral therapy can help patients to modify bad behaviors, which exacerbate their skin conditions, such as scratching and hair pulling. It is known that stress is a trigger for worsening these conditions; thus, stress reduction and psychological treatment can help to reduce and shorten episodes and ease the symptoms. Individual or group therapy may also help patients to reduce or eliminate the medications they are currently taking for their disease.

Emotions

Skin is intimately related to the emotional state in many ways. Stress causes the release of cortisol. In the short term, stress can cause hives and rashes. It can also aggravate chronic skin conditions, such as eczema, psoriasis, and systemic lupus erythematosus. Acne can be worsened by stress and anxiety by increasing oil production in the skin and slowing the ability of the skin to heal. Flushing and redness can be worsened by stress and the sun, especially in patients with systemic lupus erythematosus and rosacea. Chronic high levels of stress can weaken the ability of the skin to heal and dry out the skin. Chronic depression can also affect the skin by weakening the immune system, causing hair loss and brittle nails.

Behaviors

The skin is the largest organ of the body and as such is affected by behavioral characteristics. Tobacco use can damage the skin in the short and long term. Smoking causes vasoconstriction, which leads to ischemia, uneven skin tones, and a decreased ability to heal. Smoking also damages collagen and elastin, leading to premature wrinkles and aging of the skin. The repeated action of puckering the lips to smoke cigarettes can lead to deep perioral lines and wrinkles. Sun exposure and artificial tanning cause short-term damage to the epidermis in the form of sunburns. Long-term exposure to ultraviolet radiation causes damage to collagen and elastin, leading to photoaging. It also increases the risk for skin cancers. Alcohol use dehydrates the skin in the short term while long-term use can lead to dilated capillaries; it can also exacerbate psoriasis and rosacea.

Family and society

The views of one's family and society can influence behaviors that have an impact on disease. Smoking in the home exposes one to second-hand smoke and creates an atmosphere of acceptance and encouragement of tobacco use. This results in a higher risk of tobacco-related diseases and skin damage. Parents are the people responsible for sun protection in infants and children, and if this is ignored, the risk of photoaging is increased. The risk for skin cancers, including melanoma, is increased with each severe childhood sunburn. If, however, one is raised in a society or family that embraces smoking prevention and sun avoidance, then one will be less exposed to these dangers and more likely to practice preventive measures and seek treatment.

Societal perceptions

Over the last century, societal perceptions and scientific knowledge have changed, leading to a shift in disease treatment and prevention. In the past, physicians were in advertisements that encouraged smoking, but now the risks and diseases associated with this habit are better understood. This has led to better acceptance of preventive measures and made it more likely that patients will seek treatment. In the past, a suntan was associated with being healthy, but now the dangers of exposure to ultraviolet radiation are better known. This has led to a decrease in sun exposure and an increased use of preventive measures to block or avoid the sun. Patients have also become more knowledgeable about early treatment of skin cancers.

Occupational factors

Occupational exposures can lead to irritant contact dermatitis, allergic contact dermatitis, skin cancers, skin infections, and skin injuries. The food service industry, agriculture, cleaning, painting, construction, cosmetology, and health care are all fields in which the skin is exposed to dangerous chemicals or trauma, which may cause harm. Many fields also include outdoor work, which increases sun exposure and the risk for photoaging and skin cancers. Federal agencies, such as the Occupational Safety and Health Administration, were created to protect workers and to design guidelines for employers to decrease occupational risks. Workers should be told to wear protective clothing and eyewear and should be taught the ways in which to avoid exposures or skin trauma. It is also important that workers be instructed as to what to do in case of injury and how it should be treated. These injuries often are reported to the governing agency.

Environmental factors

Sun exposure will lead to epidermal damage and photoaging. This can be prevented by the use of sunscreen, sun avoidance, and protective clothing. Extreme temperatures can damage the skin as cold weather can lead to frostbite and ischemia. Hot temperatures can lead to dry skin. The best prevention is protective clothing or avoidance of extreme temperatures. Extremes in moisture can also affect the skin as humid climates promote the growth of fungi on the skin and dry climates disrupt the epidermal barrier by robbing it of moisture. Again, protective clothing is the best measure for prevention. Pollution and chemicals in the environment can block the pores of the skin and cause acne or folliculitis. Cleaning and protecting the skin from pollution will prevent this.

Gender

In general, women tend to be less associated with vices, such as alcohol and tobacco, but are more likely to suntan or go to a tanning salon. This influences the occurrence of skin conditions associated with alcohol and tobacco, such as rosacea, poor wound healing, wrinkles, and cancers of the oral mucosa. Women have a higher occurrence rate for photoaging, sun damage, and skin cancers due to their sun exposure. Women are also more likely to see a physician for changes in their skin, leading to early detection and treatment of skin conditions and skin cancers. Prevention and education must be tailored to men or women, as women may be more likely to listen to their physicians or read magazine articles, while men may need incentives and packaging that list the risks of their behavior.

Ethnic and cultural factors

Different ethnic groups and cultures place importance and value on certain types of behaviors and appearance. Many ethnic groups vary in the amount of melanin present in the epidermis as a result of the distance from the equator that their ancestors lived. Ethnic groups with less melanin are at higher risk for sunburns, photoaging, and skin cancers. This risk is calculated, using the Fitzpatrick scale, which assigns each patient a number from 1–6 based on their pigmentation. It can gauge the risk for melanoma and other skin cancers. Cultures that place emphasis on a dark appearance, despite having little melanin, may lead to increases in sun exposure, thereby raising the risks for sunburns, photoaging, and skin cancers.

Musculoskeletal System

Skeleton and skeletal muscle

These components of the MSS come almost exclusively from the mesoderm surrounding the notochord, beginning as paired longitudinal columns. This mesoderm is converted into the axial skeleton, its attached muscles, and the adjacent dermal coverings via the formation of paired cells called somites. Endochondral bone is created around a cartilage matrix and eventually forms the body's long bones, such as the femur and humerus. Membranous bone, on the other hand, does not require a cartilage frame, and makes up the flat bones such as those of the cranium. Skeletal muscle develops from the paired somites, which begin to appear toward the end of the third week. Eventually these give rise to skeletal muscles and the surrounding dermis, contributing to the formation of the axial skeleton as noted above. This occurs in a craniocaudal fashion, with the first somites appearing near the cranial end of the notochord. Different somites are associated with specific myotomes and dermatomes, which gradually develop the associated skin and muscles inherent to each area.

Pharyngeal/branchial arches

There are six pharyngeal arches that give rise to the musculature of the head and neck. The first arch, innervated by the trigeminal nerve's (CN 5) mandibular branch, develops into the temporalis, masseter, lateral pterygoid, medial pterygoid (mastication); tensor veli palatini, tensor tympani (tensor muscles); and the mylohyoid and anterior digastric. Arch II is associated with the facial nerve (CN VII), and yields the orbicularis oculi, orbiculare oris, buccinator (facial expression); and the stylohyoid, stapedius, and posterior digastric. The third arch is connected to the glossopharyngeal nerve (CN IX) and produces only the stylopharyngeus. Arch IV is innervated by the pharyngeal and superior laryngeal branches of the vagus nerve (CN X), giving rise to the cricothyroid and the soft palate musculature, with the exception of the two mentioned above (tensor veli palatini and stylopharyngeus). Together with the third arch, arch IV contributes to the posterior tongue as well. The sixth arch receives innervation from the recurrent laryngeal branch of the vagus nerve, and develops into the laryngeal muscles (with the exception of the cricothyroid, as noted above). Arch V is not a major factor in development of the MSS.

Integumentary system

The various parts of the integumentary system are formed from different types of embryonic tissue. From superficial to deep, the individual layers of the epidermis are: the stratum corneum, lucidum, granulosum, spinosum, and basale (which contains melanocytes). These may be distinguished by the end of the fourth month. The dermis lies just beneath the epidermis, separated by an epidermal ridge formed from a basement membrane. The only layer that actively divides is the stratum basale, which then creates the other layers, both in the womb and afterward. In the embryonic phase, the dermis is formed from the mesoderm, while the epidermis develops from the ectoderm. Melanocytes, on the other hand, while contained within the epidermis, are formed from the neural crest. The layers of the skin regenerate and are replaced every few weeks. Thick skin, such as that on the palms and soles, contains all the aforementioned layers, but thin skin (e.g., face and genitalia) develops without the lucidum layer. Between one and three months, the ectoderm begins forming stratified epithelium; at around four months it begins to yield hair, nails and the associated glands. Hair becomes detectable sometime in the fifth month. Further development of these structures continues up until and after birth. Both in and outside the womb, the three main functions of the skin are to create a barrier between one's internal structures and the environment (preventing infection), to regulate body temperature, and to protect against dehydration.

Musculoskeletal system

A mesoderm/neural crest-derived mesenchyme leads to the development of the majority of the axial and appendicular bones, starting with the formation of a cartilage matrix. Around the end of the embryonic period, the process of ossification begins to occur and continues by way of endochondral ossification, with some bones such as those of the skull undergoing a specific type known as intramembranous ossification. The fetal skull contains a neurocranium, which forms the calvaria, as protection for the developing brain; and a viscerocranium, which eventually becomes the facial bones. The remainder of the axial skeleton (spine and ribs) is formed from somite sclerotomes, which are derived from the mesenchyme. The appendicular skeleton continues to form via endochondral ossification throughout the fetal period, producing the various bones of the limbs, which harden as fetal maturation proceeds, as well as in the post-natal period. All types of joints (synovial, cartilaginous and fibrous) are derived from interzonal mesenchyme, which differentiates into different tissues, depending on the type of joint being considered. The musculature, derived from somatic mesoderm (skeletal) or splanchnic mesoderm (cardiac), matures at the beginning of the fetal stage, and then continues to grow and strengthen during the rest of the fetal period. Around weeks 21-22, the majority of the skeleton begins to grow rapidly as bones become larger and stronger. These processes continue with relatively little new occurring until birth.

Skeleton in terms of its organs (bones)

The human skeleton consists of two major divisions: the axial skeleton (skull, spine, ribs and pelvic girdle), which lies along the body's longitudinal axis; and the appendicular skeleton, which contains the rest of the bones of the appendages, or limbs. The bones within the body are stiff, hardened structures externally, containing soft marrow inside. The individual bones are joined by one of three types of joints (synovial, fibrous and cartilaginous), depending on the location. Synovial joints exist between highly movable parts of the skeleton, such as between femur and tibia/fibula; cartilaginous joints are those in locations with flexibility but a small range of motion, such as the spinal column and pelvic girdle; and fibrous joints are fixed and nearly immovable, such as those found in the sutures of the cranium. The two main functions of the skeletal system are support and movement (in collaboration with the musculature); they are also important for protection (rib cage), and to a lesser extent, sound conduction in the ear. The function of the joint spaces is to allow a certain degree of movement (depending on type) between the bones they connect.

Each skeletal muscle is attached to its associated bones via tendons at each end, between which lies the belly of the muscle. Within this belly portion, individual muscle fibers (multinucleated cells) extend longitudinally, surrounded by connective tissue called endomysium. Bundles of these individual fibers are collected into a muscle fascicle, which contains 20-80 fibers and associated endomysium, all encapsulated by another connective tissue layer known as perimysium. These fascicles are in turn grouped together to form the muscle belly, which is surrounded by a layer known as epimysium, with major vascular routes existing between the fascicles. This epimysium sheath covers the entire muscle, extending from one tendon to the other. All skeletal muscles are voluntarily controlled, though not necessarily consciously; and they generally function as flexors and extensors at joints, as well as maintaining general muscle tone surrounding the skeleton. A nerve impulse at the neuromuscular junction causes some of the microscopic motor units to fire, with the number firing dependent on demand and stimuli, producing a graded contraction of the aforementioned apparatus. These muscles may contain slow-twitch (type 1; red) or fast-twitch (type 2; white) fibers, and utilize aerobic metabolism until exhausted, at which point they switch to an anaerobic process that produces lactic acid, yielding the "burn" felt while exercising vigorously.

Smooth muscle

The individual fibers of smooth muscle contain a single central nucleus, are non-striated and have a high capacity for regeneration. This type of muscle is present in virtually all lumens of the body (intestines, vessels, bronchial tubes, etc.), as well as various other locations, and lies just beneath the endothelial lining. There are three types of smooth muscles that appear and function in different parts of the body. Multi-unit muscle is highly innervated by the autonomic nervous system and each fiber acts as a separate motor unit because of low levels of electrical coupling between cells; such fibers are found in the iris, lens, and vas deferens. In contrast, single-unit muscle, which is more common, exhibits a high degree of coupling. This allows individual contractions to be coordinated in order to contract the entire associated organ; these fibers are located in the uterus, GI tract, ureter, and bladder. Single-unit muscles also demonstrate spontaneous activity modulated by neurotransmitters and hormones. The third category, vascular smooth muscle, shares anatomical properties of both aforementioned types, depending on location and physiologic necessity. Regardless of type or location, the major function of smooth muscle is to contract and dilate various parts of the body, such as blood vessels, the gut, the eye, and the bladder, in response to autonomic and outside stimuli. The result in most cases is propulsion (peristalsis) and regulation of flow (vessels), via slow, sustained contractions.

Smooth muscle is so named because it lacks striations under microscopy, with dense bodies replacing the Z lines of skeletal and cardiac muscle. Each cell contains a central nucleus and is spindle shaped, with gap junctions at the ends of the cell for communication purposes; there are no neuromuscular junctions. While these cells do contain actin and myosin filaments, there are no transverse tubules present, and the mechanism of contraction is somewhat different. An action potential depolarizes the cellular membrane, which causes an increase of intracellular calcium (Ca) from the extracellular influx, as well as from the sarcoplasmic reticulum. However, since there is no troponin (like in cardiac and skeletal muscle), this Ca binds to calmodulin instead; this joined molecule then binds myosin light-chain kinase, an enzyme that promotes the binding of myosin and actin, to form cross-bridges. As these filaments slide past each other the muscle fiber contracts; the cross-bridge is then detached and gets ready for the next coupling, as the muscle temporarily relaxes. Innervation and stimulation occur via the autonomic nervous system, as well as hormones.

Cardiac muscle

Like smooth muscle, cardiac muscle operates involuntarily, controlled by pacemaker cells within the heart. Like skeletal muscle, cardiac muscle is composed of striated fibers and contracts with substantial force. The myocardium is basically one large muscle, divided by (and including) cardiac septae (which also include connective tissue), and is composed of muscle fibers that are smaller than those in skeletal muscle. This type of muscle is exclusive to the heart and some proximal parts of the great vessels, and is the only type of muscle that can operate independently of neurological stimulation (via the SA and AV nodes, which create their own electrical impulses and fire independently), a phenomenon known as automaticity. It is thickest surrounding the left ventricle, because this is the chamber that pumps against the most resistance and requires the most force of contraction. The myocardium is the middle layer of heart tissue, lying between the endocardium and the pericardium, which are the lining and outer sac of the heart, respectively. Papillary muscles extend inward from the endocardium and aid in valvular control. The myocardium is hormonally controlled most strongly by epinephrine, and displays an intermediate speed of contraction that is between that of smooth and skeletal muscle. The main function of the myocardium is to pump blood throughout the body.

Cardiac muscle cells are striated like skeletal muscle, though cardiac fibers are shorter and branch. They contain a single nucleus located centrally and act spontaneously, like smooth muscle. On a cellular and molecular level they are very similar to skeletal muscle, being composed of sarcomeres that contain both actin (thin) and myosin (thick) filaments and are the contractile units of the cell, running between Z lines (see skeletal muscle card for more). Compared to skeletal muscle, cardiac muscle cells contain more mitochondria and possess intercalated disks and gap junctions at the ends of cells to facilitate easy electrical transmission between cells. There is no neuromuscular junction and no entirely accepted known capacity for regeneration (though this is being further investigated). As with skeletal muscle the action potential travels into the transverse tubules, which triggers a calcium influx (mainly from the sarcoplasmic reticulum (SR) intracellularly. This calcium then binds troponin C, which moves tropomyosin aside, allowing the binding of overlapping actin and myosin filaments. As the dual filaments slide past each other during cross-bridge cycling, muscle cell contraction occurs, proportionate to the amount of intracellular calcium. Relaxation occurs upon reabsorption of calcium by the SR, which then sets up the fibers for the next round of coupling.

Cell/tissue structure

Each skeletal muscle fiber is composed of many myofibrils. These myofibrils contain longitudinal arrangements of sarcomeres, which are the basic contractile units of skeletal muscles, and exist between Z lines. Within each sarcomere are thick filaments containing myosin, and thin filaments (attached at Z lines) made from actin (as well as tropomyosin and troponin), all of which are surrounded by the sarcoplasmic reticulum (SR) and intersected by transverse tubules. The filamentous areas are divided into A bands (spanning the length of the myosin, including overlap with actin), H bands (the portion of myosin not overlapping with actin), and I bands (portion of actin not overlapping with myosin). In addition to the SR (normally known as the endoplasmic reticulum), muscles have different names than usual for cellular organelles, etc. The plasma membrane is renamed the sarcolemma, the mitochondria are sarcosomes, and the cytoplasm is known as sarcoplasm. During excitation-contraction coupling, action potentials depolarize the transverse tubules, which causes the SR to release calcium (Ca) into the muscle cell. This intracellular Ca binds to troponin C on actin filaments (beginning the cross-bridge cycle), where actin and myosin bind (facilitated by the movement of tropomyosin) and then slide over each other, driven by ATP attachment at the myosin head. Once this sliding motion produces shortening of the myofibrils, the actin and myosin detach and prepare for another cycle. This produces Ca reuptake into the SR initiatig the relaxation phase.

Endochondral ossification (longitudinal growth) begins with osteoblasts creating collagen (chondrocytes) that forms a cartilaginous frame. As calcium and phosphate are deposited on this matrix, mineralized bone is formed and osteoblasts surrounded by hardened bone become osteocytes. Under the influence of parathyroid hormone, osteocytes stimulate osteoclasts to begin resorption, allowing calcium to enter the bloodstream quickly. Calcitonin inhibits this activity, while vitamin D promotes it. During membranous ossification, the flat bones of the face, skull, and axial skeleton grow and harden without the use of a cartilage matrix. Both processes eventually result in remodeling to lamellar bone.

The long bones of the body, when viewed in longitudinal cross-section, contain an articular (hyaline) cartilage at each end. This cartilage covers the epiphysis head, or hardened end, of the bone. Further inward lies the metaphysis, which forms the neck of the bone and includes the physis, or growth plate. In between these two ends lies the main portion or shaft, known as the diaphysis, which consists of a mineralized cortex surrounding a soft medulla (the marrow cavity, containing cancellous bone). A periosteum layer surrounds the outside of all bones (except at the ends), while an endosteum layer lines the inside of these bones, separating the cortex from the medulla. Between the periosteum and the marrow lie osteocytes, which are the functional cells of the bone; they are interspersed with blood vessels and haversian canals, and exist among cement lines within the interstitial lamellae. Osteoblasts, which help form bone, and osteoclasts, which aid in resorption of bone, are also present nearby.

Joints

The function of a joint depends on its type and location. Synovial joints are potential spaces with synovial fluid inside. The fluid serves to lubricate the articulating surfaces and allows easy movement secondary to reduced friction. Each of the six types (covered under anatomy of joints) exists in specific locations, and allow for various degrees and planes of movement. Synovial joints are either uniaxial, biaxial, or polyaxial; these terms describe the number of directional movements possible within the joint (i.e., just flexion/extension vs. flex/extend and abduction/adduction). Fibrous joints serve to firmly connect two or more bony structures and allow some movement, though it is quite limited. This is because their primary purpose is stabilization of surfaces that normally remain relatively immovable, compared to the other two types of joints. Cartilaginous joints have hyaline articular cartilage separating the associated bones, which permit either substantial movement (ball and socket) or provide mainly strength and shock absorption, as well as flexibility (intervertebral discs).

There are three major classes of joints: synovial, fibrous, and cartilaginous. All facilitate the connection between two (or more) skeletal surfaces, though the morphology and functions are quite different. Synovial joints are the most common and well known joint spaces, in which a joint capsule surrounds the joint cavity. The joint cavity consists of a fibrous ligamentous capsule over a synovial membrane, which itself connects to the articular cartilage lining the ends of the bones involved. The menisci are fibrocartilaginous structures partially dividing the joint space, and associated ligaments exist within the space. There are six main types of synovial joints, so named for their shape and movement: plane (acromioclavicular), hinge (elbow), saddle (carpometacarpal), condyloid (MCPs), pivot (atlantoaxial), and ball and socket (hip). Fibrous joints are composed of fibrous tissue between two bony surfaces, allowing very slight movement, as in the cranial sutures. Syndesmosis fibrous joints contain a broader sheet of fibrous tissue between two bones, such as that between the ulna and radius. The third major type of joint is the cartilaginous joint, which consists of articular cartilage surfaces on/between two bones, and offers varying degrees of movement. Two examples are the pubic symphysis and intervertebral discs.

Tendons

Tendons are the structures that connect bones to their associated muscles, permitting movement at the joints and providing support (via muscle tone) for the skeleton. They appear as white fibrous structures that are located at both ends of skeletal muscles and continuous with the belly portion of the muscles. When a tendon is a flat sheet of tissue attaching broadly to a large muscle it is called an aponeurosis. Fibrocytes are spindle-shaped cells that comprise the majority of tendonous connective tissue, accompanied by collagenous fibers. The cellular and tissue anatomy of tendons is quite similar to that of muscles, which makes sense since the two are contiguous. Collagen fibrils are contained within collagen fibers, which are themselves enveloped in primary and secondary fascicles. These fascicles are then bunched together into tertiary fascicles, surrounded by endotenon. Groups of tertiary fascicles are likewise contained within the epitenon, which is the connective outer surface of tendons. As noted above, tendons' primary function is to connect muscles to bones, allowing the muscles to effectively move and stabilize these bony structures.

Ligaments

The anatomy of ligaments is quite similar to that of tendons, though the physiology is different. Collagenous fibers made from fibrocytes (as with tendons) are bunched together and surrounded by dense regular connective tissue, which is itself bundled and surrounded by a sheath composed of dense, irregular connective tissue. A ligament may be one of several types, though the most well-known is the articular ligament (known as a capsular ligament when involving a synovial joint), which connects two bones to form the joint space (covered separately); others types are attached to soft structures to provide support for internal organs (such as the inguinal and peritoneal ligaments). White ligaments are collagen-rich, quite strong, and relatively inelastic; yellow ligaments are composed of more elastic fibers and are capable of significant movement while still providing a large degree of strength and sturdiness. In terms of function, articular ligaments allow for movement around joint spaces and/or restrict improper movements around the same. The ACL, for instance, acts in both of these capacities. They are viscoelastic, meaning they expand and shrink as necessary depending on tension; so-called "double jointed" people have excessive elasticity within certain ligaments. This is known as hyperlaxity.

> **Review Video:** Ligaments
> *Visit mometrix.com/academy and enter Code:* **825469**

Effects of exercise and physical conditioning

Bones
Exercise and physical conditioning have definite impacts on our bones, most of which are positive if not overdone. Movement and weight-bearing activities helps to strengthen the bones by promoting growth and increased thickening; mechanical stress is the key to improving these two parameters of bone anatomy and physiology. This can be especially important for children still very actively developing, and may prevent pain and fractures to a certain extent, while reducing the odds of later chronic pain issues. Under most conditions, exercise will also make movement around a joint space easier and more fluid; but excessive workouts may eventually lead to degeneration of cartilage, eventually resulting in arthritis. For this reason, moderate exercise is almost always recommended for those with osteoarthritis, though this varies depending on patient specifics. In addition, physical conditioning will generally aid in slowing osteoporotic changes in older patients, leaving their bones less brittle and therefore less susceptible to fracture. It has also been found that those who exercise regularly can effectively reduce the level of low back pain caused by musculoskeletal strain, especially when performing low-impact activities.

Skeletal muscle
Skeletal muscle benefits greatly from exercise, which provides increased strength and better muscle tone, allowing for more efficient movement and support of the associated bones. Another primary consequence of physical conditioning is improved circulation throughout the vascular structures of skeletal muscle. This can have a huge impact and protective effect for those with ischemic injuries, compartment syndrome, venous insufficiency and muscular dystrophy, among

- 181 -

many other conditions. Likewise, conditioning also provides anti-inflammatory effects within skeletal muscles, yielding improvement in a host of chronic conditions. In terms of muscle biochemistry, regular exercise can improve aerobic conditioning and endurance, leading to an enhanced ability to work out without encountering the "burn" that comes with switching to an anaerobic process and the formation of lactic acid. This is secondary to enhanced mitochondrial capacity and respiration within the muscles, as well as an increased concentration of myoglobin. Fat oxidation is the main pathway during light exercise, with oxidation of glucose occurring during more strenuous conditioning, followed by anaerobic metabolism via glycolysis when muscles are pushed to the extreme. Aerobic mechanisms are the main metabolic routes, though anaerobic mechanisms may be utilized for short initial bursts of energy, as well as after exhaustion of aerobic capacity. Exercising also helps to prevent tears and other injuries via improved strength and vascular flow.

Cardiac muscle
Cardiac muscle effort during exercise is largely driven by skeletal muscle oxygen demand, which of course increases during these periods. In order to accommodate this elevated demand and deliver the appropriate amount of oxygen to the skeletal muscles, the myocardium utilizes several mechanisms to improve aerobic functioning. Greater amounts of oxygen are supplied to the muscles via a combination of increased cardiac output (secondary to increased heart rate and stroke volume) and increased blood flow to the lungs, allowing for an enhanced ability to carry oxygen to the locations that need it most. Physical conditioning is generally considered an important component of maintaining healthy cardiac function, and can improve one's aerobic endurance and capacity, both during exercise and at rest. However, cardiac patients with either heart failure or those who are post-MI (along with other problems) must adhere to restricted regimens, so as to not overtax the cardiovascular apparatus. Improved cardiac function is aided by vasodilation in skeletal muscle, making maximum oxygen delivery possible. Proper hydration during intense exercise is mandatory, since extreme diaphoresis can eventually reduce blood volume to an extent that muscular perfusion is compromised, secondary to reduced cardiac output.

Smooth muscle
Because of the nature of smooth muscle anatomy and physiology, it is not generally impacted long-term by endurance exercise. However, it is intricately involved in the immediate constriction or dilation of vessels as necessary to accommodate oxygenation and perfusion needs, which obviously increase during exercise. That is, while cardiac muscle provides the force necessary to drive circulation, the smooth muscle of the vasculature enables efficient delivery of blood to the tissues. Nitric oxide is an important endothelial-derived factor that drives vasodilation during times of physical stress. Similarly, during physical conditioning, the smooth muscles controlling parasympathetic-driven processes—such as that of the bladder or intestines—will usually reduce activity (and thus demand) to provide as much oxygenated blood as possible to the actively working musculature. Recently it has been found that individuals who exercise regularly also have an increased adaptive ability within their vascular smooth muscle, provided by elevated sensitivity of these muscular vessel linings to oxygen demand, and a corresponding ability to increase flow appropriately. This allows for greater and quicker responses to increased oxygenation demands of skeletal and cardiac muscle, and the greater efficiency that comes with it.

Body's ability to repair and regenerate

Bones
The variation in regenerative abilities of bone over one's lifetime mainly involves how easily trauma/fractures occur and how effectively bones affected by trauma can repair themselves via

bone remodeling. This depends substantially on whether and how soon the fracture is reduced (approximating its usual position), resulting in a fibroblast-derived, collagen-containing collar of callus that supports the approximated bone during the healing process. Upon full healing, this collar gradually calcifies and is resorbed. While children are generally more likely to suffer from fractures (especially the greenstick twisted subtype)—secondary to the combination of smaller frames, thinner bones and greater activity—they are also able to remodel and repair such bones most rapidly and without complication. This is largely because of the fact that their bones are still actively growing. In contrast, most elderly people will develop some degree of osteoporosis, or skeletal tissue atrophy, leaving the bones less dense and therefore more susceptible to fracture. This is aggravated by the fact that as people age, they become less stable on their feet, which results in many fractures, especially of the hip. Adults, depending on their ages, will lie somewhere along this spectrum. Their recuperative abilities and potential for problems will tend to decrease and increase, respectively, over time.

Skeletal muscle
Skeletal muscle is adept at repair and regeneration after injury secondary to trauma, degeneration, or strenuous exercise. Once the muscle tissue is injured, an inflammatory response brings to the area macrophages, which serve the dual purposes of phagocytosis of necrotic tissue and promotion of myogenic differentiation required for new muscle tissue. This is followed by the activation of satellite cells, which are similar to stem cells and are able to differentiate into the myoblasts necessary for the formation of new skeletal fibers. In people with severe trauma or degeneration, this capacity is insufficient to completely repair the involved muscles, leading to a combination of muscle fibers and scar tissue/fibrosis. Other than people suffering from these conditions, most children and adults have the ability to regenerate muscle fibers quite well, since the capacity for proliferation of satellite cells remains high. The extent of this repair is also diet-related, as new growth requires protein, among other things. However, as individuals age, this capacity starts to decrease for a number of reasons. Elderly people do not have this same proliferative ability for satellite cells, which means they must rely on those already present (which are generally still well-suited for this job), which can lead to incomplete regeneration. How well muscles repair themselves also depends on mechanical activity, which is lowered among older adults. In addition, a substance called osteopontin—which is more prevalent in older people—has been found to have possible down-regulating effects on this activity.

Cardiac muscle
Thinking on this topic is at a crossroads, as scientists reconsider some long-held beliefs. For many years it was thought that regardless of age, generation of cardiomyocytes was impossible outside the womb. But recent advances and discoveries in the field, relating to natural and assisted regeneration of cardiac tissues, have challenged this thinking. First, investigators began realizing that introduction of various stem cells directly into the heart did indeed result in proliferation of new cardiomyocytes. Then researchers observed unassisted natural cardiogenesis (neocardiogenesis) in young people, defined as newborns through adolescents. More recently, the same phenomenon has been observed in adults with CV disease, resulting in a paradigm shift in the cardiac research community. While the mechanism is still being elucidated, it is thought to involve a combination of intrinsic and circulating progenitor cells that stimulate new cardiomyocyte growth, as well as concurrent angiogenesis to support this new growth. Age-related factors and differences are largely unknown at this time.

Smooth muscle
Of all three muscle types, smooth muscle is best at repair and regeneration. The reason for this is twofold: the mononuclear cells involved still have the ability to divide and thus multiply; and cells

that line some blood vessels, called pericytes, can themselves divide to create brand new smooth muscle cells. This process also involves a loose connective tissue scaffold. Otherwise, while researchers have been aware of this regenerative ability for quite a while, relatively little research has taken place. It is known that certain factors (TGF-beta) are involved in and affect the signaling pathways that regulate gene expression, and therefore smooth muscle growth, but there is not much more information at this time. Also, it's important to remember that in addition to the reparative benefits of smooth muscle cell proliferation, this process is also partially responsible for atherosclerosis and hypertension.

Changes that occur over the course of one's life

Skeletal system and bones

Many bones in the body begin the ossification process while still in the womb, but do not conclude this growth and development until many months to years postpartum. This is especially true of the long bones of the body, such as the femur or humerus, which can grow until 20 years of age. Girls tend to experience fusion of the diaphysis and epiphysis a year or two before age-matched boys. During childhood and adolescence, skeletal growth leaves bones most susceptible to the effects of malnutrition and disease; but these bones also have the best regenerative ability. Normally, adulthood is a period of relatively few changes or intrinsic problems involving the bones, since development has concluded, with ossification complete and little risk of fracture during normal activities. However, as people age, they normally tend to develop various degrees of osteoporosis— skeletal atrophy resulting in loss of bone density—which leaves them open to fractures caused by falls that wouldn't likely affect a younger person (especially the hip). At this age, such fractures don't heal nearly as well as they do in a child or adult, which can lead to additional complications.

Skeletal muscles

Because of their ability to both regenerate and hypertrophy, skeletal muscles are well suited for potential growth and development throughout one's lifetime. As one ages, however, he or she does tend to experience certain changes and limitations in structure and function. In infancy and childhood, still developing muscles and tendons are increasing their muscle tone as well as their strength and capacity, either via myogenesis and/or hypertrophy secondary to mechanical workload. Adults continue to maintain tone and strength via this normal mechanical load, and may induce significant hypertrophy by such activities as bodybuilding. But in those approaching or in the midst of old age (60+), there is significant sarcopenia (reduced muscle mass and strength), which may begin as early as 40 years of age. The dual mechanisms involved in this process are a) atrophy and shortening of existing fibers, and/or b) loss of the number of fibers in a particular muscle, which results in a decreased cross-sectional area of the muscle. This process yields less contractile tissue within the muscles, which in turn leads to a natural reduction of force-generating capacity, or strength. With these decreases comes some degree of disability with respect to activities of daily living.

Cardiac muscle

After birth, cardiomyocytes and cardiac tissue do not change much, if at all, though recent findings (see regeneration card) have challenged this thinking. Still, throughout childhood and early adulthood, it is generally accepted that the myocardium doesn't normally functionally change. But from middle age through old age until death, changes first occur in cardiomyocytes before becoming obvious as myocardial tissue changes. Several factors lead to this reduction in the heart's normal and reserve capacities. In terms of cardiomyocyte aging, some of these include varied gene expression, oxidative stress and inflammatory processes, and many others. These cellular events then lead to myocardial changes that persist throughout the rest of one's life. Such changes include alteration of heart size and shape (ventricular hypertrophy causes an increase in overall size, while simultaneously reducing ventricular capacity), which yields a reduced stroke volume, making the heart less efficient. The myocardial fibers also experience delayed contraction cycles and reduced elasticity. The heart may not fill as fast or as well as previously, and changes in the pacemaker cells result in a slower heart rate. All of these changes are considered a normal part of aging, driven by intrinsic and extrinsic (diet, smoking, etc., factors which are modifiable) factors, and continue to occur until death. In fact, absent another obvious condition, most cases of "natural" death are caused by eventual heart failure, which is inevitable for those who live long enough.

Smooth muscle
During childhood (after the first few months of life, during which time there is variation in responses to circulating factors that determine muscle tone), smooth muscle changes very little, except for regeneration required by tissue disruption. But starting in adulthood, and especially in the elderly, several distinct alterations in morphology and function begin to occur. Most adults will experience some level of progressive atherosclerosis, which is partially driven by smooth muscle cell (SMC) division and hypertrophy. But there are also other changes, most of which involve vascular linings; and research has shown that the type and amount of change depends on the exact vascular bed. The proliferative ability of these cells decreases, while apoptotic activity increases, yielding less regenerative ability. During age-related vascular remodeling, SMCs also move from the tunica media to intima, resulting in a thickening of these two layers, increased luminal space, and stiffening of the vessels. The response of beta-adrenoreceptors (but not alpha) also diminishes in the elderly, which along with a reduction in endothelial-derived factors (NO, EDHF), leads to a lowered vasodilatory effect (perhaps as a response to luminal enlargement). These changes tend to occur more often in arteries than in veins, and progress as the person continues to get older.

Infections

Skeletal system
Infections of the skeletal system are divided into those involving bones directly and those involving joints. In the former category are pyogenic and tuberculous osteomyelitis (OM). Pyogenic OM is frequently caused by *S. aureus* and presents with fever, pain, and tenderness, usually at the distal femur and proximal tibia/humerus; four major routes of infection are fracture, surgery, hematogenous paths, and adjacent infection. Tuberculous OM is spread from other primary and secondary TB sites of infection (e.g., lungs) and often affects the vertebrae, hips, feet, hands, and long bones (known as Pott disease). Microbial invasion of the joints is called septic arthritis and can be divided into gonococcal, non-gonococcal, and chronic forms. Gonococcal arthritis follows contraction of gonorrhea, and is the most common arthritis in sexually active people; it is generally monoarticular at the knee and often presents with a rash and fever/chills, and it is gram negative on staining. Non-gonococcal arthritis is usually caused by either *Staph* or *Strep* species and has signs and symptoms similar to those of gonococcal; gram stain is positive. Chronic arthritides include Lyme disease, which occurs most commonly at the knee and is classified as secondary Lyme disease, appearing after the classic bull's eye rash (erythema chronicum migrans). The other example is caused by TB, though it is less common than TB bone disease.

Muscular system
Infectious myositis (IM) may be viral, bacterial, parasitic or fungal in origin, though IM in any form is relatively rare. Bacterial IM is usually secondary to muscle injury, trauma or foreign body deposition; it may be classified (according to location and causative organism) as a psoas abscess, pyomyositis, *Strep* IM (groups A and B), *S. aureus* myositis, clostridial IM, and non-clostridial myositis. Fungal IM is quite rare and almost always occurs in immunocompromised patients.

- 185 -

Parasitic infections of muscle can be caused by either helminths or protozoa, with trichinosis and cystericercosis the top two offenders. Travel history and eosinophils are keys to diagnosis. Viral IM may be mild or more serious depending on the causative bug, and often involves diffuse areas of muscle. These IMs can be categorized as benign (influenza), pleurodynic (coxsackie B), or prone to rhabdomyolysis or polymyositis. Treatment is directed by the causative microbe and clinical picture.

Inflammatory disorders

Skeletal system

In terms of inflammatory diseases of the skeletal system, the largest category is osteoarthritis, or degenerative joint disease (DJD). Of course, any infectious, autoimmune, or metabolic condition is also likely to result in inflammation. DJD is the most common form of arthritis, affecting tens of millions worldwide; it is most often the result of mechanical wear and tear, and is especially prominent at the knees (but often occurs at other sites as well), because of their weight-bearing responsibilities. DJD is usually worst at the end of the day, and symptoms tend to decrease after rest, as inflammation recedes. It is characterized by wearing down of the articular cartilage, followed by growth of bone surrounding the area (osteophytes); this process results in sclerosis, subchondral cysts, Heberden's and Bouchard's nodes (at DIPs and PIPs, respectively), and eburnation, where bone beneath the worn cartilage attains a polished appearance from constant wear. Torn cartilage and broken bone spurs cause "joint mice" on radiograph.

Muscular system

Myositis is the general term for inflammatory myopathies; those that aren't caused by infectious, metabolic, or autoimmune processes are included in this category, and generally present with a combination of inflammation, pain, and muscle weakness. The three major types are dermatomyositis (DM), polymyositis (PM), and inclusion body myositis (IBM); all three are idiopathic but suspected of being autoimmune. DM describes the combination a skin rash (usually malar or heliotrope, with Gottron's papules) and progressive muscle weakness, though the latter may be minimal or not clinically apparent; it is more common in women (as is polymyositis). PM is basically the same as DM but without the skin component, and with an association with malignancy. It presents as symmetric proximal weakness, most often at the shoulders, which limits activities of daily living such as brushing hair and putting on a shirt. T-cell mediated injury to muscle fibers is the cause of PM, which can be diagnosed by muscle biopsy. IBM affects men more than women and generally occurs after age 50. It is characterized, as with the others, by progressive muscle weakness and wasting (proximal and distal), often occurring gradually over months to years, and appearing asymmetrically. Finger and wrist atrophy are sometimes the first signs, when patients have trouble with fine-motor movements such as pinching; trouble swallowing may develop subsequently.

Seronegative spondyloarthropathies

While suspected to be autoimmune in nature, all three of these conditions have an association with HLA-B27, but test negative for rheumatoid factor and occur more commonly in males. Ankylosing spondylitis is chronic spinal and sacroiliac inflammation that may proceed to ankylosis (stiffening and fusion of the spinal column), and is sometimes accompanied by uveitis. It can also involve non-skeletal issues concerning the heart, lungs and cauda equina. Psoriatic arthritis—which is seronegative for RF but widely thought to be autoimmune—is an asymmetric arthritis that occurs alongside the psoriatic skin rash, often occurring in the feet, ankles, knees, and PIP/DIP joints. Clinical features include dactylitis ("sausage fingers") and a "pencil-in-cup" finding on x-ray. Reiter's syndrome is another disorder with a classic triad: conjunctivitis/uveitis, urethritis, and arthritis, commonly diagnosed after chlamydia or GI infection. It is most common in males between 20-40 years of age and presents as an asymmetric arthritis.

Immunological disorders

Skeletal system

There are several autoimmune disorders that involve the skeletal system (including connective tissues), as well as a few in which autoimmunity is suspected but unconfirmed. Rheumatoid arthritis (RA) is a disease that affects synovial joints, characterized by MCP and PIP inflammation (not DIP), ulnar deviation, and symmetric joint dysfunction; it involves morning stiffness, which abates with activity, and blood work is often positive for rheumatoid factor. Sjogren's syndrome (SS) is positive for ANA, SS-A, and SS-B autoantibodies, associated with RA, and most frequently seen in females between 40 and 60 years of age. Along with arthritis, SS involves dry eyes (xerophthalmia) and mouth (xerostomia), resulting in a classic triad. Lupus (SLE) is predominantly a female disease, with black females often severely affected. It tends to affect many different types of connective tissues and organs, and presents with constitutional symptoms, sometimes leading to organ failure and/or death. SLE displays positive results for several autoantibodies: ANA, anti-dsDNA and anti-Sm. Mixed connective tissue disease (MCTD) is positive for U1RNP antibodies, and can present with myalgia/arthralgia, fatigue, Raynaud's phenomenon, and possibly esophageal dysmotility.

Muscular system

Immune disorders of the muscular system often overlap with those of the skeletal system. Some muscular immunological conditions include sarcoidosis and scleroderma. *Sarcoidosis* is most common in black females and is characterized by widespread non-caseating granulomas that are immune-mediated. It often affects the lungs and may precipitate Bell's palsy; it is associated with elevated levels of IgG, ACE, and calcium. Epithelial granulomatous manifestations contain microscopic asteroid and Schaumann bodies. *Scleroderma* (progressive systemic sclerosis, or PSS) affects virtually every part of the body, causing degeneration and fibrosis of many areas, including the skin, which thickens, and the facial muscles, which results in a fixed facial expression. PSS displays positive anti-scl70 and anti-centromere autoantibodies and can sometimes present as the CREST syndrome.

Some Additional muscular immunological conditions include multiple sclerosis (MS), myasthenia gravis (MG), and Lambert-Eaton syndrome (LES). *Multiple sclerosis* MS is technically a neurologic disease (loss of myelin sheaths reduces conductive ability), but is autoimmune and frequently results in muscle weakness and spasms; it may produce visual, sensory, or motor problems. *Myasthenia gravis* MG is an autoimmune disease of the NMJ where antibodies to postsynaptic acetylcholine (Ach) receptors cause generalized weakness (worsened by muscle use), ptosis, and double vision; it is treated with AchE inhibitors. *Lambert-Eaton syndrome* LES is similar to MG in that is affects the NMJ, but different in mechanism and treatment. Antibodies to presynaptic calcium routes lead to lowered Ach and proximal muscle weakness. Unlike MG, AchE inhibitors won't solve the issue alone, and muscle use actually helps relieve symptoms.

Disorders of the MS system

Trauma to the MS system may produce skeletal fractures, soft tissue injury to muscles, and/or hemorrhage within muscles (hematoma). Such conditions may be encountered by accidental trauma or via overexertion of the involved body part (as is often the case with endurance athletes).

- 187 -

Regardless of the cause or type of problem, they are all characterized by a sustained inflammatory response aimed at healing the affected tissue, which usually leaves some level of scar tissue behind. This restorative pathophysiologic process often results in secondary injury to surrounding tissues, such as ischemic injury. Symptoms usually include various levels of pain, inflammation, and disability; treatments include both narcotic (opioids) and non-narcotic medications (acetaminophen, NSAIDs) as well as physical/occupational therapy. Extreme mechanical trauma, as is sometimes seen in car accidents, can also precipitate adult respiratory distress syndrome, which is negatively correlated with the speed of fracture reduction. Compartment syndrome occurs when there is hemorrhage into anterior or posterior compartments of the limbs, resulting in neurovascular compression that constitutes a surgical emergency.

Fractures

A fracture is defined as a break (partial or complete) in the integrity of bone tissue, and may be caused by significant trauma (traumatic) or by lesser mechanical stress in those with diseases that weaken bones (pathologic). There are several types, as well as common locations for fractures. First, fractures are considered either closed (skin intact) or open/compound (bone is visible or protrudes from skin), with compression fractures being a third type that generally involves the vertebrae. Further classification divides fractures into different types, depending on morphology and direction. A linear fracture occurs along the long axis of the affected bone; a transverse fracture is one that is perpendicular to the long axis; an oblique fracture is positioned diagonally with respect to the long axis; a spiral fracture is the result of excessive torque imposed by twisting, and may result in several different fracture lines; a comminuted fracture occurs when bone is shattered into more than one piece; an impacted fracture is present when pieces of bone are slammed into one another; and an avulsion fracture involves a piece or pieces of bone that have separated from the main bone mass. Two common fracture sites are the clavicle (middle third) and scaphoid, the latter of which may lead to avascular necrosis if not treated properly.

Sprains

Sprains are the result of either stretched (over-extended) or torn (partial or complete) ligaments, which connect bones together. Sprains are classified as grade I-III, depending on severity. They occur through falls, twisting motions, and intentional hits (as in football), and are most often seen in the ankles and wrists, with the knee being another common area of involvement. Symptoms include pain, bruising, swelling, and immobility; initial treatment generally involves resting the area, ice, compression with a bandage, and elevation (RICE), in addition to NSAIDs, while later treatment may include surgery followed by physical therapy. Two common sprains are those of the anterior cruciate ligament (ACL) of the knee and the lateral ligaments of the ankle/foot (particularly the anterior talofibular); the latter is the most common ankle trauma, resulting from traumatic inversion of the foot at the ankle, as happens when a basketball player or gymnast lands awkwardly on his or her feet.

Strains

As opposed to sprains, which involve ligaments, strains are mechanical disorders of the muscles and/or tendons brought on by excessive stress to the area that result in stretching or tearing of the concerned tissues. They are often seen in the hamstring and lower back region, although they may occur at many other anatomical locations; they are commonly caused by pulling or twisting motions (e.g., "pulling a hamstring"), often while playing sports. In contrast to sprains, strains can sometimes be the result of a chronic process, in addition to an acute injury. Symptoms include pain, swelling, spasms, weakness, and decreased range of motion. As with sprains, initial treatment involves rest, ice, compression, and elevation (RICE) and NSAIDs; serious strains may also require surgical intervention and/or physical therapy later on. Muscles affected tend to contain mostly fast-twitch fibers. Complications are usually minimal and prognosis excellent.

Separations and dislocations

Separations and dislocations are two completely different injuries, though they are often combined or confused since both involve stretching or tearing of ligaments. While they can occur at various joints, the predominant location is the shoulder, followed by the hip. Shoulder separations are ligament sprains at the acromioclavicular joint (AC joint—scapula and clavicle) that result in a widening of the space between these two bony structures, leading to pain and disability; they may be partial or complete tears. Separation at the shoulder often causes enough clavicular separation so that the distal clavicle can be seen protruding under the skin. In contrast, shoulder dislocation involves the glenohumeral (GH) joint, where the "ball" of the humerus meets the "socket" of the glenoid fossa. In a dislocation, the GH joint becomes unstable secondary to ligament sprain or tear, often at the labrum of the glenoid bone. In the majority of cases, the humerus dislocates anteriorly, though posterior and multi-directional dislocations are also possible. Symptoms common to both are pain (usually more severe in dislocations) and lack of mobility; those with dislocation also often report a feeling of the shoulder having "slipped" out of place. Common causes for both include sports injuries and falls. Dislocations must be reduced (restabilizing the GH joint); both may need eventual surgical intervention, though this is more common with dislocations than separations.

Joint injuries

The term "joint disease" encompasses a wide range of problems, including various forms of arthritis, sprains, strains, separations, and dislocations. Other than these conditions, other joint diseases that might be caused by acute or chronic injuries include bursitis (inflammation of the bursa lining the sides of synovial joints; especially subacromial), synovitis (synovial lining inflammation, common in the wrist), and tears (partial or complete) of ligaments such as the ACL (positive drawer sign) and the menisci of articular joints. The three most common locations for various joint injuries are the shoulder, ankle, and knee, followed by the wrist and elbow (nursemaid's elbow). All types of joint injuries are usually caused by either sports injuries or blunt trauma to the area, such as that seen with a severe fall. Symptoms of joint injuries include pain, tenderness, redness, swelling, and decreased range of motion. Therapeutic options differ depending on the location and severity, and may range from simple rest and immobilization to prescription of NSAIDs to surgical correction. Open joint injuries are more serious, usually involving a combination of joint components, such as bone, cartilage and soft tissue. Severe and sustained joint injuries may require partial or total replacement of that joint.

Repetitive motion injuries

Repetitive motion injury (RMI) is the result of performing the same motion repeatedly without interruption, and can be derived from occupational (computers and assembly lines) or leisure (tennis and golf) activities. It may be secondary to (or may cause) ligament sprains, muscle/tendon strains, inflammation of surrounding tissues, or any combinations thereof; nearby nerves become affected by these disturbances, yielding a host of symptoms and possible deformities. People with RMIs tend to experience pain, swelling, redness, numbness/tingling, and reduced strength/flexibility. Common locations are the hand, wrist, elbow, and shoulder; less commonly RMI occurs in the neck, back, knees, feet, and ankles. RMIs may include bursitis, tendonitis, epicondylitis, tenosynovitis, or ganglion cysts. The two most well-known examples of RMI are tennis elbow and carpal tunnel syndrome (CTS). Tennis elbow is a degenerative condition that indicates a sprain of the radial collateral ligament, resulting in small tears in the associated muscles and tendons, causing lateral epicondylitis and pain on forearm supination and wrist extension. Golf elbow is similar, but with medial epicondylitis that results in pain during pronation and wrist flexion. CTS occurs when the median nerve and nearby tendons, which travel through a narrow tunnel at the wrist, are compressed. It is a common complication of excessive computer/typing work. Treatment of RMIs primarily involves stopping or reducing the inciting factors, but may also include anti-inflammatory medications.

Impingement syndrome

Impingement syndrome (IS) concerns the muscles and tendons of the rotator cuff, located at the shoulder, and it is closely related to shoulder bursitis and rotator cuff tendonitis, which may occur concomitantly. When the narrow passage between the acromion process and humerus head—which contains the rotator cuff muscles and tendons—is compromised (via either muscle trauma and swelling, or skeletal abnormalities such as bone spurs, both of which narrow the space further), impingement (compression/entrapment) occurs, leading to characteristic findings. Under compression, these structures are squeezed and pressure increases to the point of interfering with capillary blood flow, which results in a tearing or fraying of the involved tissues; chronic cases can lead to a rotator cuff tear. This process leads to classic symptoms of pain and weakness, especially prominent when reaching behind the back or above the head. Diagnosis is mainly clinical, with radiographs used to rule out arthritis, and direct anesthetic injection used to alleviate pain, thus supporting the diagnosis. Treatment involves NSAIDs and stretching exercises; more severe cases may necessitate cortisone injections to alleviate pain and swelling.

Benign neoplasms

Bone
The most common benign bone/cartilage tumor, originating in the long bone metaphyses, is osteochondroma, which occurs mainly in men under 25, often at the distal femur and proximal tibia. Giant cell tumors, which are commonly seen at the long bone epiphyses, is so named for the characteristic giant, multinucleated spindle-shaped cells seen on microscopy. This type of tumor also tends to be seen at the distal femur and proximal tibia, but affects mostly women between the ages of 20-55; on x-ray a "soap bubble" formation can be detected. An osteoma is a neoplasm where a new piece of bone grows on an already-existing mature bone, often in the skull or face; it affects mostly men. Osteoid osteomas (OO) are tumors with a small nidus surrounded by osteoblasts and woven trabecular tissue, occurring most often in the diaphyses and metaphyses of long bones, and less commonly at the epiphyses. They generally present with dull pain, occurring more often in men between 20-30 years old. Osteoblastomas are similar to OOs, but are larger and usually are found in the spinal column. Fibrous dysplasia is a tumor where dysfunctional growth of fibrous tissue replaces bone, and may involve single or multiple bones; the classic radiograph finding is a "Chinese figures" appearance. Enchondromas are cartilaginous tumors that generally affect distal portions of the extremities and are found within medullary bone.

Muscle
There is only one major benign tumor that occurs within muscle tissue, and it is still very rare. Leiomyomas (LMs) are neoplasms of smooth muscle tissue, especially that of the uterus. They are generally less than 2 cm in diameter, and display elongated nuclei and whorls of muscle cells under microscopy. In terms of immunohistochemistry, actin and desmin antibodies are prominent. LMs

are much more common in women and are in fact the most common tumors in females. Fortunately, LMs generally have an inactive course and are easily treated and cured.

Malignant neoplasms

Bone
There are three major types of malignant bone tumors, plus bone metastases, which occur in several types of cancer. Osteosarcoma (OS) is a neoplasm that usually forms in the long bone metaphyses, and leads to tissue destruction accompanied by hemorrhage and necrosis. Most often diagnosed in teenage boys, who experience pain and swelling around the knee area, OS frequently metastasizes to the lungs first; radiograph demonstrates Codman triangle. Chondrosarcomas are malignant cartilage tumors that lead to calcification and necrosis of the involved tissue; they are most often seen in older males and usually occurs in the axial skeleton. Ewing sarcoma (ES) is another cartilage tumor that generally affects adolescent and teenage boys, who present with a painful, red, swollen mass in one of a number of locations, including the ribs, scapula, pelvis, and long bones. ES tends to metastasize early, but is responsive to chemotherapy; microscopy demonstrates Homer-Wright pseudorosettes. Metastases to bones can happen with a large number of cancers, and usually show lytic lesions on x-ray, except when the primary tumor is from the breast or prostate.

Muscle
There are two common malignancies found within muscle tissue: leiomyosarcoma (LMS) and rhabdomyosarcoma (RMS). The former is a neoplasm of smooth muscle, skin and other soft tissues; they display cigar-shaped nuclei and dense bodies under microscopy. LMSs are uncommon muscle tumors that reveal vimentin, actin and desmin antibodies upon immunohistochemical examination. The course is variable, with tumor size positively correlated with poorer prognosis. RMS is an aggressive tumor that is classified into several types, depending on tissue origin. Microscopic examination displays rhabdomyoblasts, which are considered diagnostic. RMSs most often occur in skeletal muscle, especially of the head and neck, as well as within the GU system and retroperitoneum. Antibodies to desmin, actin, vimentin, and myoglobin are seen on immunohistochemistry; treatment involves chemotherapy, radiation, and surgery. RMS is the most common sarcoma found in children and adolescents.

Osteomalacia

Osteomalacia (OM), known as "rickets" in children, literally means "soft bones." This condition is characterized by bowlegs, and is the result of poor calcification secondary to a lack of vitamin D. This defective mineralization of bony structures leads to increased calcium and decreased phosphate in the bloodstream. In children, OM can lead to craniotabes (soft, thin skull bones) and late fontanelle closure, reduced height, pigeon breast (sternal protrusion), costochondral thickening ("string of pearls"), and other skeletal deformities. In adults, OM generally leads to frequent fractures, and displays radiolucency on x-ray. Administration of exogenous vitamin D, as well as time spent in the sunlight (yielding endogenous vitamin D) can reverse the effects of OM. When renal disease is the cause of lowered vitamin D, the condition is known alternatively as renal osteodystrophy.

Osteoporosis

Osteoporosis (OP) is a condition characterized by skeletal tissue atrophy and a consequent reduction in bone density, brought about by increased bone resorption, decreased bone formation, or a combination of both. It is often a result of physical inactivity (type II), and is very common in post-menopausal women (type I) who aren't on hormone replacement therapy (controversial because of breast/uterine cancer risk). OP typically displays increased PTH and cortisol, with decreased calcium levels. Fractures are a common issue in patients with OP, especially in the vertebral column and the hips (as well as other weight-bearing joints), and healing may be more problematic than in those without OP. There is radiolucency on x-ray and DEXA scans are positive for reduced bone density. Treatment of OP consists of a healthy diet, regular low-impact exercise, and supplementation with calcium and vitamin D. In more serious cases, bisphosphonates, which counteract the effects of PTH, are often administered as a means of preventing further bone loss. Type II (senile) OP is relatively unavoidable for those who live long enough, though degree of severity may vary depending on the individual.

Osteodystrophy

The term osteodystrophy refers to any dysfunctional growth involving bone; chondrodystrophy is its equivalent involving cartilage. Most cases are directly related to renal disease, although it may also be caused by independent disruption in the metabolism of phosphorus, calcium, or both. Depending on the location and exact nature of the process taking place, osteodystrophic diseases carry a host of different names; some examples are Camurati-Engelmann disease (diaphysis) and Raine syndrome (osteosclerosis). Such disorders as achondroplasia (dwarfism) and related collagen disorders may also be classified as types of osteodystrophy, though many such diseases tend to transcend different categories. As noted, kidney failure is usually the precipitating cause, which results in the hypocalcemia and hyperphosphatemia that drives the osteodystrophic disease process. Correction of these two blood parameters through diet, supplementation, and medications will help to correct the problem, or at least slow progression.

Gout

Gout is a purine metabolism disorder that results from a buildup of uric acid in the blood (hyperuricemia), secondary to xanthine oxidase (forms uric acid) dysfunction and exogenous precipitants. It may be chronic or acute, with the latter often occurring after a protein-heavy meal or excessive alcohol consumption. Hyperuricemia leads to formation of negatively birefringent monosodium urate crystals, which are deposited within the joint spaces, resulting in extremely painful inflammation. Distribution is asymmetric, often involving only a single joint; the classic presentation is unbearable pain and swelling in the first MTP (known as podagra), brought on by as little as touching the bed sheet with a toe. Tophus formation is sometimes seen near affected joints, on the Achilles tendon, or on the ear; renal involvement may follow urate crystal deposition in collecting tubules. The gold standard for diagnosis is needle aspiration from the joint, but because it is such a painful process, many rheumatologists prefer to diagnose through pharmaceutical intervention (i.e., if the drugs stop the problem, then gout was the issue). Treatment is accomplished via a combination of NSAIDs (especially indomethacin), colchicine, probenecid, and allopurinol; prevention is aided by restricting the diet in terms of alcohol and purine-rich foods.

Pseudogout

As opposed to true gout, where sodium urate crystals are involved, pseudogout is the result of deposition of calcium pyrophosphate crystals in the joint space. For this reason, it is also known as calcium pyrophosphate dehydrate crystal deposition disease (CPPD). While the cause is unknown, pseudogout is suspected to be related to degenerative cartilage disease, since the two are often seen together. The crystals here are rhomboid in shape and weakly positively birefringent (as opposed to gout's negatively birefringent crystals). Also, in contrast to gout, pseudogout usually affects larger joints such as the knee. It is generally seen in those older than 50, and affects both sexes equally. Diagnosis may be made clinically or via aspiration of synovial fluid, and is supported via articular cartilage calcification on x-ray. Symptoms are usually similar to gout (painful inflammation of the joint), but much less severe. Treatment is accomplished using NSAIDs (indomethacin), colchicine, and/or corticosteroid injection; however, some doctors will choose to abstain from initial therapy and let it resolve on its own.

Disorders of the MSS

Metabolic/regulatory

Metabolic/regulatory diseases of the MSS can vary quite a bit in terms of clinical and laboratory parameters; but all have in common a disruption of various biochemical steps necessary for normal function. The problems may involve impaired/absent enzymatic action, hydroxylation and phosphorylation issues, uncontrolled pathophysiologic processes, or other disturbances that interrupt a certain metabolic pathway. This often leads to a buildup or deficiency of substrates or end products, which then manifests as clinical dysfunctions. Such disorders may be hereditary, and MSS pain/symptoms can also indicate systemic metabolic disease. Gout and pseudogout are two common manifestations of metabolic disruption, along with osteomalacia and osteoporosis. Scurvy is a metabolic disease that is caused by vitamin C deficiency and defective collagen synthesis; it results in disrupted bone formation and may present with bleeding gums or painful internal hemorrhage. Abnormally high PTH levels (from primary or secondary hyperparathyroidism) can lead to osteitis fibrosa cystica (von Recklinghausen disease), often displaying characteristic osteoclast-lined cystic deformities on radiograph (known as "brown tumor of bone"). Other examples include Marfan syndrome (defective fibrillin leads to elongated limbs and fingers, hyperextensible joints, and potential for aortic dissection—think Abe Lincoln) and Ehlers-Danlos syndrome (defective elastin and collagen formation leads to fragile tissues, with hyperextensible joints and frequent hemorrhages).

Structural

In the MSS, structural disorders encompass a wide range of ailments. All of them, however, involve some morphologic deformity or deficiency that leads to anatomical disruption. One example is Paget's disease of bone (cause unknown), in which one or more bones undergo enhanced osteoblast and osteoclast activity. This leads to skeletal deformities that result in painful fractures and arteriovenous shunts that may lead to high-output heart failure. It is most common in elderly people, and consists of three phases: osteolytic, mixed (mosaic bone pattern), and late. Other examples are achondroplasia (dwarfism), which leads to short stature caused by failure of long bone growth secondary to early epiphyseal sealing; and osteopetrosis (marble bone disease), in which bone density is increased because of reduced osteoclast activity. Kyphosis and scoliosis are two spinal column conditions that result in lateral deviation in the coronal plane (scoliosis) and anteroposterior deviation in the sagittal plane (kyphosis). Still other structural disorders are caused by brachial plexus lesions, which may result in a host of deformities with characteristic signs, including Erb-Duchenne palsy (waiter's tip), Klumpke palsy (claw hand when ulnar nerve involved), radial nerve palsy (wrist drop), and scapular winging.

Vascular

There are relatively few vascular disorders inherent to the MSS, though vasculitides in or around the muscle or bone will certainly lead to complications in some cases. Likewise, primary muscle or bone lesions may yield issues with the surrounding vasculature. The one major condition directly related to the MSS is avascular necrosis (aka aseptic necrosis), which can occur for a number of reasons, all of which result in fat necrosis and osteocyte death at the affected area. Some causes include fracture that interrupts flow, thrombosis, vascular compression, or any other significant vessel injury. Patients experience joint pain and dysfunction, most often at the hip/femur (Legg-Calve-Perthes disease in children) or tibial tubercle (Osgood-Schlatter disease). In many cases, the treatment involves partial or total replacement of the associated joint; once reperfusion is achieved via this or another mechanism, repair and regeneration begins, first via angiogenesis and then osteogenesis. Another vascular condition that may affect nearby bones, joints, or muscles is vasculitis (which often extends the inflammatory reaction into these tissues), which may be caused by many different etiologies. Fibromuscular dysplasia is a disease characterized by distorted smooth muscle growth, leading to stenosis and aneurysms of medium-sized vessels. In addition, Behçet's disease sometimes includes vascular complications. And of course, vascular disease of the coronary vessels may result in angina or MI, among other problems.

Systemic
Lupus (SLE), a diffuse connective tissue disorder, is the prototypic example of widespread systemic disease that affects a host of different tissue types including bones, joints, and muscles. The primary issue for many patients is joint involvement, resulting in pain and inflammation, presenting as either nonspecific arthralgias or acute polyarthritis. People who have had SLE for years may also experience joint deformities secondary to the inflammatory process, or tendon contractures. Sarcoidosis also sometimes results in fibrotic and arthritic complications. Other systemic conditions that often affect bones and/or muscles are regulatory disorders such as hyperparathyroidism—and the related increases or decreases in calcium, phosphorus, vitamin D and others—which can lead to increased osteoclastic activity resulting in bone loss and fragility. In addition, any vascular problem, whether system-wide or regional, may result in associated MSS symptoms and complications. Cardiac and cerebrovascular events may also impact muscle tissue outside the heart or brain. The former may yield referred neuromuscular pain to the shoulders, arms, neck, and/or jaws; the latter includes a wide range of potential muscular problems, including the classic presentation of trouble speaking and asymmetric muscle weakness/paralysis. Finally, hematogenous infection may occasionally seed within bones or joints, resulting in osteomyelitis.

Idiopathic conditions
Two idiopathic conditions are ankylosing spondylitis and psoriatic arthritis (PA). Despite their connections to immunological factors (HLA-B27) and disorders (rheumatoid arthritis), no clear etiology has been elucidated thus far, except for the fact that PA obviously occurs alongside psoriatic systemic disease. Spasmodic torticollis is another condition of unknown origin that results in spasms of neck muscles, and consequent rotation and tilting of the neck and head. Tendinitis or tenosynovitis may not have a known cause, but occurs mainly in older people, suggesting a connection to vascular attenuation. Dupuytren's contracture is a thickening and painless contracture of the palmar surface that may result in problems with flexion and finger dysfunction. Fibromyalgia is a condition occurring mostly in females, where there are diffuse myalgias and fibrous tissue pain, but without joint involvement or apparent inflammation. The cause is unknown but may be secondary to an infection, and may be triggered by strenuous exercise or elevated stress levels.

Degenerative diseases
There are various MSS diseases that involve some level of degeneration. Of those not yet covered, amyotrophic lateral sclerosis (ALS or Lou Gehrig's disease) is probably the most well-known. Although ALS—like many of the degenerative diseases of the MSS—is actually rooted in breakdown of different motor nerves, its effect on voluntary muscles demands its inclusion here. ALS is characterized by progressive muscle weakness, spasticity and loss of function, most often beginning

in the limbs and moving inward (limb onset), although a smaller percentage of people experience difficulty swallowing or speaking as the initial symptoms (bulbar onset). Eventually many muscular functions are compromised, leading to death from respiratory failure in most cases (Stephen Hawking is a total aberration). The muscular dystrophies are also caused by degeneration of fibromuscular tissues, but will be covered under genetic diseases. Inclusion body myositis is another example of a disorder featuring muscular degeneration. On the skeletal side, conditions such as osteoarthritis and osteoporosis are degenerative, and some elderly people (or those doing regular heavy lifting) may experience some level of degeneration of the intervertebral disks (leading to the perception that one is "shrinking").

Drug-induced adverse effects

Many different drugs may produce unwanted muscular and skeletal effects. Drug-induced myopathies may be secondary to a wide range of medications and are thought to be related to metabolic or immune dysfunction brought on by administration of the drug. Symptoms and findings include proximal muscle weakness, elevated muscle enzymes, and electromyographic and histological changes; patients may experience pain (myalgias) or may be pain-free. In extreme cases, more serious conditions such as rhabdomyolysis or neuroleptic malignant syndrome (fever, muscle rigidity, and cognitive changes) may occur. Therapy usually consists of removal of the offending agent, at which time most myopathies resolve spontaneously. Examples include vacuolar myopathies (colchicine, cyclosporine, and chloroquine) and mitochondrial myopathies (zidovudine). The major skeletal drug-induced effect is precipitation or contribution to bone loss, including osteoporosis and osteomalacia, which can be caused by a long list of medications, including seizure meds, thyroid hormone, and cyclosporine. Other conditions such as hypocalcemia or hypercalcemia may occur, which then result in related skeletal abnormalities. Finally, any drug that disrupts balance and/or alertness and thus might contribute to a fall (especially in the elderly) may impact the MSS.

Congenital/genetic disorders

Many congenital MSS disorders have a genetic component, while others do not. The muscular dystrophies (Duchenne, Becker, and seven others) are all caused by some sort of genetic mutation, which differs in each type; the dystrophin gene is often involved, and these mutations may be inherited or spontaneous in the womb. They all result in progressive muscle weakness and gait/balance issues, which eventually require a wheelchair or others' assistance in most cases. Klumpke's palsy, a non-genetic disturbance of the brachial plexus during the prenatal period or childbirth, results in muscle atrophy and sensory deficits in the arms and hands. Achondroplasia is an autosomal-dominant hereditary disorder that results in short stature secondary to premature bone closure. Genetic mutations (often autosomal dominant) that cause defective collagen synthesis often lead to osteogenesis imperfecta, or brittle bone disease, which features multiple fractures and blue sclera. Marfan and Ehlers-Danlos syndromes are similar in that they both result in hyperextensibility of joints; but they differ in causes and mechanisms. The former is an autosomal dominant congenital disorder caused by fibrillin abnormalities that yield visual, skeletal, and CV problems (aortic dissection); the latter is caused by mutations that disrupt collagen and elastin formation, leading to hemorrhage and tissue fragility.

Mechanism of action (MOA) of NSAIDs

Non-steroidal anti-inflammatory drugs have antipyretic, analgesic, and anti-inflammatory properties, driven by the inhibition of cyclooxygenase, which normally converts arachidonic acid into the prostaglandins. Conventional NSAIDs (aspirin, ibuprofen, indomethacin, and naproxen) act by inhibiting both cyclooxygenase pathways (COX-1 and COX-2) and preventing formation of thromboxane, prostaglandins, and prostacyclins, all of which mediate inflammation. Aspirin inhibits these pathways irreversibly and also has anti-platelet activity as well. COX-2 inhibitors such as celecoxib act exclusively on the COX-2 pathway, which allows for potent anti-inflammatory action while mostly sparing the gastric lining from disruption (an issue for the other forms of NSAIDs which have multiple sites of action including the GI system).

MOA of non-NSAID analgesics

There are three different types of medications that fall under this heading: acetaminophen (Tylenol), corticosteroids, and opioids. Acetaminophen acts by reversibly inhibiting the cyclooxygenase pathway, leading to antipyretic and analgesic properties, but lacking anti-inflammatory properties (in contrast to NSAIDs). It is absorbed by the GI system and processed in the liver, offering mostly CNS activity, with limited peripheral activation. Corticosteroids—via modulation of gene expression—act at the top of the inflammation cascade, by inhibiting the formation of arachidonic acid (through blockage of phospholipase-A), which is the precursor to all other inflammatory mediators. However, the occurrence of antipyretic activity is not always assured. Opioids mainly act by binding receptors within the CNS—there are four types—as well as limited peripheral activation. Of the receptor types, the mu receptor is most potently affected by opiate agonists in terms of pain reduction. The physiological effects depend on the type of medication; strong agonists such as morphine, heroin, and fentanyl have more powerful effects than moderate agonists such as hydrocodone and propoxyphene. Opiate derivatives do not possess anti-inflammatory or anti-pyretic properties, but offer potent analgesia.

Clinical uses of NSAIDs for MSS disorders

All of the NSAIDs are used to reduce pain and inflammation in MSS disorders, whether it is part of the primary disease process or secondary to another disease. The uses of aspirin depend on the dosage being administered. At low doses, such as those used after a cardiac event, there is a decrease in platelet aggregation; intermediate doses display antipyretic and analgesic properties; high doses are required to potentiate anti-inflammatory effects. Other (COX-1) NSAIDs have the same clinical uses as aspirin but generally have a more narrow dosing range; and aspirin is the only one that has anti-platelet activity. These drugs all present significant concerns of GI distress and bleeding, along with possible renal dysfunction (especially during long-term use). The COX-2 inhibitors may be used to combat any inflammation, but are most commonly used for rheumatoid and osteoarthritis. The major benefit of COX-2 medications, such as celecoxib, is the minimal risk for GI complications because of the selective mechanism that retains gastric mucosa and inhibition of gastric acid secretion. However, COX-2 medications do carry an increased risk of thrombosis.

Clinical uses of non-NSAID analgesics for MSS disorders

Acetaminophen, corticosteroids, and opiate agonists are all used in clinical practice to alleviate pain and/or inflammation. Acetaminophen is a non-narcotic analgesic used for pain relief and fever reduction, with very little anti-inflammatory effects. It is generally well tolerated with minimal adverse effects, but can be hepatotoxic at extremely high levels, requiring administration of N-acetylcysteine (Mucomyst). It is also used today in children in order to avoid the possibility of Reye's syndrome, seen with aspirin use. Corticosteroids are usually second-line therapies that are used when treatment with NSAIDs is not sufficient, though diagnostic confirmation of some disorders may mandate immediate steroid therapy. They are potent anti-inflammatories (and thus pain reducers) and are especially useful for widespread systemic diseases such as lupus or rheumatoid arthritis, but come with the substantial side effect of lowering immune function. They may also be used for direct injections into joint spaces with medication-resistant inflammation. Opioids are used for pain that is not controlled through other means, and produce a range of analgesic effects depending on the type used; none are anti-inflammatory. In addition to analgesia, opiate agonists may be habit forming. They can have serious side effects with overuse, such as respiratory depression. Naloxone can be used to reverse an overdose.

Muscle relaxants

Muscle relaxants may act at the neuromuscular junction (NMJ; peripherally acting, via acetylcholine receptors) or within the CNS (centrally acting); for the latter, inhibition of GABA receptors and calcium release are two common MOAs. Such drugs include diazepam, dantrolene, baclofen, and cyclobenzaprine, all of which may be used to mitigate muscle spasms (known as spasmolytics) from various conditions. The NMJ-mediated medications (known collectively as neuromuscular blockers) are further divided into competitive and non-competitive receptor agents. Competitive agents, such as curare and pancuronium, bind the nicotinic acetylcholine receptors and prevent depolarization, which inhibits muscle contraction at the site; high concentrations will also inhibit ion channels, which further limits muscle function. Non-competitive neuromuscular blockers, such as succinylcholine, act by attaching to acetylcholine receptors and acting as an agonist, depolarizing membranes to initiate contraction (resulting in fasciculations). However, unlike acetylcholine, they remain in the synaptic cleft, where the constant depolarization eventually results in blockage of further impulses.

For the most part, with rare exceptions, both types of neuromuscular blockers are used in surgical and intensive care situations, to paralyze muscles for intubation and ventilation, or for other paralytic purposes as necessary. They are administered parenterally because of poor oral absorption, and competitive agents have a relatively long duration of action. Non-competitive agents such as succinylcholine are shorter acting than competitive ones, and are therefore usually administered via continuous IV infusion during procedures. The spasmolytics—diazepam, cyclobenzaprine, carisoprodol and others—are generally used for chronic nonspecific pain syndromes such as fibromyalgia and neck/back pain, and provide relief from the muscle spasms thought to cause such pain. However, repeated studies have shown no solid evidence supporting their use over more traditional remedies, such as NSAIDs or antidepressants, which are commonly used for these problems.

Anti-gout medications

Besides NSAIDs (particularly indomethacin) that are used for gout, there are several specific agents used nearly exclusively for this condition. Colchicine acts by inhibiting microtubule polymerizations, which retards leukocyte chemotaxis and thus inflammation at the site. Probenecid reduces sodium urate crystal formation by inhibiting uric acid reabsorption within the kidney's collecting tubules. Allopurinol works by inhibiting the enzyme xanthine oxidase, which prevents the formation of uric acid from xanthine and thus reduces crystal formation. It also results in elevations of other medications that are normally metabolized via this pathway, including 6-MP and azathioprine.

Anti-gout medications, as one might presume, are clinically indicated in cases of true gout (versus pseudogout). They may act by reducing the inflammatory response and/or inhibiting the enzyme pathway that produces excess uric acid, and are used to a) mitigate pain and inflammation, which can be intense, and b) reduce the formation of the urate crystals that are deposited in joint spaces and cause this inflammatory response and excruciating pain. For cases of acute gout, either colchicine, indomethacin, or both are used to control inflammation and make the patient more comfortable; occasionally opioids may be given for extreme pain, but most clinicians avoid this usage. For chronic gout, once the acute inflammation has passed, patients are put on allopurinol (most common) or probenecid as maintenance medications to prevent further attacks. If/when another acute attack does occur while on these medications, the drugs used for acute gout may be added until the episode subsides. Salicylates (e.g., aspirin) should not be used for gout since they inhibit uric acid clearance; allopurinol and probenecid should not be used initially for acute attacks, since they may precipitate or worsen such acute crises.

Immunosuppressive therapies

Immunosuppressants include such medications as prednisone, cyclosporine, methotrexate, infliximab, and etanercept, which act through various mechanisms. Glucocorticoids such as prednisone offer general immunosuppression through reduction of cell-mediated and humoral immunity. Cytostatic agents—various alkylating agents, anti-metabolites, methotrexate, cytotoxic antibiotics, azathioprine and mercaptopurine—all have different MOAs, but every drug in this category acts via some form of cell division inhibition. Antibodies, whether monoclonal or polyclonal, work by occupying receptors that control some aspect of immune function. Most of the activity occurs via T-cell inhibition/destruction, with newer agents such as infliximab (anti-TNF antibody) and etanercept (recombinant TNF receptor) specifically directed at T-cell and IL-2 receptors, thus precisely regulating the immune response. Anti-immunophilins—cyclosporine, tacrolimus, and sirolimus—achieve their effect by inhibiting substances and processes that promote the immune response, such as calcineurin inhibition. Other medications are the various interferons, which decrease cytokine production and monocyte activation, and newer synthetic biologics directed at numerous receptors and/or antigens.

All of the various immunosuppressives are utilized for those musculoskeletal disorders that involve an autoimmune process, or occasionally, for inflammatory disorders of non-autoimmune etiology. Some of the autoimmune disorders (ADs) involving the MSS and targeted with these therapies include rheumatoid arthritis, lupus, multiple sclerosis, and myasthenia gravis. The goal is reduction of the immunological response that is causing severe inflammation, and these agents are used for symptomatic as well as disease progression issues. Because these medications are potent immunosuppressives, the possibility of infections is a concern during administration; many patients on long-term therapy will acquire repeat infections that last longer than in those not affected by ADs. Examples of specific drugs and their clinical uses include the use of etanercept for rheumatoid arthritis (RA), psoriasis, and ankylosing spondylitis (AS); and infliximab for RA, AS, and Crohn's disease. Drug usage is very clinician-dependent, with different doctors often preferring one drug to another.

Antineoplastic therapies

The antineoplastic agents comprise a large variety of different medicines, with various MOAs, which are used selectively depending on the type of tumor. Antimetabolites such as methotrexate act by interfering with purine and/or pyrimidine synthesis, resulting in defective DNA/RNA and thus disrupting cell division. Cytotoxic antibiotics such as doxorubicin also disrupt DNA synthesis and cellular division; the exact MOA depends on the specific agent. Alkylating agents such as cyclophosphamide work by binding several different cellular constituents, including causing the alkylation and inactivation of DNA; they often mimic the effects of ionizing radiation. Mitotic spindle poisons such as vincristine act on the cytoskeleton, interfering with microtubule function required for the completion of mitosis, thus also limiting cell division. Hormones such as

- 198 -

prednisone or estrogen act at specific receptor sites for these substances, and are thus only chemotherapeutically active when adhering to certain tissues. Additional agents (interferons, cisplatin, L-asparaginase, and etoposide) all have MOAs involving the inhibition of DNA synthesis and/or cellular division, some of which are similar to those listed above. Clinical uses are to retard progression of and hopefully eradicate tumors of the MSS. The specific agents used vary depending on tumor type and size, and prognoses are mixed. Virtually all of these medications produce some level of bothersome side effects, ranging from dizziness and nausea/vomiting to more severe consequences.

Drugs that affect bone mineralization

There are five types of drugs that are used to influence bone calcification and mineralization: calcium, vitamin D, calcitonin, bisphosphonates, and estrogen replacement therapy. Calcium (Ca) works by simply providing more raw resources to encourage bone growth and mineralization. Vitamin D, which can be attained orally (exogenous) or through exposure to sunlight (endogenous), acts in concert with Ca and phosphate by enhancing absorption and retention of these two minerals necessary for growth. Calcitonin acts via inhibition of bone resorption and increased calcium excretion, thus serving the dual purposes of reducing osteoclastic activity and removing the already-created products of this hyperactive resorption process. Bisphosphonates are pyrophosphate analogs that become included in bone formation and then reduce osteoclastic activity from inside the bone tissue. Estrogen replacement therapy acts via reduction of osteoclastic activity, which serves to maintain mineralization and prevent further bone atrophy and/or de-mineralization.

All five types of drugs that affect mineralization are used to strengthen the bone structure in those with evidence of reduced bone density, caused by either decreased osteoblastic activity, increased osteoclastic activity, or a combination of both. More specifically, calcium is used to treat osteoporosis, osteomalacia/rickets, and hypoparathyroidism; clinicians must watch for hypercalcemia. Vitamin D is employed to counteract cases of vitamin D deficiency, mainly from rickets/osteomalacia, but also possibly for those without sunlight for long periods of time; toxicity and renal impairment are concerns. Calcitonin is utilized in cases of post-menopausal osteoporosis, Paget's disease, hypercalcemia, and vertebral fractures; GI distress is a concern. The bisphosphonates are likewise used for Paget's, hypercalcemia, and osteoporosis; ocular inflammation and osteonecrosis of the jaw are potential complications. Hormone replacement therapy (HRT) with estrogen is used primarily for osteoporosis in women who are peri- or post-menopausal; concerns about HRT increasing the risk of breast and uterine cancer, along with evidence that some non-MSS benefits were exaggerated have led to the use of selective estrogen receptor modulators, which only bind bone receptors and not those in breast or uterine tissue.

Antimicrobial agents

There is a wide variation in the MOAs of the different antimicrobials used to treat MSS infections, the selection of which is strongly driven by spectrum coverage and whether the pathogen is known to be gram-positive or gram-negative. Beta-lactams (penicillin derivatives and cephalosporins, among others) work by inhibiting cell wall synthesis, as does vancomycin. Rifampin interferes with bacterial RNA polymerase, thus blocking DNA transcription. Fluoroquinolones inhibit topoisomerase II, leading to fragmentation of the DNA double helix. Clindamycin inhibits ribosomal translocation, thus preventing bacterial protein synthesis. Sulfonamides (e.g. Bactrim) inhibit the use of para-aminobenzoic acid in folic acid synthesis, thus disrupting bacterial DNA synthesis. Azoles work by inhibiting an enzyme that produces a crucial cell membrane constituent, thus stopping further fungal growth. Echinocandins act via fungal cell wall synthesis inhibition, using a MOA similar to the penicillins. Anti-helminthic medications (albendazole, mebendazole) are thought to disrupt parasitic microtubule function, thus blocking a critical part of mitosis.

Bacterial bone infections can be quite serious and hard to eradicate, thus requiring IV antibiotic treatment. Infective myositis is rare, but antimicrobial therapy is generally indicated when such infections are detected. Specific clinical uses depend on the causative organism, location of the lesion, and proven efficacy. For bacterial osteomyelitis, gram-positive infections are usually treated with one of several cephalosporins or a penicillin derivative when methicillin-susceptible, and vancomycin is used for MRSA. Gram-negative rods are treated with cephalosporins, fluoroquinolones or vancomycin. Depending on route and severity of infection, other medications may be substituted or added to the regimen. Similar or the same medications as above are administered for bacterial myositis, in addition to clindamycin in susceptible species. For fungal myositis, one of the azoles (e.g., amphotericin B) and/or an echinocandin is utilized, depending on the microbe species and route of infection. Parasitic myositis usually requires treatment with anti-helminthic agents, which aims to kill the larvae in either the GI tract (preferable) or within the muscles (less consistent results). Some parasites (e.g., Toxoplasma) are treated merely supportively, without medication, since the disease course is usually self-limited.

Therapeutic measure or modalities that may be used to treat disorders of the MSS

The particular extra-pharmaceutical treatment regimens depend on the condition to be treated. For fractures and dislocations of bones, reduction (resetting) is of paramount importance; especially with fractures, the longer the delay in reduction, the greater chance there is for less-than-ideal healing and excess scar tissue. For those with osteoporosis and other mineral-deficient disorders, a combination of a healthy diet and moderate exercise is important. Physical and occupational therapies—especially vital after major trauma or another disabling condition such as muscular dystrophy—are used to help the patient regain his or her MSS function and possibly relearn the simple activities of daily living that most people don't think too much about. Other alternative therapeutic modalities that may be of help include acupuncture, electrotherapy, thermal applications, movement therapies, and massage/manipulations. It should be noted that those alternative options listed above often rely more on anecdotal versus empirical evidence; however, there are some studies that conclude such measures are helpful.

Influence of MSS disorders in terms of disease prevention and treatment

Patient and family

MSS disorders affect both the patient and his or her family and support network. While little more than careful instruction can be offered in terms of prevention of disease, the therapeutic course, especially if it is long-term therapy, can be draining on the patient and family alike. Mere compliance with unpleasant therapies, whether pharmaceutical or physical, is a big concern for those suffering from MSS disorders. But even with good patient compliance, the stubborn resistance of some conditions to effective treatment often leaves patients feeling discouraged and defeated. As for the family, any time someone suffers from a substantial disability or disease, the impact is felt by all (if only recognized later). This is particularly relevant for MSS disorders, since they may very well limit the patient's ability to move around and/or perform daily activities. When this is the case, family members can become overburdened, which sometimes presents issues of mutual resentment between the patient and other family members.

Copyright © Mometrix Media. You have been licensed one copy of this document for personal use only. Any other reproduction or redistribution is strictly prohibited. All rights reserved.

Emotional and behavioral

These factors have differing impacts depending on the person and disease in consideration. For those with nonspecific pain syndromes such as fibromyalgia, the relentless nature of the condition and lack of definitive treatment can often result in patients becoming depressed and despondent over their situations. Such occurrences are also common in those suffering from progressive degenerative diseases, and patients in either group may be helped by both physical and mental therapies. Behaviorally, the major concern is that of intentional strenuous exercise or putting oneself in dangerous situations, and the potential such activities have for various fractures, tears, and other traumatic or exertion-induced injuries. In terms of prevention, warnings about dangerous activities are warranted. Proper warm-up before athletics is advised, as is knowledge of potential problems from contact sports (i.e., how to hit in football without hurting your opponent with an ACL tear or similar injury). Behavioral considerations in treatment of MSS disorders usually involves ensuring compliance with any prescribed medications or therapy regimens, as well as refraining from activities likely to reinjure or worsen the conditions being treated.

Society

MSS conditions, particularly seemingly (relatively) innocuous things such as low back pain and repetitive motion injuries, are responsible for massive disruptions of the workforce and lost productivity every year, costing both employers and nations billions of dollars. This cost is felt in terms of absenteeism as well as additional health care expenses. Though many MSS conditions are not very amenable to prevention, those that are must be made a priority, with proper instructions for things such as wound care and the RICE regimen for strains/sprains made readily available. The greater percentage of the population that is informed of potentially dangerous situations and how to deal with them—resulting in faster and better treatment—the more that society and country can hope to save on health care costs. Likewise, patients need to know that it is always a good idea to see a doctor earlier rather than later, since this generally reduces health risks to the patient and the monetary burden of care that might not have been entirely necessary with earlier intervention.

Environmental risk

There may be certain cases in which environmental triggers such as chemical contaminants or other offending substances are suspected to be involved in the pathogenesis of a condition (i.e., multiple sclerosis), but for the most part solid evidence is lacking as to the exact nature of such precipitants. However, there are certainly industries, environments, and occupations that pose increased risks of developing one or more MSS problems. Such risk factors and causes may be physical, psychosocial, or both. Repetitive motion injuries are very common in those who work at computers, on assembly lines, or in any other monotonous role, as the same MSS components are repeatedly stressed without time for sufficient relaxation. Frequent breaks and more ergonomic work solutions definitely help mitigate this pathology. Certainly those working in inherently dangerous professions such as logging, fishing, construction work, and emergency personnel can expect to experience statistically more accidents, leading to more MSS disability. Knowledge of CPR and basic first aid is essential in such industries, as is proper instruction on safety practices. Serious athletes also need to follow strict preparation and recuperation regimens, to minimize injuries and reduce recovery time.

Gender and ethnicity

With the exception of certain diseases such as lupus, which is highly prevalent in black women, most MSS disorders (or those that affect the MSS) do not carry inherent racial or ethnicity-based risks (aside from the fact that different types of people may engage is more or less risky activities, as dictated by local culture). In terms of gender, there may be a tendency for women to develop or report symptoms earlier than men, though this is not certain. Women do tend to develop certain conditions more than men (lupus, fibromyalgia, dermatomyositis), but the opposite is also true for men with different disorders (Reiter's syndrome, traumatic fractures, inclusion body myositis). To the extent that men are more likely to be involved in jobs and activities that carry greater exposure to inherent risks of injury, there is more likelihood that they will encounter such issues, especially those that are traumatic in nature. Also, a condition such as osteoporosis is found earlier and more often in women, because of skeletal atrophy's relation to the post-menopausal decrease in protective estrogen. There are definitely other exceptions to these rules, which are disease-specific and numerous, and therefore outside the scope of this series. In general, it can be inferred that any disease process seen more regularly in certain ethnicities and genders will naturally increase the MSS involvement that accompanies many such systemic disorders.

Respiratory System

Embryology of the airways and lungs

Like many other epithelial organs, the lungs bud off the archenteron. The respiratory diverticulation begins early, around the end of the third week of gestation. Faulty separation from the esophagus results in various types of tracheoesophageal fistulas (TEF). The primordia of the airways form a mesodermal coat that gives rise to the tracheobronchial cartilages, the smooth muscle cells of the bronchioles, and the vascular tree of the lungs, including the bronchial arteries. After separating into three principal right buds and two main parenchymal buds on the left, the lung buds undergo around 23 subsequent divisions until the normal end of pregnancy at 40 weeks. By the sixth month of gestation, only about three-quarters of these divisions have occurred. Therefore, even a week or 10 days of extra gestational time will materially increase the survival chances of a premature baby on anatomic grounds alone. A normal baby will have around 10 to 20 million alveoli, but these are not all mature air sacs, with some of them being relatively thick-walled and more acinar in character. Considerable lung maturation occurs in the first few years of life. Adults have about 500 million alveoli in each lung.

Pulmonary maturation

It is critical to understand that the alveoli are slaves to the law of Laplace, which states that the tension in the wall of a bubble or balloon is inversely proportional to the radius. Think of trying to inflate a party balloon—very difficult at first, then suddenly very easy. The alveoli are like these balloons. If water, with its extremely high surface tension, were to enter the alveoli, it would drag them to a smaller radius and therefore close them to air. Key to normal lung function is the production of pulmonary alveolar surfactant. This is a complex of proteins and lipids (including phospholipids and dipalmitoylphosphatidylcholine, with some cholesterol) that serves to lower surface tension by embedding the hydrophilic heads of the molecules in the aqueous surface and keeping the hydrophobic tails towards the air surface. Therefore, most prenatal pulmonary maturity testing is addressing the ability of the baby's type II alveolar cells (surfactant is also made by bronchiolar Clara cells) to manufacture this set of chemicals. Surfactant is stored in lamellar bodies in the secretory cells, and although it is possible to count these directly in amniotic fluid specimens, determination of the lecithin to sphingomyelin ratio is more popular. LS ratios of 1:1 suggest severe immaturity of fetal lungs, and ratios in the range of 2:1 are considered normal for term or near-term babies. Fetal lungs do not even begin to make pulmonary alveolar surfactant until the 20th week of gestation, and the LS ratios change sharply near term.

Changes that occur in the lung at the moment of birth

Just before birth, the airways are full of amniotic fluid. Much of this is expelled by the pressure exerted in the birth canal and a small amount of residual intra-alveolar fluid is absorbed over the next day or so. The first few breaths aerate much of the lung tissue, dramatically dropping its vascular resistance. This allows an alternative pathway for blood flow in the pulmonary artery. Before birth, the ductus arteriosus conveys the bulk of pulmonary arterial flow (recall that this is basically highly oxygenated umbilical venous blood) into the aorta. The ductus ordinarily remains open under the influence of maternal prostaglandin E2. Production of bradykinin by the postnatal infant lung speeds ductus closure by stimulating smooth muscle cells in the wall of this channel. Ductus closure can therefore be facilitated by use of certain nonsteroidal prostaglandin inhibitors or retarded by the administration of prostaglandins when necessitated by other congenital cardiovascular problems. The remnant ductus is the ligamentum arteriosum, a sturdy connective tissue band that is a frequent site of aortic tears in acceleration injury of the thorax.

Paranasal sinuses

The paranasal sinuses are largely absent in the newborn, or, at most, they are primordial blind pouches. Their gradual evolution during early childhood is closely correlated with the eruption of the primary and secondary dentition. At birth, the cranium constitutes approximately half of the face, with the mid-face and mandibular structures making up the other half. The addition of teeth and the rapid "invasion" of the sinus cavities into the facial bones change this geometry, such that by adolescence, the cranium amounts to only about one-third of the frontal view of the head, with the maxillary and mandibular portions equally sharing the remainder. Probably the most variable air-containing space is the frontal sinus, which can remain tiny or blossom into a pair of cavities covering most of the forehead. Because it drains inferiorly, beneath the middle turbinate, it is less likely to become occluded or infected. The ethmoids are loosely grouped into anterior, middle, and posterior air cells, and the drainage is through small ostia below the middle turbinate for the anterior group, and above it for the rest of the ethmoid air cells. Because the air cells are small and may effectively share ostia, ethmoid sinusitis may become confluent, at least on one side. The large maxillary sinuses, or antra, are intimately related to the apices of the maxillary teeth, and may therefore be involved in dental problems. Additionally, the roof of the maxillary sinus is the floor of the orbit, so "blow-out" fractures of the maxilla lead to inferior prolapse of the orbital contents. The ordinary problem facing the maxillary sinus is that its ostium is high, draining also below the middle turbinate and leading to pooling of secretions from gravity. Finally, the paired but functionally confluent sphenoid sinus(es) drain superiorly, above the variably developed superior turbinate. The sphenoid cavity provides an excellent conduit for trans-nasal, trans-sphenoidal approaches to the pituitary gland. The carotid arteries indent the lateral walls of this sinus. Sinuses lighten the skull and provide unique characteristics to the voice.

Structures that a bronchoscopist would see

The vermillion border is the junction of the redder tissue of the lip with the skin of the face. Passing over the gingiva and the incisor teeth, and then along the midline over the median raphe of the tongue, the practitioner would come to the paired valleculae, small pouches that can (uncommonly) trap foreign bodies. The epiglottis comes into view, and to either side of this are the slender pockets known as the pyriform sinuses, perfectly shaped to trap toothpicks or fish bones. Advancing the bronchoscope over the epiglottis, the practitioner will see first the false vocal cords, pink membranes overlying the glistening white "V" of the true vocal cords. Singer's nodules might be noted here. Note that the "V" points anteriorly, with the arytenoid cartilages visible as the posterior, knobby anchors of the vocal cords themselves. An awake patient who is asked to phonate will use the vagus innervation to tense the vocal cord by rotating the arytenoids, and will also move these cartilages laterally during inspiration and medially during attempted swallowing. The endoscopist advances the tube through the glottis into larynx, past the cricoid cartilage and into the trachea proper, with its vaulted ceiling of cartilage bands. The carina is reached, and it is apparent that the right mainstem bronchus is a more "direct shot" into a lung than is the left mainstem bronchus; this is the reason that foreign bodies are about twice more likely to be found in the right lung. In either lung, foreign bodies are more common in the lower lobes than in upper lobes. Only a few percent of aspirations result in bilateral lodgment.

Segmentation of the lungs

The right and left lung are similar, but not identical. There are three lobes of the right lung: superior, middle, and inferior with similarly named primary bronchi. The left lung has only superior and inferior lobes, with the lingual segment of the upper lobe being analogous to the right middle lobe. On the right, the 10 segments are:
- superior (upper) lobe – apical, anterior, and posterior segments
- middle lobe – medial and lateral segments
- inferior (lower) lobe – superior and anterior, posterior, medial and lateral basal segments.

The left lung has only 8 segments:
- superior (upper) lobe – apico-posterior, anterior, superior, and inferior lingual (variably, lingular)
- inferior (lower) lobe – superior, lateral, anterior, and posterior segments.

The oblique fissure separates upper and lower lobes on both sides, and the transverse fissure separates the upper from the middle lobe on the right. This anatomy is critical not only to the bronchoscopist, coming from within, but also to the radiologist and the surgeon, considering the lung either as a whole structure or in CT/MRI slices. Because the fissures are covered with visceral pleura, fluid can weep from the parenchyma and accumulate in these spaces.

Respiratory cycle

Normal respiratory rate in an adult is around 12 breaths per minute, which means that the respiratory cycle is only 5 seconds long. As the leaves of the diaphragm (and/or accessory muscles of respiration) contract, intrapleural pressure is decreased. This causes air passively to enter the upper airways and pass into the trachea, but the air already in the airways was never completely expelled, and it is this residual gas mixture that is mixed with incoming room air. This mixing protects the lung to some extent from the drying effect of low-humidity air, or from very hot or cold gases entering the airway, but it also means that the mixture arriving at the alveolus will be moist and enriched in CO_2, and have somewhat less oxygen than ordinary room air. Inspired gases follow the pressure differential, lagging behind it only a bit. Therefore, in a 5-second cycle, it takes about 1 to 1.5 seconds to inhale. Inhalation follows a fairly sharp muscle contraction, but exhalation is largely passive and reliant upon body wall elasticity, the pressure of abdominal organs and their contents upwards on the diaphragm, etc. Thus, exhalation takes more time than inhalation, perhaps as long as 2 to 2.5 seconds. The effect is that there is short "dwell time" for gases in the alveoli, about 0.75 seconds, and that gas exchange must be very efficient. Even very thin layers of intra-alveolar fluid (cardiogenic edema, processes related to infection, drowning) materially diminish the effectiveness of this diffusion-based system. During slower respiration (breath holding, for example), increased contact time of the respiratory gas with the alveolar epithelium compensates for decreased volume of breathing. During rapid breathing, there is increased turbulence and better mixing of inspired with expired gases.

FEV$_1$

The amount of air a person can expel from the lungs in the first second of effort after a full inhalation is referred to as the FEV_1. The predicted value is a function of age, habitus, and gender, but typical values are around 3.5-4 L for men and somewhat less (around 3-3.3 L) for women. Often, the value reported is expressed as a percent of the nomographically predicted value for the individual. The test is commonly simplified as the ability to blow out a match held 30 cm or so from the face. Inability to do this indicates rather marked obstructive lung disease and a need for more formal evaluation. Additionally, the FEV_1 is often discussed in its relationship to the FVC. Typically, most of the volume, around three-fourths of the forced vital capacity, can be exhaled in 1 second. If this ratio is decreased, it is likely that the patient has obstructive lung disease, and if it is increased, then restrictive lung disease may have adversely affected lung compliance. Typical preoperative testing of patients with mild to moderate pulmonary compromise consists of bedside spirometry and a set of resting arterial blood gases. These two determinations may suggest ways to improve respiratory function in advance of surgery, childbirth, or other repetitive stresses such as dialysis.

Ventilation

Ordinary, quiet breathing follows the general pattern called a hysteresis loop: the same pressure-volume relationships happen over and over again. Calm breathing is different from maximal ventilation. First to be considered is the minute volume, simply the number of breaths per minute times the average, or tidal volume (TV). This is quite variable, but generally around 12 x 500 mL = 6 L. Dead space refers to the air in the nasal passages, trachea, and bronchi/bronchioles that does not participate in gas exchange, a volume ordinarily of about 100 to 125 mL. In a minute, the dead space ventilation is around 12 x 100–125 mL, or about 1.2 to 1.5 L. The amount reaching the alveoli is therefore around (6 L - 1.2 to1.5 L) 5 L. Now, it is impossible to exhale all the air in the lungs (try to!); the residual volume is called the residual volume (RV), normally around 1 L or just slightly more. At the end of a normal breath, about 1 additional liter of gas can be expelled from the lungs with effort; this is the expiratory reserve volume (ERV). The ERV added to the RV is called the functional residual capacity, a number around 2 L. In addition to a normal tidal breath, it is possible to forcefully inhale much more air, the inspiratory reserve volume (IRV), averaging from 2 to about 3.5 L. IRV + ERV + TV = VC, or vital capacity, typically between 3 and 5 L for adults. (Often this is referred to as the forced vital capacity [FVC].) Total lung capacity (TLC) is the sum of VC + RV; therefore, around 4 to 6 L. (Note that the dead space *volume* is rather low, but when multiplied by the respiratory rate, the dead space *ventilation* is a much larger number.)

Modern mechanical ventilator

Ventilators have undergone steady evolution since the days of the iron lung. (There are presently about 50 individuals in the United States relying entirely on this form of external, bellows-actuated ventilation, some for over half a century!) First, modern ventilators used in ICUs allow the F_IO_2, the inspired percent of oxygen, to range from room air (about 21%) to 100% oxygen. Next, a tidal volume is chosen, usually something in the range of 500-600 mL per breath (8-10 mL/kg body mass) for normal habitus adults. The rate of breathing can usually be set from about 6 up to 30 or so. Awake patients who are anxious or in discomfort will often over-breathe these set rates, a feature allowed by setting a "trip level" of a few centimeters of water negative pressure (in other words, just the beginning of a breath) to trigger a ventilator cycle. Sophisticated ventilators can be controlled for length of inspiration, inspiratory pause, inspiratory to expiratory ratio, and so on, but these settings are typically only used by pulmonary experts. Most ventilators do allow for CPAP (continuous positive airway pressure), or at least PEEP (positive end-expiratory pressure), both measures designed to thwart the development of alveolar collapse. Many hospitals have many patients on ventilators at any one time. Power failures, such as those that occurred in New Orleans during Hurricane Katrina, necessitate crude hand bag (Ambu) ventilation for hours or even days on end.

Ventilation-perfusion match

Unlike a dog, for example, humans are both a vertical and a horizontal animal. But like a dog, human spend a portion of their horizontal time lying on the right side and a portion on the left. The erect posture presents a challenge, in that blood from the right ventricle must be pumped all the way to the apex of each lung at an average systolic pressure of only 35 to 40 torr. Of course, cephalad movement of intravascular fluid is assisted somewhat by negative forces during inspiration, but these same forces also draw blood into the lower portions of the lung. The result is that while upright, the top-most portions of the lungs are underperfused compared with the lower segments. The same thing is true for the upper-most areas of lung tissue while a person is prone, supine, or in right or left lateral decubitus position, but the differences are much less because the distance is much less between extremes. The same propositions hold for air, but in reverse. The upper segments are hyper-aerated as compared with lower segments, no matter what the position, with the effect being most noticeable while upright. This is somewhat wasteful, but necessary to achieve the type of mobilities and capacities that humans have. With 5 L of cardiac output, on average, and effective minute ventilation also of about 5 L, there is a 1:1 ventilation: perfusion (V/Q) match, but this is only an average. Some tissue areas are hypoperfused and some are hypoventilated. This becomes much more important when considering hospitalized patients and their typical semi-recumbent position in bed. In space medicine, there are no gravitational effects, so these effects are eliminated, whereas in diving medicine, there is both gravity and super-atmospheric pressure on the body wall to consider.

Gas exchange in the alveoli

The gas delivered into the alveoli is not the same gas that is inspired. It is easiest to understand gas distribution by considering the various compartments in a table. Recall that inspired water vapor varies between 0% at high altitude or in a desert to about 3.5% right over the ocean, but a typical value is about 1% of total volume and 1% of total atmospheric pressure according to Dalton's Law of Partial Pressures. Fully saturated air at 37°C is about 6.5% water, so the partial pressure of water is 0.065 x 760 torr = 49 torr. Also recall that argon constitutes almost 1% of the atmosphere.

	inspired	tracheal	initial alveolar	exhaled alveolar
pressure, torr	760	760	760	760
pN_2, torr	588	557	557	557
pO_2, torr	156	150	<u>120</u>	110
pCO_2, torr	0	0	<u>30</u>	40
pH_2O, torr	8	46	46	46
pAr, torr	8	7	7	7

Because air is not completely exhaled, there is mixing of incoming air and exhaled air in the trachea and bronchi. The degree of mixing depends on respiratory rate. Once the air is humidified, the ratios of oxygen to nitrogen remain the same, but the percent and therefore the tension of each falls because a new gas has been added to the mix (water vapor). The same thing happens again when CO_2 becomes a new component of the gas mixture. Thus, the numbers underlined in the initial alveolar column are approximate and reflect partial mixing of inhaled air with exhaled air. Only about 30% of the initially available oxygen is extracted in a single breath. This allows a rescuer in CPR to blow their own exhaled but still oxygen-rich air into a person with respiratory arrest. (Note

- 207 -

that the values will vary somewhat with the admixture of inert gases such as helium, with the administration of anesthetic gases, and when there is substantial hypercapnia.)

Histology of the upper airway

The nares are lined by hair-bearing skin that transitions into respiratory epithelium; the respiratory mucosa is ciliated pseudostratified columnar epithelium from the nasal passages far down into the bronchi. (The oral cavity is lined by stratified squamous non-keratinizing epithelium. The true vocal cord, but NOT the false vocal cord, is also covered by stratified squamous epithelium, but it is usually non-keratinizing.) Goblet cells dot the mucosa and serve the function of secreting mucus. Numerous glandular arrays lie in the subepithelial region known as the lamina propria; these also secrete mucus and immunoglobulins such as IgA. In the trachea, obvious cartilage rings are noted against a connective tissue background with small vessels and slips of vestigial skeletal muscle passing between rings. In the bronchi, the histology is very similar, except that the muscle bundles disappear completely.

Histology of the lung

Normal lung is salmon pink in color and has the consistency of a sponge or foam covered by a membrane (the visceral pleura). Pressure from retractors converts this fluffy tissue to a condensed red-purple mass with a rather dense feel. As the bronchioles get smaller, there is a gradual transition from pseudostratified columnar epithelium to columnar epithelium. Clara cells, which secrete surfactant, are noted in small bronchioles. Bronchi have cartilaginous rings (often incomplete) and elastic fibers supporting them, but they are not actively contractile. Bronchioles, however, have smooth muscle and elastin fibers surrounding them. Alveolar sacs vary in size, but typically they are around 40-60 microns. They are composed of flattened type I pneumocytes, plump type II pneumocytes (which make surfactant), and alveolar macrophages. Although the connective tissue matrix of the lung is not conspicuous, it consists of collagen and elastin fibers, which give it an intrinsic shape and the ability to recoil after expansion, respectively. There are also innumerable capillaries and arterioles and venules. On some sections of lung, arteries and veins of the systemic bronchial circulation are visible. The visceral pleura covering the lung consists of several layers of cells resembling fibroblasts covered by a single layer of mesothelial cells connected by tight junctions and resting upon a basement membrane. They have numerous microvilli and secrete lubricating chemicals such as hyaluronic acid. Vimentin and keratin are identified in visceral pleura. The important difference seen in the parietal pleura is stomata, which are open-ended lymphatic capillaries, in principle. These permit the resorption of pleural fluids and specifically underlie the ability of the pleural cavity to absorb spinal fluid when ventriculopleural shunting is performed.

Diffusing alveolar oxygen

First, there is a thin layer of surfactant through which the gas molecules must pass, followed by the inner cytoplasmic membrane of the alveolar cell, a thin layer of cytoplasm, the inner cytoplasmic membrane of the alveolar cell, a shared basement membrane, and an additional three such layers for the capillary endothelial cell. Next there is a very thin layer of blood plasma, and finally the erythrocyte cell membrane. Very small disturbances of this relationship, such as layering on a thin coating of alveolar edema fluid in congestive heart failure, can materially affect gas diffusion dynamics.

Oxygen-carrying capacity of normal, fetal, and variant hemoglobins

Hemoglobin is a metalloprotein consisting of four protein units (two alpha and two beta subunits for adult hemoglobin A), each of which binds an iron. There are four porphyrin ring complexes. The iron atom, and specifically Fe^{+2}, is the site of oxygen binding, and each hemoglobin molecule can bind up to four oxygen molecules. Upon binding, two things happen: iron is temporarily oxidized to Fe^{+3} while molecular oxygen becomes a superoxide (O_2^{-1}) species, and there is a stereo-conformational shift in the hemoglobin molecule itself. Binding of the first oxygen molecule morphs the other three molecules in the tetramer into shapes that make oxygen ligation yet more favorable. The oxygen-carrying capacity is between 1.35 and 1.4 mL O_2 per gram of hemoglobin A. In the fetus, the problem is to extract oxygen from already highly oxygenated, bright red blood. Hemoglobin F, the fetal form, has a higher affinity for oxygen than does Hgb A, so in essence, the fetus is able to "strip" oxygen from the mother. Because of the intimate association between protein chain shape and binding to the iron atom in heme, disturbances of oxygen binding may be seen in the thalassemias and in sickle cell disease (genetic conditions causing malformation of the globin chains), although in most cases the oxygen saturation is normal or nearly so. Hemoglobin binds CO at 250 times the oxygen affinity and at the same site as oxygen; the only treatment is to attempt to force O_2 onto the hemoglobin molecule by hyperbaric means. Carbon dioxide also binds to hemoglobin, but not at the central heme site; about 10% of blood CO_2 is carried this way. NO is also bound to the protein units in heme. Around 1% to 1.5% of all oxygen in the blood is simply dissolved in plasma. It makes little sense to give oxygen to a normal person because their hemoglobin is already fully saturated, and any change in the dissolved plasma portion is insignificant.

Control of respiration by the central nervous system

Respiration is under voluntary control at times, invoking higher cortical control than is usually the case. Although insults to the higher brain centers, such as a thalamic hemorrhage, produce struggling, tachypneic efforts to breathe initially, survivors of such episodes typically have rather normal breathing patterns a few weeks later. In fact, even midbrain lesions do not affect breathing very much. Lesions at the pontine level may be associated with tachypnea and hyperpnea, and very rarely, there is an inspiratory catch pattern, called apneustic breathing. Medullary lesions result in irregular and inadequate ventilator patterns, and lesions of the upper cervical spinal cord are associated with apnea and death if medical intervention is not immediate. Tumors of the roof plate of the fourth ventricle, such as medulloblastoma, rest upon the calamus scriptorius/obex region and can sometimes produce respiratory arrest with slight shifting of the tumor mass. The rare problem of Ondine's curse is a failure of central respiratory drive due to any number of brainstem problems; it can be congenital. Affected patients have fairly normal respiration when awake, but it becomes inadequate during sleep.

Carotid body and proximal aortic receptors

The carotid body is a tiny structure adjacent to the carotid bifurcation. It functions as a chemosensor, mainly detecting low blood oxygen levels, with less reactivity to CO_2, pH, and temperature. This is to be differentiated from the carotid sinus, a region of the vessel that senses blood pressure and vascular distension; surgeons usually inject lidocaine to block IX-X vasomotor reflexes, principally bradycardia and hypotension, when operating here. (Parenthetically, the author has performed several hundred carotid endarterectomies, and has never seen this structure; perhaps it is atrophic in the case of advanced local atherosclerosis.) The blood supply is from tiny regional branches of the carotid. Type I glomus cells are derived from neuroectoderm. Stimulation of these cells causes them to secrete a variety of compounds by exocytosis, including ordinary neurotransmitters, ATP, and more primitive chemicals such as substance P. They possibly act directly upon the type II, or sustentacular cells, since anatomists have had difficulty showing any direct connection with other nerve cells. At any rate, activity of these large cells leads to increased firing in the glossopharyngeal nerve; the cell bodies for these afferent fibers are located in the petrosal ganglion. The effect of lowered O_2 levels is an increase in the respiratory rate. Interestingly, respiration is not stimulated with high levels of CO as long as the plasma is oxygenated. The aortic chemosensors are similar, but they are scattered along the aortic arch and use the vagus nerve as the afferent structure.

Autonomic innervation

The trachea and bronchi contain sensory nerves that are mostly involved with coughing and associated airway sensation; some of them sense distension or distortion of the lung tissue. Sympathetic postganglionic fibers arising from the upper thoracic segments pass into mixed sympathetic/parasympathetic plexuses that lie anterior and posterior to the hilar structures. Sympathetic activation produces diminished glandular secretions in the bronchi and bronchioles, dilation of the airway, and constriction of pulmonary arterial beds. The parasympathetic innervation derives mostly from the vagus nerve; some ganglion cells are present in the nerve plexus, as well as pre- and post-ganglionic parasympathetic fibers. The effects of activation of these nerves are exactly the opposite of sympathetic stimulation. It is known that lungs of experimental animals that have been autotransplanted, thereby interrupting their nerve supply, cannot develop neurogenic pulmonary edema.

Hypoxic drive

Carbon dioxide has a molecular mass of 44 g/mole, whereas molecular oxygen has a mass of only 32 g/mole. Gases diffuse in inverse proportion to the square root of their mass, so CO_2 diffuses about 85% as fast as oxygen in a vacuum. However, gases in the body also diffuse in direct proportion to their solubility in water. Carbon dioxide is about 24 times as soluble in water as oxygen (think of a soft drink), so, overall, the actual diffusing rate in the lung is about 20 times that of oxygen. Patients with chronic obstructive lung disease hypoventilate; they are initially somewhat hypercapnic but develop renal compensation for it. They later become hypoxemic. These changes are gradual and have the effect of resetting the respiratory centers in the brain. Central respiratory triggers become less sensitive to the CO_2 levels and therefore ventilation becomes more dependent on the blood oxygen level. Although it is tempting to give patients in respiratory distress large amounts of oxygen on the theory that it "can't hurt, might help," it indeed can hurt by completely turning off the hypoxic drive to inhale. Although worsening hypoventilation is the likely effect, complete respiratory arrest can occur.

Cellular lung injury

The adult lung represents a complicated juxtaposition of epithelium upon vascular endothelium—or, alternatively, endoderm lying adjacent to mesoderm. Any number of factors external to the organism, particulates, infections, radiation, toxic fumes, etc, may injury the endothelium. Further, host factors such as age and genetics produce changes in pulmonary tissue. All of these insults are accompanied by a varying degree of macrophage and cytokine activation. Essentially, the calculus is as follows: If there is only mild inflammation and if enough epithelial cells survive, they will repopulate the basement membrane and connective tissues and establish something close to the original alveolar anatomy. If inflammatory processes predominate, then interstitial scarring and pulmonary fibrosis ensue. If the basement membranes and intrinsic lung architecture are destroyed, the alveolar pneumocytes cannot replenish alveolar anatomy, and against a damaged connective tissue framework, emphysematous regions develop.

Lymphatic drainage

Superficial lymphatic channels pass along the fissures of the lung, but end up draining centrally into the deep nodes along the bronchi and near the hilum of each side. Bronchoscopists separate the central nodes into groups for descriptive purposes. Enlargement of the subcarinal group leads to the appearance of a widened carina. Some authors have suggested that although drainage patterns are mostly unilateral, involvement of the right lower peribronchial group may signal either right or left lung problems as the source. A pair of tracheobronchial lymph ducts pass cephalad on each side, picking up contributions from the esophagus. Each drains into the jugular-subclavian junction of its side, or variably into the right accessory thoracic duct or into the thoracic duct on the left. Fetal/newborn lymphangiectasia is a severe developmental problem that severely impairs lung function at birth. Cystic hygroma (focal lymphangiectasia) is a rare problem in children, often necessitating surgical drainage. Adult lymphectasia is almost always due to occult carcinomatous blockage of lymphatic vessels.

Upper respiratory tract flora

Diphtheroids, staphylococci, and streptococci typically inhabit the anterior parts of the nasal passageways. In doctors and nurses, there is frequent colonization with MRSA due to occupational exposures; nasal mupirocin salve placed in the nares may discourage these organisms. In more posterior regions of the throat, *Streptococcus pneumoniae* and various strains of meningococcus are typical pathogenic residents. Almost everyone carries at least 1 or 2 strains of *Neisseria meningitidis* and persons coming from a different geographic region (Boy Scouts in an encampment, troops bivouacked together, etc) bring new strains whose virulence may exceed host defensive abilities. For this reason, meningococcal vaccine is recommended for students leaving for college. A new variant of *Bordetella pertussis* has come on the scene recently, leading to whooping cough outbreaks in adolescents and adults properly immunized against older strains of the organism. *Haemophilus influenzae* is a less frequent resident in the throat these days due to almost universal immunization in early childhood. The status of the dentition determines whether crypt-dwelling bacteria will be recovered during routine cultures. The normal mucociliary elevator functions in the trachea and proximal bronchi render the lower respiratory tract essentially sterile. All manner of organisms, including amoebas and water-dwelling organisms, are drawn far into the lower airways during near-drowning. Intubation gives any opportunistic organism a 7- or 8-mm wide superhighway to the deeper lung structures.

Immune defenses of the pulmonary system

Adult lungs present between 70 and 100 m^2 of delicate tissue to the atmosphere, in comparison with about 1.7 m^2 for the much tougher integument. There must be a balance between reacting to foreign antigens sufficiently to deal with them protectively, but not to such a degree as to interfere with respiratory function. The mucociliary elevator, which is rendered useless by cigarette smoke, is now known to be stimulated by the release of NO from pulmonary capillaries. Immunoglobulin A is a regular component of tracheobronchial secretions. Alveolar macrophages probably have the ordinary assignment of reacting to bacteria, viruses, and microparticulates in the lower airways; encapsulated bacteria such as *Klebsiella* can gain footholds because the macrophages cannot digest the slime coats of the organisms. Both T and B lymphocytes are resident in the lung interstitium.

Polymorphonuclear granulocytes are normally absent from the alveoli, but large numbers can be recruited in response to infections. The other granulocytes, eosinophils, and mast cells, and to some extent basophils, are normal cellular constituents of the lung; they are extremely important in allergic disease and in the component of anaphylaxis involving the lung.

Chest radiograph

Radiologists develop a systematic approach to reading a chest radiograph. It is important to remember that besides the heart and lungs, portions of the neck, the clavicles, the shoulders, the chest wall, the diaphragm, and portions of the upper quadrants of the abdomen are visible, as well as numerous monitoring or therapeutic devices, such as pacemakers and their wires, NG tubes, ET tubes, central IV lines, and the like. Also, a breast shadow may be missing in mastectomy patients. Many radiologists develop a paradigm wherein the peripheral structures are first examined in some definite and repetitive order: left before right or vice versa, usually upper structures before lower. This helps them avoid missing important findings that would not be sought out on a radiograph of the chest. A good place to start with pulmonary findings is to begin in the trachea, noting the position of an ET tube, if there is one, air in the mainstem bronchi, the development of air bronchograms in the case of consolidative processes, or the sometimes subtle evidence of air trapping. The hilar width is noted, as well as any lymph node enlargement, distortions around the aorta, or masses in the thymic region. Next, there is orderly examination of the parenchyma of each side, looking for atelectatic or pneumonic areas, nodules, Kerley B lines suggestive of heart failure, and the like. The appearance of the pleural spaces and the costophrenic angles is examined, along with the domes of the two hemidiaphragms. Finally, attention is directed to the cardiac shadow, and this is most conveniently thought of in terms of the circulatory pattern of blood entering the chest: sequentially, inferior vena cava and superior vena cava, right atrium, right ventricle, pulmonary outflow tract and pulmonary artery, then the lung small vessel beds, then pulmonary veins, left atrium, left ventricle, and finally the aortic shadow. Acceleration injuries often tear the aorta at the ligamentum arteriosum, obscuring the aortopulmonary window.

Spirometry

It is common for anesthesia services to request that a few basic spirometric parameters be established before putting a patient to sleep. The respiratory therapy department typically takes care of this assignment. Modern bedside spirometers are reasonably inexpensive and can produce attractive graphics for the patient's chart. Although the numbers are useful by themselves, they are even more helpful if there are older, baseline measurements against which to compare. The patient is usually told to take a few normal breaths, followed by the deepest breath possible. This air is then expired into the device as forcefully and as long as possible. The FEV_1 and FVC are determined and compared with nomograms for the patient's habitus and gender. The test mainly establishes how much obstructive lung disease is present; the degree is proportional to the diminution of the FEV_1/FVC below a ratio of 0.8. Because patients have trouble understanding and doing the test for a variety of reasons (weakness, confusion, somnolence from medications, etc), replicate runs are needed. Sometimes the test is repeated a few minutes after the administration of bronchodilating drugs such as beta-adrenergic agonists. When combined with a sample of arterial blood gases and determination of plasma bicarbonate levels, much is known about the baseline respiratory status of patients.

Arterial blood gas specimens

Arterial blood gases can be obtained from indwelling arterial catheters after the first small sample of blood (which is diluted with flush fluids and heparin) is discarded. The sample itself must be heparinized and submitted promptly for laboratory examination. Alternatively, radial artery puncture is fairly easy and safe (if Allen's test for palmar arch patency shows a competent ulnar artery). Occasionally femoral or other arteries must be accessed. Three determinations are made: pO_2, pCO_2, and pH. Respective normal ranges are 95-105, 38-42, and 7.35-7.45. Determination of hypoxemia is straightforward. The partial pressure of carbon dioxide is interpreted in light of the pH. Elevated CO_2 levels with low pH indicate a component of respiratory acidosis. High CO_2 levels with elevated pH indicate chronic respiratory compromise with compensatory metabolic alkalosis. Low carbon dioxide tensions with lower pH indicate a metabolic acidosis with attempts to correct the situation by hyperventilation. Finally, low CO_2 levels with higher pH demonstrate a respiratory alkalosis.

Respiratory quotient of 0.8

The RQ really has nothing directly to do with breathing; it is a term relating to metabolism. It refers to the number of carbon dioxide molecules produced by combustion of a foodstuff, divided by the number of molecules of O_2 used to do so. Pure carbohydrates have a value of 1.0, but other foods, including fats, have lower values, down to around 0.7 or so. Many respiratory physiology questions assume an RQ value of 0.8, and there is a broad misconception that this means that unequal volumes of gas are exchanged in the lung. This is not the case. If excess gas was absorbed, the alveoli would tend to collapse in each cycle of breathing, and if excess gas was liberated, the alveoli would swell if the glottis was closed, causing embarrassment of the pulmonary circulation. Instead, there is an (essentially) equimolar exchange of oxygen and carbon dioxide in the alveoli.

Oxygen extraction ratio (OER)

OER refers to the use of oxygen in tissues compared with the delivery to tissue, expressed as a fraction. Normal tissue OERs average 0.25, but tissues such as a tendon are well below this, while the brain (about 0.33-0.35, but perhaps as high as 0.42 in cortical regions) and heart (0.6) are far above this number. It is important to differentiate tissue hypoxia from hypoxemia. As an example, a patient with normal lungs but a hemoglobin of half-normal (say, 7 g/L) will have close to 100% saturation of the hemoglobin and probably a compensatory tachycardia to increase the circulatory rate of the "diluted" blood. Assuming for simplicity that the system only carries 0.5 times the oxygen it once did, then the heart will begin to dysfunction because it is below its tissue requirements, and the cortex of the brain will be next to suffer. This patient is not hypoxemic, but may have tissue hypoxia. This underlies the clinical thrust to optimize tissue blood flow and to transfuse below a certain hemoglobin level, in order to increase tissue delivery of oxygen. The lungs are working perfectly in these situations; it is the delivery system that is faulty, not the oxygen diffusion/capture mechanism.

Calculating the A-a O_2 difference

This refers to the alveolar-arterial difference in O_2 content, and it is principally used to estimate the amount of shunting and ventilation/perfusion (V/Q) mismatch in the lung. Normal intra-alveolar gas has a pO_2 somewhere around 110-120 torr, in contrast with a normal (optimal) arterial blood pO_2 around 100-105 torr. Simple subtraction yields a difference of about 10 torr. Values as low as 5 torr may be present in young, non-smoking normal people; the value tends to increase slightly with age. High values correlate with right-to-left shunting of blood, or expressed alternatively, only some of the blood volume gets saturated. This occurs commonly in the situation of ventilation-perfusion mismatch. The hemoglobin in blood flowing through over-ventilated lung cannot be saturated higher than 100%, whereas the hemoglobin passing through underventilated or unventilated lung certainly is not well saturated. The result is a low blood pO_2. (Alveolar oxygen tension is still considered to be normal for calculation purposes, but this is untrue because it is only normal in the normally ventilated air sacs.)

Airway emergencies

Perhaps only uncontrolled hemorrhage exceeds airway issues in terms of terror for the physician. The causes for sudden airway compromise are many: aspiration of food, vomitus, or foreign bodies, trauma to the face or throat, infections such as quinsy (peritonsillar abscess), tumors, dislodgment of endotracheal or tracheostomy tubes the list goes on and on. Add to this acute allergic reactions and sudden CNS or cardiac events necessitating immediate artificial ventilation, and it becomes obvious that this process must be thought out well in advance. The Heimlich maneuver, consisting fundamentally of sudden abdominal compression, is widely credited with saving many lives by expulsion of a foreign body or food from the upper airway. As a general rule for children, their trachea is the diameter of their fifth finger. The rule of thumb for adults is about a 7 mm tube for small women, a 7.5 to 8 mm internal diameter tube for most adults, and an 8.5 mm ID tube for large men. Depending on the clinical situation (possible fractured C-spine or advanced spinal arthritis), it may not be possible to extend the patient's head very much. Then, too, internal distortions of the throat (swollen tongue, large adenoids, broken mandible, fractured larynx) may make identification of the glottis nearly impossible. Progression to a surgical airway must be considered if a patient's arterial oxygen saturation begins to slip below around 90% (correlating with a pO_2 of about 70-75 torr). A transverse skin incision for cricothyroidotomy is easiest and puts the operator in a capacious portion of the airway. Lower incisions may complicate placement of a tracheostomy because of bleeding from the thyroid isthmus. Large bore (12G, 14G needle) tracheostomy with high-flow oxygen administered through a catheter may buy some time and also gives the operator a clear pathway to the tracheal lumen. Literally seconds count in these often desperate situations. Once the airway has been established, it must be very firmly secured with tape or umbilical ties for several days, until it is no longer needed, or until some degree of epithelialization of the tract has occurred.

Virus infections of the upper airway

You are tired from studying for the Step I exam, worried, haven't been sleeping well, and now, just a few days before the test, you identify that annoying scratchy feeling in your throat, associated with a little malaise and just a hint of fever. "Oh no, not me, not now!" you think. Rhinovirus, influenza/parainfluenza viruses, coronavirus, adenovirus, and respiratory syncytial virus are the main agents causing the common cold. Viral attachment involves the intercellular adhesion molecule 1 (ICAM-1) receptor. As everyone knows, the symptoms will last several days, and they are more fatiguing and annoying than actually debilitating. The upper respiratory tract probably has a stereotypic response, releasing pro-inflammatory cytokines. Patients immunized against the seasonally prevalent strain of "the flu" may nonetheless develop attenuated cases of influenza because they are partially protected against a different antigen package. In this case, they may have an illness intermediate in severity between a mild cold and serious influenza. Nasty-tasting zinc interacts with the ICAM-1 receptor, possibly interfering with virus uptake and proliferation. Nasal decongestants such as oxymetazoline and phenylephrine help alleviate the stuffy nasal symptoms, but beware—rebound rhinitis medicamentosa occurs after about 3 days of receptor saturation, and then the patient is "addicted" to nose spray for a long time. The main medical issue with colds (apart from absenteeism from work and school) relates to their occurrence in patients who already have diminished lung function, neuromuscular problems such as multiple sclerosis or myasthenia gravis, or other generally sick persons. These individuals are much more likely to develop secondary bacterial infections of the upper or lower respiratory tracts, or both. Prophylactic antibiotics are to be considered, although their use is controversial.

Sinusitis

Infections of the sinuses are very common problems, more so in patients who smoke or use the nose for recreational drug absorption, or in those with other problems affecting the airways, such as allergies, prior facial injuries, tumors, and the like. Typical presentations include regional pain (variously described as headache or face pain); distinct feelings of fullness; nasal discharge, sometimes foul-smelling; fever; and malaise or other constitutional symptoms. Occlusion of the ostia of the paranasal sinuses in simple colds is common, and time plus decongestants are typically all that is required. In more complicated cases of bacterial sinus infections, the full complement of symptoms may develop, and sharp pain to palpation of the face is noted. Then, too, there is always the threat of meningitis from cephalad spread of infectious material either through emissary veins or as phlegmons from adjacent osteomyelitis. Skull radiographs are rarely used, but they are often diagnostic. CT scanning of the facial structures shows the degree of involvement of specific sinuses, but this modality is expensive. Cultures often show mixed flora; both gram-positive (staphylococcal and pneumococcal) and gram-negative (*Moraxella spp.*) organisms are common pathogens. Diabetic patients notoriously develop (and usually quickly die of) fungal sinusitis with *Mucor* species, an extremely aggressive problem requiring urgent surgical debridement and antifungal medications. For the majority of patients, appropriate oral antibiotics suffice, sometimes combined with decongestants, gentle lavage of the nasal passageways, and occasionally needle, endoscopic, or surgical drainage of pus under pressure.

Atelectasis

Atelectasis occurs when alveoli in a region of the lung collapse without being inflamed or infected; it is a purely mechanical process. This can be due to bronchiolar or bronchial obstruction, in which case the gases in the isolated segment are gradually absorbed. Much more commonly, it simply results from hypoventilation of a segment, either due to compression from external pressure (pleural effusions, masses in the abdomen pressing upwards) or from a combination of unchanging posture and inadequate respiratory excursions. Atelectasis is very common in hospitalized patients who hypoventilate because of sedation, pain, or conditions producing obtundation. Atelectasis typically occurs in multiple small (usually basilar) segments of the lung simultaneously. Auscultation discloses sounds variously described as crackling or rhonchi; they represent airways snapping open during the forceful inhalation that the physician has requested the patient to perform. Low-grade fever often accompanies uncomplicated atelectasis. Treatment includes incentive spirometry, frequent postural changes, coughing even though surgical incisions may ache, and ultimately walking about in the room on or the ward. Atelectasis is important because persistently collapsed segments of lung tend to become infected either hematogenously or from the tracheobronchial tree. In other words, atelectasis is the first step on the pneumonic path into the morgue. Additionally, there is V/Q mismatch in the atelectatic segments. This is one of many essentially preventable complications in everyday medical practice.

Viral pneumonia

Viral pneumonia is sometimes extremely virulent. In the pandemic that swept the world in 1918, now known to be due to H1N1 influenza virus, soldiers who felt only a mild illness at morning roll call were cyanotic by afternoon and dead before the next morning. Host defenses in young people, particularly, are very strong, which means that very substantial cytokine release occurs in the alveoli. This leads to pulmonary edema and even parenchymal hemorrhage. Viral pneumonias are not always this serious, but they tend to involve both lungs symmetrically. Treatment is largely supportive, although antiviral agents such as acyclovir (herpetic pneumonitis) or ribavirin (RSV) can be considered. Bacterial pneumonia usually is slower in onset, days as opposed to hours, and it more commonly affects those with preexisting lung disease or elderly patients. Aspiration underlies many cases, but some arise from COPD and bronchiectasis. The treatment consists of appropriate antibiotics based on sputum stains and culture results, and sometimes bronchoscopy to assist with opening of major airways.

Primary atypical pneumonia

Mycoplasma is the lead suspect in a mild to moderate case of pneumonia occurring in a healthy individual when the symptoms are both constitutional and pulmonary. Chronic productive cough occurs, but it is not necessarily the predominant feature of the disease. Low- to medium-grade fever, poor appetite, diminished energy levels, malaise, and myalgia may predominate, leading the physician initially to suspect a viral tracheobronchitis. The patient feels ill but seems paradoxically fairly well. Examination of the lung fields often discloses nothing specific. When the symptoms do not clear after a week or more, primary atypical pneumonia (PAP) must be considered. It is often lobar and the chest radiograph opacity may be strikingly dense and large. Empiric treatment with azithromycin or tetracycline usually results in fairly prompt resolution of symptoms. The idiomatic condition, PAP, is not to be confused with pneumonias caused by less common organisms. PAP is known as "walking pneumonia."

Pneumocystis infection in AIDS patients

This organism was previously classified as a protozoan, but recently it has undergone a taxonomic shuffle; it is now officially a ubiquitous fungus living permanently in the yeast form. Normal people have developed immunity to this organism, but the vicissitudes of HIV/AIDS reopen the doorway for infection. The organism produces interstitial inflammatory changes and severe hypoxemia. Confirmation via bronchoscopy is often needed, because the sputum is notoriously thick. The organism tends to clump together, which is more or less unique for pathogenic fungi. Polymerase chain reaction (PCR) may also be used to establish the character of the infection. These patients appear quite ill. Supplemental oxygen is always needed, and chemotherapy includes trimethoprim-sulfamethoxazole with a kitchen sink of possible simultaneously administered agents, including Dapsone (which is ordinarily used for leprosy) and the antimalarial drug primaquine. Steroids are usually coadministered to decrease treatment-associated inflammation. Other systems may be involved, including, rarely, the central nervous system (meningitis).

Coccidioidomycosis

Valley Fever is an airborne fungal disease. It lives in the desert soil in the American Southwest (think retirement communities like Prescott, Arizona, or Palm Springs, California). Under dry conditions, it is relatively dormant, but rains rejuvenate the fungus and it sheds spores into the air. These are inhaled and begin to establish infection as a rather pedestrian fungal pneumonia. Fever and cough are the nonspecific initial symptoms; muscle and joint aches and a skin rash signal something unusual to the astute clinician. Many cases are self-limited and patients do not see a physician. In some cases, the chest radiograph will show infiltrates, often in the upper lobes. Proof of infection from sputum cultures is ideal. The disease should be treated if the patient has persisting fever or constitutional symptoms because it can become invasive. An infectious disease expert should be consulted, since the antifungal regimen itself is toxic and poorly tolerated by some patients.

Histoplasmosis and blastomycosis

Histoplasmosis and blastomycosis are fungal diseases that begin as inhalation pneumonias. *Histoplasma capsulatum* is believed to be acquired mostly through exposure to soil or bird droppings containing the organism. Many cases are self-limited, leaving only a granulomatous mark on the chest radiograph. When pneumonia develops, it is nonspecific, with cough, low-grade fever, and malaise as the main symptoms. The aggressive form of the disease is associated with widespread dissemination. The author once performed craniotomy and cranial nerve/meningeal biopsy to establish an otherwise completely elusive diagnosis, later confirmed by antigen (histoplasmin) testing. Systemic antifungal drugs administered over long periods may be curative. Both cutaneous lesions and symptoms of fungal pneumonia occur in blastomycosis. The organism can sometimes be identified on sputum stains, and specific antigen testing is available as well. The yeast form of the fungus secretes a protein adhesin appropriately named BAD-1; this substance interferes with immune reaction to the fungus and it is considered to be a necessary virulence factor. In both diseases, lung biopsy, mediastinal lymph node biopsy, or other tissue specimens may be needed to establish a diagnosis. Both conditions are much more aggressive in HIV patients.

Pulmonary anthrax

Concerns about bioterrorism have rejuvenated interest in this almost-vanished disease. Rare exposures to the extremely infectious spores occur chiefly in persons who have used imported animal products or who have cared for or consumed affected animals. Person-to-person transmission, per se, does not occur; it is the spores that are contagious. A person may transmit spores on their clothing, in secretions from the deep, purple ulcers of cutaneous anthrax, potentially in vomitus or fecal material from the GI variety, and their entire body is a spore repository when they die of the disease. Extreme quarantine measures must be instituted under the guidance of senior infectious disease specialists and experts from the CDC. Pulmonary anthrax initially presents as nothing more than an aggressive community-acquired pneumonia. One differentiating feature is the appearance on chest radiographs of confluent mediastinal adenopathy. Confusion, dehydration, and vascular collapse can occur in less than a day. Early treatment with combined oral and antibiotic regimens, particularly ciprofloxacin, doxycycline, and penicillin, is required. A monoclonal antibody (raxibacumab) directed against a common component of both the edema toxin and the lethal toxin has just become available. Vaccination is preventative. Because of the rapid progression and high lethality of the disease, prophylactic treatment of persons possibly exposed is just as rigorous as treatment of those known to have the illness.

Legionnaires' disease

Unusual outbreaks of pneumonic illnesses due to *Legionella* species have been identified retrospectively as far back as the time of World War II. Cough, dyspnea, fever, and sharp constitutional symptoms arose in a group of older persons attending an American Legion bicentennial celebration in Philadelphia in 1976. The causative organism, a gram-negative, facultatively aerobic, intracellular pathogen, lives in moist soil and water. Inhalation from hotel lobby fountains, misting devices, and air conditioning systems of large buildings has been reported, with occasional illnesses being traced to potting soil, gardening, etc. Chest radiographs often demonstrate large pneumonic infiltrates with pleural effusions. A peculiar feature of the disease is that the pleural fluid collections often appear or enlarge after days of appropriate antibiotic (erythromycin) therapy. It is believed that pulmonary macrophages serve as the primary host cell for the invasive bacterium. Mortality rates are fairly high, as the disease preferentially affects elderly or immune-compromised persons. A less severe illness known as Pontiac fever is also traceable to *Legionella* spp. Proof of the diagnosis can be established in three ways: culture, identification of *Legionella* antigens in the urine, or a rise in antibody titers.

Tuberculosis (TB)

Like other smart bacteria, tubercle bacilli have developed considerable resistance to antibiotics over the past decades. Multidrug-resistant (MDR) and extensively drug-resistant (XDR) strains have emerged and they are both potential public health nightmares. The mainstay of treatment is a combination of isoniazid (INH) and rifampicin. The recommended dosage of INH is 5 mg/kg/day in adults and 10 mg/kg/day in children. INH is hepatotoxic, so patients taking this drug should avoid alcohol for the duration of treatment (months). Rifampicin may also be hepatotoxic; it is administered once a day in a standard 600 mg dose for ordinary-sized adults. Pyrazinamide in dosages of 20-25 mg/kg/day and ethambutol in doses of 15 mg/kg/day are usually added during the first few weeks of treatment. Pyrazinamide is also hepatotoxic and it can also cause arthralgias. Among these drugs, ethambutol has the unusual potential adverse effect of optic nerve damage. Directly observed therapy (DOT) means just what it says—either the patient comes to the clinic, 7 days a week, week after week to take the drugs under observation, or else the public health nurse goes to their house every day. Quarantine was recommended for recent XDR cases, but there is no applicable civil law to limit the movement of contagious patients; compliance is voluntary.

This is no quick or easy task. Screening for exposure with traditional purified protein derivative (PPD) skin testing involves intradermal inoculation of tuberculosis antigens and observation over 2 days to measure the degree of induration of the tissue. Patients who have never had any exposure to the TB bacillus have no reaction (but this is also true for patients who are anergic), whereas those with prior exposure develop various degrees of induration in rough proportion to how active the disease is. A person who was previously PPD negative and who now converts the test to positive presumptively has active tuberculosis. PPD evaluation requires reporting back at least once to a trained observer/reporter. Many of the patients who have TB are the least capable of keeping follow-up appointments or participating in complicated treatment plans. (Measurement of interferon-gamma release by white cells has recently become available as an expensive but faster alternative.) If active tuberculosis is suspected, several different morning sputum samples must be collected, stained with acid fast technique, and carefully examined for tubercle bacilli. The specimens are also sent to the reference laboratory (often a county lab in many metropolitan areas) for culture on special media such as Lowenstein-Jensen agar. Unfortunately, under ideal conditions, it still takes weeks for colonies to grow. Modern PCR techniques do allow earlier confirmation, but they are not in common use. A baseline chest radiograph is obtained. Treatment is begun while awaiting test results, and close contacts of the patient should be screened as well.

One need only go to great literature or famous paintings to learn of the malignant and chronically debilitating nature of TB. The disease is mostly spread by droplet inhalation from other affected humans, although certain strains can also be transmitted from animals to humans. It begins as a lung infection, typically in the upper lobes. In the vast majority of people, the waxy-coated bacilli are either destroyed by the immune system, or remain dormant in local lymph nodes. The radiographic appearance of a (usually calcified) tubercular nodule with an associated enlarged lymph node is called a Ghon complex. In individuals with poor cellular immunity, or perhaps just in unlucky normal patients, the disease begins to spread within the bronchial system; it will ultimately disseminate itself everywhere in the body. Night fevers, sweating, loss of weight, chronic cough, and hemoptysis all occur. In fact, torrential and terrifying endobronchial hemorrhage is the means of death in some tubercular patients. The infection can establish itself anywhere in the body: in a bone or joint, in the eye, or as a tuberculous abscess of the brain, or as disseminated miliary tuberculosis in the lung fields. HIV-positive patients are particularly likely to develop not only the primary disease, but every manifestation of it as well.

Lung abscess

Lung abscesses can develop from hematogenous sources, as would occur, for example, if a septic embolus lodged in a bronchial arteriole. Of course, almost all abscesses of the lung develop in the setting of pneumonia, and many are related to aspiration of bacteria from the mouth. Pus-filled alveoli and small bronchioles have rich arterial supply (albeit with low oxygen tension) and there is little tissue "counter-pressure" to serve as a containment force. The delicate background stroma of the pulmonary parenchyma is no match for aggressive, rapidly dividing bacteria, and it is not until more central bronchial and vascular structures are reached that any serious mechanical barrier to spread is encountered. Lung abscesses can contain more than one organism; anaerobes are common. Patients can be treated empirically with antibiotics that match the sensitivity profile of sputum aspirates or blood cultures. Needle drainage or placement of catheters into larger abscesses can be done under radiographic control, or, alternatively, some abscesses can be drained or at least sampled by needles passed through a bronchoscope. Resolution of large, solitary abscesses usually leaves a scar in the involved tissue, with some local bronchiectasis and parenchymal fibrosis.

Pleurisy

Pleurisy (almost no one uses the correct term, "pleuritis") is simply inflammation of the visceral pleura, the parietal pleura, or both. The parietal pleura has a considerable segmental sensory nerve supply, so any condition that irritates this membrane is likely to be painful. Patients describe aching, dull feelings, and sometimes sharp pain. Because inspiration is faster, it hurts more than expiration, and patients may demonstrate an "inspiratory catch" as the lung moves over the chest wall. This leads to splinting and diminished respiratory minute volume. It may be helpful occasionally to consider blocking several intercostal nerves with long-acting topical blocking agents, such as bupivacaine. Pleurisy is diagnosed by inspection and by auscultation (where the examiner hears a rub or squeak, similar to the sound produced by rubbing dry fingers together). A needle tap of the pleural space will usually demonstrate a thin, serosanguineous fluid that should be cultured for infectious processes and examined microscopically to rule out malignant cells. Many cases of pleurisy "just" represent pneumonic processes extending to the surface of the lung and resolve spontaneously when the infection is controlled.

Cat and dog dander

The family pet is a source of inhaled allergens, which fortunately affect a minority of people. Proteins known as Fel d I (from felines) and Can f I and d II (from dogs) are blamed for pulmonary irritation. Flakes of epidermis as well as proteins in animal saliva, tears, etc, all enter the "respiratory environment" and persist there for long periods of time, essentially only being diluted away by repeated cleaning, even after the animal has been removed from the home. (This is analogous to being able to detect cocaine on almost any US currency!) Rare individuals develop hives after being licked by a dog or cat. The proteins elicit immunoglobulin elevations in humans. Formal allergy testing is advisable.

Pollen

Palynologists (pollen experts) will tell you that those plants whose pollen is distributed on the wind (as opposed to insect or bird carriers) account for the majority of seasonal allergic complaints. Although this is a minor nuisance for most people, severely affected patients can be absolutely miserable and nonfunctional. Each microscopic grain of pollen contains numerous plant proteins as well as other structural features, such as complex carbohydrates and protective waxes. After initial exposures, patients manufacture mast cell–bound immunoglobulins that react to the seasonally inhaled particles, producing histamine release. The main treatment is antihistamine medications with the occasional additional need for nasal steroids. Cross-reaction between specific allergens may be noted. Certainly, patients with reactive airway disease or asthma are much more sensitive to pollens, which may trigger severe respiratory crises; they should carry epinephrine pens. Desensitization by controlled administration of proven allergens over long periods of time may be helpful in management.

Anthracosis

Coal dust is not soot or carbon black from a lamp, and it is not the same as the black tars collected by cigarette filters. Coal is a metamorphic stone, and anthracosis results from inhalation of this particulate debris, churned into very small pieces by high-speed drills used in the coal and adjacent stone trapping it. Some of the inhaled material contains silicates, so there is always a concomitant element of silicosis. Pulmonary alveolar macrophages ingest this material, secrete cytokines, and, ultimately being unable to digest the material, end up as masses of black, fibronodular tissue. Small emphysematous areas alternate with scarred regions, leading to a honey-combed arrangement of tissue with both obstructive and restrictive features on pulmonary testing. Note that city dwellers may have blackened lung tissue, but this is often more limited to the peripheral lymphatics; in other words, they are breathing nanoparticles of carbon, not stone dust.

Sarcoidosis

Sarcoid, or sarcoidosis, is an immune disorder with protean manifestations, but it is often first diagnosed as a pulmonary disease. The etiology remains elusive. There is some tendency to familial/ethnic clustering, but many environmental exposures remain on the list of possible causes. Noncaseating granulomas develop in the presence of bilateral hilar adenopathy. Initial vague constitutional symptoms provide little in the way of simplifying a differential diagnosis, and chest CT, bronchoscopy, mediastinoscopy, and node or lung biopsies may be needed to help establish a diagnosis. Monocytes, macrophages, and T-helper lymphocytes all participate in granuloma formation; increased levels of tumor necrosis factor alpha and gamma interferon have been documented. Many cases resolve spontaneously, or at least progress very slowly. Troublesome symptoms are sometimes, but not always, helped by oral steroid administration over fairly long periods. Sarcoid can progress to chronic interstitial fibrosis and it is fatal in 5%-10% of all cases.

Idiopathic pulmonary fibrosis

This is a diagnosis of exclusion. It is fairly difficult to think of and exclude every other possible cause of a gradually sclerosing lung condition. The primary pathology in this condition is proliferation of bland interstitial fibrosis affecting many areas of both lungs simultaneously. Patients in the second half of middle age complain of gradually worsening dyspnea. There is nothing specific on examination. Spirometry may show an increased FEV_1/FVC ratio, indicative of a restrictive component. Radiographs show streaky opacification of the lungs fields bilaterally, and CT of the chest is usually helpful in portraying the distribution of the honeycomb pattern. Interestingly, if the diagnosis is in question, pathologists often ask for open lung biopsy specimens, since transbronchial biopsies do not provide enough tissue for them to ascertain a pattern. There currently are trials of immuno-modifying agents, but lung transplantation is the more definitive therapy. Men and women are equally affected by this unusual and uncommon illness.

Reactive airway disease

This term often includes the concept of asthma, because the bronchioles in that condition are overreactive in comparison with normal individuals. The term encompasses unusual sensitivity to extremely cold air, or to single-breath exposure to irritants such as H_2S, molds or pollens, or even perfume. An occasional individual will develop sustained coughing with or without rhinitis and accompanying signs of a true allergic response. Laryngospasm requiring intubation is possible. As unusual as it may seem, certain individuals are severely affected by allergy to the vapors from cooked shellfish, possibly due to the inhalation of heat-stable invertebrate tropomyosin. In a similar vein, inhalation of peanut oil used in cooking may produce anaphylaxis in peanut-allergic persons. Reactive airway disease is therefore not exactly a diagnosis, but a description of symptoms induced by something that is inhaled.

Byssinosis

Byssinosis, a rare occupational respiratory disease, is also called "cotton lung" or brown lung disease. The lungs in byssinosis are not discolored, and there is little specific about the histology of the bronchial and pulmonary tissues in these patients. Any changes that have been advanced have been discounted as being due to coexistent factors such as cigarette smoking. One would expect pulmonary interstitial fibrosis from chronic dust exposure in cotton mill, hemp factory, and similar workers, but it is lacking. Byssinosis has also been called "Monday lung" or "holiday lung," since it seems to present its most severe dyspneic episodes on first returning to work after a few days of absence. Patients complain of chest tightness and difficulty breathing. The examination is usually fairly normal, but testing may show some obstructive component. Some studies have suggested that a soluble factor in the dust of certain plant products may release histamine. Other workers have suggested that endotoxin release from certain bacteria growing on cotton fibers might be to blame. At present, the nature of the condition remains elusive, although it is a definite occupational diagnosis and a real health concern. Affected persons should change jobs if possible.

Farmer's lung and silo-filler's disease

Silo-filler's disease develops after inhaling fumes from silage. Silage, meaning plant materials harvested within the last 3 weeks and stored in sealed facilities, undergo fermentation and liberate NO_2 gas, which is heavier than air. Exposure to high concentrations of this gas can incapacitate workers in a matter of minutes, whereas lighter exposures may result in mild illness days later. The gas forms nitric acid on contact with water vapor, so essentially this is an acid-vapor injury of the lung tissue. Acute pulmonary edema necessitating oxygen administration, steroids, and even ventilator support may occur. Farmer's lung is a constellation of dust and mold exposure problems experienced by agricultural workers. The term "allergic alveolitis" perhaps best summarizes the medical condition. The condition is principally a type III hypersensitivity disorder, with immune complex deposition in the lung occurring after repeated exposures to certain Actinobacteria (a group of Gram-positive bacteria) living on crops of any sort. Symptoms vary from mild and chronic to acute and asthma-like in presentation. Slow deterioration of lung function may occur, and it is fatal in some cases. Direct exposure must be discontinued; actually moving off the farm may be necessary.

Asthma

Having a child with asthma may resemble living under a mythological curse. The child has recurrent, terrifying, life-threatening episodes of severe dyspnea, leading parents to spend many an anxious night in the emergency department. There is certainly a genetic component to asthma, and most affected children have attendant allergies and skin rashes. Boys are more affected than girls. Asthma attacks may occur in the setting of ordinary viral illnesses, but more commonly, minor exposures to environmental contaminants such as smoke or pollen may unpredictably trigger an attack. For this reason, asthma is often included under the moniker of "reactive airway disease." Whatever the exact cause, the pathophysiology involves bronchiolar smooth muscle contraction leading to expiratory wheezing and air trapping: bronchospasm. The lungs show changes of chronic inflammation, including gland hyperplasia, basement membrane alterations, and a plethora of immune cells in high numbers. There is also excessive mucus production. Alternatively phrased, it is a dynamic but chronic obstructive lung disease. In fact, one of the diagnostic criteria involves the demonstration of material change in spirometric parameters over a few days. Management involves inhaled corticosteroids, such as beclomethasone, and sometimes long-acting beta agonists and immune response modifiers.

An asthma attack is frightening for the patient and health care professionals, and sometimes fatal. If prophylactic routines have been observed, this represents a breakdown in attempted therapy and a need to step up the intensity of interventions. Calm breathing is difficult in this alarming situation, but quiet breathing of warm, humidified air may help and indeed may abort progression of the attack. Albuterol, a short-acting beta-2 agonist, is administered via "rescue inhaler" in metered doses. This drug has replaced epinephrine, which could be used as an alternative in an emergency. Attacking the opposite side of smooth muscle physiology, anticholinergic muscarinic blocking drugs may be tried. Oral or intravenous steroids are usually administered at this time as well. The symptoms the patient is experiencing are probably as good an indicator of success of treatment as arterial blood gases or spirometric studies. Although the problem is in the small airways, in certain rare cases, chemical paralysis and tracheostomy are life-saving when all else has failed.

> ➤ **Review Video:** Asthma and Allergens
> *Visit **mometrix.com/academy** and enter **Code: 799141***

Adult respiratory distress syndrome (ARDS)

ARDS is a constellation of findings, rather than a specific condition. The general setup for developing ARDS is as follows: An older patient has had 1 or more physiological stresses over the prior few days, such as a broken hip with surgery, or a documented septicemia with a gram-negative organism, or perhaps a substantial burn. Gradually it becomes apparent that the patient has lung trouble of some sort; the patient has developed a shallow tachypnea, is febrile, and is confused. (Sounds like pulmonary embolism? Good, but not this time.) Auscultation of the chest reveals some rales and crackles that were not there half a day ago. A chest radiograph is obtained, and it shows bilateral basilar infiltrates. By the time someone decides to put a pulse-oximeter on the patient, or to obtain blood gases, they are almost in respiratory crisis. Intubation follows.

Placement of a pulmonary wedge catheter shows that the patient is not fluid overloaded. They are difficult to ventilate, requiring higher than expected pressures and PEEP, and the A-a O_2 difference is marked. Steroids are administered, with no immediate effect noted. Institution of broad-spectrum antibiotics after obtaining blood cultures is probably the most important step directed at the origin of the problem. The mortality rate is very high, with multisystem organ failure being a common cause of death. The underlying pathology is usually overwhelming sepsis

Management of breathing in an acute quadriplegic patient

The phrenic nerve fibers arise principally at spinal cord levels C3, 4, and 5. Patients who damage the cord at or above these levels have immediate respiratory muscle paralysis and are instantly *in extremis*. They require immediate and expert airway management, and, specifically, they must undergo intubation without significantly extending the neck, because the spine is presumptively unstable *and* there is some chance that the cord injury may recover spontaneously; don't make it worse. Ventilatory support will be needed. Persons who damage the cord below this level may nonetheless develop respiratory impairment in several ways. Injured cord tissue swells, and ascending edema of just a centimeter or so may cause significant respiratory impairment. Increasing dyspnea in such a patient suggests a need for airway management before it becomes an emergent problem. Hematomyelia, or hemorrhage into an area of damaged cord tissue, may cause a similar phenomenon. Atelectasis begins immediately; aggressive lung physiotherapy is indicated if the patient can cooperate. Frequent turning to drain secretions is needed. Early mobilization in halo devices or early surgical stabilization of the spine diminishes the chances of pneumonia. Finally, these patients are at substantive risk for pulmonary embolism due to limb paralysis, so prophylactic low-dose subcutaneous heparin administration and external compression of the legs is absolutely indicated.

Pulmonary oxygen toxicity

The only element more electronegative than oxygen is fluorine. Oxygen in molecular form is a very strong oxidizer, other forms such as singlet oxygen (O^0), peroxides (O^{-1}), superoxides (O_2^{-1}), and ozone (O_3) exist at normal physiological conditions. At one time, the Earth had an atmosphere that was as much as 35% oxygen, but all modern mammals have evolved in times when the percentage of O_2 was very close to its present level. Oxygen toxicity is not observed with administration of excess oxygen below about 40%; atelectasis is encouraged, however, because the oxygen is rapidly cleared from alveoli, lowering their volume. Long-term administration of oxygen at levels over 40%-45% at normal atmospheric pressure hyper-oxygenates the tissues to some extent, but it is probably not hazardous over shorter periods of time (12-24 hours). In normal persons, exposure to these levels at ambient pressure may lead to cough or unpleasant airway sensations. Exposure to higher concentrations at high pressures occurs in ventilated patients and in hyperbaric medicine (therapeutic and diving). Oxygen causes a chemical alveolitis, which develops into pulmonary edema. In premature infants who are ventilated for weeks to months, it leads to bronchopulmonary dysplasia. Small, individual hyperbaric chambers are used to treat diving decompression, but also chronic nonhealing wounds, synergistic gangrene, and other aggressive infectious processes. Here, it is only the patients who are at risk for pulmonary oxygen toxicity. Some civilian and military facilities have large (operating-room size) tanks where hyperbaric states can be created. Medical and nursing personnel who are exposed to these conditions, along with their patients, may develop oxygen toxicity. Besides the pulmonary problems, affected persons can develop ocular and CNS problems, including seizures.

Chlorine gas

Molecular chlorine, Cl_2, was used against (mostly Canadian) troops in World War I. Although gas warfare is illegal under international law, there is concern about its use by terrorists, because railroad tank cars full of liquid chlorine routinely sit on spurs adjacent to metropolitan water treatment facilities. The most likely case to be seen in the emergency department relates to industrial, water purification, and swimming pool use. The practice of putting pump motors and chlorine tanks in pits adjacent to swimming facilities makes serious exposure a real risk, because the gas is heavier than air. Chlorine gas is somewhat soluble in water, which reduces its immediate irritant effects in the upper airways and perpetuates inhalation. The gas combines with water to produce both hypochlorous and hydrochloric acid. It is believed to induce oxygen-free radical formation, but the mechanism is not clear. It is a strong oxidizing agent in its own right, however. Symptoms include airway irritation, lacrimation, cough, wheezing, and ultimately pulmonary edema due to transudation of fluid from damaged capillaries. The absorbed hydrochloric acid can produce a hyperchloremic <u>metabolic</u> acidosis. Respiratory support with or without steroid administration constitutes the main axis of care. Aerosolized bicarbonate or other inhaled bases have been advocated by some workers. Persons with asthma or other preexisting lung disease are more affected than normal individuals, given the same exposure level. Death from accidental exposure is quite rare, but serious intoxications can produce chronic pulmonary problems.

Exposure to aerosolized Teflon or Teflon pyrolysis products

Probably every reader has anti-stick cookware in their kitchen. Teflon is polytetrafluoroethylene, or PTFE. It is widely used in industry and even vascular grafts are made of modified PTFE. Because the covalent bonding is so strong in the material, it is probably safe in ordinary use. Teflon begins to break down at temperatures above about 200°C, and it decomposes rather completely around 260°C, temperatures easily achieved on any kitchen stove if a pan is allowed to boil dry. Aerosolization of microparticles occurs, and these have been linked to the development of acute pulmonary edema in humans, pulmonary edema and hemorrhage in other mammals such as experimental rats, and sudden death in caged pet birds, including parrots. In 1 reported inadvertent industrial exposure, a middle-aged man developed bilateral lower lobe pulmonary edema within 1 hour of exposure, but the condition resolved spontaneously over 2 weeks. Some patients develop a self-limited flu-like illness referred to as "Teflon fever." There has also been recent attention to the toxicity of PFOA (perfluorooctanoic acid), which is another fluorocarbon used in the manufacture of Teflon; a variety of ills have been mentioned as possibly linked to PFOA, and none are lung-related.

Management of an episode of severe bronchitis

Extremely cold, dry, mid-continental winter air is enough to initiate an episode of bronchial irritation in a healthy person. The airways react with narrowing and increased mucus production; coughing begins. Inadequate hydration at these times means that the secretions are thick and difficult for the mucociliary elevator to deliver to the upper airway. If the process is arrested here by breathing warm, moist air from a clean nebulizer, it might end soon. Unfortunately, if coughing and cold air exposure continue, the sharp inspiration at the end of a coughing episode draws in bacteria that would not normally be in the trachea during quiet respiration. The development of a bacterial tracheobronchitis is now common. Dry coughing turns into sustained episodes of coughing, productive of increasingly purulent and foul-smelling sputum. Fatigue, low-calorie intake, and chest wall pain from tussive episodes that can last 30 minutes turn an annoying problem into a true medical illness. The chest radiograph would likely remain normal, and all that is heard on exam are coarse airway sounds. Hydration, nutrition, suppression of the cough reflex with dextromethorphan, use of guaifenesin as an expectorant, and quiet breathing of warm, humidified air are needed to treat most cases. If there is low-grade fever, then brief use of a broad-spectrum antibiotic such as amoxicillin should be considered. The patient should be instructed to cover their nose and mouth with a "ski mask" for the duration of the winter, so as to warm and humidify air before it reaches their glottis.

Nanoparticles

Large, visible particles in the air, such as fly ash from incinerators, usually pose little pulmonary risk because they are filtered out of the airways on the turbinates or in the trachea and proximal bronchi. Before the advent of modern protective respirators, firemen would cough out and vomit soot for a day or more after a major fire. It is what you can't see that is problematic. The alveoli are on the order of 40 to 60 microns in size; particles (including viruses) ranging in size from about 1 micron to 10^{-9} m are loosely called nanoparticles. Some of these entities occur in association with natural phenomena such as lightning and perhaps volcanism or meteor impacts, but many are man-made, either intentionally or accidentally. Many carbonaceous particles exist in the atmosphere near any large city; a special concern is that absorption of volatile organic compounds may occur on their surfaces. Recent thinking analogizes this to breathing in activated charcoal, which is presaturated with all manner of carcinogens, mutagens, and other harmful chemicals. For example, in Houston, you are breathing in CO and soot while sitting in a traffic jam, but you are also taking in benzene, pentane, phenol, toluene, formaldehyde, and other chemicals associated with petroleum refining, all absorbed by or adsorbed to a small carbon particle. People who live immediately adjacent to major highways or near manufacturing facilities may be at unusually increased risk of intoxication through their respiratory epithelium.

Common respiratory illness from various locations

All of these individuals have been near an active volcano. VOG is the colloquial term for volcanic origin smog, although it may also stand for volcanic out-gassing. Volcanoes in pyroclastic (Plinian) eruption eject enormous amounts of hot silicates high into the atmosphere (sometimes as high as the stratosphere), where they are distributed locally, regionally, or sometimes worldwide. These microscopic particles are essentially glass- or sand-like in character. Rare individuals who survive near these eruptions suffer thermal injury to the lungs and inhale large volumes of the dust. Pulmonary silicosis can result. Because the body has no enzymatic means of digesting silicates, these microparticles that have been ingested by macrophages persist as irritants, ultimately leading to lamellar scarring. This presents on chest radiographs as a micronodular process mnemonically resembling "ground glass." (Rescue workers around the 9/11 site have developed interstitial pulmonary fibrosis in part due to inhalation of similar materials.) But individuals 1,000 or more kilometers away can also be affected, depending on where the dust drops to the ground. Particularly, persons with asthma, COPD, or other pulmonary problems may be sickened by these distant events. Volcanoes also emit SOX-NOX gases: SO_2, SO_3, mixtures of the five combinations of nitrogen with oxygen, and H_2S. Sulfurous and sulfuric acid as well as nitrous and nitric acid are formed in the airways and on alveolar membranes; additionally, the nitrogen oxides are directly toxic to intermediary metabolic pathways.

Chronic obstructive lung disease (COPD)

COPD includes chronic bronchitis, bronchiectasis, emphysema, and certain diseases caused by occupational exposures, such as mining. It is often associated with smoking of cigarettes. The unifying characteristic is a diminished FEV_1 to FVC ratio, signifying air trapping. It is important to recall that during inspiration, negative forces pull open smaller bronchioles, but the reverse happens during expiration —they are compressed. Damaged small airways tend to collapse, delaying the emptying time of the pulmonary tree. Emphysematous areas do not "spring" down to smaller spheres because the elastic fibers in their walls are missing. Chest inspection often shows an expanded thoracic cage in an almost universally thin patient (who has used all their calories trying to breathe). Percussion shows resonance. Auscultation often discloses a variety of wheezes and gurgles associated with larger airway disease, and areas with diminished aeration due to emphysema; expiratory wheezes and whistles can sometimes be heard across the room. Early on, the patients are relatively pink, although they are somewhat hypoxemic on formal ABG testing. Chest radiographs show substantial hyperinflation due to air trapping, and CT of the lungs may help show where the areas of most significant emphysema are. There is some enthusiasm for "blebectomy" or "bullectomy," surgical resection of useless areas with advanced emphysema so that more normal lung may expand into the available space. General support with bronchodilators, mucolytics, and expectorants, immunization against pneumococcus and seasonal influenzas, and antibiotic treatment of bronchitic episodes will increase life quality. The conditions all tend to progress, however, leading to limitations of mobility and the necessity to use supplemental oxygen in the outpatient (home) setting.

Ventilator lung

Artificial ventilation became available in hospitals in the mid-1960s, and a decade later, sustained artificial ventilation was common in ICUs everywhere. The process is certainly life-saving, but it is not without risks, including the risk of injuring the lung with the ventilator itself. Respiratory gases have difficulty entering closed or severely narrowed bronchioles or alveoli, preferentially seeking the path of lowest resistance—the ones already open. This leads to overdistension and excessive ventilation of some lung tissue; intermittent opening of airways in other segments, followed by closure during the expiratory cycle; and failure entirely of certain areas to be ventilated at all. V/Q mismatch is common. But as the process continues, actual alveolar damage may occur, with diminished surfactant production, rupture of alveoli with microhemorrhages, etc. Patients may become "harder to ventilate," requiring ever higher inspiratory and end-expiratory pressures. "Failure to wean" from the ventilator is common is such patients after a week or more of respiratory support. The best strategy for prevention is cautious use of pressure support as ventilator use is instituted, bronchoscopy to open closed major airways, antibiotic use as needed for associated pneumonias, and, above all, avoidance of turning up the ventilator controls to achieve slightly better blood gas numbers. Note that this is not the same as ARDS.

Restrictive lung disease

Restrictive lung disease is almost, but not quite, synonymous with pulmonary fibrosis. A number of conditions cause intrinsic lung scarring, from prior severe infection to toxic gas exposure. Extrinsic causes include ankylosing spondylitis, severe kyphoscoliosis, and diseases with pleural thickening. Whatever the cause, the forced vital capacity is diminished and the work of breathing is materially increased. In a sense, simple obesity with the development of Pickwickian syndrome is an example of restrictive lung disease. If the problem is extrinsic to the lung tissue, some form of therapy may be devised, but if intrinsic and progressive, respiratory failure will ensue. Some individuals may be candidates for lung transplantation.

Negative inspiratory force pulmonary edema

Negative inspiratory force pulmonary edema is a rather unusual problem. In this situation, a strong inspiratory effort fails to draw air into the lungs, resulting in sustained negative intra-alveolar pressure. Examples of the rare clinical situations that lead to this are inadvertently closed valves on closed-loop anesthetic machines or complete airway occlusion that might occur with a heavy object crushing the soft tissues of the nose and mouth. As the patient struggles to pull in air, fluid from pulmonary capillaries instead is drawn into the alveoli. If the situation is recognized and relieved, the airway is filled with pink, frothy, proteinaceous fluid that is rapidly cleared by suction and by natural reabsorption into the pulmonary capillary bed. Neurogenic pulmonary edema (NPE) is quite common in severe head injury. The appearance of the sputum is identical, but the mechanism producing the fluid is completely different. It is probable that disturbances in hypothalamic blood flow or oxygenation underlie this problem, which is caused by severely increased sympathetic tone in pulmonary venules. This raises the pulmonary capillary pressure and fluid is passively extruded into the alveoli. In the situation of combined head and facial injury, it may be unclear which process is operative. The occurrence of NPE is considered to be a morbid sign of head injury.

Small, unilateral pneumothorax

Spontaneous, small pneumothorax occurs occasionally in young patients, probably as the result of rupture of a small, superficial bleb. The symptoms vary, and may be confused with the onset of bronchitis or a minor respiratory tract infection. Cough and some chest discomfort are almost universal. Physical examination may not be revealing if the air collection is small. There is little disturbance of ventilation, so the patient may not seek help for several days, usually because their symptoms are not getting better. Radiographs disclose the problem if they are read carefully. Treatment options include simple observation, administration of oxygen, and head-up positioning (the former with the idea that oxygen will be better absorbed from the pleural space than inert nitrogen), or placement of a small conventional chest tube or a small catheter under radiographic control. Chest tubes are typically connected to a device that includes a "water seal," meaning that any air collected from the pleural space is allowed to bubble to the other side of a column of water, where it cannot return. If no suction is applied, then the order is written to connect the tube to "water seal." If suction is applied, then an order is written specifying a certain amount of negative pressure, such as "chest tube to -20 cm H_2O pressure." Chest tubes will collect small amounts of serosanguineous pleural fluid as well, and these can either drain under gravity or be mechanically stripped along a soft section of rubber tubing in the system. When a chest tube is removed, the patient is asked to hold their breath and perhaps to slightly Valsalva; the tube is then suddenly withdrawn from the chest while a Vaseline-impregnated pressure dressing is simultaneously applied over the incision and the tunneled track. (Slow removal would simply allow room air to pass into the first exposed ostium in the tube, and then back into the chest cavity.) Recurrent pneumothorax, or a collection that is refractory to thoracostomy drainage, may require either thoracoscopic repair or thoracotomy.

Tension pneumothorax

If the trachea, bronchi, or lung tissue are torn in such a way as to produce a flap-valve arrangement, then with each inspiration, air is drawn into the pleural space, but with each expiration, it is trapped. This leads very rapidly to accumulation of extra-pulmonic air under considerable pressure. Shift of the lung, the mediastinum, and the trachea to the opposite side occur within minutes, and the heart itself is displaced, with attendant compromise of cardiac filling. The blood pressure begins to fail. The hemithorax with the trapped air is hyper-resonant to percussion, and breath sounds there are distant or absent. Prompt drainage by chest tube leads to an immediate improvement in the patient's condition. Paramedics are often equipped with one-way valves incorporated into a needle; when they insert the needle, there is typically a gush of air. Such treatment only relieves the high pressure and shifting, and definitive treatment for the residual large pneumothorax is still required.

Chylothorax

Iatrogenic injury to the thoracic duct near the point where it enters the junction of the left jugular and the left subclavian vein is the most common cause of chylothorax. Cancer, radiation injury, blunt chest trauma, and congenital malformations of the lymphatic system may also create this problem. Chyle consists of fluid rich in chylomicrons and lymphocytes. The diagnosis is made by chest radiograph and thoracentesis; the laboratory will usually be able to confirm that evacuated fluid is chyle by performing fat stains on it. Chronic evacuation of chylothorax by chest tube depletes the lymphocyte population, but if a leak did respond to short-term thoracostomy drainage by ebbing spontaneously, the patient and treating team would be far ahead. If the locus of the leak is unknown, lymphangiography may disclose it. If the leak follows, for example, a subclavian catheter placement or similar intervention, early exploration and thoracic duct ligation is usually recommended. If the patient is given a large amount of oral mayonnaise on the evening before surgery, intestinal lacteals will have sufficient time to package these chemicals and turn the chyle milky white. This greatly helps surgeons find the tiny thoracic duct and ligate it. Repair of this delicate, diaphanous vessel is impractical.

Hemothorax

Following an assassination attempt, former President Ronald Reagan immediately developed a large and persistent hemothorax due to splintering of the 7th rib by a bullet, and fairly brisk oozing of venous blood from the hole in the left lung parenchyma. Placement of two chest tubes failed to stem the hemorrhage, and prompt thoracotomy saved his life. Hemothorax occurs after penetrating trauma such as this, but also in response to blunt trauma, and occasionally due to hemorrhage from tumors or inadvertent puncture of large vascular structures during therapeutic attempts. Because blood clots, large bore chest tube placement is essential; multiple tubes may be needed. In President Reagan's case, a 500 mL clot covered the hole in the lung and prevented it from coapting to the pleura (which might have been enough to stem the flow of blood). High negative pressure suction (-30 to -40 cm of water) is often used. If blood flow does not materially diminish in the first few hours of closed drainage, thoracotomy may be needed. Auscultation of the involved side usually discloses faint breath sounds, and percussion may elicit dullness. X-rays usually disclose hazy opacity of much of a lung field, due to posterior layering of the blood. Intrapleural blood is an excellent culture medium.

Resection of large emphysematous blebs or pneumonectomy

Amazingly, patients tolerate removal of a whole lung fairly well. Typically, this is done for cancer, although fungal infections, severe and unusual traumatic problems, and, rarely, congenital problems are the cause for operation. If patients are free of significant COPD, there is low mortality. Arterial blood gases hardly budge from normal limits, and measures such as the FEV_1 show less than a 50% decline. Essentially, the other lung gradually inflates to occupy more space, but not the entire opposite hemithorax. The resection field fills with pleural fluid, and the heart, mediastinum, and abdominal contents shift over a period of months to fill in the space. Because of this large dead space, bronchopleural fistula is an especially feared complication, as there are potentially liters of space for pus to occupy. Cardiac function is immediately impacted, with right ventricular end-diastolic volume rising measurably. Ordinarily, patients maintain a normal blood pressure. When large blebs are resected, the surrounding lung parenchyma expands to fill the void. Pulmonary artery resistance may actually be lowered if mass effect is relieved by the resection. Oxygenation usually improves because V/Q mismatch is partially corrected.

Thoracoplasty

Thoracoplasty was once a common operation for tuberculosis; in fact, surgical residents who were rotated through TB hospitals in the 1950s gained considerable familiarity with the apical regions of the thoracic cavity by performing these operations on a daily basis. The idea was to reduce the aeration of tuberculous cavities by collapsing the chest wall against that portion of the lung, and also to reduce the pleural space, where a tuberculous empyema could form. It is conceptually similar to bullectomy or lobectomy as performed today. Several (as many as 8) ribs were removed through an extrapleural approach; this produced considerable deformity of the chest wall and shoulder. Interestingly, modern use of this procedure persists in the management of very advanced TB in the third world, and with reasonably good results. The advent of antibiotics that were effective in treating tuberculosis made the operation essentially obsolete; however, a procedure similar to this is sometimes needed when resecting chest wall neoplasms such as a fibrosarcoma. Today, only master surgeons have any familiarity with the procedure at all.

Superior sulcus lung tumor

In 1924, Pancoast originally separated out lung cancers of the superior sulcus based on the unusual constellation of clinical findings. These masses have usually invaded adjacent structures at the time of diagnosis. Involvement of the subclavian artery or vein, the brachial plexus, the vagus and phrenic nerves, and the ascending sympathetic chain have all been described. Horner's syndrome (ptosis, miosis, and anhydrosis of the face) may be seen. Superior vena cava syndrome has also been reported. Invasion of the chest wall in this confined space is fairly common. Most of these are squamous cell or adenocarcinomas, but they are difficult to resect because of attachment to the vital structures named above. Treatment is often palliative.

Pleural mesothelioma

Asbestos is a highly useful silicate mineral that causes a specific pneumoconiosis disease and has been linked to malignant mesothelioma. Since asbestos is no longer used in most countries, exposure is limited to persons demolishing asbestos-containing structures such as buildings, boilers, and ships. There is little particularly special about the gradual pulmonary interstitial fibrosis that is produced. Perhaps the only unusual feature is the development of parietal pleural plaques visible on routine chest radiographs. Pulmonary function testing shows progressive restrictive disease. Mesothelioma is incontrovertibly linked to asbestosis. The exact mechanism producing neoplasia of mesothelial cells is unknown, but it is clear that asbestos fibers alter the function of macrophages. Mesothelioma presents as an enlarging, peripherally based mass with or without a pleural effusion. Biopsy by needle, thoracoscopy, or open technique leads to definitive diagnosis. There are many cellular markers for this unique tumor. Cisplatinum chemotherapy has some utility in management of the disease, but over half of all patients die within a year of diagnosis.

Squamous cell carcinoma

Bronchogenic carcinoma of the lung is divided into adenocarcinoma (about one-third of all tumors), squamous carcinoma (around one-quarter), and oat cell cancer (about one-fifth), with the remainder being mixtures of cell types. Adenocarcinoma frequently metastasizes, whereas squamous cancer of the lung may remain local for longer periods of time. If a local nodule is discovered and there are no lymph node metastases on chest CT, the disease is stage 1; if only local lymphatics are involved, stage 2 disease exists. Certainly stage 1, and possibly stage 2 disease, is amenable to surgical treatment. As far as cancer causation, the horse is out of the barn. Immediate smoking cessation is still critical to achieving a surgical result and long-term palliation, however. Perhaps as little as 1 week of chest physiotherapy, with or without bronchodilator drugs, may substantially improve pulmonary function. The ability to successfully undergo lobectomy or even pneumonectomy is obviously directly correlated with preoperative pulmonary status. Therefore, every effort should be made to "clean up" the lungs in advance of an operation. Chemotherapy generally does not work well for these tumors. Radiotherapy may offer long-term palliation, however.

Small cell carcinoma

These tumors are commonly called oat cell carcinomas because the stained sections show monotonous sheets of fairly primitive cells with large nuclei and almost no cytoplasm. They are nonetheless often endocrinologically active, producing the so-called paraneoplastic syndrome. In these situations, patients may often present with unusual problems, such as sudden-onset oliguria and hyponatremia mimicking the syndrome of inappropriate antidiuretic hormone secretion; it is the tumor that is making a vasopressin analogue. Conditions resembling myasthenia gravis may occur, causing weakness. In fact, bizarre neurologic symptoms in a smoker who has a normal CT of the brain are often due to these paraneoplastic problems. Chemotherapy and radiotherapy are the mainstays of treatment, but survival at 5 years is quite unusual.

Carcinoma of the larynx

The archetypal patient with squamous cell carcinoma of the larynx is a very heavy smoker in their early 60s; concomitant heavy alcohol ingestion is common. Complaints include a change in the voice, hoarseness, pain in the throat, a full sensation or a lump in the throat. All these symptoms should lead at least to indirect laryngoscopy. Any abnormalities noted (eg, asymmetry of the vocal folds, a nodule on the vocal cord) should then prompt direct laryngoscopy with biopsy. CT of the neck is a common next step, to assess the degree of nodal spread. Depending on the TNM stage of the tumor, surgery and/or radiotherapy are the next steps. Chemotherapy has little role in the management of most of these tumors. Laryngectomy with tracheostomy is sometimes a dreadful necessity. Because of the heavy smoking history, these patients are at risk to develop carcinoma of the lung, and even other cancers of the oral cavity as well.

Lymphangitic bronchial carcinomatosis

Malignant tumors usually metastasize to the lungs and present as nodules, but this is not always the case. Occasionally patients have hazy, micronodular chest radiographs and similar CT scans, done for the indication of malaise, dyspnea, or tightness of the chest. This pattern is not highly specific, but it suggests either an inflammatory/infectious process or spread of malignancy through the pulmonary lymphatic tree. The diagnosis is clarified usually by bronchoscopy; either transbronchial needle biopsy or bronchoalveolar lavage, or both, may disclose malignant cells. Obviously this represents a very advanced stage of metastasis, no matter what or where the primary tumor may be. Chemotherapy and/or radiotherapy would ordinarily be used to palliate symptoms. As an additional note, a primary lung tumor will occasionally disseminate itself through the bronchial tree; this condition can be diagnosed with certainty by bronchoscopy.

Pulmonary embolism

Thromboembolic disease is one of the most stealthy and frequent killers in the hospital setting. Even mild compression of venous drainage in an unconscious or sedated patient for just a couple of hours is sufficient to initiate thrombus formation. Then, too, certain individuals inherit defective blood coagulation proteins, making them susceptible to spontaneous thrombosis; it is probably mostly these people who have trouble after long air flights. Thrombosis generally occurs in the veins of the legs, although thromboembolism from the upper extremities has been reported in association with peripherally inserted central catheter lines and similar foreign bodies. Low-grade fever is common; pain in surgical incisions may be reported by patients, rather than aching in their calf. Unwillingness to move around in bed or oversedation of patients is common. If prophylactic doses of heparin were ordered to be given subcutaneously, one or more may have been missed. Mild dyspnea is sometimes noted. Quite often, the patient is not diagnosed until they have a massive and fatal embolism while walking to the bathroom. Careful examination of the calves, checking for calf pain on forceful plantar flexion (Homans' sign), and determination of blood gases may all be life-saving, but they require a high index of suspicion. Doppler flow studies and other examinations may disclose propagative thrombotic disease before it is too late. Heparinization and concomitant coumadinization are required when the diagnosis is established.

Once venous thrombosis has been established, it is necessary to do everything possible to prevent proximal propagation of the clot and to prevent it from dislodging and traveling to the lung. Small, recurrent emboli actually cause pulmonary hypertension. A large, single embolus may produce acute tachypnea, hemoptysis, chest pain, and acute respiratory embarrassment. A huge Y-shaped saddle embolus is sufficient to cause immediate right-sided heart failure and underperfusion of both lungs. The systemic pressure immediately falls to zero because the left circulation is empty. Death is instantaneous, or nearly so. In addition to anticoagulating a patient, consideration may be given to thrombolysis by administering tissue plasminogen activator. The problem, naturally, with all these interventions is that they tend to produce bleeding. Patients who have undergone major surgery or who have had major trauma are predisposed to develop clots in their legs, but also are likely to bleed into injured tissues when anticoagulant or thrombolytic therapy is begun. Damned if you do, damned if you don't; the physician must walk a tight therapeutic tightrope for several days. Placement of filters into the vena cava seems to be less popular now than a decade ago. Finally, interventional radiologists may be able to snare out large clots in more proximal pulmonary arterioles, or to deliver lower doses of tissue plasminogen activator (tPA) directly onto a thrombus or embolus.

Parasitic lung infections

Amebic abscess of the lung due to *Entamoeba histolytica* is a rare problem, occurring usually in the context of a juxtaposed liver abscess and trans-diaphragmatic pleural extension. Schistosomiasis may involve the lungs by lodgment of trematode eggs that cause enough immune reaction to initiate fibrosis, ultimately leading to right-sided heart failure. Paragonimiasis is due to infestation of the lung fluke, which comes to human hosts via incompletely cooked fish; the organisms produce interstitial scarring similar to that in schistosomiasis. Dirofilariasis, mosquito-borne heartworm infestation, is a common veterinary problem, but it can involve humans. The adult worms preferentially live in the pulmonary artery and the right heart; they are deadly if untreated. It is not just Fido who is being cared for by monthly heartworm prophylaxis.

Renin-angiotensin-aldosterone system

Sensing lower blood pressures, the renal juxtaglomerular apparatus secretes the enzyme renin. Hepatically produced angiotensinogen, a pro-hormone, is converted to 10 residue angiotensin I, which is then presented to the lung and back to the kidney. Although the main source of angiotensin-converting enzyme (ACE) is the endothelial cells of the lung, the kidney is also able to produce this protease enzyme. ACE cleaves a dipeptide from angiotensin I to make the active agent elevating blood pressure, angiotensin II. Interestingly, ACE is one of the three natural enzymes that lyse bradykinin, a vasodilator. A strange factoid concerning ACE is that it is often elevated in pulmonary sarcoidosis, but it may not be the endothelial cells of the lung that produce it in this instance.

Metabolic acidosis

Creation of an acidic blood pH ordinarily stimulates the breathing control centers in the brain to cause faster and deeper respiratory excursions. An example would be the tachypnea that accompanies aspirin poisoning or diabetic ketoacidosis. A problem arises when there is incomplete respiratory compensation, as in cases with CNS disease or sedation. Consider the Henderson-Hasselbalch equation, which states that the blood pH is effectively the pK_a for carbonic acid (6.1) plus the log of the number indicated by the HCO_3^{-1}/CO_2 ratio. Now, the concentration of carbon dioxide is approximately 0.03 x the arterial pCO_2, or 0.03 x 40 = 1.2 mEq/L and normal bicarbonate is about 26 mEq/L, a ratio of about 22. The log of 22 is 1.3, so normal blood pH is 6.1 + 1.3 = 7.4. If hypoventilation raises the pCO_2 from 40 to 50, then the new blood becomes:

- pH = 6.1 + log 26/1.5 = 6.1 + log 17.3 = 6.1 + 1.2 = 7.3. So an easy rule of thumb is that for each 10 torr rise in arterial CO_2, there is a decrease of 0.1 pH units in the blood. A metabolic acidosis that cannot be corrected by the lungs rapidly becomes a disaster.

Respiratory acidosis

Simply put, hypoventilation creates CO_2 retention. Recall that carbon dioxide diffuses better across alveolar membranes than oxygen. Room air contains only 0.04% carbon dioxide, essentially none. Inspired air has a pCO_2 level near zero, but this fresh air soon mixes with residual air in the airways. Depending on ventilation rate, the initial alveolar pCO_2 might be very low, or it might be 30 torr, reflecting low tidal volumes and a low respiratory rate. The pulmonary arterial pCO_2 is about 46 torr, so prompt degassing of carbon dioxide from the alveolar capillaries still occurs. When very slow, shallow respiration occurs, the alveolar tension of carbon dioxide may actually climb to blood levels. Since the gas is diffusing passively, it will rapidly come to a new equilibrium. Gradually, the CO_2 levels in the blood and alveoli rise. This ordinarily stimulates respiratory rate and depth, but it cannot do so in the presence of sedatives, nor can it alone overcome obesity. If the process is slow, the kidneys respond by secreting a more acidic urine to compensate for the respiratory acidosis. CO_2 levels rise demonstrably in the air of a medical school classroom (true!), and they are chronically high in limestone (karst) caves. The Apollo XIII astronauts were subjected to acute CO_2 poisoning because the lithium hydroxide scrubbers were in the other compartment of the space vehicle; until they could make repairs, they were irritable, confused, and clumsy with carbon dioxide levels around 6% to 7% in the air.

Cystic fibrosis

Cystic fibrosis is an autosomal recessive disease caused by a disorder of the chloride channel in many cells in the body, including the liver, pancreas, and lungs. It affects up to 1 in 2,000 to 3,000 children of European descent. There are many variations of the genetic defect, and therefore there is a wide spectrum of severity as life goes on. Most diagnoses are established as part of the newborn screening routinely conducted by hospitals in the United States. Once the diagnosis is established, the child should be followed by a CF team at a children's hospital. The pulmonary issues are conceptually straightforward: the disease produces COPD because thick mucus cannot be cleared from the airways. Repeated instances of segmental or lobar collapse can occur, as well as repeated episodes of pneumonia. Bronchiectasis becomes a later feature of the disease. Many young patients are on chronic prophylaxis against *Pseudomonas*, *Staphylococcus,* and other opportunists. Meticulous care may stave off serious symptoms for a decade or more. Ultimately, lung transplantation may be considered, but the long-term prognosis is still poor.

Helping a patient understand emphysema

Discuss this disease with the patient and her family, so that all concerned parties understand the gravity of the situation. If the patient is still smoking, then every available asset should be employed to help her stop. If the emphysema is in early stages, smoking cessation could lead to a degree of reversal of laboratory findings and symptoms. Vaccination against seasonal influenza and pneumococcal pneumonia is necessary. Meticulous attention to the avoidance of contact allergens, such as animal allergens and house or agricultural dust, is very important. Pets may have to find a new home. Air conditioning the living space (with frequent filter cleaning) may lessen symptoms. If there are strong seasonal exacerbations (for example, pine pollen in Atlanta), then trips away or even changing permanent residence could be tried, if feasible. Bronchodilators and expectorants may help. Postural drainage and chest physiotherapy conducted by family members also could lessen the impact of the illness. Most likely, a chest CT, baseline pulmonary function testing, and perhaps an early consultation with a pulmonologist would be in order. In more advanced cases, thoracic surgical consultation for resection of severely emphysematous tissue might be considered. Whatever the starting point, it is important that the patient and family understand that the disease is likely to progress and rob the individual of her vitality. All that can be hoped for is lessening of symptoms and slowing the rate of progression. Ultimately, oxygen will probably be needed, and the patient will develop end-stage lung disease.

Alpha-1 antitrypsin deficiency

The protein known as alpha-1 antitrypsin is a protease inhibitor that is the main component of the electrophoretic alpha-1 grouping. It functions as an inhibitor of proteases and particularly elastase; tissues gradually loose background connective tissue support, and particularly lung tissue. This leads to emphysema. The gene for this protein is on chromosome 14, and the most serious form of the condition is manifest in homozygous recessive states. Cigarette smoke renders normal amounts of this protein less active in proportion to the amount smoked; the specific effects in a given patient also depend on the exact gene product he is making. Although donor protein can be administered intravenously, treatment is exceedingly expensive. Ongoing research examines the effects of delivering modified protein by inhalation.

Lung transplantation

Two related issues limit lung transplantation: availability and limited graft longevity. In the United States, somewhere around 1,600 to 1,800 lung or heart + lung transplants (for those with cor pulmonale due to pulmonary hypertension) are performed yearly. The technical issues are not daunting: vascular anastomoses, plus either tracheal (bilateral transplant) or bronchial suturing (either staged bilateral lung transplant or single lung transplant). Approximate size match is important, and of course tissue compatibility. The ordinary problems with immune suppressed patients are experienced. Five-year survival is only around 50%, as opposed to 85% or more for kidney transplantation. Death is due to repeated graft rejection in most cases, with gradual accumulated damage to the transplanted tissue.

Smoking

Cigarette smoking has acute and chronic effects. As early as the 1960s, it was shown that epithelial ciliary beat rate decreased 20% to 100% in experimental animals exposed to cigarette smoke. This fact, coupled with the acute irritative effects of smoke, mean that excess mucus produced responsively in the airways will be cleared slowly, with difficulty, or not at all. Cigarette smoke contains CO, so blood levels of this chemical rise immediately. The immediate effects of the hundreds of chemicals ordinarily in tobacco are inestimable. Sometimes, tobacco or marijuana leaves are contaminated with insecticides or other agricultural products. Inhaling paraquat, a defoliant used by governments to destroy marijuana plants, produces immediate pulmonary edema. Of course, in most instances, there is no discernible adverse effect from smoking one, two, or a hundred cigarettes. Over the long term, direct damage to alpha-1 antitrypsin molecules prevents them from exerting a protective shield for elastin fibers. Once these fibers undergo proteolysis, emphysema ensues. The wide variety of chemical agents in the smoke include carcinogens, so cigarette smoking accounts for about two-thirds of lung cancer cases, with exposure to radioactive radon gas causing or contributing to the other one-third. Second-hand smoke affects sensitive adults and particularly young children. It is associated with reactive airway complaints and asthma.

Incentive spirometry

Inexpensive bedside incentive spirometers are found on all wards of the hospital. Typically, these devices require a patient to suck in air as forcefully as possible in order to float a small ball against gravity in a clear tube; the device uses the Venturi effect to lift the ball. The lightweight unit is easily made into a game or a toy for pediatric use. On the other end of the age spectrum, even poorly motivated, sedated, or elderly, confused patients can usually be encouraged to "play the game" and lift the ball to a designated level a few times in several sessions each day. The idea is to use normal inspiratory force to open atelectatic lung or to prevent the development of alveolar collapse completely. The use of forced expiration (blowing to keep the ball suspended) is less common. In addition to the directed pulmonary treatment, there is the shifting and resettling in the bed or chair, further helping the patient's lung function. One very famous cardiovascular surgeon simply had the nurses remove all pillows from the patient's bed, in the belief that minor discomfort and shifting around to find a more tolerable sleep position achieved much the same thing. At any rate, oversedation and failure to encourage deep breathing contribute to respiratory complications in hospitalized patients.

Oxygen administration

Oxygen administration is not as simple as it seems, and rather than being overly scientific about the process, most clinicians are content to adjust delivery depending on the effect seen in the patient's clinical status or blood gas profile. This is similar to over-engineering the construction of a house, rather than calculating the strength of supporting beams. Nonetheless, some basic issues need to be reviewed. Room air is 21% oxygen, and at sea level (760 torr), this means that the partial pressure of oxygen at the nares is about 159 torr. Let's use 150 as an easy way to remember the numbers. It is not until one reaches an altitude of 3,600 m above sea level that the pressure falls to 500 torr, and therefore to an inspired oxygen partial pressure of 105 torr. Therefore, in almost every clinical situation except on a mountainside, in an airplane, or in space, the oxygen in ambient air is overly plentiful to saturate hemoglobin completely if the circulation and lungs are normal. Loose-fitting oxygen masks with perforations in the sides probably do not deliver oxygen at concentrations above about 25%, no matter how high the flow is set. With face-fitting masks, concentrations on the order of 28%-30% can be achieved. Quite often, pressurized air or oxygen is used in nebulizers to deliver drugs such as albuterol or isoproterenol. Here, a Venturi effect is used to diminish the pressure over a reservoir of fluid containing a dissolved medication. Mechanical ventilators with closed, unidirectional circuits (non-rebreathing) can deliver very high oxygen concentrations in intubated individuals.

Jet ventilation

Instead of the gentle sighing of a normal ventilator, patients undergoing jet (high-frequency) ventilation are surrounded by a buzzing machinery noise. The idea of high-frequency ventilation is to deliver essentially a constant stream of respiratory gas into the alveoli by shortening the delivery time to about 20 milliseconds, sharply decreasing the tidal volume, but simultaneously increasing the rate to around 100-150 breaths per minute. This has the overall effect of lowering the pressures needed to deliver fresh gas into the alveoli, and the technique essentially blasts out gas from the previous alveolar filling by laminar flow principles. The process does not work with very small endotracheal tubes, and as expected, the problems associated with it are pneumothorax, pneumomediastinum, and the like.

Extracorporeal membrane oxygenation (ECMO)

ECMO is only considered in extreme situations where lung function is severely compromised but is expected to recover, or when it is anticipated that the patient can be rescued by lung transplantation in just a few days. It goes without saying that this is an advanced technique for an experienced team. An extracorporeal pump circulates blood from the right half of the circulation through an oxygenator and then returns the blood either to the right side of the heart (veno-venous technique) or into a major artery (veno-arterial technique). ARDS is the most common cause for ECMO in the adult setting, and prematurity is probably the most common reason for using ECMO in children. Either the whole patient or the system must be heparinized, so bleeding is a major complication, as are problems with the lines themselves (e.g., infection, damage to vessels from huge indwelling lines). The most feared complication is central nervous system involvement from multiple micro-emboli ("pump brain") or major occlusive stroke. However, because the process is only considered in the very sickest patients, there is actually little to lose and something to gain.

Pathogenesis and management of high-altitude pulmonary edema (HAPE)

HAPE is a condition known mostly to aviation medicine experts, emergency physicians, and alpinists. It is probably identical in pathogenesis to neurogenic pulmonary edema; specifically, it is produced by hypoxemia affecting the hypothalamus. Here, increased sympathetic tone produces slight outflow obstruction in the pulmonary circulation, and when coupled with diminished intra-alveolar pressure, varying degrees of pulmonary edema can occur. The condition is believed to be aggravated by youth, with occasional hiking/climbing families or parties reporting that the youngest member turned blue abruptly around the 3,500-3,800 m level. Indeed, the author discovered that his own apathy and confusion at 3,780 m was accompanied by mild cyanosis. Climbers are therefore encouraged to take with them acetazolamide, a diuretic that tends to ameliorate mild cases, and steroids such as dexamethasone, which probably act centrally. Of course, the best treatment is simply to return to lower altitudes. Paradoxically, excellent hydration may be important in staving off an episode. Gradual acclimation to higher altitudes in the form of dwelling in base camps for a few days makes the condition less likely. Those who develop this condition once are prone to develop it again under similar circumstances. Rapid ascent up a mountain on a gondola or even a bus by persons with diminished pulmonary reserve should be discouraged, as they are at risk of a true medical crisis.

Bleomycin

Bleomycin refers to a family of large-molecule antibiotics produced by certain *Streptomyces* species. It is used principally as an anti-neoplastic drug because of its ability to break DNA strands; the most common diseases for which it is prescribed are testicular cancer and Hodgkin disease. The main side effect of this drug is the induction of pulmonary fibrosis due to activation of the proinflammatory interleukins 18 and 1-beta (also known as catabolin). There is some consideration that bleomycin may sensitize lung tissue to oxygen toxicity, and a number of patients receiving the drug would ordinarily receive supplemental oxygen during surgery or other procedures. Because of its ability to induce severe inflammation, bleomycin has been administered into the pleural space in order to induce pleurodesis—scarring together of the visceral and parietal pleura.

Drugs that can be administered down an endotracheal tube

The list of drugs is short: LEAN stands for lidocaine, epinephrine, atropine, and naloxone. (Some sources also list diazepam (Valium) and vasopressin.) The assumption is that there is fairly prompt but imperfect absorption from the airway and alveolar spaces, but this is speculative. Doses are around 2-4 mg/kg for lidocaine, and around 2-2.5 times greater than the IV dose for the other three drugs. Only L, E, A, and N are approved for pediatric use. As noted, these should only be given in this way when ordinary IV access cannot be obtained.

Social factors that led to an increase in smoking in women

About 34% of US women were smoking in 1965, and the current rate is half of that. The factors leading to smoking in women are complex and not limited to the population of the United States. Once more the province of men (57% were smokers in 1965, and 21% now), the general expansion of gender rights after World War I, as well as the incorporation of many women into the work force during World War II, introduced the practice of smoking. Smoking can be a structured social event marking the times of a day, such as the "smoke break" at work. There was also an aggressive campaign to market cigarettes to women in the late 1960s, which extended through the next decade. The rugged male smoker stereotypes were cast against softer images of women smoking "slim" cigarettes in thinly veiled sexual innuendo. Perhaps all the present stresses in the modern world contribute to this unfortunate habit, such as political-social, economic, and family issues. Paradoxically, concern for the well-being of children exposed to second-hand smoke has possibly lowered the smoking rate in parents of both genders. Whatever the cause, both men and women who smoke are 25 times as likely to die of lung cancer as nonsmokers, around 22-25 times as likely to develop COPD, about 2-3 times as likely to have an ischemic coronary event, and twice as likely to have a stroke.

Smoking cessation

The hardest thing in the world to change is a habit. Raw nicotine alkaloid is an extremely poisonous compound, with laboratory deaths reported within seconds of inadvertent cutaneous contact. In the ordinary single milligram doses absorbed over a few minutes while smoking a cigarette, it is a highly addictive stimulant of the parasympathetic nervous system. The chemical causes a variety of pharmacologic effects, including release of epinephrine from the adrenal medulla and endorphins from the brain. Only about 15% of established smokers are ever able to quit entirely. Graphic, gory depictions of smoker's lung or emphysematous patients struggling to breathe as they tell people to quit smoking probably have little effect on the majority of smokers, and particularly younger ones. Self-help groups similar to AA may have some positive effect, substituting nonsmoking social contact for those that occur in smoking contexts. Since smokers have been expelled from the workplace and restaurants, however, the social bonds that do form between the banished may be quite important. The use of nicotine patches to withdraw patients gradually from the smoking process may spare the lungs, but abuse of the patches to get nicotine highs is a known problem. At the very least, strong family support is needed to help people attempting to quit, and they may also need psychotherapy or psychoactive medications.

Cardiovascular System

Embryonic development of the cardiovascular (CV) system

The CV system starts forming near the end of the third week, with the heart beginning to beat on day 21 or 22. Initially, angiogenesis takes place at the cardiogenic mesenchymal area of the yolk sac, opposite the stalk. This occurs via angioblast clusters known as blood islands, which flatten themselves to form an early endothelium template. From here, two paired endothelial heart tubes are formed, which later join together to establish a primitive single heart tube. While blood formation begins at this time in the allantois and yolk sac endothelium, the embryo does not start producing its own blood until the 5th week, at the same time that the conduction system starts taking shape. Partitioning of the primitive heart tube starts in the 4th week, and will eventually lead to formation of the chambers and septae; at the same time, aortic arch derivatives begin developing into what will eventually become the aorta and arteries.

Development of the CV system as the fetus matures

As the heart continues to grow and mature beyond the embryonic stage, so does the rest of the fetal circulatory system. The major changes during the fetal stage involve circulation and the shunting of blood from one area to another, in order to perfuse the necessary regions of the body, while concomitantly reducing flow to areas that are not yet mature enough (such as the lungs). Highly oxygenated blood is transported to the fetus' inferior vena cava via the umbilical vein and the ductus venosus, which is controlled by a sphincter. At the same time, the foramen ovale shunts well-oxygenated blood directly from the right atrium to the left atrium, largely bypassing the lungs, in order to adequately perfuse the rest of the maturing body. Finally, the ductus arteriosus provides a shunt between the pulmonary trunk and the aorta for any blood that makes its way to the right ventricle. This blood is moderately saturated with oxygen and it encounters high pulmonary vascular resistance, resulting in a strengthening of the right ventricle and simultaneous minimization of pulmonary blood flow, which allows the lungs to mature without the burden of having to be fully functional.

Perinatal changes that occur in the CV system of the mature fetus/newborn

As the fetus enters the world to become a neonate, several important changes begin occurring almost immediately. With the first and subsequent breaths, the lungs expand and being working on their own, resulting in a reduction of pulmonary vascular resistance and concomitant increase in pulmonary blood flow. Along with the closing of the ductus venosus, this ensures adequate circulation to the alveolar capillaries, via the right ventricle. As the pressure difference between right and left reverses, the higher pressure on the left leads to the closing of the foramen ovale against the septum secundum, and a constriction of the ductus arteriosus (DA), which no longer needs to provide oxygenated blood to the aorta directly from the pulmonary trunk. Often, as a result of this rapid pressure shift, the DA will remain open for several days, during which time small amounts of blood are shunted in the opposite direction from that in the womb, with flow now following the pressure gradient from left to right, or aorta to pulmonary artery. Finally, the umbilical artery constricts at birth, to prevent excessive blood loss back into the placental region.

Anatomy and physiology (A & P) of the four heart chambers

The human heart contains four chambers: the right atrium (RA), right ventricle (RV), left atrium (LA) and left ventricle (LV); the ventricles are separated by the interventricular septum, while the atria are separated by the interatrial septum. In addition, the atrioventricular septum separates the right atrium from the left ventricle. The RA receives deoxygenated blood from the vena cavae, as well as coronary venous blood through the coronary sinus, which is then pumped through the tricuspid valve (three leafs) into the RV. (Both atrioventricular valves are attached to the ventricular walls by chordae tendinae attached to papillary muscles, which help support the valves and prevent regurgitation.) The RV empties through the pulmonic semilunar valve into the pulmonary artery. On its return from the lungs, well-oxygenated blood travels through the four pulmonary veins into the LA, and then travels through the mitral/bicuspid (two leafs) valve, into the LV. From here, the LV pumps blood through the semilunar aortic valve and into the aorta, for distribution throughout the body. The walls of the LV are considerably thicker and more muscular than those of the RV (excepting the shared septum), to accommodate the pressure required to pump against systemic vascular resistance. Also, the valves on the left side of the heart are much closer to each other than are those on the right.

Heart valves

There are four major heart valves: mitral/bicuspid (MV), tricuspid (TV), aortic valve (AV) and pulmonic valve (PV); there is also a smaller valve located at the opening of the coronary sinus. The MV contains an anterior and posterior leaflet, and separates the left atrium and left ventricle, preventing backflow from the latter into the former. The TV has three leaflets (anterior, posterior and septal) and separates the right atrium from the right ventricle, again preventing backflow from latter to former. The semilunar AV has three semicircular cusps and lies at the superior aspect of the left ventricle, separating the left ventricle from the aorta. At the aortic root, closing of the AV yields the three sinuses of Valsalva; the left and right sinuses lead to the corresponding coronary arteries, while the third is a non-coronary sinus. The PV, also semilunar and with three cusps, separates the right ventricle from the pulmonary artery. It has more fragile cusps than the AV, and no related coronary arteries. Notably, the right-sided valves are considerably further apart from each other than the corresponding left-sided valves.

Cardiac cycle

During the cardiac cycle, blood that enters the right atrium via the vena cavae is passed through the tricuspid valve into the right ventricle, before being pushed through the pulmonic valve into the pulmonary artery. At this point, blood travels to the lungs for oxygenation at the alveolar capillaries, before resuming its journey through the heart via the pulmonary veins, which drain into the left atrium. Blood is pushed from the left atrium through the mitral valve, into the left ventricle. From here, the blood is forced through the aortic valve and into the aorta, from which it travels through the rest of the body. This trip from entry into the right atrium through exit from the left ventricle completes one full cardiac cycle.

Diastole and systole

For the cardiac cycle to proceed, the chambers and valves must alternate contracting and relaxing, and opening and closing, respectively. This occurs nearly simultaneously on both sides of the heart (and should be assumed in the descriptions below of the left side). The cardiac cycle is generally divided into two parts: ventricular diastole and ventricular systole. During the former, both atria contract (atrial systole), closing the semilunar valves, and both ventricles begin receiving blood through the AV valves, down the pressure gradient from atrium to ventricle. When the ventricles become filled and pressure equalizes, they begin to contract, closing the AV valves, and proceeding through isovolumetric contraction, until ventricular pressure is greater than aortic pressure, which forces open the aortic valve, allowing blood to flow to the systemic vasculature. At the point where the pressure in the aorta becomes greater than that in the left ventricle, the semilunar valves close. In the time between the aortic and pulmonic valves closing and the reopening of the AV valves, there is a period of isovolumetric relaxation, which occurs just before the pressure in the ventricles dips below that in the atria, and the AV valves open and begin a new cycle. On a normal EKG, atrial systole begins at the start of the P wave, while ventricular systole begins at the start of the QRS complex.

Heart sounds

The two main heart sounds are S1 and S2, which are further divided into M1 and T1, and A2 and P2, corresponding to the closing of the four heart valves. During ventricular systole, the pressure increase in the ventricles forces shut the AV valves, with the mitral closing (M1) just before the tricuspid (T1); this dual closing produces S1, or the "lub" part of the heartbeat. As the ventricles empty and they enter diastole, the pressure gradient forces the semilunar valves closed, with the aortic shutting (A2) just before the pulmonic (P2), and the two producing the familiar "dub" sound. The two semilunar valves closing can sometimes be distinguished, which results in audible splitting of S2 into its components.

Cardiac conduction during normal sinus rhythm

The heart, unlike other muscles in the body (which require an outside source of electrical impulse) can generate its own electrical current (automaticity or intrinsic rhythm), leading to the action potential that causes muscular contraction. During normal sinus rhythm, this impulse begins in the sinoatrial (SA) node, also known as the heart's pacemaker, located on the upper wall of the right atrium. This first impulse starts atrial contraction, forcing the blood into the ventricle. From here, the impulse is sent to the atrioventricular (AV) node, located in the lower right atrium, which delays excitation briefly, allowing the ventricles to completely fill. After pausing momentarily, the AV node fires, leading to ventricular contraction and ejection of blood from the ventricles. In certain situations, if the SA node fails to fire, the AV node will take over, which maintains the heartbeat, albeit at a slower rate.

Hemodynamic principles of the CV system

Normal circumstances

The CV system and its hemodynamics are based on pressure, flow and resistance throughout the cardiac cycle and within vasculature. Blood flows down the pressure gradient throughout the body, from areas of high pressure to areas of lower pressure. Arteries are under far more pressure than are veins, which contributes to this directional flow, and ensures that oxygenated blood flows smoothly from the heart, and that deoxygenated blood returns smoothly to the heart. The equation $v = Q/A$ tells us the velocity of blood flow (v - cm/sec), based on the blood flow (Q – ml/min) and cross-sectional area (A – cm^2) of the vessel. Blood flow (Q) is also called cardiac output, and can be found with the equation Q = pressure difference / R, where mean arterial pressure minus right atrial pressure yields the numerator (delta P – mm Hg), while the denominator (R – mm Hg/ml/min) is the total peripheral resistance. This formula is analogous to Ohm's law in physics (I = V/R), where Q equals the current I, delta P equals the voltage V, and R equals resistance in the wire. In addition, Reynolds number tells us whether flow will be turbulent (high) or laminar (low), and capacitance describes how distensible the vessels are, with veins having a higher capacitance than arteries. Changes in cross-sectional area and vessel diameters, via vasodilators or vasoconstrictors, are the main way that the CV system regulates blood flow and blood pressure.

Systemic circulation

The primary objective of the systemic circulation is to deliver oxygen and nutrients to the cells and tissues of the body, while removing carbon dioxide and waste. In order to do so efficiently, there must be adequate blood flow throughout the body. This requires a large enough pressure gradient between areas of high pressure (arteries) and areas of low pressure (veins). The highest pressure is found in the aorta, while the lowest pressure is in the vena cava. As blood flows from the arteries → arterioles → capillaries → venules → veins, pressure and resistance changes occur, whereby the arterioles have the highest systemic resistance, and therefore experience the largest drop in pressure during systemic circulation. Mean arterial pressure is the average pressure in the arteries over a period of time, and can be found by multiplying cardiac output times total peripheral resistance. The largest proportion of blood volume, owing to the low pressure, exists in the venous system. Capillaries have the largest total cross-sectional area of all the vessels, which combined with their single cell walls, allows for the greatest amount of gas and nutrient exchange. In the systemic vasculature, resistance is parallel, which means that the total systemic resistance is lower than within any specific artery.

Pulmonary vasculature

Unlike the rest of the body, the roles of the pulmonary circulation, in terms of arteries and veins, is reversed. While the pulmonary *artery* delivers *deoxygenated* blood from the right ventricle to the lungs for gaseous exchange and oxygenation, the pulmonary *veins* deliver *oxygenated* blood to the left atrium. Blood flow within the pulmonary circulation, as a result of an afterload that is far lower than in the systemic circulation, occurs against less resistance from the corresponding vessels, allowing greater flow to and from the lungs. However, when pulmonary wedge pressure is estimated to determine right atrial pressure, the pressure in the lung's capillaries are found to be slightly higher than that of the atrium. The resistance against flow from the lung's vessels is known as pulmonary vascular resistance (PVR). Problems within the pulmonary circulatory loop, such as pulmonary hypertension, can radically alter blood flow to and from the lungs, and requires an alteration in systolic pressure. Many factors can affect the hemodynamics and flow of the pulmonary vessels, including cardiac output.

Coronary vessels

Although all hemodynamic parameters are important, those of the coronary vasculature are especially significant, since these vessels feed the heart muscle itself. For this reason, reductions in their diameter (whether via CAD or otherwise) can seriously affect blood flow and perfusion to various areas of the heart. In some cases, this results in partial or complete blockage of the coronary arteries, which may lead to a heart attack (MI). As with the rest of the CV system, increased oxygen demand, whether because of exercise or pathology, results in utilization of the coronary flow reserve (CFR) to increase flow to the coronary vessels. The coronary microcirculation (capillaries) handles the functional duties of this system, and can be affected by not only normal CV variables, but also by the pressure and contractility of the heart itself, as these tiny vessels lie embedded within the myocardium. This is thought to be by design and a crucial part of control of these arteries and veins.

<u>Blood volume</u>
In addition to the formula using pressure and resistance, cardiac output (CO) can be measured using the equation CO = stroke volume (SV) x heart rate (HR), where SV is the volume of blood pumped from the ventricle with each beat of the heart. SV is the largest factor affecting pulse pressure (PP), which is the difference between systolic and diastolic pressures (pressure while the heart is contracting and relaxing, respectively). The largest proportion of blood resides in the venous system, because of the low pressure and high capacitance. The volume of blood in the veins is known as unstressed volume (because of the low pressure), while that in the arteries is known as stressed volume, owing to the increased pressure in this system. Hypovolemia can result in reduced blood pressure and flow, which can become critical when there is too little to perfuse various bodily tissues. In contrast, hypervolemia can result in pressure increases, which can produce vascular accidents such as stroke or aneurysm when not compensated for by normal physiological mechanisms.

Differences in circulation in specific vascular beds within the body

There are three different general vascular beds in the body: pulmonary, systemic and coronary. When referring to "beds", we are mainly referring to the capillaries, where diffusion occurs; this diffusion is regulated by hydrostatic and oncotic forces. The systemic bed can be further divided into the microvasculature found in and around specific organs (e.g. renal bed, cerebral bed, dermal bed, etc.) or type of tissue (e.g. skeletal muscle). Each vascular bed has somewhat unique properties that help promote efficient functioning, and each experiences different levels of oxygen saturation and various pressure changes. Of particular note are the beds of the coronary, cerebral, pulmonary and dermal systems, as well as those for skeletal muscle, which are designed to maximize physiological demands. For example, the cerebral circulation maintains tight endothelial seals (blood-brain barrier), while the GI system contains wide endothelial spaces, allowing for easy transfer of large molecules. All vascular beds maintain blood pressure and flow via both intrinsic (local) and extrinsic (hormonal) regulation.

Structure and function (A & P) of the heart muscle

The myocytes that make up cardiac muscle tissue contain contractile units called sarcomeres, which operate using a sliding filament mechanism involving actin and myosin. Intercalated disks join the ends of these cells, where spaces called gap junctions allow for low resistance passage of electrical current and action potentials, which are then transmitted intracellularly via t tubules. This excitation of the myocytes leads to calcium influx, aided and somewhat controlled by the sarcoplasmic reticulum, which leads to contraction (by removing inhibition of filamentous interaction) of the individual cells and heart muscle. This is known as excitation-contraction coupling, and the strength of this contraction depends directly on the level of intracellular calcium. Not surprisingly, the t tubules are better developed in the ventricles than the atria, to accommodate the difference in contractility required in the respective chambers.

Cell/tissue metabolism within the CV system

Cardiomyocyte metabolism is almost entirely aerobic under normal conditions, with only approximately 1% performed under anaerobic conditions. These cells contain an abundance of mitochondria, which serve the dual purposes of ATP production and calcium homeostasis, allowing for sustained forceful contraction of the muscle fibers. Myoglobin molecules are also abundant within cardiac tissue, which results in efficient use of oxygen by the heart cells and tissue; this oxygen-rich environment is further aided by an excellent blood supply. Cardiac tissue uses fats and carbohydrates (primarily glucose) in roughly a 60/40 division under normal circumstances to produce the energy necessary to function, mostly as ATP. During exertion, glucose metabolism increases within the cells and tissues, to accommodate needs for increased perfusion and oxygen consumption. Myocytes are terminal cells designed to last an entire lifetime, though either ischemia or apoptosis can lead to a shortened lifespan.

A & P of the CV system

Using an almost exclusively aerobic metabolic mechanism, cardiac cells and tissue demand on enormous amount of continuous oxygen supply, without which they can only perform anaerobically for a short time before becoming infarcted and necrotic. For this reason, cardiomyocytes are rich in myoglobin molecules and mitochondria, which cater to this immediate oxygen need. Oxygenation of the heart and brain will always take precedence in an oxygen-poor environment, as the body attempts to maintain perfusion to the most vital organs. Consumption of oxygen depends directly on the muscular tension of the ventricles, which relates to the contractile force and cardiac output required at a given moment. It is increased in situations where there is an increased afterload, enlarged heart size, heightened contractility (via inotropics or otherwise), or a need for elevated heart rate, such as during exercise.

A & P of vascular smooth muscle

While cardiac muscle is very similar in structure and function to skeletal muscle, the smooth muscle that lines the vasculature of the body is distinctly different in both areas. This is a result of the nature of its job compared to that of the other two types. Vascular smooth muscle (VSM) is non-striated, though it still utilizes primarily actin and myosin to effect contraction. Although there are two types of smooth muscle, single-unit and multi-unit, VSM is composed almost entirely of the former type, which allows for contraction of entire muscle sheets in a given area, which is known as a syncytium. The primary role of VSM is to regulate vasoconstriction and vasodilation within the CV system, via alpha-receptors, in order to control blood pressure and volume. The arteries have much more VSM than do the veins, because of the differences in the functions they must perform (i.e. arteries must maintain greater pressure to ensure circulation). As opposed to skeletal and cardiac muscle, VSM displays substantially increased contractility, which permits rather wide changes in vessel diameter while still retaining initial elasticity.

Biochemistry involved in normal CV functioning

Under normal aerobic conditions, the heart utilizes ATP (and to a lesser extent, creatine phosphate) as its major energy source, derived via oxidative phosphorylation within the mitochondria that are abundant in cardiomyocytes. The mitochondria achieve both ATP production and intracellular calcium regulation via the hydrogen electrochemical gradient, which is made possible by electron transport within these organelles. Increased intracellular calcium stimulates the Krebs cycle, which produces the needed ATP used for immediate cardiac demands. Myosin ATPase activity is responsible for muscle contraction and requires approximately ¾ of the ATP-derived energy created during this process. During periods of starvation, where usual nutrients are scarce, the CV system can utilize lactate, which is converted to pyruvate and eventually yields a large amount of ATP to be used for energy purposes when it can't be amassed using normal nutritional routes.

Endocrine or exocrine secretory function

In addition to responding to numerous outside neural and hormonal control mechanisms, the heart also plays a role in this regulation itself, secreting atrial natriuretic peptide/hormone (ANP/H). ANP is secreted by the atria in response to increases in atrial pressure. Locally, ANP may have a modest effect in limiting hypertrophy of the cardiac tissues, but most of its effect occurs outside the heart itself. ANP is released in order to combat increased arterial blood pressure, using a variety of mechanisms. Within the CV system, it relaxes vascular smooth muscle, which leads to lowered total peripheral resistance; in the renal system, it increases salt and water excretion, leading to a reduction in overall blood volume and cardiac output. These two mechanisms, in addition to inhibition of renin and countering of aldosterone, serve to help lower systemic blood pressure.

Secretory function of the endothelium

Besides the well-known purposes of endothelial cells (ECs) in the CV system (maintaining integrity of endocardial and vessel walls; gatekeeping, or regulating permeability to water, blood cells, peptides, lipids and many other substances; containing receptors for all sorts of purposes), it also serves a distinct secretory function as well. Endothelium-derived relaxing factor (EDRF) is produced by the ECs and serves to relax vascular smooth muscle locally, lowering pressure. Nitric oxide is one example. EDRF acts by producing cGMP, and can be stimulated/enhanced by the presence of circulating acetylcholine, which produces the expected anticholinergic effect of lowering blood pressure and resistance. ECs also regulate blood flow by altering the nature of its surface molecules, to range from prothrombotic to anti-thrombotic.

Microcirculation

The microcirculation, or capillary networks, have several unique features not found in the rest of the vasculature. Arterioles and metarterioles branch out into capillary beds, which eventually come together again to form venules. At the arteriole/capillary junction there is a smooth muscle sphincter (precapillary sphincter), separating the two structures. Unlike the rest of the CV system, capillaries do not contain any muscle tissue, consisting only of single endothelial cells (ECs) attached to a basement membrane. For this reason, capillary blood flow is controlled almost entirely by constriction or dilation of these sphincters, as well as that of the arterioles that precede them. There are small spaces between the ECs known as clefts or pores, which allow for movement of various substances across the capillary walls, facilitating gas exchange and diffusion of nutrients and waste. Depending on size and solubility, particles may cross this barrier using simple diffusion, pinocytosis or other means. Fluid exchange is governed by the Starling equation, and may result in net movement into or out of the capillary lumen.

Lymph flow

The lymphatic system runs roughly parallel to and complements the circulatory system, although unlike blood vessels, the lymphatic vessels form an open rather than closed system. Each vessel is lined by endothelial cells, which are surrounded by smooth muscle tissue, which itself is surrounded by a fibrous adventitia. The main role of the lymphatic vessels (particularly the lymphatic capillaries) is to reabsorb any extracellular/interstitial fluid that has been left behind after capillary filtration separating blood cells from plasma. While the majority of this fluid is actually reabsorbed directly by the venous system, any excess is taken up by the lymphatic system, for eventual return to the closed circulatory system, helping to maintain proper blood volume. In addition to fluid, the lymph that flows from the interstitial spaces may contain other particles, such as proteins and cells, targeted for reentry into the systemic circulation. One-way valves within the walls of lymph channels ensure that fluid cannot escape back into bodily tissues; when this system reaches capacity and can no longer absorb this extra fluid, edema results, which may be caused by increased filtration and/or occluded lymphatic ducts.

Atherosclerosis

Atherosclerosis, or "hardening of the arteries", is a phenomenon where fatty deposits of oxidized LDL particles initiate a monocytic inflammatory response in the arterial wall, sending macrophages to the area for the purpose of removing these lipid substances. When these immune cells prove incapable of performing this job successfully, they tend to rupture, leading to further deposits of oxidized LDL (and continuation of this cycle), and eventual formation of an atheroma, which is the central portion of an atheromatous plaque. As a chronic and mainly asymptomatic process, this buildup of plaques continues to occur, slowly occupying more and more luminal space of the arteries. Older plaques tend to begin calcifying as well (i.e. hardening), leading to further obstruction and dysfunction. Occasionally areas distal to an atherosclerotic-derived stenosis will become ischemic, resulting in positive symptoms. However, the major clinical concern in patients with atherosclerosis is eventual thrombus formation that can produce thromboembolic events such as stroke.

Normal neural control

Heart
The sympathetic and parasympathetic branches of the autonomic nervous system, based in the medulla, control immediate cardiac function by altering the heart rate (chronotropic effects) and conduction velocity (dromotropic effects). The former is accomplished by altering the SA node firing rate; the latter involves manipulation of AV node conduction velocity, with a consequent change in the PR interval. The parasympathetic system has negative chronotropic and dromotropic effects, decreasing heart rate and slowing conduction velocity (which increases PR interval), via the neurotransmitter acetylcholine, which acts at muscarinic receptors. Sympathetic impulses have positive chronotropic and dromotropic effects, leading to increased heart rate and AV node conduction velocity (decreasing the PR interval); they are modulated by norepinephrine acting at beta-1 receptors. Contractility is also affected by autonomic innervation, increasing under sympathetic influence and decreasing in the atria during parasympathetic control. Together, the two branches work to adjust to the changing demands placed on the CV system during times of rest versus activity.

Blood vessels and blood volume
Neural vascular regulation focuses on maintaining arterial blood pressure over the short term, primarily utilizing the baroreceptor reflex to effect moment-to-moment changes in pressure. The baroreceptors detect stretch levels of the artery walls at the carotid sinus and aortic arch, and direct the vascular system to respond accordingly. They are particularly sensitive to rapid changes in pressure. Lowered arterial pressure reduces stretch, which then slows firing of the carotid sinus nerve, indicating to the vasomotor center that it must raise arterial pressure. This is accomplished by decreasing parasympathetic impulses to the heart, while increasing sympathetic regulation of the heart and blood vessels. The result is an increase in pressure mediated by increased heart rate and contractility (yielding greater cardiac output), as well as arteriolar and venous vasoconstriction. Acting as a negative feedback loop, the baroreceptor reflex reduces these efforts once mean arterial pressure is restored to approximately 100 mm Hg. Additionally, chemoreceptors in the sinus and arch locations respond to slight decreases in oxygenation levels,

occurring as a result of the pressure drop, and further signal the vasomotor center to increase pressure (and thus oxygenation). An increase in arterial blood pressure causes the opposite sequence of events, via increased parasympathetic and decreased sympathetic stimulation.

Hormonal regulation

Heart

Hormones play a large role in regulation of the CV system, but mostly on tissues other than cardiac muscle. Their main effects are potentiated via changes in vessel diameter, as a means of controlling pressure and volume; these effects will be covered elsewhere. Epinephrine (adrenaline) does act on beta-1 receptors in the heart muscle to increase heart rate (and restart the heart in cases of asystole), but this is mostly in its capacity as a neurotransmitter in vivo, rather than a hormone (as when pushed IV in an emergency). Otherwise, hormonal control of the heart is minimal compared to that of the vessels and blood volume. Experimentally, adrenergic and thyroid hormones have been shown to influence growth of myocytes, but this is only in developmental stages and has only been demonstrated in the laboratory.

Blood vessels and blood volume

With the exception of acute hemorrhage, hormones are normally used for long-term regulation of blood pressure via alterations in blood volume. There are several mechanisms by which this takes place, but the most important is the renin-angiotensin-aldosterone system (RAA system/axis), which responds to reduced renal per-fusion pressure by increasing blood volume. Detection of low pres-sure in the afferent arteriole stimulates renin secretion, which helps convert angiotensinogen to angiotensin I (Ang I) in the plasma; Ang I is then converted to the physiologically active angiotensin II (Ang II) in the lungs, via angiotensin converting enzyme (ACE). Ang II performs two functions that help increase blood volume and pressure. First, it stimulates aldosterone produc-tion in the adrenal cortex, which leads to increased retention of sodium chloride (and thus water) by the kidneys; and it also causes vasoconstriction of arterioles. Together, these actions help to raise volume and resistance, which serve to increase blood pressure to desired levels. Another hormone, antidiuretic hormone (ADH, or vasopressin), is involved in pressure regulation only in cases of hemorrhage. ADH is released from the posterior pituitary in response to detected volume/pressure drops, and acts to constrict arterioles and reabsorb water, both of which aid in bumping up blood pressure via volume effects. In addition, there are other hormones (bradykinin, histamine, serotonin and prostaglandins) that act as vasodilators and vasoconstrictors in specific areas and circumstances.

Neural regulatory response of the CV system

Postural changes

Upon standing from a supine or sitting position, venous blood pools in the lower extremities, decreasing blood volume and venous return, which leads to reduced cardiac output (via lowered stroke volume). The baroreceptors in the carotid sinus detect a rapid fall in blood pressure, which causes the vasomotor center to respond with compensatory mechanisms that enhance sympathetic outflow while decreasing parasympathetic impulses. The net result is an increase in heart rate and total peripheral resistance, which serves to raise blood pressure back to normal. This response is an attempt to correct the orthostatic hypotension that occurs upon standing. If one rises too quickly while dehydrated, at high altitude or with impaired baroreceptor reflexes, he or she may experience syncope because of the lack of cerebral perfusion pressure (since the brain is furthest away from the pooled venous blood).

<u>Exercise</u>
The neural response to exercise is composed of an anticipatory branch and a reactive branch. Initially, in response to the expectation of exercise, the sympathetic system is stimulated, increasing outflow to the heart and vessels, with a resultant rise in heart rate, stroke volume and cardiac output. At the same time, there is an increase in venous return, providing larger stroke volume; and there is increased arteriolar resistance in secondary areas not crucial to the effort (skin, GI, kidneys, etc.), which reduces blood flow to these regions and increases flow where it is needed most. Once exercise has begun, active skeletal muscles produce metabolites such as adenosine, potassium and lactate, which act as vasodilators at the arteriolar level. This dilation effect allows for greater blood flow (hyperemia) and oxygenation of active areas, and yields an overall drop in total peripheral resistance.

Hormonal regulatory response of the CV system

<u>Postural changes</u>
Hormonal responses within the CV system are generally slower than those controlled neurally, which means they play less of a role in the immediate or rapid responses required after a postural change. While they begin to act once reduced arterial pressure is detected, the fact that they are slower than their neural analogues makes their effects much less potent, especially at first. However, changes in posture do cause increases in several active hormones relevant to the CV system, including prostaglandins, renin, angiotensin II, aldosterone, vasopressin and norepinephrine. A decrease in atrial natriuretic peptide occurs at the same time. These changes are usually noticed over the span of minutes rather than seconds, in contrast to neural responses that act much more quickly. Also, increases are not always linear and may be biphasic or multiphasic. As a result, their effects are markedly milder, but appear to have some impact in maintaining the hemodynamic adjustments initially achieved via neural mechanisms, particularly regarding cerebral hemodynamic homeostasis. The frequency of postural changes obviously affects how impactful such slower hormonal influences are.

<u>Exercise</u>
Even though neural regulation is much more important than hormonal on a moment-to-moment basis during exercise, the CV system does respond to hormone release upon exertion, albeit more slowly than via autonomic mechanisms. When exercise is undertaken, epinephrine and norepinephrine are released to accommodate the increased perfusion and oxygenation demands on the CV system, acting on beta-1 receptors in the cardiac muscle and alpha-receptors on the vessels. In addition, levels of angiotensin II, renin and aldosterone all increase (mildly at first, and then more prominently after significant exertion); aldosterone increases fastest, followed by renin, and then angiotensin II. Still, the response by the CV system to these changes is considerably slower and less potent than those potentiated by neural control. Plenty of other hormones are released and become active during exercise – testosterone, growth hormone and cortisol are a few examples – but none demonstrate significant effects directly on the CV system.

Repair and regeneration processes in the CV system

Cardiomyocytes are terminal cells, meaning they do not grow into other types of cells, and do not regenerate in adults. This means that once the heart muscle experiences ischemic or cardiomyopathic injury sufficient for necrosis, these cells will not heal, and the respective area of the myocardium will become non-functional, with the formation of scar tissue. This scar tissue does not contribute to muscle contraction, which affects pumping ability. The vessels of the CV system do have certain repair mechanisms capable of mending endothelial injuries, but these repairs also pose other threats within the system. At the start of ischemic injury to the heart, marrow-derived stem cells do rush to the site in an attempt to repair/regenerate, but in limited numbers and among the chaos of the inflammatory and necrotic processes, they are incapable of effecting any reparative changes. Research has shown new cardiomyocytes may be grown from both adult and embryonic stem cells lines, and that there may indeed be a stem cell mechanism innate to the heart muscle as well. The latest of this research has even shown success with this method using one's own heart stem cells, which are removed during bypass surgery and re-seeded in the heart when their number grows to one million cells.

Changes the CV system undergoes at various stages of life

From birth through old age, the CV system undergoes a number of normal changes, based on "physiological" age, rather than "chronological" age (making separation into stages difficult). As we age, the SA node loses cells, which results in a slower intrinsic rhythm and lowered heart rate. There is also reduced elasticity and increased stiffness throughout the CV system, particularly in the arteries, which affects the aorta and leads to an increase in systolic blood pressure, which itself results in left ventricular hypertrophy, as the heart tries to maintain cardiac output in the face of increased resistance. The valves, especially the aortic, calcify and stiffen, producing an expected murmur. ECG changes commonly occur (possibly leading to dysrhythmias), and capillary walls thicken somewhat. Baroreceptors become less sensitive, which results in a greater tendency to experience orthostatic hypotension. These changes tend to occur on a continuum, taking place gradually throughout the lifecycle, and are somewhat dependent on age, diet, exercise and lifestyle, in addition to genetics.

Infectious disorders

Many microbes have the possibility of causing infection within the CV system, including viruses, fungi and bacteria (including parasites). Within the heart itself, the two major conditions that result from microbial seeding are myocarditis (muscle) and endocarditis (endothelial lining), the latter of which includes valvular disease. Infection of the valves (usually by bacteria) is particularly common in patients with valve replacements, and especially in those with artificial valves. This is also frequently the site of initial infection in rheumatic fever from Strep, which can develop into rheumatic heart disease if not treated with antibiotics. Myocarditis is most often viral in nature, although it may also be caused by a variety of infectious agents. Pericarditis (outer sac) can also be caused by microbes, as can vasculitis, though these generally experience a wider range of etiologies.

Inflammatory disorders

Inflammatory CV disorders, much like inflammatory conditions in general, can have a huge variety of causes and consequences, depending on the offending agent or event. Infectious and immunological etiologies are covered elsewhere, while we focus here on general principles of inflammation in the heart and vessels. Anything CV-related ending in -itis can be considered an inflammatory disease: endocarditis, myocarditis, pericarditis, and vasculitis. In addition, many related conditions are known or suspected to be at least partially a result of a prolonged inflammatory response, including atherosclerosis, MI and CVA. Depending on the specific disorder, inflammation may be traumatic, iatrogenic, metabolic, dietary, or secondary to stress; inflammation also occurs after a MI or other cardiomyopathy, in an attempt to restore function. Of course this inflammatory response, especially as a reaction to a specific insult, is meant to be protective and restorative, but it also takes its toll physiologically; this is particularly true of chronic inflammation.

Immunologic disorders

There are two basic classes of cardiovascular immune disorders: those caused by autoimmunity (including allergies), and those enabled by immunodeficiency. The former often manifests as one or more vascular disorders, including MI, CVA and atherosclerosis, all of which are believed to be susceptible to the prolonged effects of cytokines, proteases, autoantibodies and many more immunomodulators. In addition, several autoimmune diseases have been linked to increased CV morbidity, including lupus, rheumatoid arthritis, antiphospholipid syndrome and Sjögren syndrome, among others. Rheumatic heart disease is an autoimmune disease that occurs chronically after initial Strep infection. As with other sources of inflammation, autoimmunity can yield endocarditis, myocarditis and pericarditis. With immunodeficiency, whether via HIV (which has become more common) or otherwise, the CV system, along with the rest of the body, becomes much more open to opportunistic infections. Such infections range from manageable to deadly, and may be caused by a long list of potential pathogens.

Trauma

The most obvious type of cardiac trauma in terms of pathology and effect is a direct puncture or laceration, which can have a range of effects, from minimal through fatal, usually depending on internal blood loss and or myocardial damage. Blunt cardiac trauma (as in a car accident) usually results in myocardial contusion, and may have other deleterious consequences as well. Abnormalities that may result from blunt trauma include dysrhythmias, wall motion dysfunction, and in the worst-case scenario, septal or wall rupture. The last category may induce cardiogenic shock, depending on the size and location of the lesion. Other types of pressure-related traumas (the extreme example being caught in a constrictor snake's grip) may also result in rupture of parts of the vasculature. Pulmonary trauma can make it difficult to oxygenate the tissues, and cerebral trauma can affect the vasomotor center in the medulla. Finally, any trauma that causes a massive hemorrhage will greatly affect the CV system, tanking cardiac output and leading to hemorrhagic shock.

Mechanical disorders

The most well known mechanical disorder is heart failure, which is actually the culmination of other inciting mechanical disorders that occurred previously. The list of potential disorders is long, as is the list of possible causes, but they can be broken down into two categories: cardiomyopathies (defects involving ventricles) and valvular disease. Cardiomyopathies can result from any insult to the myocardium that affects pumping ability, or they may be idiopathic; a common cause is an MI, where some parts of the muscle become non-functional. These disorders are generally divided into dilated congestive (ventricular expansion/stretching, usually left, reducing contractility), hypertrophic (ventricular wall thickening, reducing stroke volume) and restrictive (ventricular wall stiffening, reducing diastolic filling). Valve disorders are categorized by the specific valve involved (mitral, tricuspid or aortic) as well as the structural/functional defect. Prolapse describes a valve that has one or more leafs protruding into the atrium, which prevents full closure during systole; it often results in regurgitation, where there is backwards flow during systole from ventricle to atrium. Stenosis occurs when there is a narrowing of the valve space, leading to an obstruction of flow across that valve.

Neoplastic diseases

CV neoplasms can be divided into benign and malignant primary lesions, as well as secondary malignant metastatic tumors. Malignant tumors are exceedingly rare and are seen mainly in children, with sarcoma (soft tissue tumor) being the most prevalent; other examples include primary lymphoma and pericardial mesothelioma. Benign tumors are still quite rare, with the most common being myxoma (women>men; usually in left atrium); others seen less often are certain types of fibroma, elastoma, myoma, teratoma, lipoma and hemangioma, among others. Metastases to the heart from primary carcinomas of the lungs, breast and kidneys are common, as are those from leukemia, lymphoma and melanoma. Prognoses with CV metastases are generally poor. Finally, vascular tumors (including those related to or surrounding vessels) are variants of sarcoma, and range from benign to intermediate to malignant. Benign forms include hemangioma, lymphangioma and glomus tumor. Neoplasms of intermediate severity include hemangiopericytoma and hemangioendothelioma, while angiosarcoma and Kaposi's sarcoma (commonly seen with HIV) are considered malignant.

Metabolic and regulatory disorders

The main metabolic disorder that contributes hugely to CV disease and dysfunction is actually a cluster of problems known as metabolic syndrome (MS). The definition varies a bit according to the agency cited, but MS is generally present when a person is found to have some combination (differs based on criteria list) of obesity, hypertension, dyslipidemia and elevated fasting glucose. Having MS can greatly contribute to development of diabetes (itself a risk factor) and coronary heart disease (CHD), as well as other CV abnormalities, including atherosclerosis and CVA. Regulatory CV disorders are based on autonomic disturbances (including receptor problems), hormonal imbalance or rhythmic dysfunction. The issue is usually one of maintaining the appropriate heart rate, force of contraction and/or blood pressure. The most common of these disorders is actually quite normal, especially for the elderly, and is known as orthostatic hypotension, whereby BP temporarily drops in response to standing. If this affects cerebral perfusion to a large enough degree, the person may faint; but it is otherwise generally self-limited. Other regulatory conditions involve problems with the SA node, as well as longer-term issues with the renin-angiotensin-aldosterone axis.

Dysrhythmias

A dysrhythmia (*not* arrhythmia, which means no rhythm) is any electrical disturbance within the heart that results in a rhythm other than normal sinus. It can be the result of a problem anywhere along the electrical circuitry of the heart, including the SA node (pace-maker), AV node, bundle of His, Purkinje fibers, bundle branches or fascicles; and may produce tachycardia, bradycardia or another irregularity, such as flutter or fibrillation, among others. In all varieties, the effect of a dysrhythmia is impaired conduction and prevention of proper blood flow to a greater or lesser degree, in addition to potentiating possible thromboembolic complications. Clinically, patients range from being completely asymptomatic (sub-clinical disease) to having palpitations to experiencing life-threatening hemodynamic instability. Atrial fibrillation is the most common dysrhythmia, exhibiting an irregular and disordered rhythm, while atrial flutter is similar in effect but with different pathology. Both involve reentrant circuit issues and display charac-teristic ECG changes, and are known as supraventricular because they occur above the level of the ventricle. Ventricular dysrhythm-ias, in contrast, originate because of problems within the circuitry of the ventricles themselves, and include ventricular tachy-cardia and ventricular fibrillation. Of the many other types of rhythm disturbances possible, some of the more common include partial or complete

- 250 -

heart block, ectopic beats, narrow/wide QRS syndrome and sick sinus syndrome, all of which display unique ECG tracings.

Systolic dysfunction

Having dilated (congestive) cardiomyopathy (majority of cardiomyopathies) is the main cause of systolic dysfunction (trouble with ventricular contraction), which often leads to heart failure if it cannot be treated successfully. It is a problem of reduced inotropy/contractility within the left ventricle, which results in decreased stroke volume and ejection fraction, as well as increased preload, and end diastolic volume and pressure. There are many possible precipitants of dilated cardiomyopathy and systolic dysfunction, with alcohol/cocaine abuse, viral myocarditis, Chagas' disease, Beriberi, doxorubicin toxicity and peripartum myopathy topping the list. Some clinical findings are an S3 heart sound, heart dilation on echo, and a classic "balloon" shape on chest x-ray. Treatment includes inotropic medications like digitalis (to increase contractility), as well as beta agonists, arterial vasodilators and diuretics (all of which aid in reduction of various volumes, loads and pressures).

Diastolic dysfunction

Either hypertrophic cardiomyopathy (HC) or restrictive/obliterative cardiomyopathy (RC) can eventually lead to diastolic dysfunction (DD) of the heart, where there is a defect/problem filling the ventricles with sufficient blood. However, DD generally has a better prognosis for most patients than does systolic dysfunction. DD is defined as clinical heart failure signs and symptoms, without evidence of systolic dysfunction (meaning the patient has an ejection fraction > 45%), though stroke volume is still reduced. It must be distinguished from the systolic variant before treatment begins. In HC, a thickened interventricular septum blocks outflow from the mitral valve, leading to a ventricular filling defect. Half of the cases are inherited in autosomal dominant fashion, and it is most often the cause of sudden cardiac death among athletes. Clinical findings include an S4 sound, apical electrical impulses and systolic murmur, all in the context of normal heart size on x-ray with ventricular hypertrophy on echo. Treatment involves the use of beta-blockers and myocardial calcium channel blockers. In RC, which is less common, the pathology is somewhat different, but the effect is much the same. Causes include sarcoidosis, amyloidosis, hemochromatosis and other forms of fibrosing disease.

Low-output heart failure

Most progressive cardiac disease results in left or right-sided low-output heart failure (LOHF), where there is a decreased ability of the heart to pump sufficient blood to meet the tissue metabolism requirements, resulting in problems with peripheral circulation. Except in cor pulmonale, right-sided failure is usually secondary to left-sided failure. LOHF may be seen in both systolic and diastolic dysfunction, and is determined to be present when the ejection fraction is < 45%. It may be acute or chronic, and has a long list of possible causes, which vary somewhat according to specific pathology and timing. Some of the more prominent etiologies include cardiomyopathy, coronary artery disease, hypertension, diabetes, infection, inflammation, valve disease, certain drugs, dysrhythmias and (especially in an acute case) myocardial infarction. Some common signs and symptoms are tachycardia, tachypnea/dyspnea, fluid overload with edema (because heart can't keep up with venous return), orthopnea, jugular venous distention and rales/crackles (resulting from pulmonary edema). It is normally diagnosed via echo showing reduced stroke volume and ejection fraction, along with angiography, ECG and blood tests, as corroboration or investigation into a cause. Treatment centers on improving cardiac output and reducing workload, while decreasing patient symptoms and discomfort. Medications used may include ACE inhibitors, beta-blockers, diuretics, vasodilators and aldosterone antagonists; dietary changes, including lowered salt intake, are also recommended.

High-output heart failure

In contrast to low-output heart failure, which comprises the majority of cases, high-output heart failure (HOHF) exists when ventricular function, stroke volume and cardiac output remain normal, with an ejection fraction > 45%, but clinical signs and symptoms of failure are present. Seen mostly with diastolic dysfunction, it is caused by an increase in blood volume or cells, which may be the result of a number of conditions or scenarios, and leads to increased circulatory demand. This increase leads to inefficient circulation of the entire volume through the vascular system, and effective HOHF. Some common situations that may lead to HOHF include fluid overload secondary to infusions, hyperthyroidism, anemia, hepatomegaly, Paget's disease, septic shock, kidney disease and arteriovenous fistulae or malformations. The result is a lowered vascular resistance, which makes maintaining arterial blood pressure and proper circulation difficult. Treatment focuses on correcting or ameliorating the underlying pathology if possible, and reduction of blood volume, easing afterload and demand crises. It is vital to distinguish from low-output heart failure, since the use of vasodilators in the face of HOHF will likely further complicate blood pressure stabilization.

Differences between low-output and high-output heart failure

Most heart failure is categorized as low-output heart failure (LOHF), as most significant cardiac disease, if not treated or treatable, eventually result in a reduced stroke volume, ejection fraction (< 45%) and cardiac output. This reduced output separates LOHF from its counterpart, high-output heart failure (HOHF), where those same parameters remain normal, but the patient exhibits signs and symptoms of heart failure. Both states present with roughly the same symptoms – including dyspnea, tachycardia, orthopnea, and pulmonary and lower limb edema – as the pathophysiological effects are quite similar, despite different mechanisms. As opposed to LOHF, HOHF involves an increase in blood volume, which is realized via a number of pathways, including infusions, renal/hepatic disease and hyperthyroidism, among others. While ventricular function remains normal or even higher than normal, the increased blood volume in HOHF leads to systemic circulatory and pressure problems. One of the main differences is in diagnosis and treatment, since the two must be distinguished before therapy begins. The reason for this is because some of the medications prescribed for LOHF may adversely affect HOHF patients, and to a lesser extent, vice versa.

Cor pulmonale

When it is not secondary to left-sided heart failure, right-sided heart failure is most often the result of a pulmonary-derived cardiac problem known as cor pulmonale (CP). CP may be caused by primary lung disorders (especially COPD, tissue loss, primary pulmonary hypertension and pulmonary embolus), abnormal chest wall/cavity structure, fibrotic disorders (scleroderma) or a decreased respiratory drive with subsequent alveolar hypoventilation and hypoxia (which further constricts pulmonary vessels, adding to the effects). Regardless of the cause, CP virtually always features right ventricular enlargement and pulmonary artery hypertension, which leads to an increased afterload on right ventricular contraction.

The most common symptoms are exertional dyspnea/syncope and substernal anginal pain; signs include systolic lift, a loud second pulmonic sound and exertional fatigue, as well as possible tricuspid/pulmonic murmurs and edema. Other clinical findings are enlarged right heart and pulmonary artery on imaging and ECG (showing RV hypertrophy) and a gallop rhythm with prominent S3 and S4. Diagnostic testing and determination is essential, since underlying conditions may hide CP, and it may be mistaken for left heart failure. Treatment is of variable efficacy, depending heavily on resolution of underlying causes. In the absence of that possibility, diuretics may be used but also may cause respiratory alkalosis, and oxygen via nasal cannula should be administered constantly. Other measures include possible use of pulmonary vasodilators, and the potential need for anticoagulation in the event of venous thromboembolic events (occur more often in CP).

Pulmonary hypertension

Pulmonary hypertension may develop secondary to a host of non-primary causes, but when there is no other clear etiology, a diagnosis of primary pulmonary hypertension (PPH) is generally made (often leading to cor pulmonale). PPH is a very rare disorder of unknown cause, seen more in women, that affects small and medium-sized pulmonary arteries, and almost always eventually results in right ventricular failure. It characteristically displays hyperplasia and hypertrophy of vessel walls, and consequent stenosis of the lumen, increasing blood pressure; the chief symptom is exertional dyspnea that becomes progressively worse. In order to make a diagnosis of PPH, all other potential causes of cor pulmonale must be excluded, utilizing a battery of tests that may include an echo, pulmonary function tests, V/Q scan and/or cardiac catheterization, in addition to others. While vasodilators are successful in radically lowering pulmonary artery pressure in some patients, this is the exception rather than the norm. Empiric treatment with long-term anticoagulation is sometimes added to the medication regimen because of the tendency for PPH patients to develop silent thromboses or emboli (which may or may not be the precipitant of the PPH itself) and for the purposes of counteracting venous stasis effects from right heart failure.

Systemic hypertension

Systemic hypertension (HTN) refers to increased arterial blood pressure in the systemic circulation and it is hugely prevalent worldwide. It is known as the "silent killer", since many patients remain asymptomatic until the effects of HTN on various end organs begin to take hold. Even then, symptoms are generally non-specific and varied, while none are pathognomonic for HTN. It may be categorized as primary/essential HTN (90%) or secondary (usually a result of kidney disease). One can have systolic, diastolic or combined HTN, which are defined as a BP measurement > 140/90 mm Hg (on at least two different occasions), according to which of these indices are elevated. Primary HTN involves an increase in both cardiac output (via increased venous return) and/or total peripheral resistance (via vasoconstriction), and is believed to be influenced most heavily by the sympathetic nervous system and renin-angiotensin-aldosterone axis. Risk factors include obesity, aging, diabetes, smoking and genetic predisposition; blacks are at greater risk than whites, who are at greater risk than Asians. Treatment involves several types of antihypertensive medications, including possibly beta-blockers, calcium channel blockers, diuretics and ACE inhibitors; lifestyle changes are necessary. Complications of untreated hypertension include atherosclerosis, left ventricular hypertrophy, CHF, CVA, renal failure, aortic dissection and retinopathy; malignant HTN is a rapidly progressive form of severe HTN that constitutes a medical emergency.

Ischemic heart disease

Ischemic heart disease (IHD), or coronary artery disease (CAD), describes a state where one or more coronary arteries become partially or totally occluded (stenosis vs. complete blockage), resulting in a lack of perfusion and consequent ischemia of the myocardium. The offending mechanism is the inability of the coronary arteries to adequately meet cardiac output and myocardial oxygenation demands; the effect without resolution can lead to infarction and necrosis of tissue. IHD can present either acutely or chronically, though most acute MI sufferers, especially in the absence of illicit drugs or other extreme factors, probably have some degree of chronic IHD as well. It is most often a result of chronic accumulation of lipid materials within the arteries and atherosclerosis, though it may also be driven by coronary artery spasms. There are four major potential manifestations of CAD: angina pectoris, myocardial infarction (MI), sudden cardiac death and chronic IHD. Angina occurs when there is > 75% occlusion and has several variants; symptoms include substernal chest pain with radiation to various areas. MI generally involves an acute thrombosis of one or more coronary arteries and causes myocardial cell death if not resolved; symptoms are variable but may be similar to angina. Sudden death is defined as fatality within one hour of the start of symptoms, and usually derives from a lethal dysrhythmia. Chronic IHD gradually progresses towards CHF over many years.

Acute myocardial infarction

An acute MI is the result of coronary artery occlusion (LAD>RCA> circumflex), usually via acute thrombosis, that is significant enough to cause infarction of the surrounding tissue. Symptoms may include one or more of the following (it can be be asymptomatic): crushing chest pain, diaphoresis, dyspnea, nausea/vomiting, left arm or jaw pain/radiation, and other adrenergic symptoms, such as tachycardia. MI can be diagnosed using a combination of ECG (especially within six hours of onset) and enzyme measurements (CK-MB, troponin 1 and AST). Enzymes may be elevated, and ECG changes depend on the location of the infarct, but generally show either ST elevation or depression, and/or pathologic Q waves (which remain after the acute episode). Transmural infarcts affect the entire wall thickness, tend to do more damage, and display ST elevation; subendocardial infarcts typically involve < 50% of the ventricle wall, and display ST depression. Acute empiric therapy may include oxygen, morphine, nitroglycerin, beta blockers and thrombolytics (if within the time range); the patient may be told to chew an aspirin tablet immediately, to potentiate anticoagulant effects. Chronic treatment focus on reducing or removing inciting factors such as hypertension or atherosclerosis/hyperlipidemia, monitoring progress, and substantial changes in diet and lifestyle. Possible complications of MI include dysrhythmia/arrhythmia, cardiogenic shock, ventricular wall rupture, aneurysm, pericarditis, and left ventricular failure with pulmonary edema.

Systemic hypotension and development of hypotensive shock

Hypotension is defined as a state where blood pressure (BP) has fallen below the minimum needed to maintain proper circulatory function and tissue perfusion. As BP is the single most important vital sign, hypotension and hypotensive shock can be medical emergencies. All forms of shock are hypotensive by definition, regardless of mechanism; the end result is always BP that is too low, yielding a lack of adequate tissue perfusion. There are three mechanisms by which shock can occur: hypovolemia, poor cardiac function and vasodilation. While all shock is hypotensive, each case is labeled according to the presumed cause, of which there are five: hemorrhagic (hypovolemic), cardiogenic, neurogenic (leading to cardiogenic), anaphylactic and septic (both vasodilatory). Regardless of the cause, the main object of treatment is to increase blood pressure to normal levels as soon as possible, since inadequate perfusion quickly leads to tissue ischemia and death. Specific therapy depends somewhat on the inciting factor and mechanism, but all involve finding a way to quickly stabilize vitals. The most crucial of these is first stopping further blood loss if possible. Among many other possible interventions are fluid infusion, cardiac restoration, vasopressors and assisted ventilation. Without prompt attention, all versions of shock can rapidly proceed to death. Lay people are almost never referring to actual hypo-tensive shock when they refer to someone as "in shock", but rather to a state of delirium and confusion following a trauma or tragedy.

Cardiogenic shock and hemorrhagic shock

Cardiogenic and hemorrhagic shock is two of five recognized types of shock, with the other three being neurogenic, anaphylactic and septic. Cardiogenic shock refers to hypotension pre-cipitated by an abnormality in cardiac function and output, which lowers BP and reduces the amount of oxygenated blood available to body tissues. In contrast, hemorrhagic shock is a form of hypo-volemic shock, where because of some injury or defect (other than cardiac) there is not enough blood volume in the system to ensure adequate BP and circulation. Both types result in similar clinical pictures: weak or absent peripheral pulses, tachycardia, cold and cyanotic extremities, increased capillary refill, tachypnea/hyper-ventilation and mental status changes. Both require immediate stabilization of vital signs. With cardiogenic shock, therapy centers on correcting or treating any cardiac defects if possible (such as following the protocol for acute MI), as well as fluid infusions and pharmacological vascular management to restore blood pressure. Hemorrhagic shock, which involves either an external or internal massive bleed, should be treated first and foremost by stopping the bleeding, since other rescue efforts (including CPR) will be meaningless without adequate blood volume to maintain pressure. With an external wound, the object is to find the site and stop or reduce the blood flow; suspected internal bleeding requires prompt surgical attention in an attempt to discover the culprit and resolve the issue. Both types, as with all shock, have the same end result if not resolved: death.

Dyslipidemias

A dyslipidemia (also known as hyperlipoproteinemia, because of the way lipids travel coupled to proteins in the plasma) is any of a number of disorders that results in elevated levels of cholesterol (VLDL/LDL/IDL/HDL) and triglycerides (TGs) in the blood, as a result of altered or overwhelmed metabolism and/or disordered regulation. Dyslipidemias are found to be either familial or exogenous (fairly rare). There are several reasons this can occur, with diet and heredity being two major influences; and there are myriad possible mechanisms that may contribute to this increase. Their effect on the CV system is mostly via formation of atherosclerotic plaques in the arteries, which in the worst-case scenario can lead to MI and CVA, or similar manifestations; other less lethal problems such as peripheral artery disease may also occur. Atherosclerosis leads to stenosis of the vessel lumen, which hampers the body's ability to properly perfuse tissues. In the absence of major acute cardio or cerebrovascular incidents, dyslipidemias can still be recognized by several characteristic signs, including atheromas (vessel wall plaques), xanthomas (skin and tendons) and corneal arcus lipid deposits. Medical management carries several options, which include pharmacological agents to lower lipid levels, stents to open severely occluded arteries and procedures such as endarterectomy, to remove the blockage.

Aneurysms

An aneurysm, which is a bulging/ballooning of a vessel wall, can have several common causes; a ruptured aneurysm is a medical/surgical emergency. A few common types are: arteriovenous fistula (secondary to trauma, results in high-output heart failure), atherosclerotic (secondary to chronic atherosclerotic disease; usually abdominal aortic aneurysm, or AAA), berry (congenital; cerebral arteries, especially circle of Willis; danger of subarachnoid hemorrhage), dissecting (secondary to hypertension and common with Marfan syndrome; usually aortic arch), syphilitic (secondary to tertiary syphilis; ascending aorta and/or aortic root/valve), and infectious (secondary to bacterial infection; abdominal aorta). All have the potential for rupture, which is why many are surgically fixed prophylactically. Also, it is worth noting that AAAs are notorious killers, since pain is not felt in most cases until serious damage has been or is about to be done; a midline abdominal bulge with a strong pulse is a key sign. This has earned it the following refrain: most patients don't know they have it until they're dead. Quick intervention is obviously essential.

Reducing hypertension using antihypertensives

Hypertension (HTN) is mediated by two mechanisms: increased cardiac output (CO) and increased total peripheral resistance (TPR); specifically, arteriolar resistance is increased, while venous capacitance is lowered. Untreated, HTN can lead to CHF, MI, CVA and renal damage. Therefore, the goal of antihypertensive therapy is the reduction of one or both of these measures via various medications. Blood pressure is regulated primarily by two different systems: the baroreceptors, which control immediate changes in BP via modulation of sympathetic and parasympathetic outflow and corresponding changes in vasoconstriction and cardiac output; and the renin-angiotensin-aldosterone axis, responsible for longer-term control, via constriction or dilation of the vessels (renin-angiotensin), increasing resistance, as well as by changing blood volume by controlling renal sodium absorption (aldosterone). Thus antihypertensives' mechanisms are centered on countering these control measures, at the cardiac, renal and/or vascular level. Patients are generally started on one agent from among the major classes, and additional medications may be added as needed. While most people are treated with one or more of the specific antihypertensive types covered elsewhere, specific circumstances may call for other meds such as prazosin, hydralazine or diazoxide.

Common disorders of the CV system

Congenital
Several common CV disorders are present at birth, some of which resolve on their own, while others require intervention. Here we examine some of these congenital conditions. Atrial septal defect (ASD): primum or secundum (more common) depending on location along septum, causing left-to-right shunting, may be asymptomatic for decades and more common in females. Patent ductus arteriosus (PDA): failed closure of ductus arteriosus (DA) because of premature birth and/or hypoxemia, with constant/machinery murmur, second most common. Coarctation of the aorta: infantile is proximal to PDA, while adult is distal to subclavian artery, symptom levels depend on stenosis of vessel (lower limb cyanosis in infants, upper limb HTN in adults) and may be asymptomatic, seen in Turner syndrome males. Tetralogy of Fallot: four defects seen together (overarching aorta, ventricular septal defect (VSD), pulmonary stenosis and RV hypertrophy) causing right-to-left shunting and cyanosis with "boot-shaped heart" on x-ray, squatting relives symptoms. Transposition of the great vessels: distinct pulmonary and systemic circulations because of aorta connection to RV and pulmonary artery connection to LV, cannot support life without concomitant shunt, cyanosis at birth, common with diabetic mothers. VSD: hole along ventricular septum can be membranous or muscular, with left-to-right shunt and murmur (with small defect, which may resolve spontaneously), most common congenital defect.

Vascular
There are quite a few fairly common vascular disorders other than aneurysms, which are discussed separately; here we consider some of the most commonly seen conditions. Churg-Strauss: vasculitis affecting small and medium arteries, associated with eosinophilia and asthma. Henoch-Schönlein purpura: IgA-mediated vasculitis in smaller vessels, often seen in children with an URI.

Kaposi sarcoma: viral origin, involving cutaneous and visceral vessels, mainly in immunodeficient patients. Kawasaki disease: necrotizing inflammation in all vessels, with systemic symptoms, usually in children. Rendu-Osler-Weber: autosomal dominant inheritance, small vessel dilation with GI bleeding, seen in Mormons. Polyarteritis nodosa: necrotizing breakdown of media layer, caused by antineutrophil antibodies (p-ANCA), in small and medium arteries, often with Hep B infection. Takayasu arteritis (pulseless disease; aortic arch syndrome): stenotic inflammation of aortic arch with loss of carotid, ulnar and radial pulses, often in Asian women.

Temporal arteritis (giant cell): temporal artery inflammation presenting with headache and visual problems, usually in elderly and showing elevated ESR. Thromboangiitis obliterans (Buerger disease): full-thickness inflammation of small and medium vessels, presents with Raynaud phenomenon, found in heavy smokers of Jewish ethnicity. Von Hippel-Lindau disease: autosomal dominant inheritance, affects visceral vessels with hemangioblastomas and cysts, predisposes to renal cell carcinoma. Wegener granulomatosis: necrotizing granulomatous lesions of lung and kidney small vessels, caused by c-ANCAs, often presents with nasal septum ulcers. Finally, lack of movement or failing valves in the elderly can lead to stasis of the blood in the lower limbs and deep venous thrombosis (DVT), which can itself result in a pulmonary embolus.

Systemic
Many systemic diseases may adversely affect the CV system; here we consider some of those most commonly seen and their possible consequences. Diabetes mellitus: atherosclerosis, coronary artery disease (CAD), restrictive cardiomyopathy and MI. Hyperthyroidism: sinus tachycardia, fatigue, systolic hypertension (HTN), palpitations and increased cardiac output (CO) with high-output failure. Hypothyroidism: lowered CO/HR/BP/pulse pressure, bradycardia and cardiomegaly. Marasmus/Kwashiorkor: thin flabby heart with reduced CO and systolic BP. Malignant carcinoid (elevated serotonin): coronary artery spasms and right-sided dysfunction. Obesity: elevated CO and blood volume, HTN, CAD and myocardial hypertrophy. Pheochromocytoma: HTN, LV hypertrophy and myocardial necrosis. Rheumatoid arthritis: coronary arteritis and pericarditis. Systemic lupus erythematosus (lupus, or SLE): pericarditis, endocarditis (Libman-Sacks) and antiphospholipid syndrome. Thiamine deficiency: dilated cardiomyopathy, systolic murmur, S3 sound, tachycardia and high-output cardiac failure.

Genetic
Despite the fact that they are technically lipid metabolism disorders, the familial dyslipidemias are one category of inherited CV conditions, and include hyperchylomicronemia (high chylomicrons), hypercholesterolemia (high LDL with fewer receptors), combined hyperlipidemia (high LDL and VLDL), dysbetalipoproteinemia (high IDL and VLDL) and hypertriglyceridemia (High TGs, possibly with high VLDL and/or chylomicrons, depending on variant). There are three additional genetic disorders of the heart itself: hypertrophic cardiomyopathy (can lead to failure), Marfan syndrome (high risk of aortic dissection because of aortic insufficiency) and long Q-T syndrome (can lead to torsade de pointes). Additionally, there are several inherited congenital diseases that can result in CV complications: Down syndrome (ASD, VSD, septal defect with endocardial cushion effect), Turner's syndrome (coarctation of aorta) and 22q11 syndromes (tetralogy of Fallot, truncus arteriosus). Other congenital disorders without a genetic component but passed down from the mother are rubella (septal defects, PDA, pulmonary artery stenosis) and complication from diabetic mothers (transposition of great vessels).

Idiopathic
There are several CV disorders that may be labeled as idiopathic when no obvious cause is found. Ventricular tachycardia and premature ventricular contractions may appear without a known

cause, and can result in other serious conduction abnormalities. Idiopathic heart failure occurs in a certain percentage of cardiac patients, though it can usually be linked to one or more factors/conditions. All three main types of cardiomyopathy (dilated, hypertrophic and restrictive) may be idiopathic in the absence of an obvious etiology, though restrictive is most likely to be so, as opposed to the other two. Finally, idiopathic thrombocytopenic purpura (ITP), while technically a coagulation disorder, can greatly affect the CV system and its clotting abilities, owing to decreased platelets in response to anti-platelet antibodies.

Drug-induced adverse effects
While many systemic agents can cause problems with the CV system, there are several types that frequently do so. Oral contraceptives, with high levels of estrogen and progestins can lead to thrombotic events and complications. Interestingly, while high levels of these substances are considered thrombogenic, lower levels such as that found in hormone replacement therapy appear to have a cardioprotective effect. Several other pharmaceuticals may lead to cardiac toxicity, cardiomyopathies (also caused by chronic alcohol abuse) and altered cardiac function: doxorubicin and daunorubicin (antineoplastic), lithium and tricyclic antidepressants. Both class IA (quinidine) and class III (sotalol) antiarrhythmics can lead to torsade de pointes, which is a particularly unstable conduction disorder. Digitalis, which is used to treat many dysrhythmias, can also cause most of them, though this incidence has decreased. Sympathomimetics and phenothiazines may also contribute to certain dysrhythmias. Other agents can lead to hypertension (steroids), hypotension (phenothiazines), arterial spasm (ergot alkaloids), ischemic disease (contraceptive steroids) and even heart failure (beta-blockers).

Degenerative
The term "degenerative cardiovascular disease" describes any CV-related condition where there is chronic anatomical and physiological breakdown occurring. Depending on where you search, such diseases are categorized and listed in different ways, but most are driven by atherosclerosis and hypertension, which serve to wear down the associated structures. Major examples of these types of disorders include essential hypertension, coronary artery disease, cardiomyopathies, cerebral vascular accidents, rheumatic heart disease, angina pectoris, valvular disease and certain congenital heart diseases. Myocardial infarction may also be precipitated by such degeneration. Because these are chronic conditions, degenerative CV disease is generally found in adults who are middle-aged and older. Preventive measures include eating a healthy diet and getting regular exercise, along with lipid lowering medications. However, some of the above conditions, such as congenital disease, may not respond to such interventions, depending on the mechanism of pathology.

Mechanism of action (MoA) and specific uses

Coronary and peripheral vasodilators
Vasodilators act via relaxation of the smooth muscle of vessels, resulting in lowered resistance and blood pressure. They may be direct-acting or enzymatically driven, and may produce selective (arteries vs. veins) or balanced dilation. They are most often used to treat hypertension, angina and heart failure. In addition, the term "vasodilators" is an overarching term used to describe drugs from different classes that all achieve similar effects, through varied mechanisms. Examples of direct-acting agents are hydralazine and minoxidil, which dilate mostly arteries and arterioles; minoxidil specifically dilates resistance areas (arterioles) but not capacitance vessels (venules). Sodium nitroprusside and diazoxide are used in emergency situations; nitroprusside dilates both arterial and venous systems, while diazoxide dilates specifically arterioles. There are other vasodilators such as nifedipine and verapamil, which are calcium channel blockers and will be covered separately.

Antiarrhythmic drugs

The goal of antiarrhythmic therapy is to either decrease or remove an aberrant electrical rhythm, until the patient is electrophysiologically stable. There are four major classes, with class I being further divided into a, b and c. Different drugs are used to correct certain rhythms, and many have more than one use; they mainly act by altering various phases of the myocardial action potential. Class I drugs all work by blocking sodium channels, and include quinidine and procainamide (IA – ectopic, ventricular and reentry dysrhythmias), lidocaine and phenytoin (IB – ventricular, especially during MI), and flecainide and propafenone (IC – ventricular, especially PVCs). Class II agents are beta-blockers, including propranolol (lowers chance of sudden death), esmolol (short-acting, for surgical dysrhythmias) and metoprolol (partial agonist, reduces bronchospasm). Class III medications act by blocking potassium channels; examples are bretylium (V-tach and V-Fib) and amiodarone (refractory tachyarrhythmias). Class IV are calcium channel blockers, and include such drugs as nifedipine (mostly vascular effect), diltiazem and verapamil (both for atrial fib and flutter). Finally, digoxin/digitalis, which is in its own category, acts by shortening the myocardial refractory period, while extending that of the Purkinje fibers. It is used for atrial flutter and fib; toxic levels can cause V tach or fib.

ACE inhibitors in combatting hypertension (HTN)

Angiotensin converting enzyme (ACE) is responsible for producing angiotensin II, an extremely powerful vasoconstrictor. ACE inhibitors are therefore aimed at blocking the actions of this enzyme, preventing 1) constriction, and 2) subsequent stimulation of aldosterone secretion (thus limiting retention of sodium at the kidney). This inhibitory action results in decreased peripheral resistance while leaving cardiac output unchanged. In addition, ACE inhibitors act by increasing levels of bradykinin. The combined effect of these two mechanisms is peripheral vasodilation. These agents can be used in a range of hypertensive situations, but tend to work best in young white people. They are effective in combatting HTN in those patients who also suffer from CHF, as opposed to beta-blockers. Along with calcium channel blockers, ACE inhibitors are drugs that can be utilized in patients with most CV-related comorbid disorders, whereas others have more restrictions. Examples include captopril, enalapril and lisinopril.

Calcium channel blockers in combatting HTN

Calcium influx into the smooth muscle of the vasculature causes vasoconstriction and increased peripheral resistance, leading to an increase in blood pressure. Therefore, calcium channel blockers (CCBs) act by inhibiting this action, which produces reduced vascular muscle tone and resistance, leading to a decrease in hypertensive pathology, via vasodilation. A benefit of using CCBs is that they are natriuretic, meaning there is usually no need for an additional diuretic under most circumstances. As with ACE inhibitors, CCBs can be used in most clinical HTN situations, with a few exceptions. Unlike some other antihypertensives, they may be used in patients with asthma, angina, diabetes and peripheral vascular disease. Examples include verapamil, nifedipine, diltiazem and nicardipine.

Diuretics in combatting HTN

The renin-angiotensin-aldosterone axis can contribute to hypertension (HTN) by two different mechanisms: production of angiotensin II and consequent elevated resistance, and release of aldosterone, causing retention of renal sodium. ACE inhibitors work on the first mechanism, while diuretics are the main tools used to combat the second. They work by increasing renal excretion of sodium and water, which decreases extracellular volume and results in lowered cardiac output. The most common and effective are the thiazide diuretics, such as hydrochlorothiazide; they are sometimes used in conjunction with potassium-sparing diuretics such as spironolactone. Thiazides also counter the retention of sodium and water potentiated by some of the other antihypertensives, meaning they are often a good choice for combination therapy with beta-blockers and ACE inhibitors. They should not be used in patients with diabetes or hyperlipidemia, and usually work best in black or elderly people.

Beta antagonists in combatting hypertension (HTN)

Beta-blockers achieve their antihypertensive effect via three different mechanisms. First, they lower stimulation of beta-1 receptors on the myocardium, which decreases cardiac output. They also reduce production of renin, which in turn decreases production and release of both angiotensin II (lowering peripheral resistance) and aldosterone (decreasing blood volume). Additionally, it is thought that they may inhibit sympathetic output from the CNS, further enhancing these effects. Beta-blockers are useful in addressing comorbid conditions that exist along with HTN, such as certain tachyarrhythmias, angina, glaucoma, migraine headaches and previous MI. They are most useful in young white patients, being less effective in blacks and the elderly. Having certain conditions – asthma, COPD, CHF and others – makes these agents contraindicated because of negative effects on these diseases. Examples include propranolol, esmolol and labetalol, all of which have the same or similar MoAs.

Agents used to combat hypotension and shock

There are several different agents that may be used to fight hypotensive shock, in an effort to stabilize the patient. The inotropic vasopressor catecholamine drugs – norepinephrine (NE), dopamine (DOP) and dobutamine (DOB) – are most frequently used for this purpose, in an attempt to quickly increase blood pressure and perfusion. They act in similar but slightly different ways, all through adrenergic stimulation. NE affects mainly alpha-receptors, causing increased resistance via vasoconstriction. DOP stimulates both alpha and beta receptors, as well as its own dopaminergic receptors, achieving most of its effect via beta-1 receptors on the heart, which induces inotropic and chronotropic effects; alpha receptors may cause vasoconstriction at high concentrations, and renal arterioles are dilated to prevent kidney damage during intervention. DOB acts directly on beta-1 receptors, stimulating increased cardiac contractility and cardiac output. In terms of therapeutic uses, NE is used almost exclusively for shock; DOP is used to treat shock and refractory CHF; DOB is used mostly for increasing cardiac output in CHF, though it may be chosen as a second-line therapy for shock.

Drugs that lower lipid/cholesterol levels

Drugs that aid in decreasing lipoprotein levels act using one or more basic mechanisms: reduced production of lipids, increased catabolism within the plasma, and/or enhanced excretion from the body. They are selectively used for the various dyslipidemias common in patient populations, along with lifestyle changes. The medications commonly known as "statins" – lovastatin, simvastatin, pravastatin and others – are HMG-CoA reductase inhibitors, and act by preventing the formation of mevalonate, a cholesterol precursor, which serves to lower LDL and triglycerides (TGs) while raising HDL levels. Niacin works via inhibition of lipolysis and reduction of circulating VLDL; it also works by lowering LDL and TGs while raising HDL. Bile acid resins – cholestyramine, colestipol and colesevelam – all act by interfering with reabsorption of bile acids in the intestine, which forces the liver to use cholesterol to make more. They cause a decrease in LDL, along with mild increases in HDL and TGs, and they tend to be used secondarily because of their side effects. Cholesterol absorption blockers – ezetimibe – have a MoA that prevents intestinal reabsorption of cholesterol, and lower LDL while having no effect on HDL or TGs. The "fibrates" – gemfibrozil, clofibrate, bezafibrate and fenofibrate – stimulate the action of lipoprotein lipase, which helps to clear TGs from the system. They potently lower TGs, while having more modest effects on decreasing and increasing LDL and HDL, respectively.

Anticoagulants

There are three major drugs traditionally used as anticoagulants: heparin, warfarin/Coumadin and dicumarol. In addition, there are newer drugs such as Xarelto and Pradaxa, which are factor Xa inhibitors and direct thrombin inhibitors, respectively. Heparin is an indirect-acting agent given IV, with an immediate effect that acts by binding to antithrombin III, which then inhibits formation of several clotting factors, including thrombin, which serves to reduce clot expansion. It is used for treatment and prevention of deep vein thrombosis (DVT) and pulmonary embolism (PE), as well as during the initial phase of a developing MI. The other two – warfarin and dicumarol – are known as coumarin anticoagulants and are taken orally with slower action, making them suitable for long-term treatment. They both act by inhibiting vitamin K functionality, which is a required cofactor at points along the clotting cascade; this results in reduced clotting ability. These medications are commonly used to reduce the chances of thrombus formation, as well as preventively for those who have already experienced a thrombus or embolism. Clinical uses are for atrial fibrillation, artificial valves, DVT and PE; other possible uses include as a post-MI prophylactic measure, although this is controversial.

Reversal of anticoagulants is used when there is suspicion or findings of increased bleeding as a result of anticoagulation therapy. For the coumarin anticoagulants – warfarin and dicumarol – reversal is accomplished via doses of vitamin K, which is the cofactor required for certain steps in the clotting cascade. Adding this vitamin in large enough doses stops the anticoagulation effect and allows coagulation to proceed normally. Vitamin K is used to treat bleeding tendencies, but may take up to 24 hours to reach full effect. Therefore, immediate needs must be met by using either prothrombin complex concentrate (PCC) or fresh frozen plasma (FFP). Heparin reversal requires IV infusion of protamine sulfate; dosing depends on the amount of heparin given. Factor Xa inhibitors such as Xarelto and Arixtra can be reversed via either PCC or recombinant activated clotting factor VII (rFVIIa). Direct thrombin inhibitors such as Pradaxa and Angiomax can be reversed using rFVIIa, PCC, desmopressin or aminocaproic acid, while antifibrinolytics should be reserved as a last resort. In addition to these agents, removal of the anticoagulant from the system may be accomplished by dialysis, hemoperfusion or plasmapheresis. Finally, anti-platelet drugs can be reversed using desmopressin or via infusion with platelets.

Thrombolytic agents

The thrombolytic medications all act in similar ways, by converting plasminogen to plasmin, which then acts to inhibit fibrin by hydrolysis, resulting in dissolution of clots. The kinases – streptokinase (SK) and urokinase (UK) – have systemic fibrinolytic activity (which may cause bleeding problems), while tissue plasminogen activator (tPA) tends to work only on the clot and local surrounding area, making it more selective and less apt to result in bleeding complications. All types should be used as early as possible after clot formation, to avoid a buildup of resistance to their effects. These medications were originally intended as "clot busters" for use in deep vein thrombosis (DVT) and pulmonary embolism (PE), but have since been expanded to treat acute peripheral thromboembolism, acute MI, and to unclog shunts, stents and catheters that have become seeded with coagulants, forming thrombi.

Antiplatelet agents

The anti-platelet medications are all used to prevent platelet aggregation (and are thus also known as platelet aggregation inhibitors) and thrombus formation, and are used in a variety of clinical situations. Aspirin is probably the most well known and acts by inhibiting cyclooxygenase, which prevents formation of thromboxane A2; uses include prevention of transient ischemic cerebral attacks and reduction of recurrent MI and mortality in the post-MI state. Other thromboxane inhibitors, such as dipyridamole and picotamide, inhibit phosphodiesterase (PDE) and/or block platelet receptors; they may act by preventing adhesion of platelets to the endothelial surface. They are used to treat multiple conditions, including angina, MI prevention and embolus prevention for those with artificial valves. Adenosine diphosphate inhibitors (ADPs) block P2Y receptors; some examples are clopidogrel and ticagrelor. PDE inhibitors, such as cilostazol, block the actions of PDE, which results in prevention of cAMP and cGMP inactivation, which in turn prevents platelet activity and thrombus formation. Glycoprotein inhibitors, such as abciximab, eptifibatide and tirofiban, work by blocking receptors for these substances on the platelet surface; they are often used during interventional cardiac investigations such as angioplasty, and may be used selectively for acute coronary syndrome. Prostaglandin (prostacyclin) analogues, such as beraprost and treprostinil, achieve their effects by binding platelet surface receptors, preventing activation.

Inotropic agents

Inotropic agents are mostly used to treat CHF, acting to increase contractility of the heart muscle, in an attempt to boost cardiac output. Some are also used to combat hypotensive shock. Cardiac glycosides, such as digoxin and digitoxin, have dual MoAs: they increase intracellular calcium, which increases systolic force; and they enhance contraction efficiency by reducing diastolic volume. They are often used in CHF and hypertensive heart disease, and are the main positive inotropes. Other types of inotropic medications include beta agonists, such as dopamine and dobutamine, which act to increase cardiac contraction and rate via elevated calcium levels, while simultaneously causing vasodilation. Certain antiarrhythmics, such as amrinone and milrinone may be used as alternatives to the above-mentioned agents, and act by increasing calcium concentrations, which enhance contractility. They are most often used for short-term CHF management. Vasodilators, such as captopril and nitroprusside, work by dilating both arterial and venous vessels, which yields reductions in preload and afterload, reducing the workload of the heart in failure.

Immunosuppressive agents

Immunosuppressive medications are generally used either to combat certain cancers or to treat autoimmune diseases (via reduction of humoral and cellular responses), in an attempt to reduce symptoms and signs. For autoimmune disorders, they may be utilized for diseases that are not primarily cardiac in nature, but which may have cardiac manifestations, such as lupus. However, their main function within the cardiovascular system is to blunt immune reactions following heart transplant, where there is significant risk of transplant rejection. Azathioprine and mercaptopurine, which inhibit early lymphocyte production, affect both branches of the immune system and are particularly useful for this purpose. Some of the other agents used are methotrexate (anti-metabolite folate antagonist), cyclophosphamide (alkylating agent affecting T-cells), prednisone (corticosteroid hormone that reduces lymphocytic activity) and antibodies (monoclonal and polyclonal).

Antimicrobial agents

Antimicrobials are generally used for endocarditis, myocarditis, or pericarditis. They are of course also used to treat infectious vasculitis and phlebitis. A patient with bacterial endocarditis may be treated with vancomycin or ceftriaxone (cell wall synthesis inhibitors) empirically, and by those agents as well as penicillin (cell wall) and/or aminoglycosides (likely protein synthesis inhibitors), depending on the organism. Myocarditis is most often viral, and may be treated with antivirals, which mostly inhibit viral replication, though this is controversial. When pericarditis is infective, it may be treated with penicillin, cephalosporins or more specific agents once the microbe is identified. Infectious vasculitis may be treated with cephalexin, while infectious phlebitis, which is very rare, would require empiric treatment with ceftriaxone or vancomycin. Infectious arteritis is almost unheard of, except in horses, which sometimes develop equine viral arteritis.

Antineoplastic agents

Most cardiac tumors are benign, with myxoma much more common than others; it generally responds to surgical excision. Malignant primary cardiac tumors are rare, with sarcomas being the most common, occurring predominantly in the pediatric population. Much more common are metastases to the heart from other primary neoplasms. When chemotherapy is required, it of course depends on the type of cancer. Sarcomas are often treated with Adriamycin (doxorubicin), which acts in three ways: inhibiting DNA/RNA synthesis, blocking transport through the cell membrane and formation of oxygen free radicals that selectively destroy tumor tissue. Other chemotherapy agents sometimes used are cyclophosphamide (DNA cross links cause apoptosis), vincristine (disrupts microtubule spindle and stops mitosis in metaphase), methotrexate (various mechanisms lead to lowered DNA/RNA synthesis and apoptosis), and dacarbazine (alkylating agent that probably inhibits DNA synthesis). There may be others used by oncologists, depending on the clinical and histiologic findings, but these are among the most common. When a cardiac tumor is metastatic, the type of primary tumor dictates the choice of chemotherapy and/or radiation.

Antiparasitic agents

There are several parasitic infections, from protozoa and helminthes, which may have cardiac manifestations. By far the most common is Chaga's disease (American Trypanosomiasis, caused by T. *cruzi*). It is usually treated with nifurtimox (MoA unknown but thought to interfere with DNA synthesis in parasites and/or produce superoxide radicals harmful to the bug) or benznidazole (likely inhibits RNA and protein synthesis in the parasite). Sleeping sickness (African Trypanosomiasis) is treated with pentamidine (possibly disrupts mitochondrial function), sulmarin (possibly inhibits enzymes involved in cellular respiration and glycolysis), melarsoprol (likely inhibits production of ATP by inactivating pyruvate kinase) or eflornithine (inhibits cell division preferentially in parasite). For amoebiasis, metronidazole (likely causes parasitic DNA strand breakage) or related compounds are used, as well as paromomycin (protein synthesis inhibitor) and iodoquinol (MoA unknown). Toxoplasmosis is usually only treated in immunodeficient patients, with either sulfa or aminoglycoside antibiotics. Cysticercosis responds to albendazole or derivatives (helminthic-specific enzyme inhibition leading to reduced ATP production; also used for echinococcosis and trichinellosis) or praziquantel (MoA unknown, but induces contraction and paralysis of the parasite).

Antianginal agents

There are several classes of drugs commonly used to treat angina, including nitrates, calcium channel blockers and beta-blockers. The goal of antianginal therapy is threefold: to directly relax the coronary arteries, providing more oxygen to match the myocardial demand; to relax cardiac oxygen demand; and peripheral vasodilation to lower peripheral resistance. The nitrates – nitroglycerin, isosorbide dinitrate and amyl nitrate – relax coronary smooth muscle, likely via elevated cGMP within the cells. Calcium channel blockers – nifedipine, verapamil and diltiazem – stimulate vasodilation in both the coronary and systemic vasculature, via blockage of calcium flow into the muscle cells, causing them to relax. Beta-blockers, chiefly propranolol, act by inhibiting beta-1 receptors on the heart, which results in reduced cardiac activity and output. These drugs are especially useful in reducing severity and frequency of angina episodes.

Drugs used to treat peripheral artery disease (PAD)

PAD occurs most often because of atherosclerotic occlusion of the arterial system in the extremities, resulting in intermittent claudication. The goal of therapy is to a) reduce painful claudication attacks, and b) address the underlying atherosclerotic process. Drugs used to treat this condition and help reduce painful episodes include vasodilators (MoA covered elsewhere), such as calcium channel blockers or beta-blockers (which may also worsen the condition). Quite frequently anti-cholesterol medications, such as statins that interfere with HMG-CoA reductase, are used to stop or reverse accumulation of lipids in the arterial lumen. Depending on the presence of comorbid conditions, other agents may be prescribed, such as antihypertensives (MoA elsewhere), various diabetes medication and/or blood thinners (to reduce the risk of clot formation that may occur with poor circulation; MoA elsewhere). It is especially important to be vigilant with diabetes drugs, since the disease already presents its own vascular issues in the extremities. Cilostazol is another agent that is quite useful for managing the pain of claudication episodes, and works by dual mechanisms of vasodilation and anticoagulation.

Drugs utilized to control bleeding

Bleeding, whether from surgical fibrinolysis, use of anticoagulants or because of intrinsic pathology such as hemophilia, must be attended to promptly. If the cause is hemophilia, the treatment is an infusion of the missing clotting factors, usually VIII or IX, from a human donor. If bleeding is because of something other than this natural disease state, other measures are used. For patients in a fibrinolytic state (most often after GI or prostate surgery), either aminocaproic or tranexamic acid may be utilized, which inhibit activation of plasminogen. Bleeding complications from heparin are treated with protamine sulfate, which neutralizes the negatively charged heparin with its positive charge, resulting in a stable complex with no anticoagulant properties. When the cause of bleeding is administration of longer-term anticoagulants, such as warfarin, vitamin K is used to treat it, simply overloading and reversing the inhibition of the vitamin's activity in the clotting process. Vitamin K's effects are generally not fully realized for 24 hours, making it important to monitor these patients closely over that period.

Drugs utilized to treat anemia

There are several different types of anemia, but regardless of the etiology or pathology, the goal of therapy is to increase the amount of hemoglobin, and therefore oxygen, available to the body's tissues. Most anemias and the reduced hemoglobin plasma level that defines them are the result of a low number of circulating RBCs, whether because of blood loss or impaired production, making the restoration of proper levels the therapeutic objective. With iron deficiency anemia, a lack of a suitable iron plasma level leads to hypochromic microcytic anemia. Whether from blood loss or inadequate intake, the treatment is dietary iron supplementation, usually in the form of oral ferrous sulfate, which provides sufficient iron available to bind the hemoglobin molecule. Megaloblastic anemia is caused by either folic acid and/or vitamin B12 (cyanocobalamin) deficiency. Folate depletion leads to lowered purine and pyrimidine synthesis with impaired DNA and cell replication, usually caused by malabsorption or increased demand (pregnancy). B12 deficiency often develops secondary to poor absorption or low dietary intake, and impairs cell replication by means similar to folic acid; it also causes pernicious anemia. Either type of anemia requires supplementation of one or both of these substances, since they are both important in production of blood cells. Anemia caused by end-stage renal disease may be alleviated using recombinant human erythropoietin, usually formed in the kidney, to the marrow, for RBC proliferation.

Drugs used to combat inflammatory conditions of the heart

For the most part, the same anti-inflammatory or immunosuppressive drugs used for other local and systemic inflammation are used to treat inflammatory conditions of the CV system. When needed, standard medication such as ibuprofen or naproxen is generally prescribed, but the selection of agent is up to the treating physician and depends on the condition being treated and any complicating factors. For pericarditis, an additional medicine is available and has good efficacy.

Colchicine, which was originally prescribed (and still is) for treatment of acute and chronic gout, has become a mainstay of pericarditis treatment in the last decade or two, with studies suggesting it be the drug of choice, often along with another agent, for acute pericarditis. For infective disorders, such as bacterial endocarditis, antibiotics are added to the regimen, which helps remove the inciting microbe and calm inflammation. Problems such as coronary artery disease that are suspected of being driven by chronic inflammation may be addressed with anti-inflammatory agents as well as those aimed at preventing further lipid-induced damage. Autoimmune disorders that affect the CV system, which are touched on elsewhere, are often treated with a combination of drugs that interfere with synthesis of inflammatory mediators (naproxen, ibuprofen, cox-2 inhibitors) and immunosuppressants that blunt the body's abnormal response to autoantigens.

Non-pharmacologic treatment

Hypotensive shock

All shock is, by definition, hypotensive shock, regardless of mechanism or cause. However, the specific reason for shock does influence somewhat the non-pharmacologic (as well as pharmacotherapy, for that matter) measures taken to reverse it. Most obviously, the first action in hemorrhagic shock, is stopping the massive bleeding contributing to it – without this action, other efforts will be mostly useless. This type of shock also requires rapid infusion of fluids, whether blood products or normal saline / Ringer's lactate. More generally, the patient should initially be kept warm with leg elevation (to enhance venous return and improve cardiac output if possible). If CPR is needed, the airway should be cleared and it should be initiated ASAP (after controlling any significant external bleeding), since every moment becomes critical. Oxygen therapy, with assisted ventilation if necessary, should also be started ASAP, since the basic deficit in shock is hypoxemia. Once the patient is stabilized, vitals and rhythms must be closely monitored for changes. In the event of pericardial tamponade secondary to cardiogenic shock, pericardiocentesis must be performed to maintain adequate filling and pumping of the heart.

Heart failure

Aside from pharmacotherapy, CHF management involves a range of measures intended to change environmental as well as systemic contributing factors. These therapies are also based on the specific etiology and pathophysiology. Oxygenation is required, whether via nasal cannula or ventilator; and rest is always prescribed, in order to reduce heart rate and cardiac workload, and should be with elevation of the head. Systemic factors such as fever, thyrotoxicosis, hypertension and anemia must first be addressed and corrected before restoration of heart function can really be effective. Avoiding excess salt and alcohol intake is also key to reducing and preventing damage. Electrical cardioversion may be employed to resolve dysrhythmias that may be contributing to the CHF. Finally, in conjunction with pharmacotherapy, compliance must be addressed and maintained in order for the patient to realize maximum benefit from prescribed medications.

> **Review Video:** Congestive Heart Failure
> *Visit **mometrix.com/academy** and enter **Code: 924118***

Chemical versus electrical cardioversion for abnormal rhythms

When the heart rhythm is anything other than normal sinus rhythm (NSR), either chemical or electrical cardioversion (or occasionally both) may be used in an attempt to restore NSR and proper heart function. The most common dysrhythmia amenable to conversion is atrial fibrillation, followed by atrial flutter. Chemical or pharmacological cardioversion involves the use of appropriate antiarrhythmics, chosen from one of four classes (covered elsewhere) depending on

- 265 -

the specific rhythm abnormality. Regardless of drug choice, the goal is to take the patient out of his or her dysrhythmia and into NSR. In contrast, synchronized electrical cardioversion (so called because it should occur in most cases in synchrony with the R wave on the ECG) uses electrodes or traditional paddles, placed on the chest or chest and back, to shock the heart back to NSR. This shock effectively "resets" the heart by causing all myocardial cells to contract at once, interrupting the aberrant rhythm and hopefully restoring NSR. While A fib and A flutter are the most commonly cardioverted rhythms, many other rhythms may be treated this way as well, depending on the clinical and electrophysiological situation.

Inflammatory conditions

In a way, there are two types of inflammatory CV conditions: those ending with –itis, caused by infection, trauma, autoimmunity or other factors; and chronic atherosclerotic and ischemic disease, where inflammation is highly suspected as a major contributing component. Though this remains to be definitively proven, there is a high correlation of inflammation with MI or CVA, both of which display elevated inflammatory markers; and those with chronic inflammatory disease are likely to have increased risk of coronary artery disease and MI. Endocarditis, myocarditis and pericarditis are covered elsewhere in this series, and are generally treated with antimicrobials and/or anti-inflammatory drugs. Non-infective causes of these and similar disorders may be autoimmune, as with lupus, which can affect virtually every part of the heart, or sarcoidosis, which may asymptomatic. Scleroderma is an autoimmune disorder that often causes cardiovascular damage via inflammation and fibrosis, which contributes to mortality. Other vascular disorders such as Wegener's, Kawasaki and giant cell arteritis are covered elsewhere, and comprise but a few of the many possible vasculitides affecting the CV system.

Treating heart disease

Common procedures
Cardiac procedures are quite common, whether they are intended to diagnose and/or treat disease. One of the most common therapeutic procedures is cardiac catheterization with angioplasty and possibly stent placement, which is used to treat atherosclerotic disease of the vessels and/or stenotic valvular disease, among other purposes. A similar intervention is called atherectomy, where a rotating head at the tip of the catheter shaves plaque from the arterial wall. Artificial heart valve replacement is used to treat valvular disease, where several options for a substitute exist; the new valve may come from another human being or an animal such as a pig, or it may be completely synthetic. Bypass surgery is another option for those with severely clogged coronary arteries. Arteries or veins from another part of the body (autografts) are used to create new unblocked vessels, replacing the old atherosclerotic coronary arteries. This is performed as an open-heart procedure. Ablation is a procedure where a catheter with an electrified tip is used to destroy a very specific area of the heart that is responsible for causing the aberrant rhythm; it is used for several dysrhythmias, such as atrial fibrillation. Heart transplant surgery is exactly what it sounds like: a matched donor heart replaces the patient's original model; it carries a sizable risk of transplant rejection. Cardioversion to correct certain dysrhythmias has been covered elsewhere.

Lifestyle changes
While specific pathologies may require or prohibit some of them, there are certain lifestyle changes recommended to all cardiac patients, as ways to live a "heart-healthy" life. The single most important is probably cessation of smoking if applicable, but there are several others. Losing weight is never a bad thing, but obesity puts extra demand on the heart, which means that obese patients are gradually hurting their heart with each beat. Thus losing weight is mandatory in these

patients. A "heart-healthy" diet is also suggested, which means lots of leafy greens, fiber and lean protein, while omitting/limiting fried food or food with high fat content, as well as excess salt and processed foods. Getting proper exercise is very important, as this improves the aerobic function of the heart and its ability to adequately perfuse tissues, and it can lead to reductions is cholesterol, blood pressure and of course, weight. If weight reduction and exercise don't accomplish the task themselves, hypertension and hypercholesterolemia may be addressed with medications to lower these indices. Proper management of diabetes and compliance with treatment regimens is one of the keys to cardioprotective lifestyle changes for those with the disease. A decrease in alcohol intake and stress are also necessary components of living healthily with heart disease. For heart failure, some additional recommendations include monitoring daily fluid intake, getting enough rest, avoiding caffeine and adhering to sexual restrictions, as directed by the clinician.

Ablation and pacemakers

Ablation and/or pacemakers are indicated for problems with the electrical rhythm of the heart, where the cardiac conduction circuits function abnormally and require assistance to return to normal sinus rhythm (NSR). Ablation involves passing a catheter equipped with an electrode at the tip through a vein and into the right atrium (frequently the location of the lesion), at which point the physician seeks the suspected dysfunctional tissue causing the dysrhythmia. The tip is then electrified and used to destroy this tissue very selectively, without damaging the rest of the heart. The end result is hopefully ablation of the offending tissue and re-establishment of normal conduction pathways and NSR. When ablation doesn't work, especially after repeated attempts – or for situations directly indicating one – a pacemaker may be required to correct the problem. It is a battery-operated device inserted inside the chest or worn externally that takes over control of the "pacemaker" job usually handled by the SA node (or AV node), in an attempt to correct a number of dysrhythmias and conduction blocks, as well as other disorders affecting the rate and rhythm.

Impact of emotional health on CV disease treatment and prevention

When someone is not emotionally healthy, whether chronically or acutely, the inherent psychological distress involved can lead to several problems regarding CV disease treatment and prevention. High stress levels correlate positively to increased inflammation, which is strongly suspected of playing a large role in chronic atherosclerotic disease. Thus stress management is nearly always advised, regardless of method, both for preventive and therapeutic purposes. Also, elevated stress levels lead to elevated levels of adrenergic activity, which places an additional workload on the heart and may add to hypertension concerns. Severe anger or anxiety can even lead to electrical disturbances in the heart. Furthermore, someone who is actively suffering from psychological issues is much more likely to forget or refuse to take medication, yielding major compliance problems in certain patients. This is especially dangerous with cardiac patients, in prevention and treatment. Being in an unhealthy psychological state can make recuperation from procedures more difficult as well. And chances are decent that patients in this population will be diagnosed with comorbid conditions, both mental and physical, which may complicate such preventive and therapeutic efforts. Conversely, recent research has shown that emotionally healthy and happy people are less likely to experience disease states, and they recover quicker from cardiovascular incidents and interventions.

Impact of behavioral factors on CV disease treatment and prevention

Whether it's for purposes of prevention or treatment, the patient must ultimately implement behavioral recommendations made by a clinician, and it is up to him or her to remain vigilant.

When diagnosed with CV disease, the single most important injurious behavior that needs to stop immediately is smoking. Since factors like obesity, hyperlipidemia and hypertension also make it harder for the heart to function and/or recuperate, a healthy diet low in fat and high in fiber, with low salt intake and adequate exercise, is usually recommended, except under certain circumstances. And compliance with any medication regimen for these conditions is absolutely essential; not complying can result in major problems, especially in the future. If the patient has diabetes, tight glucose control is crucial, since peripheral circulation is likely already poor. Use of alcohol and/or illicit drugs, especially over long periods, can lead to a number of problems involving the heart, including dilated hypertrophy (alcohol), coronary artery spasm (cocaine) and dysrhythmias (several).

Impact of heart disease on the patient, patient's family, and society

Depending on the patient and specific disease, the impact of heart disease may range from largely inconsequential to life-altering and disabling, or even death. Some patients with atrial fibrillation may be asymptomatic for their entire lives, while others will present with near-constant symptoms, necessitating frequent trips to the doctor/hospital. Having to endure cardiac symptoms along with lifestyle changes (including increased office and hospital visits) and potential pharmacological and procedural interventions results in a reduced quality of life, which in turn leads to major depression in a sizable portion of this patient population. In addition, patients with heart disease, especially those who have had an MI or suffer from CHF, may have to adjust to changes in activities of daily living, and accept that certain limitations now apply to everyday routines, including being able to go/return to work. Heart disease may also limit allowable sexual activity, which can further distress the cardiac patient. And the patient may learn to play the "sick role", whereby he or she becomes comfortable with being tended to, and continues to play this part after being cleared for normal activity.

The family of a patient with heart disease experiences their own challenges in dealing with such conditions, and serious pathology can often lead to problems with family dynamics. If the patient is partially or largely incapacitated by his or her illness, he or she will require assistance from family members in many regards. This often places a great strain on those helping, as well as their relationship with the patient. The family unit at its best will function as a close support system for the patient, though this support may vary and come at a price of resentment, as family members are forced to adjust to new roles and responsibilities. Another major impact on the family of heart disease patients is the potential for monetary trouble, particularly for those without insurance, or for whom the patient is the regular breadwinner. Trying to keep the family together and functioning under these circumstances becomes doubly difficult. Furthermore, genetically related family members may now begin to worry about their own susceptibility to heart disease, increasing anxiety levels. And having to care for an ill family member often leaves other members of the family vulnerable to neglecting their own health. If things get bad enough, family counseling, to help everyone get through the experience, is often suggested.

As more and more people worldwide (but especially in the U.S.) become obese, hypertensive, diabetic and/or hyperlipidemic, the impact on local and global society cannot be overstated. Economically, heart disease costs the U.S. hundreds of billions of dollars annually, much of it spent treating conditions that are largely preventable, or at least ameliorable. Part of that estimate includes lost productivity from days absent from work, which greatly affects our economy's efficiency. Those living in poorer communities, where prevalence of disease is higher while availability of care is lower, feel a particular strain, as this situation leads to more extensive and expensive treatments for emergent conditions that might have been avoidable or less severe. In terms of morbidity and mortality, heart disease is the number one killer for both men and women in the U.S., making it a societal problem as much as an individual one, as virtually everyone knows several people in their community with cardiac disorders. The trend of rising heart disease rates also indicated that as a society, nutritionally and in terms of physical activity, we are headed in the wrong direction.

Risk factors that may affect CV disease treatment and prevention

Occupational
Almost any occupation can be considered to put its workers at risk for CV disease, based on the fact that stress and anxiety are well-recognized contributing factors, and nearly everyone experiences some degree while at work. The exact nature and impact of occupational risk factors for CV disease is largely unclear or hasn't been investigated thoroughly. However, exposure to certain workplace toxins such as carbon disulfide, nitroglycerin and carbon monoxide have been linked with an increased incidence of heart disease. Other possible factors that are suspected but unconfirmed include extreme heat or cold (for those working in such environments), as well as secondhand smoke from fellow workers. Some probable risk factors that are still unproven to date are loud noise (leading to hypertension), shift work (disrupting circadian rhythms) and either too much or too little exertion/activity. That is, while a sedentary lifestyle is generally associated with increased risk, in certain situations, strenuous exertion can increase risk of MI. Finally, research has demonstrated that a high workload combined with a low level of job control may indeed be an especially potent occupational factor.

Environmental
Environmental cardiology is a relatively new field that examines the impact the environment may have on CV disease prevention and treatment. Researchers are fairly certain that air toxins and pollutants, as well as some foods, contribute to CAD and other pathologies, likely through inflammatory states, though the pathway is unclear. Cardiac abnormalities can include conduction and contractility disruptions. One of the biggest risk factors present in the surrounding environment is that of secondhand tobacco smoke, which is correlated with increased CV morbidity and mortality. In general, the environmental impact of such offending substances is directly related to the amount in the air and the exposure to this pollution. Living in an unstable home situation can also present significant challenges and stress, increasing CV risk. Expectant mothers who expose themselves or are exposed to drugs, alcohol, cigarette smoking or infection are at increased risk for delivering a baby with some form of cardiac pathology.

Discuss gender and ethnicity
Anyone of any age may be affected by heart disease, with males and females being almost equally impacted (males slightly more), particularly by CAD. This is important, since CV disease is still largely thought of as a "man's" disease by much of the lay public, meaning more education is needed. Despite the possibility of cardiac disease at any age, the risk increases with age, starting prominently at age 45 for men, and 55 for women. In terms of ethnicity and race, there is a definite hierarchy regarding morbidity and mortality, which may reflect genetic as well as lifestyle differences. However, in each group, heart disease and stroke are still the number one killers for that group. Blacks overwhelmingly suffer from more heart disease than any other race/ethnicity, with more related deaths; unfortunately they are also often the least educated about CV disease, which presents problems in attempting preventive measures. After blacks come Pacific Islanders, who are closely followed by whites in terms of mortality from CV disease. Hispanic, Asian and American Indian people fall below whites, and are all somewhat clustered together in terms of incidence and prevalence of CV mortality.

Gastrointestinal System

Embryonic/fetal development of the gastrointestinal system

At 4 weeks, the embryo consists of a layer of simple ectoderm epithelium covering the mesenchyme. The gastrointestinal system begins to develop at 5 weeks. Between 4 and 8 weeks, a wall forms between the trachea and the esophagus, which have developed from the same tissue. At 10 weeks, the intestines rotate. In the first trimester, the esophagus begins peristalsis. Between 11 and 14 weeks, the liver begins to produce red blood cells. Between 15 and 18 weeks, the pancreas and liver produce fluid secretions, including bile from the liver. During the second trimester, gastroesophageal reflux can be seen. By week 21, the fetus has begun swallowing amniotic fluid. Toward the end of the third trimester, the fetus begins to form meconium, which is a waste product.

Changes in the gastrointestinal system after birth

The first change to occur after birth is the way in which the newborn takes in food, which is now through the mouth; thus, the digestive system must adjust to new substances. The organs of digestion grow quickly after birth; the stomach weighs 1 ounce after birth and increases to 3 ounces by the end of the first week. The newborn stool changes in the first few weeks, beginning as meconium, which is black and tar-like, and changing to a yellow-green color. The gastrointestinal system is also populated by intestinal bacterial florae, which are necessary for digestion throughout life. Initial passive immunity is gained through the maternal immunoglobulins from breast milk. The use of antibiotics in the newborn has been shown to affect the gut microbial population in adulthood. Premature infants are at high risk for necrotizing enterocolitis, presumably due to the initiation of enteral feedings. Forty percent of afflicted infants require intestinal resection.

Errors in fetal development that result in problems after birth

Errors in fetal development, involving the common wall of the trachea and esophagus, can result in tracheoesophageal atresia and fistulas. The fetus is unable to swallow or may be at high risk for aspiration after birth. Congenital hypertrophic pyloric stenosis is caused by overgrowth of the fetal longitudinal muscles, resulting in stenosis at the pylorus, which prevents substances from passing into the small intestine. The annular pancreas is formed when the dorsal and ventral fetal pancreatic buds encircle the duodenum blocking it. Meckel's diverticulum is a blind pouch off the ileum, resulting from part of the yolk sac failing to degenerate. Malrotation of the midgut as it retracts back into the abdominal cavity can result in obstruction and volvulus, where the intestines twist and become obstructed. Imperforate anus results when the fetal anal membrane fails to break down in which case it must be surgically removed and reconstructed to allow fecal passage.

Differences between adult and fetal gastrointestinal systems

In the fetus, the small intestine grows at a linear rate and then at a sharply increased rate for the last 15 weeks of gestation. Postnatally, this rapid growth continues until 1 year of life and then continues at a linear rate until adulthood. In the fetus, nutrition is gained through the placenta, whereas in the adult all nutrition is enteral or taken via the alimentary canal. In the fetus, the digestive system musculature is functioning insofar as the fetus swallows amniotic fluid and makes meconium. The fetal intestines grow at such an exponential rate that initially they are located outside of the ventral wall, and it is only later in fetal development that room in the abdominal cavity is available. The intestines then rotate and move back inside as the ventral wall closes. In the adult, there are no external remnants of the intestines.

Alimentary canal

The alimentary canal consists of the entire digestive tract through which food passes upon entering until leaving the body. It is during this passage that nutrients are absorbed and digestion takes place. Food enters the mouth, passes through the pharynx and esophagus and then enters the stomach. From the stomach, it enters the small intestine, passing to the large intestine and making its way to the anus where the indigestible products are expelled. The alimentary canal allows digestion and absorption of nutrients through the mucosal walls of the various organs of the alimentary canal, but it also allows the hormones, enzymes, and bile salts that are produced by digestive organs to work on the food while it is moving through the body. This allows an even greater absorption of nutrients from food.

Liver and biliary system

The liver is responsible for the production of bile. After hepatocytes produce bile, it travels through ducts to the common hepatic duct. The gallbladder lies tucked underneath the liver and stores approximately 50% of the bile produced by the liver. The cystic duct drains the gallbladder, and when it joins the common hepatic duct, it is called the common bile duct, which empties into the duodenum. When fats enter the duodenum, the gallbladder contracts, releasing bile into the duodenum. Bile consists of waste products from the liver, bile salts, and cholesterol. Bile salts help to emulsify fats, facilitating their absorption through the intestinal walls. Bile is then excreted in feces. The biliary system eliminates waste products from the liver and aids in the emulsification and absorption of fats.

Salivary glands and exocrine pancreas

Salivary glands are located in the oral cavity and include two parotid glands located in the cheek region, two submandibular glands located along the inner surface of the mandible, and multiple sublingual glands located in the floor of mouth. Salivary glands function as exocrine glands and release amylase when food is eaten. They also produce saliva, which helps to decrease the bacterial load in the mouth and provide moisture. The pancreas also has an exocrine gland function. It is located in the curve of the duodenum and lies below the stomach, extending to the spleen. The main pancreatic duct channels digestive enzymes to the duodenum through the common bile duct. These enzymes exist as zymogens, an inactive form, until they enter the duodenum. These enzymes aid the digestion of carbohydrates, fats, proteins, as well as neutralize acids via bicarbonate.

Motility, digestion, and absorption

Motility of the food bolus is controlled by the muscles of the gastrointestinal (GI) tract through two processes. The smooth muscles control peristalsis, which moves the food bolus, and the longitudinal muscles control segmentation, which mixes the food bolus, ensuring maximal absorption of nutrients. Digestion is facilitated by enzymes, which are secreted in the oral cavity, stomach, and intestines. These enzymes, in addition to bile salts produced in the liver and stored in the gallbladder, cleave the complex proteins, carbohydrates, and fats into smaller components, which can be absorbed through the GI mucosal walls. Absorption is the major function of the small intestine as the loss of fluids leads to dehydration. The GI system secretes 8 L, and approximately 2 L are ingested, most of which is reabsorbed. Absorption can be active or passive via facilitated diffusion. Glucose, galactose, amino acids, calcium, iron, folic acid, ascorbic acid, thiamin, and bile acids are transported actively. Fructose, riboflavin and vitamin B_{12} (in combination with intrinsic factor) are transported passively.

Gastrointestinal hormones

Gastrointestinal (GI) hormones, which have endocrine functions, are secreted by various organs and travel through the bloodstream to have distant effects on target cells. The GI tract is the largest endocrine organ, and the hormones secreted by it are referred to as the enteric endocrine system. These cells are found spread out throughout the GI system next to mucosal cells. Because their apical surface faces the GI tract, these cells can sample the GI tract composition and act appropriately. Three major enteric endocrine hormones are gastrin, cholecystokinin, and secretin. Gastrin is secreted by the stomach and controls the secretion of gastric acid in the stomach. Cholecystokinin is secreted by the small intestine and controls the secretion of pancreatic enzymes and bile. Secretin is secreted by the small intestine and leads to secretion of bicarbonate-rich fluids from the pancreas and liver.

The enteric neural system regulates the gastrointestinal tract and is divided into two systems: the myenteric plexus and the submucosal plexus. The myenteric plexus, also known as Auerbach's plexus, is located between the external longitudinal and internal circular muscle layers, and the submucosal plexus, also known as Meissner's plexus, is located between the circular muscle layer and the submucosa. The myenteric plexus targets the smooth muscle of the gut to promote intestinal motility. The submucosal plexus targets the mucosa and submucosa and is poorly understood. It is thought to work in an inhibitory fashion in the stomach, but it works in conjunction with the myenteric plexus in the intestine. Both systems are under primarily autonomic control but can be influenced by conscious control.

Secretory products

Salivary and gastrointestinal
Saliva is produced by the salivary glands of the oral cavity. It is 99.5% water; the remaining 0.5% is composed of electrolytes, mucus, enzymes, glycoproteins, and antibacterial components. The enzymes include amylase, which helps to break down starches, and salivary lipase, which helps to break down fats. The antibacterial components include secretory immunoglobulin A, lactoferrin, lysozyme, and peroxidase. In the stomach, gastric juice is secreted under the action of gastrin. Gastric juice contains mostly water, with small amounts of hydrochloric acid and digestive enzymes; these enzymes include rennin, pepsin, and gastric lipase. Rennin is found in young mammals and helps to convert milk protein into insoluble curd. Pepsin helps to convert proteins into peptones and proteoses. Gastric lipase digests fats into fatty acids and glycerol. All of these enzymes must be activated by hydrochloric acid.

Pancreatic and hepatic
The pancreas is responsible for secreting bicarbonate, which helps to neutralize the food bolus as it travels from the stomach. It also secretes enzymes, such as trypsinogen, chymotrypsinogen, elastase, carboxypeptidase, pancreatic lipase, and amylase. Trypsinogen is the inactive form of trypsin, which can cleave the peptide bond after an arginine or lysine, where it helps to digest proteins and activate more trypsin. Chymotrypsinogen is the inactive form of chymotrypsin, which is activated by trypsin and then breaks down peptides and polypeptides. Elastase also helps to break down proteins. Carboxypeptidase helps to break down peptides and proteins. Pancreatic

lipase helps to break down fats, while pancreatic amylase helps to digest carbohydrates. The liver secretes bile, which contains bile salts that aid in emulsifying lipids in the small intestine.

Hepatocytes

Hepatocytes are the cells that make up the liver, and they contain more rough endoplasmic reticulum and mitochondria than other cells. They are also the storage vesicles for glycogen, lipids, hemosiderin, and vitamin A. Hepatocytes are responsible for the synthesis of bile salts, cholesterol and phospholipids, which together make up bile. Bile aids in the digestion of lipids. The hepatocytes synthesize proteins, such as albumins, globulins, fibronectin, and prothrombin. The metabolic functions include gluconeogenesis and the deamination of amino acids to urea. Gluconeogenesis involves the formation of glucose from non-carbohydrate precursors. Liver cells also contain peroxisomes, which are involved in the breakdown of hydrogen peroxide. Hepatocytes are responsible for detoxifying the blood and inactivating dangerous substances. Liver cells are also capable of regeneration.

Gastrointestinal system

Repair

The esophagus can repair itself if there is no food or liquid that passes through it. If the damage is due to gastroesophageal reflux, the esophagus may repair itself with more acid-resistant cells, leading to Barrett's esophagus. The stomach is lined by protective mucus. This mucus can repair itself, but if the stomach acid has eroded the stomach itself, the mucus will be unable to protect it, resulting in an ulcer. Medications that raise the pH of the stomach acid can aid in the repair process. The colon can heal itself if the damage is the result of a short-term disease process. Chronic diseases, such as Crohn's and ulcerative colitis, prevent the colon from healing itself unless medications are taken to suppress the disease process. Surgical repair is usually needed for perforations in the gastrointestinal (GI) tract as these often result in a fistula. A fistula will only heal if the GI contents and liquid are not traveling through it.

Regeneration

True regeneration and not merely repair of the gastrointestinal system is only possible in the liver. Scientific research is exploring the use of growth factors and other drugs to stimulate regeneration elsewhere but so far they are still experimental. Hepatocytes technically do not undergo regeneration but rather undergo compensatory growth; however, this means that as little as 25% of the liver can regrow to an entire functioning liver. Hepatocytes retain the ability to re-enter the growth phase and begin mitosis anew. This is controlled by p75 receptors, and there may be liver stem cells that can differentiate into hepatocytes or cholangiocytes. This remarkable potential of the liver has expanded the role of liver transplantation so that living donors can be used. This is especially useful as infant recipients only need 20% of an adult liver, and both donor and recipient will eventually grow a fully functional liver.

Changes associated with aging

Soon after birth, the gastrointestinal (GI) system is capable of handling all of the types of foods it will encounter throughout life. Starting in the fourth decade of life, disease processes begin to develop, which can impair the functions of the GI system. Some of these changes are related to obesity, such as gastroesophageal reflux, diabetes (pancreatic disease), gallbladder disease, and peptic ulcer disease. Starting in the fifth decade of life, the rates of certain cancers begin to increase. These include stomach cancer, liver cancer, pancreatic cancer, and colorectal cancer. These rates can also be influenced by lifestyle habits, such as alcohol consumption, fatty food consumption, lack of fiber in the diet, and high consumption of red meat. Vascular disorders, such as hypertension and atherosclerotic disease, can impair blood flow to the GI system, impairing the absorption of nutrients. By the seventh decade of life, salivary and gastric fluid secretion slows, making it harder to digest and absorb nutrients.

Normal bacterial composition

The human gut contains the largest collection of microbial flora. These organisms are vital in aiding digestion and can be thought of as an organ in and of themselves. Somewhere between 300 and 1000 different bacterial species live in the gut. Most are anaerobic bacteria, but in the cecum, aerobic bacteria can be found in large populations. Gastrointestinal bacteria assist in fermenting unused energy substrates, regulating the development of the gut, preventing the growth of harmful and pathogenic bacteria, training the immune system, and producing vitamins for the host and hormones that lead to lipid storage. The Human Microbiome Project has sought to identify the human gut microbial flora and has found that most bacteria are of the genera *Bacteroides*, *Clostridium*, *Fusobacterium*, *Eubacterium*, *Ruminococcus*, *Peptococcus*, *Peptostreptococcus*, and *Bifidobacterium*. These bacteria are in a sensitive balance, and the same bacteria can cause disease when they increase disproportionately or become present outside the gut.

Cellular components

The epithelial cells, or enterocytes, lining the gastrointestinal tract are joined by tight junctions that form an epithelial monolayer that prevents the passage of large molecules. The intestinal villi contain enterocytes, which are replaced every 3 to 6 hours to prevent or minimize pathogen colonization. The intestinal mucosa is over 25% lymphoid tissue, which is known as gut-associated lymphoid tissue. Lymphocytes are present between the intestinal epithelial cells and also in organized follicles known as Peyer's patches. M cells preferentially bind to foreign cells and bring back their antigens to lymphoid follicles where antibodies can be quickly synthesized. Autophagosomes in the cells assist in deactivating the pathogenic bacteria or other substance by signaling to lysozymes to break them down with enzymes so that they can no longer cause harm to the host.

Infections

Gastrointestinal infections are characterized by inflammation of the stomach or small and large intestine, which results in diarrhea, vomiting, pain, and cramping of the abdomen. These infections can be caused by viruses, commonly rotavirus in children and norovirus in adults, or bacteria. The other causes include a disruption in the normal proportions of bacteria as a result of antibiotics or the introduction of new bacteria from food or water that is contaminated with fecal material. Viral causes are usually short-lived, but bacterial causes may persist and require antibiotic treatment. Many bacteria produce exotoxins, which cause inflammation and impair the absorption of water in the intestines. This can very quickly lead to dehydration from diarrhea and vomiting; hydration with electrolytes remains the most important aspect of treatment. In severe cases, hospitalization with intravenous fluids is necessary.

Bacterial infections

Bacterial infections of the gastrointestinal (GI) system are commonly acquired through food or water contaminated with fecal material or by food that has been left unrefrigerated. Some foods commonly associated with illness include raw or undercooked meat, poultry, seafood, eggs, raw sprouts, unpasteurized milk, soft cheeses, and fruit and vegetable juices. The most common bacterial infections include *Escherichia coli*, *Shigella*, *Vibrio cholerae*, *Campylobacter*, and *Salmonella*. In the elderly and those undergoing antibiotic treatment, *Clostridium difficile* is a common cause of GI infection. Bacterial GI infections present with nausea, vomiting, diarrhea, abdominal pain, cramping, and loss of appetite. Bacterial GI infections tend to present with bloody diarrhea, not watery diarrhea, and fever is sometimes present. In later stages of the infections, patients present with signs of dehydration, such as loss of turgor, fatigue, decreased urine output, high heart rate, and low blood pressure.

Some bacterial infections, such as those related to food poisoning from unrefrigerated foods, are short-lasting and can be managed with judicious use of fluids to prevent dehydration. Over-the-counter medications to control diarrhea, such as loperamide, can also be used. More serious infections, such as those related to fecal contamination of food or water, require antibiotic treatment as they can be long-lasting. Drinking fluids with electrolytes, known as oral replacement therapy, is crucial, and in severe cases, hospitalization with intravenous fluids may be required. The most common complications are related to dehydration, but certain species of *Escherichia coli*, known as 0157:H7, can result in anemia or renal failure. Hemolytic uremic syndrome is caused by the exotoxin produced by *E. coli* 0157:H7, which damages the intestinal lining, allowing the bacteria to enter the bloodstream and cause kidney damage.

Viral infections

Viral gastrointestinal infections can be spread easily and quickly among groups of people spending large amounts of time together; for example, children in day care and passengers on cruise ships are at high risk. The most common viruses responsible for infections include rotavirus, norovirus, enteric adenovirus, and astrovirus. These viruses cause inflammation in the small and large intestines, which decreases the ability of the intestines to absorb water. Rotavirus tends to affect children and norovirus tends to affect adults. Viral gastrointestinal infections tend to present with watery diarrhea, vomiting, abdominal pain, and cramping. Dehydration can present as fatigue, loss of turgor, sunken eyeballs, low blood pressure, high pulse, inability to produce tears, decreased urine output, and in young infants, sunken fontanelles. Sufferers may remain infectious long after their symptoms have dissipated.

Most viral infections run their course over a short period of time, and nutritional support is all that is needed to prevent dehydration. However, children are at especially high risk of suffering the complications of dehydration because of their low blood volume. Oral fluids should be given with electrolytes to replace those lost through diarrhea and vomiting. Over-the-counter medications, such as loperamide, to control diarrhea can be used by adults but should be avoided in children. In serious cases and more often with children, hospitalization with intravenous fluids may be needed if symptoms of dehydration appear. Signs of dehydration include a decrease in wet diapers, fatigue or sleepiness, low blood pressure, rapid pulse, and a lack of tear production. Without nutritional support, death can result. The vaccine for rotavirus should be given to all children, especially those entering day care.

Fungal infections

The gastrointestinal (GI) tract contains a multitude of bacteria, fungi, and viruses, which exist in a steady state. However, if one population decreases, another population would no longer be in check and could increase. This is what can happen after antibiotic use as the antibiotics affect the GI bacteria as an unintended consequence. With a declining bacterial population, fungi, such as the yeast *Candida*, can begin to increase, leading to fungal gastroenteritis. *Candida* can also affect the oral cavity and esophagus, causing pain with eating and leading to weight loss. Upon examination, the affected areas appear erythematous and covered by a cheese-like material that is easily scraped off the mucosal surface. If this is examined under the microscope, characteristic fungal hyphae are apparent. Immunocompromised individuals are also at risk for fungi infections, such as those with *Histoplasmosis capsulatum*, *Mucorales* species, and *Paracoccidioides brasiliensis*.

Fungal gastrointestinal infections can be diagnosed by obtaining a sample of the affected area, either directly or via endoscopy. This sample can be examined under the microscope for the appearance of fungal hyphae, but often this is a clinical diagnosis made by viewing erythema, mild edema, and a white cheesy substance covering the mucosa. Unlike leukoplakia, this substance can be easily scraped off. The affected patients' stool can also be examined microscopically. Immunocompromised patients, such as those with uncontrolled diabetes or HIV, should invoke a high suspicion of fungal disease when presenting with gastrointestinal symptoms. Treatment centers around antifungal medications. These are often taken orally in the form of troches for oral cavity disease and pills for stomach or intestinal disease. In serious cases, intravenous antifungal medications may be required. The overuse of antibiotics and use for long periods of time can also contribute to a high risk for fungal infections.

Parasitic infections
Parasitic infections of the gastrointestinal system are not uncommon and are found more commonly in persons who have traveled to areas with parasitic infestations, children in day care, homosexual men, and after environmental disasters in which the water sources have become contaminated. The most common parasitic infections involve *Giardia lamblia*, *Entamoeba histolytica*, *Cryptosporidium* species, *Strongyloides* species, and *Schistosoma* species. Schistosoma species are more likely to affect the stomach. Parasitic gastrointestinal infections present as gastroenteritis with cramping, abdominal pain, bloating, flatulence, and diarrhea. These parasites can also cause anemia and may travel to the lung, causing cough, or to other organs. In children, fussiness and restlessness may be seen. Diagnosis is made by stool sample or by applying tape to the anus overnight to check for eggs.

Mycobacterial infections
Mycobacterial infections of the gastrointestinal (GI) system tend to occur in immunocompromised people, such as those infected with *Mycoplasma avium intracellulare* (MAIC) in AIDS and HIV patients. Infections of the GI tract are commonly concurrent with systemic infection. The duodenum is frequently involved and can be covered in white patches. Workup for GI mycobacterial infections includes upper endoscopy, sigmoidoscopy, liver biopsy, bone marrow aspiration and biopsy, stool and blood cultures for MAIC, and D-xylose absorption tests. The D-xylose absorption test is not diagnostic of mycobacterial infections; it only indicates malabsorption. These infections typically present with nausea, anorexia, malabsorption, diarrhea, fatigue, weight loss, and fevers. Treatment centers around the use of multiple antimicrobials for at least 1 year. These may include macrolides, ethambutol, and rifamycins. Aminoglycosides can also be used, including streptomycin and amikacin.

Factors that impair system defense
The gastrointestinal (GI) system has multiple defense mechanisms; if any of these defense mechanisms are damaged or altered, opportunities result for pathogens to cause disease. The stomach is one of the first areas of defense with a highly acidic environment maintained by gastric juice. The stomach is protected from the acidic environment by a mucous layer, which can cause erosion and the entry of bacteria if it is disrupted. If the environment is not maintained at an acidic level, then ingested pathogens are not destroyed. The intestines have a tight cellular lining that prevents the entry of pathogens, but if this lining is compromised from disease or injury, then pathogens and GI flora may enter the bloodstream. Peristalsis, copious GI secretions, and the frequent shedding of epithelial lining cells dilutes and moves pathogens through the GI tract quickly so that there is no opportunity for colonization.

Crohn's disease

Crohn's disease is a form of inflammatory bowel disease, as differentiated from irritable bowel syndrome. It can affect the gastrointestinal (GI) tract anywhere and is an autoimmune disease in which the immune system mistakenly attacks the body. It can be related to both genetic and environmental factors and usually begins between the ages of 15 and 35. Crohn's disease is characterized by fatigue, weight loss, abdominal pain, cramping, diarrhea, and constipation. Crohn's disease is also characterized by failure to thrive and fistulas and abscesses along the GI tract. There is no cure for Crohn's disease, and treatment centers on suppressing the immune system. Medications can include aminosalicylates, corticosteroids, azathioprine, 5-mercaptopurine, and infliximab. Antibiotics may be needed to treat infections and abscesses. Surgery is necessary to treat fistulas and to perform bowel resection in severe cases.

Ulcerative colitis

Ulcerative colitis is a form of irritable bowel disorder that affects the large intestine and rectum. It is not known exactly what causes ulcerative colitis, but a family history and Jewish ancestry increase the risk of having it. This disease has two age peaks at 15–30 and 50–70 years of age. Symptoms can include bloody or pus-laced feces, diarrhea, fever, abdominal pain, cramping, and weight loss. Diagnosis is usually made by a colonoscopy with biopsy to show crypt branching with an increase in inflammatory cells in the lamina propria. Patients with ulcerative colitis are at an increased risk for colon cancer so must undergo routine colonoscopy screenings with biopsies. Medical treatment can include aminosalicylates, corticosteroids, azathioprine, 5-mercaptopurine, and infliximab. Colectomy may be required if medications are unsuccessful or if precancerous or cancerous changes are identified. A colectomy is curative for ulcerative colitis. There is also an association between ulcerative colitis and ankylosing spondylitis.

Malocclusion

Malocclusion occurs when the teeth of the mandible and maxilla do not line up properly. Occlusion is the terminology for the correct alignment of the teeth and is defined as the mesiobuccal cusp of the upper first molar in alignment with the buccal groove of the mandibular first molar. This is referred to as a class I occlusion. A class II occlusion is when the upper first molar is in an anterior position, and a class III occlusion is when the upper first molar is in a posterior position. Malocclusion may develop from genetic factors, prolonged bottle use, prolonged thumb sucking, and a lack of masticatory stress during development. Malocclusion puts unequal stresses on the jaw, which can lead to temporomandibular joint problems and arthritis. It can also lead to difficulties with the mechanical digestion of food as the food will not be ground down effectively for the enzymes to reach maximal surface area. Orthodontic or orthognathic treatment is necessary to correct malocclusion. This can involve braces, retainers, or surgery where the mandible or maxilla is broken and reset in a more anatomical position.

Obstruction

Obstruction of the bowel is defined by mechanical or functional obstruction that prevents the normal passage of a food bolus; it occurs anywhere in the small or large intestine or rectum. This condition is a medical or surgical emergency as normal peristalsis does continues to mobilize towards the obstruction. Also, the gut flora acts on the food bolus, producing gases and liquids, which combined with the increasing food bolus, leads to high pressures proximal to the obstruction. Once the pressure reaches a threshold (this is different for different areas), the bowel

- 277 -

ruptures, spilling its contents into the sterile peritoneal cavity, which leads to peritonitis as the bowel contains a large amount of bacteria that overloads the body's defenses. This may lead to organ failure and sepsis, which carry a high mortality rate.

Perforation

Perforation of the gastrointestinal (GI) tract can occur as a result of internal or external forces. Medical conditions, such as Crohn's disease or bowel obstructions, can lead to bowel perforation and potential fistulas and peritonitis. Peritonitis can lead to organ failure and carries a high risk of death, which makes it a surgical emergency. Perforation can occur anywhere along the GI tract from the esophagus to the anus. Blunt trauma, which is trauma that does not pierce the skin, can result in esophageal, stomach, and intestinal perforation. Underlying medical conditions, such as stomach ulcers, may predispose to this condition. Bowel perforation may present on abdominal x-ray or computed tomography scan as free air under the diaphragm or extravasation of contrast material. Bowel-wall thickening, free fluid, and mesenteric infiltration may be seen with blunt trauma injury and partial thickness injuries. All patients with blunt trauma must be evaluated with a high suspicion for bowel perforation so as not to miss this surgical emergency.

Hiatal hernia

A hiatal hernia occurs when the stomach protrudes above the diaphragm, entering the thorax. This is commonly due to a loosening of the diaphragm muscle. There are two different classes of hiatal hernia. Class I is referred to as a sliding hiatal hernia and is the most common. This occurs when the entire gastroesophageal junction slides superiorly, bringing the stomach into the thorax. Class II is referred to as a rolling hiatal hernia and occurs when the stomach rolls alongside the esophagus into the thorax. This condition does not change the position of the gastroesophageal junction. Both types can lead to gastroesophageal reflux as a result of the loosening of the diaphragm muscle around the gastroesophageal junction. Though a hiatal hernia can present with a variety of symptoms, including shortness of breath, chest pain, dysphagia, odynophagia, most cases are asymptomatic. A patient may suffer from gastroesophageal reflux without symptoms, and left untreated, gastroesophageal reflux can predispose patients to esophageal cancer.

Inguinal, femoral, and abdominal wall hernias

A hernia describes when an organ, in this case the bowel, or the fascia covering it penetrates through the cavity containing it, in this case the abdominal cavity. A hernia can develop in many area of weakness in the abdominal wall. An inguinal hernia develops along the pubic bone as fascia and possibly intestine migrate through the internal inguinal ring. The inguinal hernia is the most common type of hernia and can extend into the testicles in men. These hernias present as a bulge in the lower abdomen that becomes more apparent with standing. Femoral hernias develop through the femoral ring, which is located along the upper thigh region. Abdominal wall hernias can occur anywhere along the abdominal wall, but areas of weakness, such as the umbilicus, are more prevalent. An incarcerated hernia occurs when the intestine becomes stuck in the ring through which it pushed. This can lead to bowel obstruction and necrosis, which is considered a surgical emergency.

Esophageal, intestinal, and colonic diverticula

A diverticulum is defined as the outpouching of a hollow or fluid-filled structure in the body. If it involves all layers of the organ, it is called a true diverticulum; otherwise it is known as a false diverticulum. An esophageal diverticulum can develop in three distinct areas: the pharyngoesophageal area, the midesophageal area, or the epiphrenic area of the esophagus. Zenker's diverticulum, which develops through the cricopharyngeal muscle, is the most common. Intestinal diverticula occur as small false diverticula covered by mucosa and submucosa in the small intestine; these are far less common than colonic diverticula. Colonic diverticula, or diverticulosis, are common in adults over 50 years of age and may have a genetic predisposition. They occur more commonly in people who consume a low-fiber diet. All diverticula may trap food particles, especially seeds and nuts, resulting in diverticulosis. This can lead to inflammation and obstruction of the diverticula. In colonic diverticula, this can develop into diverticulosis with a risk for perforation and peritonitis.

Carcinoma

Colon
Colon cancer is one of the leading causes of death in the United States. Nearly all colon cancers start in the intestinal glands in a colon polyp. Colon polyps are benign outgrowths in the lining of the colon that become more common with age. The only way to visualize such growths is through a colonoscopy, which also enables physicians to biopsy these polyps. This remains the best way to catch colon cancer early when treatment is more successful. Colon cancer risk is related to family history; a history of inflammatory bowel disease; and a diet high in fat, low in fiber, and with red meat products. Treatment centers on surgery to remove the cancerous portion; this may involve a small biopsy or a colon resection. More advanced stages are often treated with chemotherapy and radiation.

Liver
Liver cancer, otherwise known as hepatocellular carcinoma, originates from the liver cells, or hepatocytes. The risk factors for hepatocellular carcinoma include: age over 50, male sex, history of hepatitis B or C, history of hemochromatosis, autoimmune disease, and most commonly, a history of chronic alcohol abuse, leading to cirrhosis. Hepatocellular carcinoma presents with signs of liver failure, including jaundice, easy bruising or bleeding, ascites, and abdominal pain. If caught early, the disease is treatable with surgical resection, but only 10%–20% of the liver can be resected and if the disease extends beyond these borders, it will recur. A liver transplant may be an option for patients whose disease is confined to the liver, but there is long waiting list for these transplants. Chemotherapy and radiation are not as successful as in other cancers because many of the patients have underlying cirrhosis of the liver.

Stomach
Gastric cancer most commonly comes from the epithelium that originates in glandular tissue, giving it the name adenocarcinoma. It shows predominance in Japan, Chile, and Iceland, although it is unknown if this is related to regional diets of salted, cured, and smoked foods. It is common in men over 40, those with a family history of gastric cancer, those with a history of chronic atrophic gastritis, those with *Helicobacter pylori* infection, and smokers. Unfortunately, many cases are asymptomatic or have symptoms that can easily be dismissed as related to gastroesophageal reflux or heartburn. The majority of cases are diagnosed in the late stages hampering treatment. Gastrectomy or surgical removal of the stomach can be curative if the cancer is locally contained. Chemotherapy and radiation can be palliative when used alone or can help in treatment after gastrectomy.

Esophageal

Carcinoma of the esophagus is not common in the United States and can be divided into two types: squamous cell carcinoma and adenocarcinoma, depending on the cell type from which it is derived. Squamous cell carcinoma of the esophagus is more common in patients who smoke and drink heavily. Esophageal adenocarcinoma frequently develops from changes in the esophagus known as Barrett's esophagus. Barrett's esophagus results when the lower esophagus is exposed to a high acid environment for long periods of time, such as in untreated gastroesophageal reflux. The esophageal cells are then replaced by cells that are more acid-resistant. If caught before it spreads beyond the esophagus, the treatment of choice is surgical resection or esophagectomy. Chemotherapy and radiation are useful for palliative treatment. Regular screenings of those at high risk with esophagogastroduodenoscopy and biopsies can catch the disease early.

Rectal

The rectum is part of the large intestine, approximately the last 6 inches, ending in the anus. Rectal cancer is defined separately from colon cancer because of the presence of different types of cells. The upper part resembles the colon but with longer, more widely spaced crypts, more abundant lymphatic tissue, and no teniae coli in the muscularis externa. The rectum then transitions to the anus and contains longitudinal folds known as the column of Morgagni and anal valves. Simple columnar epithelium in the upper part of the rectum transitions to non-keratinized stratified squamous epithelium as it becomes the anal region. Rectal cancer can present with blood in the stool, weight loss, loss of appetite, and generalized abdominal pain and discomfort. Endoscopy with biopsy is the best diagnostic test, and survival is good if the cancer can be entirely removed with surgery.

Gastrointestinal lymphomas

Gastrointestinal (GI) lymphomas are not common, but when present, are most commonly located in the stomach. Patients are at high risk if they are over 60, immunosuppressed, have HIV, or have *Helicobacter pylori* infection. These patients may present with weight loss, fatigue, abdominal pain, and loss of appetite. Endoscopy with biopsy is necessary to distinguish this from other adenocarcinomas of the GI tract, and because of its propensity for submucosal invasion, laparotomy may be necessary. Most GI lymphomas are non-Hodgkin's type of B-cell origin. Treatment involves chemotherapy with the CHOP (cyclophosphamide [Cytoxan], hydroxy doxorubicin [Adriamycin], vincristine [Oncovin], prednisone) regimen. Low-grade lymphomas, known as MALT (mucosa-associated, lymphoid tissue), are treated with antibiotic therapy to eradicate *H. pylori*. Radiation therapy may be used for MALT tumors that are *H. pylori* negative. Surgery may be necessary to deal with complications, refractory cases, and recurrences.

Neoplasm

A neoplasm is defined as the abnormal growth of tissue; this can be either malignant or benign. Gastrointestinal (GI) neoplasms usually present with pain, weight loss, and bleeding, which can be detected in the stool. Risk factors for GI system malignant neoplasms include *Helicobacter pylori* infection, Barrett's esophagus, ulcerative colitis, colonic polyps, smoking, alcohol consumption, and a diet high in fat and red meat. Ulcerative colitis and dietary factors also contribute to the growth of benign colonic polyps. Most neoplasms are asymptomatic though some may present with abdominal pain and discomfort, weight loss, loss of appetite, and blood in the stool. Fecal occult tests can be done at home and serve as a screening tool to detect blood in the stool. Patients may then undergo upper or lower endoscopy to visualize the areas and to take biopsies of anything that looks suspicious. Benign neoplasms may require surveillance with endoscopy, and malignant neoplasms are often treated with surgery, chemotherapy, or radiation therapy.

Metastatic disease is defined as the spread of disease from one organ to another non-adjacent organ and is most commonly used to refer to malignancies. Malignant cells have lost the ability to stop cell mitosis and continue to grow, producing a tumor. Metastasis can occur through the blood, hematogenously, or through the lymphatic system. The gastrointestinal (GI) system has an extensive blood supply network so that the absorption of nutrients and fluids can be most effective. There is also a shunting of blood from much of the GI system to the liver for detoxification. This also means that the liver is a common site of metastases, especially from colon cancer. Because of the proximity of many GI organs, direct spread can also occur from one organ to another. For instance, stomach cancer can spread to the liver, pancreas, and esophagus because of its location near these organs.

Motility disorders

Motility of the gastrointestinal (GI) system is controlled by peristalsis, which is largely controlled by the autonomic nervous system. If peristalsis is not functioning properly, the food bolus will not move down the GI tract. Achalasia is an esophageal disorder where the esophagus does not empty into the stomach. It can be caused by nerve damage, neoplasms, and parasitic infections. Gastroparesis is a condition where the stomach does not empty its contents into the duodenum. Nerve damage from surgery, neoplasm, or diabetes is a frequent cause. Gastrointestinal reflux where the stomach contents travel backward up the esophagus is often due to a weakening of the sphincter between the stomach and the esophagus. Ogilvie syndrome is a pseudo-obstruction of the colon in severely ill patients. The exact etiology is unknown, but it can lead to megacolon. Constipation occurs when the intestinal contents do not mobilize to the rectum, anus, and then outward. This can be due to a low-fiber diet, consumption of too few fluids, or medications.

Malabsorption disorders

Malabsorption disorders of the gastrointestinal system can have serious side effects as the body does not receive the vitamins and nutrients it needs to function properly. This may lead to malnutrition or anemia. Celiac disease is an autoimmune disorder that causes blunting of the small intestinal villi in response to the ingestion of gluten. This causes malabsorption of many nutrients and vitamins by the small intestine. Whipple's disease is an infectious disorder cause by the bacterium *Tropheryma whipplei*. It leads to diarrhea, joint pain, and weight loss; it can be cured by antibiotics. Lactose intolerance is a common disorder in Asian patients due to a deficiency of the enzyme lactase. This leads to diarrhea, bloating, and gas when lactose in ingested. Inflammatory bowel diseases, such as Crohn's disease, can lead to malabsorption due to the inflammation of the small and large intestines, which lowers the surface area thereby impeding absorption. Systemic sclerosis is associated with malabsorption, most commonly with gastroesophageal reflux, which can lead to strictures.

> **Review Video:** Lactose Intolerance
> Visit *mometrix.com/academy* and enter *Code:* **672651**

Hepatic failure

Liver failure is the breakdown of the liver and its ability to perform its metabolic and synthetic functions. Liver failure can be classified as acute or chronic. Acute liver failure is frequently due to toxic ingestion of poisonous mushrooms, drug or alcohol overdoses, or trauma. Chronic liver failure is associated with cirrhosis, chronic alcohol intake, fatty liver disease, hepatitis B or C, or chronic toxic ingestion. The body can cope with chronic liver failure for much longer periods of time until almost all of the liver's function is destroyed. Acute liver failure produces a sharp increase in toxic by-products that the body cannot handle. Both conditions lead to ascites, encephalopathy, jaundice, constipation, and a rise in liver function tests. These toxic by-products build up in the blood and lead to mental instability and organ failure.

> **Review Video:** Liver Failure
> *Visit **mometrix.com/academy** and enter **Code:** 762010*

Cholelithiasis

Cholelithiasis or gallstones are a frequent problem for many people. The risk factors for gallstones include being overweight, over 40, female, and pregnant. Gallstones are crystallized stones of cholesterol most commonly. They can also be composed of bilirubin. Most gallstones are asymptomatic. However, when a stone travels into the cystic or common bile duct, it can cause obstruction with accompanying pain known as biliary colic. If the stone does not pass, jaundice, upper right quadrant pain, fever, nausea, and vomiting may develop. Surgery is the best option for those patients with chronic gallstones. Open cholecystectomy may be done if previous abdominal surgery has been performed or scarring is present. However, most patients can undergo laparoscopic cholecystectomy, which has a much shorter recovery period. Endoscopic retrograde cholangiopancreatography can also be performed without any major incisions.

Nutritional disorders

Nutritional disorders can involve too much or too few nutrients and vitamins. Overeating can lead to obesity, which causes many disorders. Obesity is associated with diabetes, hypertension, obstructive sleep apnea, osteoarthritis of the knees, and hypercholesterolemia. Overconsumption of vitamins, specifically fat-soluble vitamins, and iron can lead to severe side effects, including liver problems and death. Lack of protein in the diet can lead to kwashiorkor and marasmus, which may lead to long-term physical and mental impairments. A deficiency of calcium or vitamin D, which is needed for the absorption of calcium, will lead to osteoporosis or rickets. These conditions make the malformation of bone and fractures more likely. Iodine deficiency in adults can lead to an enlargement of the thyroid called goiter. In children, it can lead to permanent intellectual disability.

Portal hypertension

Portal hypertension is hypertension or high blood pressure in the portal vein due to dysfunction of the liver, most commonly cirrhosis. The blockage and decreased flow in the portal vein lead the blood to be shunted to other surrounding vessels in order to drain from the gastrointestinal tract. This leads to varices across the abdomens that enlarge to shunt blood from the esophagus and stomach. These varices were not designed to handle such large volumes, so that they strain the vessel wall and are prone to rupture. These ruptures can lead to blood in the stool or vomiting blood. The blood that travels through these varices bypasses the liver, leading to the accumulation of toxic by-products. This can lead to ascites (fluid in the abdomen), encephalopathy (mental status changes), and a decreased ability of blood to clot because of a lack of clotting factors.

Esophageal varices

Esophageal varices are dilated blood vessels in the submucosa of the esophagus, most commonly in the lower third of the esophagus. The most common etiology of esophageal varices is portal hypertension, which causes blood to be shunted around the liver, usually due to liver cirrhosis. Esophageal varices are prone to rupture and bleeding, which can lead to hematemesis. This is because these vessels are usually 1 mm in diameter but can become dilated up to 2 cm in diameter. These varices can be diagnosed by endoscopy, and therapeutic endoscopy is the treatment of choice when bleeding develops. In emergencies, volume resuscitation should be conservative so as not to exacerbate portal hypertension. Banding of the vessels, sclerotherapy, or balloon tamponade can be performed via endoscopy. Further treatment should center on treating the underlying cause (i.e., the portal hypertension).

Hemorrhoids

Hemorrhoids, also known as piles or rectal lumps, are swollen veins in the lower end of the gastrointestinal tract. These veins become dilated and prolapse through the external anal sphincter and can be felt and seen outside the body. The most common etiologies are straining while having a bowel movement, pregnancy, childbirth, anal infections, sitting for long periods, portal hypertension, or constipation. Hemorrhoids can present with pain, bright red blood in the stool or on the toilet paper, or tender lumps near the anus. A stool guaiac shows the presence of blood in the stool, and further workup should include a lower endoscopy to examine the source of bleeding. Hemorrhoids can be relieved with the use of stool softeners, hemorrhoid creams, warm sitz baths, and soft cushions in the shape of a doughnut for sitting. Surgery may be done for intractable cases and involves banding of the hemorrhoids to block blood flow through them.

Anal fissures

An anal fissure is a tear or rip in the mucosa lining the lower rectal/anal region. Anal fissures can be caused by constipation and passage of firm stool or frequent diarrhea. They are common in infants, women after childbirth, and patients with Crohn's disease. Anal fissures often present with bright red blood in the stool or on toilet paper. The fissure can sometimes be seen if one spreads apart the tissue and sees a crack in the middle of the skin. A rectal examination is sufficient for diagnosis if the fissure is detected. Treatment involves treating the underlying condition. For constipation, stool softeners, an increase in fluid intake, and an increase in fiber intake can be used. For diarrhea, over-the-counter medications can be taken. With these measures, anal fissures will in most cases resolve on their own. People who develop anal fissures are at high risk for recurrences.

Ischemia

Bowel ischemia can be either mesenteric ischemia, which is a loss of blood supply to the small intestine, or ischemic colitis, which is loss of blood supply to the colon or large intestine. Bowel ischemia is more common in the elderly population. The decrease in blood supply can be due to a systemic hypotension or to local factors, such as vascular compression or a blood clot. Three phases have been elucidated: hyperactive, paralytic, and shock. The hyperactive phase can present with abdominal pain and bloody stools, and the paralytic phase presents with absent bowel sounds, no stools, and diffuses abdominal pain. The shock phase occurs when fluids begin to leak though the bowel lining into surrounding tissue and can lead to shock. Ischemic colitis and chronic mesenteric ischemia can resolve without treatment. Acute mesenteric ischemia is a surgical emergency and the cause of obstruction must be removed.

Angiodysplasia

Angiodysplasia is a small vascular malformation in the gastrointestinal tract. It occurs most frequently in the cecum or ascending colon and can present with positive fecal occult blood testing; it may cause anemia. Angiodysplasia can be difficult to find but is usually diagnosed by endoscopy. If endoscopy is negative, but there is still high clinical suspicion, arteriography of the mesenteric arteries can be done to look for extravasation of contrast. Embolization can also be performed at the same time. Although angiodysplasia is thought to be common, in patients with bleeding disorders, it can become problematic. In severe cases, blood transfusions are necessary. Endoscopy with cauterization or embolization via angiography may be possible, though bowel resection may be necessary in limited cases. In cases in which these treatments cannot be used, systemic estrogen can be used to increase coagulability.

Thromboses

Thromboses in the gastrointestinal (GI) tract can significantly decrease or completely cut off blood supply to an area of the GI tract supplied by that vessel. The mesenteric vessels are the primary blood supply to the intestines, and therefore, thromboses in these vessels can have serious consequences. Mesenteric artery thromboses are a medical emergency and have a high mortality rate. Patients with a long history of smoking, uncontrolled diabetes, and vascular disease are at high risk. Patients present with abdominal pain that is out of proportion to the findings on clinical exam. Arteriography is useful for diagnosis, as it will show lack of filling in all or part of the mesenteric artery. Surgical intervention with thrombectomy or vascular bypass is necessary in acute cases. Thromboses of the mesenteric vein may present with a slower onset of symptoms, over 7–10 days, and the underlying hypercoagulable state should be corrected. Surgery is only necessary for bowel infarction or perforation.

Vasculitis

Vasculitis involves inflammation of the vascular system. It is often an accompaniment to systemic disorders, such as systemic lupus erythematosus and polyarteritis nodosa. Vasculitis occurs when the immune system mistakenly recognizes the gastrointestinal tract as foreign and begins to attack it. Patients may present with acute abdominal pain, positive fecal occult blood testing, or peritonitis. These patients may mimic those with acute mesenteric ischemia so a high level of suspicion should be raised in patients with no source of embolization. Diagnosis involves a workup for the systemic condition, such as laboratory tests and possibly a biopsy via endoscopy. Computed tomography scans show non-specific inflammation of the bowel. Treatment is the same as that used to treat the systemic diseases, such as anti-inflammatory medications (e.g., steroids) and medications to suppress the immune system. Cytotoxic drugs include azathioprine and cyclophosphamide; rituximab also helps to dampen the immune response.

HIV/AIDS

HIV is the virus that causes AIDS, which leads to a compromised immune system and serious infections. Gastrointestinal (GI) tract symptoms that can accompany HIV/AIDS include diarrhea, odynophagia/dysphagia, anorectal disease, and Kaposi's sarcoma and GI lymphomas. Diarrhea can be linked to bacteria, such as *Campylobacter*, *Giardia*, or *Clostridium difficile*. A stool culture is useful to identify infectious etiologies. Lower endoscopy with biopsy can identify cytomegalovirus infections. Odynophagia and dysphagia can result from infectious processes and are best diagnosed with upper endoscopy with biopsy. Anorectal disease can be diagnosed on careful physical examination and is most frequently due to anal fissures or hemorrhoids. Medical treatment is the treatment of choice because surgery is usually only successful in patients in the early stages of AIDS. Kaposi's sarcoma is not fatal and can be managed conservatively, while GI lymphomas can metastasize and are treated with chemotherapy and radiation.

Diabetes mellitus

Patients with diabetes mellitus can have dysphagia, early satiety, reflux, constipation, abdominal pain, nausea, vomiting, and diarrhea. These symptoms can be worse with a longer course of disease and poor glucose control. Diabetics suffer from dysfunction of the peripheral nervous system, and this can affect the gastrointestinal system, which is largely controlled by the autonomic nervous system. This can lead to motility, absorption, and secretion disorders. Diabetic gastroparesis is due to nerve dysfunction and can prolong emptying of the stomach, leading to bloating, early satiety, and gastroesophageal reflux. Peptic ulcer disease can be related to *Helicobacter pylori* infection, and treatments include antibiotic and proton pump inhibitor therapy. Oral and esophageal *Candida* infections are more common in diabetics and can be treated with antifungal therapy. Pancreatic exocrine dysfunction occurs in up to 80% of patients with diabetes mellitus type I and to a lesser extent, in those with type 2.

Hyperlipidemia

Hyperlipidemia is a condition characterized by an increase in fatty substances in the blood. These substances may include cholesterol and triglycerides. These fatty substances can deposit in organs, causing dysfunction. In extreme cases, pancreatitis or inflammation of the pancreas can develop. Fatty liver disease can also be caused by high cholesterol and triglyceride levels. Pancreatitis can present with nausea, vomiting, and abdominal pain and can be life-threatening. Patients are often kept on intravenous antibiotics and kept from taking any nutrition by mouth until it resolves. Fatty liver disease can cause scar tissue to build up in the liver, impairing function. In severe cases, it can lead to liver failure. Treatment for hyperlipidemia involves a healthy diet, exercising, and not smoking. Medications called statins can also be added to lower cholesterol and triglycerides.

Idiopathic eosinophilic gastrointestinal disorder

Eosinophilic gastrointestinal disorder is an idiopathic disorder characterized by abdominal pain, eosinophilic infiltrates, the absence of any etiology for the eosinophilia, and no eosinophilic infiltration in any other organs. The disease most often involves the stomach and small intestine, and patients frequently have a history of food allergies or other atopy. Children can present with failure to thrive and delayed puberty, while adults can present with abdominal pain, diarrhea, and dysphagia. Work-up should include a complete blood count with differential, which may show peripheral eosinophilia. These patients also have high alpha$_1$-antitrypsin in their stool, indicating protein loss. Oral glucocorticoids may be helpful in treatment as well as elimination of any foods implicated in allergy testing. Surgery is only useful in cases of pyloric stenosis or small intestine stenosis and is not curative. Disease can recur after treatment, and conservative measures are advocated.

Purpura

Henoch-Schönlein purpura is a type of vasculitis that is characterized by purpura in the gastrointestinal tract. It can also cause a characteristic rash, joint pain, and kidney problems. It is more common in children and adolescents, and gastrointestinal (GI) symptoms include abdominal pain, nausea, vomiting, and bloody stools. The GI symptoms typically appear about a week after the rash. Henoch-Schönlein purpura is postulated to be caused by an overactive immune response to viruses, medications, chemicals, insect bites, or immunizations. In rare cases, the GI purpura can develop into intussusception and bowel obstruction that can cut off the blood supply to the bowel. Bowel obstruction is a medical emergency and frequently needs immediate surgical attention. This can also lead to inflammation of other organs, including the pancreas. Henoch-Schönlein purpura usually resolves on its own, but medical attention may be needed for the complications of the disease, including bowel obstruction and gastrointestinal bleeding

Degenerative hepatic disease

Degenerative hepatic disease can be due to a number of conditions, but the ultimate result is dysfunction or a complete lack of hepatic function. Conditions that can contribute to degenerative hepatic disease include the following: Wilson's disease, a genetic disease that is characterized by dysfunction in copper metabolism; cholestasis, which causes backup of the bile salts and triglycerides produced by the liver; autoimmune hepatitis; viral hepatitis; hemochromatosis, a genetic disorder of iron metabolism; and steatosis or fatty liver disease. These conditions lead to cirrhosis and scarring of the liver, which slowly reduce the functional capacity of the hepatocytes. Liver damage caused by degenerative hepatic disease is irreversible, and medical treatments can merely lessen the side effects from the toxic substances. A liver transplant is the only real treatment or cure for this disease.

Cocaine

Cocaine is drug that has both medical and abuse potential. It acts as a serotonin, norepinephrine, dopamine reuptake inhibitor that is a nervous system stimulant and a topical anesthetic. Cocaine use can have disastrous consequences, especially in those who swallow packets of large quantities of cocaine to smuggle it. Due to the vasoconstrictive effect of cocaine on the alpha-adrenergic receptors of the mesentery, acute bowel ischemia is a common adverse effect. Depending on the length of time of the ischemia, bowel necrosis, gastropyloric ulcerations, and bowel perforations can occur. Cocaine can also cause mesenteric vascular thromboses due to platelet aggregation, leading to bowel ischemia and perforation. Acute hepatotoxicity and hepatocellular necrosis has also been seen with cocaine toxicity. Concurrent alcohol use in cocaine users may sensitize the liver to damage by cocaine. Cocaine also reduces salivary secretions and causes bruxism.

Prednisone

Prednisone is a corticosteroid used to treat inflammatory conditions. The side effects seen with this medication are directly proportional to the dosage and length of time the medication is taken. The gastrointestinal (GI) manifestations of prednisone include vomiting, nausea, abdominal pain, bloating, diarrhea, or bloody stools. Prednisone can also reduce the normal intestinal flora, leading to overgrowth by other bacteria or fungi. One serious consequence can be a *Clostridium difficile* infection, which must be identified and treated. Stool culture is the only method of diagnosis. Abdominal pain, peptic ulcers, mouth sores, stomach pain or bloating, and hepatitis steatosis are also seen with prednisone use. It can also worsen gastroesophageal reflux. Prednisone use can also raise blood glucose levels in diabetics, making the GI complications of diabetes worsen.

Anti-cancer drugs

Chemotherapy drugs target rapidly dividing cells, and through different mechanisms, cause cellular apoptosis. Cells of the bone marrow, digestive tract, skin, and hair follicles all consist of rapidly dividing cells that are targeted unintentionally by these drugs. Nausea, diarrhea, constipation, and vomiting are common side effects of chemotherapy. Severe cases can lead to dehydration and malnutrition. Medications or hospitalization with intravenous fluids may be needed to treat these side effects and prevent complications. There is also a transdermal patch of granisetron that can be applied for 7 days during chemotherapy treatments to control nausea and vomiting. These symptoms should also raise a high suspicion of typhlitis or inflammation of the cecum, which is infectious and can be a medical emergency. There are also indirect side effects of chemotherapy, such as an increased risk of infection as a result of granulocytopenia and an increased risk of gastrointestinal bleeding as a result of thrombocytopenia.

Acetaminophen

Acetaminophen is a common over-the-counter medication used to treat headaches, muscle aches, fever, and joint pain. At high doses and with chronic use, serious side effects can develop. Overuse of acetaminophen can cause nausea, vomiting, abdominal/stomach pain, extreme fatigue, or jaundice. There is a risk of upper gastrointestinal bleeding and perforation. This risk is increased when acetaminophen is used in combination with other anti-inflammatory drugs. Acetaminophen can also have toxic effects on the liver when taken in high doses. Hepatotoxicity may range from transient rises in liver enzymes, such as transaminase, to fulminant hepatic failure. People who are chronic alcohol drinkers or suffer from underlying liver cirrhosis are at greater risk of liver damage due to acetaminophen because of the small hepatic reserve available. The risk is also higher in people who have been fasting.

Esophageal atresia

Esophageal atresia is a condition in which the esophagus does not develop or recanalize properly. During fetal development, the esophagus is a solid tube; it becomes hollow before birth. If this does not occur properly, the esophagus is not fully patent, and food cannot pass through it. This condition can occur in conjunction with a tracheoesophageal fistula, which leads to aspiration and pneumonia. Esophageal atresia is usually detected shortly after birth when the infant attempts to feed for the first time and begins choking and coughing or becomes cyanotic. Diagnosis involves attempting to pass a feeding tube down to the stomach, which is not possible with this condition. This condition is a surgical emergency because oral feedings are not possible and can potentially lead to lung infections. Malnutrition and dehydration develop quickly without surgery or intravenous hydration.

Meckel's diverticulum

Meckel's diverticulum is a congenital condition in which there is a small pouch on the wall of the lower intestine. It is a true diverticulum, composed of all three layers of the intestinal wall. Many patients are asymptomatic, but some may present with abdominal pain or bloody stools. It is a vestigial remnant of the omphalomesenteric duct and is usually located near the ileocecal valve. Meckel's diverticulum may contain gastric or pancreatic cells, which can lead to the development of gastric ulcers. This condition may cause anemia from gastrointestinal bleeding, volvulus, intussusception, bowel perforation, or peritonitis. Sometimes, it is mistaken for appendicitis. These symptoms may not develop until adulthood even though the condition has been present since birth. If complications arise, surgery may be needed to remove the diverticulum and reattach the two remaining intestinal ends.

Intestinal malrotation

Intestinal malrotation is a congenital error in the rotation of the midgut during development. As the midgut returns into the abdominal cavity during gestation, it rotates. However, if this rotation is not precise or not in the right direction, abdominal contents can end up in non-anatomic positions. For example, the small bowel is on the right side, the cecum is near the epigastrium, fibrous bands lie across the duodenum, and the ligament of Treitz is more inferior and to the right. The midgut is also more prone to volvulus because of the narrow base of the small intestine. This condition makes patients more prone to the following: acute and chronic midgut volvulus, acute and chronic duodenal obstruction, internal herniation, and superior mesenteric artery syndrome. All of these complications can lead to bowel ischemia and perforation.

Hirschsprung's disease

Hirschsprung's disease is a congenital condition in which the autonomic nerves are missing from a part of the large intestine so that peristalsis is impaired, leading to a blockage of the large intestine. Without the nerve signals, the bowel musculature does not receive any signals to contract, and peristalsis does not occur in that area. The food bolus cannot move past this area and creates an obstruction, which leads to bowel enlargement and risk of perforation. In mild cases, this can lead to constipation, growth retardation, and abdominal swelling. Infants can present with failure to pass stool, vomiting, poor weight gain, and poor feeding. -Treatment involves surgery to remove the diseased area of bowel and usually the rectum. Usually this is a two-stage operation over the first year of life. Without surgery, patients run the risk of bowel perforation.

Celiac disease

Celiac disease is a condition of unknown etiology in which the consumption of gluten causes damage to the lining of the small intestine. Gluten is found in products such as wheat, barley, and rye. Consumption of gluten leads to a flattening of the villi of the small intestine. These villi are finger-like projections that increase the surface area of the small intestine to maximize absorption of nutrients and vitamins. With damage to the villi, proper absorption of nutrients and vitamins is compromised and can lead to malnutrition, failure to thrive, and growth retardation. This condition can present with abdominal pain, bloating, weight loss, diarrhea, nausea, vomiting, fatigue, mouth ulcers, or signs of vitamin deficiencies. Blood tests to look for anti-tissue transglutaminase antibodies or anti-endomysium antibodies can be used to diagnose celiac disease. Treatment involves life-long avoidance of gluten and gluten products.

Congenital biliary atresia

During fetal development, ducts develop by recanalization, whereby the solid tube is transformed into a hollow duct. If there are errors in development, these ducts can be atretic or not functional. If this occurs in the biliary system, congenital biliary atresia can develop. This atresia can occur in the common duct, the hepatic duct, or the right and left hepatic ducts. This can decrease or block the flow of bile from the gallbladder and liver. Most infants present with jaundice, but some may present with dark urine and light-colored stool. There is no medical treatment for this disorder, and without proper bile drainage, liver damage can occur. This is considered a surgical emergency. During surgery, an intraoperative cholangiogram is done to confirm lack of flow through the bile ducts. The Kasai procedure, or hepatoportoenterostomy, is considered the standard of care and involves attaching the small intestine to the exposed liver surface under the porta hepatis. This will allow drainage of the bile ducts from the liver.

Peptic ulcer disease

Gastroesophageal reflux occurs when stomach acid travels back up into the esophagus. This causes damage to the esophagus and can cause cellular changes known as Barrett's esophagus. This condition raises the risk of esophageal cancer. Medical treatment is often attempted before surgical options. Medical treatment centers around a clarithromycin-based triple therapy or triple therapy for short. Gastroesophageal reflux has many causes, which require three medications to treat it effectively. This triple therapy consists of two antibiotics to kill *Helicobacter pylori*, the bacteria that can cause ulcers, and a proton pump inhibitor to reduce the acid volume in the stomach. Typically, the antibiotics include clarithromycin to stop the growth of *H. pylori* and amoxicillin to kill the *H. pylori*. This triple therapy is taken for 14 days or more as research has shown this to be the minimum treatment time needed to reduce gastroesophageal reflux.

Antacids, anti-histamine blockers, and proton pump inhibitors

Gastroesophageal reflux or heartburn is a common condition that affects adults in industrialized nations. Many medications, both over the counter and prescription, can be used to treat reflux. Antacids are over-the-counter medications made of chemical compounds that neutralize stomach acid. They work immediately and can be taken at the first symptoms of heartburn. However, they do not change the volume of acid in the stomach; they merely raise the pH. Anti-histamine blockers, such as ranitidine, work to block the H_2 receptors in the stomach, which prevents stimulation of the stomach cells to produce more acid. This can lead to a decrease in the volume of acid produced but will not change the pH of the stomach acid. Drugs, such as omeprazole, a proton pump inhibitor, block the production of hydrogen/potassium ATPase in the gastric parietal cells, which, in turn, blocks the final step in acid production, lowering the acid volume in the stomach.

Drugs commonly used to alter gastrointestinal motility

Gastrointestinal motility issues can result in constipation, diarrhea, bowel obstruction, and possible bowel perforation. Cholinergic agonists can be used when the parasympathetic system is being suppressed. Neostigmine blocks the enzyme, which degrades acetylcholine, and bethanechol is a muscarinic stimulant. Prokinetic agents stimulate motility. Tegaserod is a serotonin receptor type 4 partial agonist. Metoclopramide blocks dopamine receptors and sensitizes nerves to acetylcholine, and cisapride promotes acetylcholine release into synapses. These drugs enhance peristalsis. Methylnaltrexone blocks opioid receptors, which relieves constipation. Antidiarrheals, including a loperamide, diphenoxylate, an atropine and diphenoxylate combination known as Lomotil, and a difenoxin and atropine combination known as Motofen, act on intestinal wall muscles slowing motility. Erythromycin binds to and activates motilin receptors.

Many different classes of medications are used to treat gastrointestinal motility disorders. These include: cholinergic agonists, prokinetic agents, opioid antagonists, antidiarrheals, and antibiotics. Cholinergic agents can relieve excessive parasympathetic suppression in cases where the parasympathetic suppression is blocking signals for peristalsis. This can then relieve obstruction. Prokinetic agents improve or stimulate gastrointestinal motility and are used in patients with constipation-predominant symptoms and irritable bowel disease. Opioid reversal agents or antagonists are used to block the opioid receptors. These can be used to treat constipation in patients taking narcotics who are unresponsive to laxatives. Antidiarrheal medications slow intestinal motility and cramping. Antibiotics act as prokinetic agents to treat gastroparesis. The type of medication prescribed should be tailored to the specific condition from which the patient is suffering.

Fluid replacement

Fluids can be replaced orally, intravenously, or injected into the subcutaneous tissue. However, intravenous fluid acts the fastest. Fluid must be replaced with an ionic content that is identical to the body's composition; it cannot be hypo- or hypertonic as this leads to cellular apoptosis. Fluid replaced orally is called oral replacement therapy and is used in cases of severe diarrhea to make up for fluid losses and prevent dehydration. Pedialyte is the brand name of a form specialized for children to be used during episodes of vomiting or diarrhea. Intravenous forms of fluid replacement include lactated Ringer's solution and dextrose 5. Total parenteral nutrition is an intravenous form of nutrition that can be used in patients who cannot take any nutrition by mouth. Blood transfusions are used when a patient has suffered severe blood loss as other fluids will not replace lost oxygen-carrying capacity.

Diarrhea, vomiting, blood loss, sweating, or fluid shifts, such as with ascites, can cause fluid loss that has to be treated. Without proper fluid, the organs cannot function, and severe fluid loss can be fatal. The proper electrolytes are needed as cells move these ions across cell membranes to generate energy. Fluid also allows the blood to flow smoothly and oxygenate all the organs and cells in the body. As fluid volume drops, the heart rate will increase, and blood pressure will drop to maintain blood flow to all areas of the body. Fluid replacement can be used orally for minor cases of dehydration from diarrhea, vomiting, or sweating. In severe cases of dehydration or fluid loss due to hemorrhaging, the intravenous route is the most advantageous. However, in cases of blood loss, the fluid dilutes the blood volume and does not replace lost oxygen-carrying capacity, which may require a transfusion.

> ➤ **Review Video:** Blood Transfusions
> *Visit **mometrix.com/academy** and enter **Code: 759682***

Pancreatitis

Pancreatitis is an inflammation of the pancreas. It can present in both acute and chronic forms. Without treatment, it can lead to pancreatic abscess, pancreatic pseudocyst, and peritonitis. Pancreatitis can present with abdominal pain, nausea, vomiting, steatorrhea, pain when reclining, and fever. The most common causes associated with chronic pancreatitis are long-term alcohol consumption and repeated episodes of acute pancreatitis. Calcium deposits in the pancreas may be seen on imaging. Acute pancreatitis can also be caused by long-term alcohol consumption, autoimmune diseases, blockage of the bile ducts, or trauma or injury to the pancreas. Treatment for both forms of pancreatitis involves nothing by mouth, intravenous or total parenteral nutrition, fluids, and antibiotics. Surgery may be needed to eliminate the underlying cause if possible or to drain fluid around or in the pancreas.

Pancreatic replacement therapy

The pancreas secretes about 64 ounces of fluid into the duodenum every day. This fluid helps to digest fats, proteins, and carbohydrates, and without it, the proper absorption of vitamins and nutrients may not be possible. Some conditions, such as cystic fibrosis, chronic pancreatitis, pancreatic cancer, pancreatic resection, and a total pancreatectomy, compromise or eliminate the ability to produce pancreatic enzymes. These patients typically present with steatorrhea (i.e., oily stools that float on the water due to excess fats). This can lead to malnutrition, and pancreatic replacement therapy is used. Pancreatic replacement therapy consists of a mixture of digestive enzymes, including lipase, protease, and amylase that are derived from a porcine pancreas, and is available in capsule form. Pancreatic lipase helps to break down fats, pancreatic protease helps to digest proteins, and pancreatic amylase breaks down carbohydrates.

Hepatic failure

Hepatic failure is the termination or decrease of the liver's ability to perform its metabolic functions. It can present in both acute and chronic forms. Acute hepatic failure can result from acute alcohol poisoning, toxic ingestions, infections, and overdoses. It leads to coagulopathy and mental status changes, known as encephalopathy. Chronic hepatic failure is more commonly linked to long-term alcohol consumption with cirrhosis or hepatitis infections. It can lead to the slower onset of hepatocellular dysfunction with coagulopathy and encephalopathy. Both conditions can also lead to jaundice, ascites, and clay-colored stools. Treatment is designed to minimize the symptoms, such as medications for the encephalopathy, drainage of the ascites, transfusions, or medications to control the coagulopathy. The only cure is a liver transplant, which may take years on a waiting list.

Biliary disease

Biliary disease can affect the function of both the gallbladder and liver. When the formation of bile is not in the correct ratio, bile salts can crystallize, leading to gallstones. Bile stasis and gallbladder hypomotility can also contribute to gallstone formation. Gallstones are common in women, those over 40, and overweight patients. Their formation is thought to be due to diet and genetic factors, such as decreased bile acid secretion. Gallstones can present with colicky right upper quadrant pain, jaundice, nausea, vomiting, and weight loss. Treatment can be symptomatic or definitive. Most cases of gallstones will resolve on their own after the stones have passed. Intravenous fluids and pain medications may be necessary to wait this passage out. In cases of recurrent gallstones or infection of the gallbladder, surgery via a cholecystectomy may be necessary to remove the gallbladder.

Anti-inflammatory drugs

Anti-inflammatory drugs include steroids and non-steroidal medications. Steroids like prednisone work by irreversibly binding glucocorticoid receptors. This can lead to immune suppression and a reduction in inflammation. They are often used to treat inflammatory bowel diseases, such as Crohn's disease, and autoimmune hepatitis. Chronic use, however, can lead to bone loss, constipation, pancreatic edema, nausea and reduced wound healing. Non-steroidal medications, such as aspirin, naproxen, and ibuprofen, also have anti-inflammatory effects. They work by non-selectively inhibiting the enzyme cyclooxygenase. They can be used to treat such conditions as inflammatory bowel disease, though caution should be exercised as they can increase the propensity for gastrointestinal bleeding. Aspirin is the only non-steroidal medication to inhibit platelet aggregation irreversibly and can be used to treat vascular disorders, such as mesenteric arterial thromboses.

Immunosuppressive drugs

Immunosuppressive drugs are used to treat autoimmune conditions and to prevent rejection in patients who have had organ transplants. Patients who have undergone a liver transplant due to hepatic failure and patients who suffer from autoimmune gastrointestinal diseases, such as Crohn's disease and ulcerative colitis, may use these medications. Immunosuppressive medications can be categorized as glucocorticoids, cytostatics, antibodies, or drugs acting on immunophilins. Glucocorticoids act by suppressing cell-mediated and humoral immunity. Cytostatics act by inhibiting cell division and replication. Antibodies work by binding to antigens and preventing recognition of a foreign material by the body. Drugs that act on immunophilins inhibit calcineurin, leading to a decrease in transcription of interleukin-2, which normally stimulates T cells. Other drugs, such as interferon, opioids, tumor necrosis factor binding protein, and small biologic agents, can also be used for their immunosuppressive effects.

Antineoplastic drugs

Antineoplastic drugs are used to treat cancers and work by inhibiting cell division. Antineoplastic drugs work by targeting rapidly dividing cells, which can be neoplastic cells, but can also be cells of the gastrointestinal tract, hair follicles, and skin cells. Chemotherapeutic drugs can be classified as: alkylating agents, antimetabolites, anthracyclines, plant alkaloids, topoisomerase inhibitors, and other antitumor agents. They all work to impair cell division. Alkylating agents, such as cisplatin and carboplatin, work by forming covalent bonds with specific groups on sensitive molecules. Antimetabolites, such as azathioprine and mercaptopurine, can take the place of purine or pyrimidine molecules in the synthesis of DNA. Anthracyclines, such as doxorubicin, are antibiotics derived from streptomyces that intercalate between base pairs in DNA and RNA and can also block topoisomerase. Plant alkaloids, such as vincristine and vinblastine, bind to tubulin, inhibiting the synthesis of microtubules needed for cell division. Topoisomerase inhibitors, such as amsacrine, interfere with proper DNA supercoiling.

Antimicrobial drugs

An antimicrobial agent is a compound that kills or inhibits the growth of bacteria. Antibiotics are produced by nature. Antimicrobial agents can be classified as bacteriostatic, bacteriocidal, or bacteriolytic. Bacteriostatic antimicrobials can only halt the growth of bacteria. These include tetracycline, trimethoprim, and chloramphenicol. Bacteriocidal antimicrobials are able to kill bacteria and include daptomycin, fluoroquinolones, metronidazole, and nitrofurantoin. Bacteriolytic antimicrobials induce cell destruction by cellular lysis and include the beta lactam classes of antibiotics, such as penicillin derivatives and cephalosporins. Beta lactam antibiotics are recommended for pancreatitis, *Helicobacter pylori* infection, uncomplicated peritonitis, and uncomplicated intra-abdominal infections. Metronidazole, a nitroimidazole antibiotic, is used in cases of *Clostridium difficile* and *Giardia lamblia* infections. However, caution should be used in patients with diarrhea as most cases will resolve on their own, and antibiotics can worsen diarrhea.

Antiparasitic drugs

Antiparasitic drugs are used to treat parasites, including worms. Mebendazole and albendazole are antiparasitic medications used to treat common nematode infections. These medications work by binding to tubulin, preventing microtubule formation necessary for cell replication. Praziquantel is used to treat cestode and trematode infections. It works by increasing the cell membrane permeability of the worm, leading to a loss of calcium ions, paralysis, and death. Niclosamide is used to treat beef, fish, and dwarf tapeworms. It works by inhibiting oxidative phosphorylation in the mitochondria of the worms, leading to death. Primaquine is used to treat liver parasites, specifically *Plasmodium vivax* and *Plasmodium ovale*. Ivermectin is used to treat intestinal helminths. It works by opening a chloride channel, and the influx of chloride is toxic to the helminth. Nitazoxanide is used to treat intestinal protozoa, such as *Cryptosporidium* and *Giardia* species. It works by interfering with anaerobic metabolism for the protozoa.

Massage and biofeedback therapy

Biofeedback therapy involves monitoring vital signs or muscle activity while the patient is taught relaxation techniques. These techniques can be used to reduce stress and alter vital signs to reduce the symptoms of diseases. Four gastrointestinal conditions are difficult to treat with conventional medicine, and biofeedback can be helpful in controlling symptoms. These conditions are: irritable bowel syndrome, constipation and fecal incontinence in adults, and encopresis in children. Results from scientific studies are varied, but some do show a benefit in case-controlled studies using biofeedback, especially in adult fecal incontinence and encopresis in children. Massage therapy has been advocated to assist in gastrointestinal conditions like constipation and autoimmune diseases that worsen with stress. Massage can help to reduce abdominal pain and increase the number of bowel movements, but medications may still be necessary.

Psychological treatments

Functional gastrointestinal disorders are disorders that have no physical etiology. Psychotherapy can be beneficial in these cases as there is often a psychological component. Anxiety and depression can exacerbate many conditions, such as abdominal pain and irritable bowel syndrome. Anxiety disorders, mood disorders (e.g., depression), and somatoform disorders represent the most common psychiatric diagnoses associated with gastrointestinal symptoms. A history of abuse, especially sexual abuse, is also seen in patients with functional gastrointestinal disorders. Eating disorders, such as anorexia and bulimia, can lead to gastrointestinal symptoms, but psychological treatment is needed for resolution.

Medications and surgeries are often prescribed but can worsen the conditions or cause complications. A negative workup should direct the questioning to psychological aspects, which, if dealt with by a professional, may relieve the gastrointestinal symptoms.

Emotions

Stress and anxiety affect all people, and stress can be mental or physical. Stress and anxiety activate the body's flight or fight response, which has a variety of physical effects. The motility of the gut speeds up considerably in order to release any passage of bowels or vomiting, which might hamper the flight or fight response. Common gastrointestinal symptoms due to stress are heartburn, indigestion, nausea, vomiting, diarrhea, constipation, and associated lower abdominal pain. Stress is known to exacerbate inflammatory bowel diseases, such as ulcerative colitis and Crohn's disease. Irritable bowel syndrome is less well understood, but it exhibits increased stress responsiveness in the gut with increased colonic motility. Some diseases, such as dyspepsia and irritable bowel syndrome, are known as functional gastrointestinal disorders because emotions and stress play a primary role.

Behaviors

The behaviors that a patient exhibits, including the food and other substances ingested, can have both immediate and long-term effects on the gastrointestinal system. Diets high in fat and red meat and low in fiber can lead to constipation in the short term. In the long term, the same diet can increase the risk for colon cancer and can increase the predisposition to develop diverticulosis and as a consequence, diverticulitis and peritonitis. Smoking can cause vasoconstriction, which in the short term has a negative effect on digestion and, in the long term, can lead to vascular problems, such as mesenteric thrombosis and an increased risk for pancreatic and hepatic cancers. Chronic alcohol consumption in the short term can lead to alcohol poisoning, whereby the liver cannot detoxify the alcohol at a sufficient rate. In the long term, it can lead to cirrhosis, liver failure, and liver cancer.

Family and society

The views of one's family and society can influence behaviors, which can have an impact on gastrointestinal disease. Having family members or close friends who smoke make it more likely that a person will also smoke. Smoking increases the likelihood that a person will develop vascular disease, which can impact nutrition absorption and bowel perfusion. Smoking also increases the risk of developing pancreatic and hepatic cancers as well as colon cancer in women. Smokers are more likely to suffer from peptic ulcer disease and gastroesophageal reflux as smoking weakens the sphincter between the stomach and the esophagus. Smoking can interfere with the liver's ability to detoxify ingested substances and can enhance the toxic effects of alcohol. Alcohol consumption is influenced by one's family, and society and can have negative impacts on disease occurrences. Chronic alcohol consumption can lead to cirrhosis, which increases the risk of developing hepatic cancer and hepatic failure.

Occupational factors

Occupational factors can influence the gastrointestinal system in a negative fashion, can be detrimental to worker productivity, and can contribute to sick leave. Shift workers and those in high-stress jobs suffer a disproportionate number of gastrointestinal symptoms. These symptoms can include gastroesophageal reflux, diarrhea, constipation, and peptic ulcer disease. Shift workers must work during the nighttime hours, and this disrupts their circadian rhythm. The body can interpret this disruption as a stress and respond with a flight or fight response, involving the release of cortisol. Additionally, to remain awake during hours when the body naturally wants to sleep, the patient may eat high-sugar and high-fat foods in larger amounts than usual in an effort to remain awake. These foods contribute to gastrointestinal symptoms. Workers at high risk should be carefully monitored, as many peptic ulcers are asymptomatic. Medications to control symptoms should also be prescribed and recommended for high-risk workers.

Environmental factors

The environment in which one is raised can influence the gastrointestinal system and the prevalence of certain diseases. For reasons that are poorly understood, industrialized nations have a much higher percentage of people who suffer from gastroesophageal reflux, peptic ulcer disease, Crohn's disease, diverticulosis, and fatty liver disease or steatohepatitis. It is postulated that the dietary changes that coincide with industrialization may contribute to these diseases. As societies move farther away from agriculture, the diet becomes more focused on low-fiber, high-fat foods (e.g., red meat) and away from fruits and vegetables. In addition, more time for leisure and more disposable income lead to higher rates of smoking and alcohol consumption, which, in turn, lead to constipation, diverticulosis, fatty deposits, cirrhosis of the liver, and gastroesophageal reflux.

Gender

Gender can influence the occurrence, treatment, and prevention of gastrointestinal diseases. Women are more likely to suffer from autoimmune diseases, such as Raynaud's disease, which can have gastrointestinal complications, such as gastroesophageal reflux and achalasia. Twice as many women as men suffer from irritable bowel syndrome; this may be compounded by different perceptions of pain in women. Women are also more likely to suffer from constipation and bloating. Dyspepsia is also more common in women, in addition to cholelithiasis and primary biliary cirrhosis. Women may also have different responses to medical treatment, such as their decreased response to triple therapy, which is thought to be due to a higher bacterial load in women. Men have a higher rate of colonic polyps and colon cancer. Women are more likely than men to participate in screening for gastrointestinal diseases, which may lower the incidence and raise the survival rate in women, especially for colon polyps and colon cancer.

Ethnic and cultural factors

Ethnic and cultural factors influence the occurrence, treatment, and prevention of gastrointestinal diseases. Dietary habits differ among ethnic and cultural groups, which lead to greater risks for gastrointestinal disorders. Diets high in fat and red meat and those low in fiber may predispose to higher rates of colon cancer, diverticulosis, and gastroesophageal reflux. The acceptance and promotion of smoking and alcohol consumption in certain ethnic and cultural groups may also raise the risks for certain gastrointestinal disorders. Smoking is linked to vascular disorders, including mesenteric ischemia and thromboses. Chronic alcohol consumption leads to cirrhosis of the liver and increases the risk for liver carcinoma. When treating patients from different ethnic or cultural groups, there may be language barriers that interfere with the understanding of instructions and medication use. These must be addressed so that treatment or preventive measures can be followed correctly.

Societal perceptions of the gastrointestinal system have changed

Over the last century, societal perceptions and scientific knowledge has changed and advanced, leading to a shift in disease treatment and prevention. Peptic ulcer disease and gastroesophageal reflux have been chronic problems over the last century, but our understanding of them has advanced significantly. For much of the last century, the etiology of these diseases was unknown, and therefore, no successful treatment could be developed. Physicians used to recommend drinking milk to coat the stomach, not knowing that milk actually increases acid production. With the landmark research that identified the *Helicobacter pylori* bacteria underlying many cases of peptic ulcer disease, treatment was revolutionized. Currently, there is successful triple therapy that incorporates antibiotics to treat the bacteria along with newer medications (e.g., proton pump inhibitors, H_2-blockers) designed to lower acid production in the stomach.

Renal/Urinary System

Urinary system

The urinary system is responsible for fluid and electrolyte homeostasis, and its development involves the formation and regression of several intermediate organs, which may have once played a critical role in human life. The intermediate mesoderm gives rise to three structures: the pronephros, mesonephros, and metanephros. The pronephros, also known as the "first kidney," forms from epithelial buds that originate from the intermediate mesoderm adjacent to the mesonephric duct. This structure regresses by day 24 or 25 of fetal development. The mesonephric duct, which forms from an invagination and epithelialization of intermediate mesoderm on either side of the vertebral column, gives rise to the mesonephric tubules. Approximately forty tubules are produced, but only twenty remain at the end of the fifth week of growth. At this point, differentiation occurs into units that resemble nephrons, with a Bowman's capsule and a glomerulus. The renal corpuscles are formed between 6 and 10 weeks and begin producing urine. At 10 weeks, they regress and cease to function.

Development of the metanephros (the adult kidney) begins with the ureteric buds in the sacral region, which originate from the mesonephric ducts around day 28. Each bud differentiates into multiple lobes, which eventually form two functional components. The collecting portion comes from the ureteric bud and ultimately turns into the ureter, renal pelvis, major and minor calyces, and collecting ducts. The excretory portion is the metanephric blastema, a part of the sacral intermediate mesoderm. This eventually develops into the glomerulus, proximal convoluted tubule, loop of Henle, and distal convoluted tubule.

Kidney

The kidney consists of a cortex, medulla, papillae, calices, and a renal pelvis. The outer part is called the cortex. The inner portion of the kidney is known as the medulla, which contains multiple papillae. Each papilla drains into a calyx, and the calyces drain into the renal pelvis, like spokes on a wheel. The renal pelvis empties into a ureter, which carries urine to the bladder. The hilum of the kidney is found at the medial aspect and is where the renal artery, vein, and pelvis enter and exit the kidney. The *renal artery* is posterior to the *renal vein*, which is anterior to the *renal pelvis*. (A useful pneumonic is VAP, anterior to posterior.) The left renal vein crosses over the aorta to join the inferior vena cava, whereas the right renal vein is much shorter and has a direct course.

Ureters

The ureters are tubular structures that originate from each renal pelvis and run inferiorly to the urinary bladder. They carry urine from the kidneys to the bladder. Their entire course is located in the retroperitoneum with an average length of 25–30 cm. Upon entering the pelvis, the ureters run from lateral to medial while crossing over anteriorly to the bifurcation of the common iliac arteries. Each ureter runs alongside the gonadal vessels (i.e., ovarian in females, testicular in males). The blood supply to the ureters is segmental; that is, gonadal arteries proximally and internal iliac, superior, and inferior vesical arteries distally. Generally speaking, the blood supply to the ureter is medial above the pelvic brim and lateral once it travels below.

Glomerular filtration barrier

The components that make up the glomerular filtration barrier include: epithelium made up of podocytes (foot processes), a basement membrane composed of heparan sulfate, and the endothelium of the capillary, which contains fenestrations. The basement membrane contains a negative charge due to the heparan sulfate molecules. Glomerular filtration rate can be estimated by measuring the creatinine clearance.

Nephron

The nephron is the primary unit of the kidney. There are over 1 million nephrons in each kidney. The nephron is a long tubule the end of which is Bowman's capsule, which encapsulates a tuft of capillaries called the glomerulus. The glomerulus and Bowman's capsule are known collectively as the renal corpuscle, which does the primary job of filtering blood and producing urine. The parts of the nephron that are located in the cortex are the glomeruli, the proximal convoluted tubule, the distal convoluted tubule, and the proximal portion of the collecting duct. The outer portion of the medulla contains the thick ascending loop of Henle, whereas the inner portion is made up of the thin ascending limb and the papillary collecting duct.

Glomerulus and juxtaglomerular apparatus

The nephron, the primary unit of the kidney, is composed of a glomerulus interspersed with a series of tubules. The glomerulus is a tuft of capillaries sandwiched between an afferent arteriole and efferent arteriole. Endothelial cells line the tubules that make up a significant portion of the nephron. The juxtaglomerular apparatus is composed of juxtaglomerular cells and the macula densa; the juxtaglomerular cells are smooth muscle cells that make up part of the afferent arteriole and secrete renin in response to changes in blood pressure, increased sympathetic tone, and decreased sodium concentration. These cells are also the main source of erythropoietin. The macula densa is a component of the distal convoluted tubule that responds to changes in sodium concentration, which, in turn, decreases the glomerular filtration rate.

Proximal convoluted tubule

The proximal convoluted tubule is vital to the function of the nephron, removing water, salt, sugar, and other nutrients from urine and performing approximately 60% of the reabsorption of filtrate. The filtrate composition and the percentage of total reabsorption in the nephron are listed below:
- Sodium (65%): The sodium ion is the only ion that is reabsorbed through active transport in the proximal convoluted tubule.
- Potassium (65%): Reabsorption occurs through simple diffusion in the proximal convoluted tubule.
- Calcium (65%): Most of the calcium is absorbed in the proximal convoluted tubule and the ascending loop of Henle.
- Bicarbonate (90%): There is no maximum limit to its reabsorption.
- Water (80%): Reabsorption occurs transcellularly and paracellularly via passive transport.
- Phosphate (80%): Reabsorption occurs via a sodium–phosphate cotransporter.
- Glucose and amino acids (100%): Reabsorption is dependent on passive sodium reabsorption.

The proximal convoluted tubule can be divided into early and late segments. The early portion can adjust its ability to reabsorb filtrate as a response to changes in glomerular filtration rate. The late segment is where secretion of drugs and toxins, which cannot cross the membrane, occurs. The last major function of the proximal convoluted tubule is the formation of ammonia from glutamine. This serves as the primary mechanism to acidify the urine.

Loop of Henle

The loop of Henle is made up of three distinct components serving slightly different functions. When taken as a whole, the loop of Henle reabsorbs 25%–30% of the filtered sodium, creating an interstitial gradient that is ultimately responsible for the concentration of urine. The loop of Henle is made up of the:

- Thin descending limb: Minimal active transport takes place here. There is very high water permeability. The nephrons in the renal cortex have short, thin, descending limbs, whereas those in the medulla have long ones.
- Thin ascending limb: There is no active transport, and it is impermeable to water. It is highly permeable to sodium and urea, which are passively reabsorbed down the osmotic gradient.

Thick ascending limb: It is completely impermeable to water. There are medullary and cortical portions. This is where the sodium is reabsorbed via secondary active transport down the gradient created by Na^+-K^+ ATPase pumps. The specific transporter responsible is the $Na^+/K^+/2Cl^-$ co-transporter. The process of sodium reabsorption in this segment is critical to creating the interstitial gradient that drives urine concentration.

Distal tubule

The primary function of the distal tubule is sodium and calcium reabsorption. It is composed of the distal convoluted tubule and the connecting tubule. The major functions include:

- Sodium reabsorption: The distal convoluted tubule reabsorbs most of the remainder of filtered sodium (5%–10%). This occurs via a Na^+/Ca^+ co-transporter. The reabsorption of sodium in the distal convoluted tubule can be upregulated in response to more tubular sodium. The connecting tubule also reabsorbs sodium, but does so mainly in the presence of aldosterone.
- Calcium reabsorption: The distal convoluted tubule is responsible for a small, but important portion of calcium reabsorption (10%–15%). This occurs passively via a gradient created by low, free, intracellular calcium. Calcium in the cell is bound by binding proteins called calbindin, a process that is somewhat regulated by parathyroid hormone and vitamin D.
- Magnesium reabsorption: This occurs via active transport and is responsible for approximately 5%–10% of intraluminal magnesium reabsorption.

Collecting tubules

The collecting tubules are composed of a cortical component and a medullary component. The cortical collecting tubules have two functional units: principal cells and intercalated cells. Principal cells are mainly responsible for the reabsorption of water via aquaporins. Aquaporins are channels that are low at baseline but can be upregulated in response to antidiuretic hormone (ADH). The process of inserting preformed aquaporins into the luminal membrane under the influence of ADH is what creates highly concentrated urine. The principal cells can also reabsorb sodium, potassium, and chloride via passive transport and specialized luminal channels.

Intercalated cells

Intercalated cells have two different functions: hydrogen ion (H^+) secretion and bicarbonate (HCO_3^-) secretion. The main process that occurs in these cells is dictated by the enzyme carbonic anhydrase, which combines water with carbon dioxide to create H^+ and HCO_3^-. In type A intercalated cells, H^+ is secreted into the collecting tubule under acidemic conditions. Bicarbonate is sent into the systemic circulation via HCO_3^-/Cl^- transporters, thereby increasing extracellular pH. Type B intercalated cells respond to alkalemia and serve the exact opposite function, secreting H^+ into the bloodstream and HCO_3^- into the collecting tubule.

Countercurrent multiplication in the nephron

The human kidney can concentrate urine up to a level of 1200 mOsm/kg, which may be necessary in cases of severe body volume depletion. In contrast, in states of fluid overload, the urine can become quite dilute, with an osmolarity as low as 50 mOsm/kg. The process of urinary concentration is completely dependent on the kidney's ability to create an interstitial osmotic gradient. This occurs through a complex mechanism called countercurrent multiplication, which is poorly understood. The main step occurs in the ascending loop of Henle through the reabsorption of sodium and water impermeability, creating a relatively hyperosmolar medullary environment. The efficiency of this process is highest in nephrons with long, thick, ascending loops of Henle. At the same time, urea is absorbed via the collecting duct, further contributing to the concentration of the interstitium. Maintaining the interstitial hyperosmolarity is paramount to achieving maximal urinary concentration and occurs through two important mechanisms: the reabsorption of water in the collecting duct via antidiuretic hormone–sensitive aquaporins and the hairpin turn in the vasa recta, minimizing solute loss from the interstitium.

Metabolic acidosis

Metabolic acidosis is a physiologic state characterized by low arterial pH and reduced serum bicarbonate (HCO_3^-) concentration. It primarily results from the following pathologic processes: increased production of acid, HCO_3^- loss, and decreased renal acid excretion. The most common processes responsible for the creation of acid are lactic acidosis, ketoacidosis, and any acid state that results from the ingestion of a variety of agents (e.g., methanol, ethylene glycol, salicylates, chronic acetaminophen intake). Bicarbonate loss can result from proximal renal tubular acidosis, after an ileal conduit (replacement bladder created by the small intestine), and most commonly from diarrheal illness. The average diet has 50–100 mEq of acid a day that the kidney has to process. If the glomerular filtration rate is decreased, then there is decreased excretion of acid. Distal renal tubular acidosis is another condition that causes decreased renal acid excretion.

Metabolic alkalosis

Metabolic alkalosis is a physiologic state characterized by high arterial pH and excessive loss of hydrogen in the urine or intestinal tract. It can also occur as a result of increased serum bicarbonate (HCO_3^-), secondary to either increased alkali intake or stable serum HCO_3^- in the setting of low intravascular volume (contraction alkalosis). Hydrogen is lost from the intestinal tract most commonly from vomiting or from removal of gastric acid through nasogastric suction. Acid can be lost in the urine as a result of hyperaldosteronism or loop diuretics. Another mechanism for

- 299 -

metabolic alkalosis is through an intracellular shift of hydrogen ions from the intravascular compartment to the intracellular compartment, most often in the setting of hypokalemia. Contraction alkalosis results from loss of HCO_3^--free fluid, during vomiting, for example, with resultant volume depletion that causes a relative increase in plasma HCO_3^-.

High anion-gap metabolic acidosis

Increased serum anion gap occurs as a result of the accumulation of a strong acid along with a fall in bicarbonate (HCO_3^-), with no change in serum chloride. The causes of anion-gap (normal anion gap = 3–10 mEq/L) metabolic acidosis can be remembered through a simple mnemonic: MUDPILES
- **M**ethanol
- **U**remia
- **D**iabetic ketoacidosis
- **P**ropylene glycol
- **I**soniazid
- **L**actic acidosis
- **E**thylene glycol
- **S**alicylate poisoning

However, more recently the mnemonic GOLDMARK has been created to fit with more modern causes of anion-gap metabolic acidosis.
- **G**lycols (ethylene glycol, propylene glycol)
- **O**xoproline
- **L**-lactate
- **D**-lactate
- **M**ethanol
- **A**spirin
- **R**enal failure
- **K**etoacidosis

Renin–angiotensin–aldosterone system

The kidney secretes renin from the juxtaglomerular apparatus (JGA), located in the afferent arteriole, when a drop in blood pressure is detected. Specific stimuli for renin release include stretch receptors in the afferent arteriole, sympathetic activity in the JGA, and fluid composition reaching the macula densa. The macula densa is a group of specialized cells lining the distal convoluted tubule, which sense changes in the plasma sodium concentration. Renin converts angiotensinogen to angiotensin I in the liver. Angiotensin I is converted to angiotensin II by angiotensin-converting enzyme in the lung capillaries. Angiotensin II has many actions. It is a potent vasoconstrictor, causes aldosterone to be released from the adrenal cortex, causes antidiuretic hormone to be released from the posterior pituitary, and stimulates the hypothalamus to produce thirst. The goal of the angiotensin system is to increase intravascular volume, thereby increasing blood pressure. Aldosterone, which has been released from the adrenal cortex, works to decrease sodium and water excretion, further increasing extracellular volume.

Vasopressin/antidiuretic hormone (ADH)

Vasopressin, otherwise known as antidiuretic hormone (ADH), originates in the hypothalamus (supraoptic and paraventricular nuclei) and is secreted into the portal capillaries in the median eminence. Its primary role in the kidney is to increase the permeability of the collecting duct, which promotes water reabsorption. This occurs via V2 receptors in the kidney. The V2 receptor upregulates a protein kinase that, through a series of events, leads to the production of more water channels called aquaporins. The aquaporins are stored in the cytoplasm, move to the cell surface, and combine with the cell membrane when stimulated by ADH. Aquaporins allow the movement of water into cells along the gradient, thereby not requiring any adenosine triphosphate for this process to take place.

Micturition

The process of micturition (urination) is complex, involving the coordination of several neuronal pathways, and is incompletely understood. However, the role of the bladder can be broken down into two phases: filling and emptying. During the filling phase, peristalsis of the ureters 1–5 times/minute, helps move urine from the kidneys to the bladder. Since the ureters enter the bladder at an oblique angle, urine is prevented from refluxing during peristaltic waves. The emptying phase is the active stage of micturition. The detrusor muscle, a circular smooth muscle that makes up a major part of the bladder wall, contracts during urination. Fibers from the detrusor muscle encircle the first portion of the urethra, creating an "internal urethral sphincter." The urethra has a membranous portion as well, with an external urethral sphincter, composed of skeletal muscle. The detrusor muscle is controlled by the autonomic nervous system, making it involuntary, whereas the skeletal muscle of the membranous urethra is innervated by the somatic nervous system and is under voluntary control. During micturition the detrusor muscle contracts and the pelvic floor muscles relax to eject urine from the bladder and urethra.

Aldosterone

Aldosterone is secreted from the adrenal cortex (zona glomerulosa):
- When triggered by angiotensin II and low blood volume.
- In response to an increase in plasma potassium (K+).

Aldosterone acts on the distal convoluted tubule of the kidney and regulates the reabsorption of sodium (Na+) in exchange for K+ and hydrogen (H+) in the intercalated cells of the collecting tubule. Its effect is to increase Na+ reabsorption, as well as chloride reabsorption, and to increase the secretion of K+ and H+. It also acts on the principal cells to increase the number of Na+/K+ adenosine triphosphate pumps to allow for increased Na+ reabsorption.

Other various hormonal effects on fluid homeostasis

Renin is released from the juxtaglomerular apparatus (JGA) in response to low blood pressure and blood volume. It converts angiotensinogen to angiotensin I, which is then converted to angiotensin II by angiotensin-converting enzyme (ACE) in the lungs. Angiotensin II acts at the efferent arteriole of the JGA to cause vasoconstriction, which increases the glomerular filtration rate (GFR), and thus increases sodium (Na+) and bicarbonate reabsorption. Atrial natriuretic factor (ANF) is secreted from cardiac muscle cells and exhibits its effect on the JGA, when increased atrial pressure is detected. Atrial natriuretic factor increases GFR and Na+ excretion. It has the opposite effect of aldosterone on fluid balance. Antidiuretic hormone or vasopressin is secreted from the posterior pituitary; as a response to a decrease in blood volume and an increase in plasma osmolarity, it increases water reabsorption in principal cells.

Erythropoietin

Erythropoietin is primarily produced in the kidney, with some production occurring in the liver as well. Erythropoietin aids the progenitors of red blood cells in their growth and differentiation. The kidney senses oxygen tension, and when low levels are detected, indicating hypoxia, the kidney stimulates increased synthesis of erythropoietin, thereby increasing red blood cell mass and oxygen-carrying capacity to counteract the hypoxia. Normal production of erythropoietin depends on adequate renal function. In chronic kidney disease, patients become anemic in part because of a decrease in functioning renal mass. Patients with anemia due to chronic kidney disease are treated with exogenous erythropoietin or red blood cell transfusion. In untreated patients with chronic kidney disease or end-stage renal disease, the anemia can lead to worsening neurologic and cardiac function.

Vitamin D

Vitamin D is a fat-soluble vitamin. It is produced by the skin or ingested through one's diet. These versions of vitamin D are inactive and require conversion to their active form, 25-hydroxylase [25-(OH)] vitamin D, by the liver. After passing through the liver, 25-OH vitamin D enters the circulation, carried by vitamin D–binding protein, and exits into the kidney's proximal tubule. Once in the proximal tubule, it is converted into its most active form, $1,25\text{-}(OH)_2$ vitamin D. This conversion is regulated by the parathyroid hormone and serum levels of calcium and phosphate. Its most important function is to increase intestinal uptake of calcium. Its other functions include intestinal phosphate absorption, bone resorption through its effects on osteoclasts, and feedback inhibition of parathyroid hormone.

Prostaglandins

Prostaglandins are made from cell membrane phospholipids through the action of several enzymes (e.g., phospholipase, cyclooxygenase, lipoxygenase). At baseline, prostaglandins have no function in regulating renal perfusion. However, in hypotensive physiologic states accompanied by renal hypoperfusion, their primary function in the kidney is vasodilation. They counteract the vasoconstriction initiated by angiotensin II, norepinephrine, and vasopressin. Prostaglandins protect the kidney against ischemia. Secondary functions of prostaglandins include increasing the release of renin, stimulating water excretion, and increasing sodium excretion. Nonsteroidal anti-inflammatory drugs (NSAIDs) block cyclooxygenase, an important step in the production of prostaglandins. As a result, NSAIDs can contribute to acute kidney injury through renal ischemia or extended periods of uncontrolled vasoconstriction.

Electrolyte management

Parathyroid hormone is secreted from the chief cells of the parathyroid, in response to low plasma calcium concentration. It acts on the kidney to cause increased calcium reabsorption from the distal convoluted tubule, as well as decreased phosphate reabsorption at the level of the proximal convoluted tubule. It increases 1,25-vitamin D (cholecalciferol) production via stimulation of 1-alpha hydroxylase, which eventually works to increase calcium reabsorption from the intestines via a protein called calbindin.

Changes that occur to renal function with advanced age

Aging affects many organs, but as patients get older, the kidney happens to be one of the most sensitive. With increasing age, there is a progressive decline in the number of nephrons, along with scarring of the glomerulus and interstitium. Age-related changes to the kidney begin to take place in the fourth decade of life and accelerate after the age of 65. Glomerular filtration begins decreasing after 40 years of age, affecting men disproportionately. A lower renal blood flow is also a hallmark of aging as a result of increasing renal vascular resistance. Protein losses in the urine, in the form of microalbumin and albumin, are yet another manifestation. The presence of microalbuminuria is a risk factor for cardiovascular disease and associated mortality. Additionally, there is impaired fluid and electrolyte homeostasis, with dysregulation of sodium and water balance.

Pyelonephritis

Pyelonephritis is a urinary tract infection specifically affecting the kidney. It is much less common than cystitis, which is an infection of the bladder. Pyelonephritis most often begins as a urinary tract infection, which spreads to the bladder and eventually travels via the ureter to the kidney. However, pyelonephritis can also start in the kidneys, though rarely, after seeding from the bloodstream or lymphatics. Pyelonephritis presents with all the symptoms associated with cystitis (e.g., dysuria, frequency, hematuria), but additionally, flank pain, chills, costovertebral angle tenderness, and fevers. In severe cases, patients may arrive at the hospital in septic shock and renal failure. Treatment involves oral antibiotics for clinically well individuals but also intravenous antibiotics for patients with more severe disease. Antibiotics should only be initiated after urinalysis and urine culture are sent for sensitivity testing.

Renal and perinephric abscesses

Renal and perinephric abscesses are relatively uncommon infectious complications of an upper urinary tract infection. A patient who develops this condition is at high risk of morbidity and mortality. Renal abscesses are contained within the renal capsule and renal parenchyma, whereas perinephric abscesses are adjacent to the kidney in Gerota's fascia (i.e., the layer that encapsulates the kidney) and associated retroperitoneal fat. Infections usually start as a urinary tract infection that eventually spreads retrograde to the kidneys, causing pyelonephritis. However, the renal and perinephric spaces can also be seeded hematogenously in patients with certain comorbidities, such as diabetes, nephrolithiasis, and urolithiasis. Computed tomography scan is the best imaging test to diagnose a renal or perinephric abscess. Early antibiotic therapy and percutaneous drainage are the primary means of treatment. Purulent fluid from the abscess cavity should be sent for culture to identify organisms and to help guide decisions about antibiotic therapy.

Urinary tract infection

A urinary tract infection can either present as cystitis (i.e., an infection of the bladder) or as pyelonephritis (i.e., an infection of the kidney). The primary organism responsible for these infections is *Escherichia coli* in up to 90% of patients. Other possible microbes include: *Enterobacter, Proteus mirabilis, Klebsiella* pneumonia, and rarely other gram-negative/gram-positive species. There are many choices for antibiotic therapy, but the best options include nitrofurantoin, trimethoprim-sulfamethoxazole, or fosfomycin. Some clinicians advocate the use of fluoroquinolones; however, increased antimicrobial resistance has become an issue.

Nephrotic syndrome

Nephritic syndrome is a disorder of the glomerulus associated with hematuria, proteinuria (much less than is seen with nephrotic syndrome), and dependent edema. Other signs and symptoms include oliguria, azotemia, hypertension, and red cell casts. It is caused by an inflammatory disorder affecting either the renal system primarily or in conjunction with a systemic disease process. Etiologies include the following:
- Postinfectious (streptococcal) glomerulonephritis
- Membranoproliferative glomerulonephritis
- Lupus
- Hepatitis C
- Cryoglobulinemia
- Vasculitides, including polyarteritis nodosa, Wegener's, Henoch–Schönlein purpura, Goodpasture's syndrome, thrombotic thrombocytopenic purpura, hemolytic uremic syndrome [i.e., infectious endocarditis, IgA nephropathy (Berger's disease), hereditary nephritis (Alport's syndrome)]

In this disease process the negative charge barrier of the glomerular basement membrane is affected. Nephrotic syndrome is manifested by proteinuria in the severe range (> 3.5–4 grams protein/day), generalized edema (peripheral and periorbital), low albumin levels, and hyperlipidemia. Urine may appear foamy. Etiologies include the following:
- Diabetic nephropathy
- Minimal change disease
- Focal segmental glomerulonephritis
- Membranous glomerulonephritis
- Amyloid deposition
- Lupus

Treatment is affected by the etiology, which can require a renal biopsy to make a definitive diagnosis. Standard treatment involves dietary restriction (i.e., limiting protein and salt intake) and diuretics. In severe disease, the use of steroids may be required. Complications may include hypercoagulability, thrombosis, and infection.

Membranous nephropathy

Membranous nephropathy is a common cause of nephrotic syndrome in patients without diabetes. Membranous nephropathy appears as nonfocal glomerular basement membrane thickening under the microscope. While it can be associated with hepatitis B, lupus, various malignancies, and the use of nonsteroidal anti-inflammatory drugs, most cases are idiopathic. Signs may be as subtle as elevated serum creatinine with asymptomatic proteinuria, but a definitive diagnosis can only be made by kidney biopsy. All patients should be screened for occult malignancy, antinuclear antibodies, and hepatitis B and C antibodies. More in-depth pathologic testing reveals diffuse granular immunoglobulin G and complement deposits. Electron microscopy shows subepithelial deposits, as well as mesangial and subendothelial deposits. Membranous nephropathy can also occur in association with other renal pathologies, including diabetic nephropathy, rapidly progressive glomerulonephritis, focal segmental glomerulosclerosis, and immunoglobulin A nephropathy.

Immunoglobulin A nephropathy

Immunoglobulin A (IgA) nephropathy is the most common type of primary glomerulonephritis and one of the major causes of end stage renal disease worldwide. Looking at renal tissue from patients with IgA nephropathy under the microscope reveals proliferation of mesangial cells in the glomerulus with deposition of IgA antibody complexes. The incidence of IgA nephropathy is higher in Asians, specifically the Japanese, with prevalence rates as high as 20%–40%. It affects men three times as often as women. Some patients present with transient or episodic macroscopic hematuria, which often occurs shortly after the resolution of an upper respiratory infection (1–2 days). It can also be associated with other infections, such as gastroenteritis or urinary tract infections. Along with hematuria, patients may have systemic symptoms, including fevers, weakness, muscle aches, and abdominal pain. Other patients have asymptomatic hematuria and proteinuria. Very rarely do patients have proteinuria without hematuria. There is no cure, and treatment focuses on supportive care and controlling disease progression to end stage renal disease.

Tubulointerstitial injury

Several mechanisms can explain how tubulointerstitial disease worsens renal function in the human kidney. One theory is that obstruction from inflammation and fibrosis blocks the flow of urine and increases the pressure of the renal tubule. The end result is a decreased glomerular filtration rate. Another thought is that capillaries adjacent to the renal tubule are damaged, resulting in a relatively ischemic state in the tubulointerstitial space. The increase in vascular resistance affects blood flow through the arterioles in the glomerulus. A third concept is that as a result of tubulointerstitial injury, the feedback loop in the glomerulus has gone awry. Edema and a worsening inflammatory condition develop in the interstitial space, which results in disruption in the autoregulation of renal blood flow. Tubulointerstitial nephritis can cause a disassociation between the glomerulus and renal tubule, which subsequently become atrophic and nonfunctioning.

Acute interstitial nephritis

Acute interstitial nephritis is a renal disease of sudden onset caused by renal tubule and interstitial inflammation and edema. It is one of many etiologies of acute renal failure and is mainly caused by drug hypersensitivity. Antibiotics are the major drug offenders, especially cephalosporins and penicillins. Nonsteroidal anti-inflammatory drugs and diuretics can also result in acute interstitial nephritis. The other causes of acute interstitial nephritis are infectious and autoimmune in nature. Bacteria, viruses, and other organisms may lead to acute interstitial nephritis. Bacterial infections include diphtheria, *Escherichia coli*, and species of *Legionella, Staphylococcus, Streptococcus, Campylobacter, Yersinia*, and *Brucella*. Viral causes include cytomegalovirus, HIV, herpes, Ebstein–Barr virus, polyomavirus, and hantavirus.

Chronic tubulointerstitial nephritis

Chronic tubulointerstitial nephritis is characterized by several pathologic features: atrophic cells in a dilated renal tubule, fibrosis of the interstitium, flattened epithelial cells, and infiltration of lymphocytes, macrophages, and B cells between tubules. The basement membrane is often thickened. The abnormal process eventually progresses to fibrosis and sclerosis of the glomerulus and tubule, with thickening of renal arterioles. There is no vasculitis. Patients present with renal insufficiency (elevated creatinine) and can also have other associated symptoms, such as nocturia, malaise, and weakness. Half of patients are hypertensive at diagnosis. Anemia is also a common finding in these patients. Chronic tubulointerstitial nephritis can be caused by drugs, metabolic disorders, autoimmune diseases, bacterial or viral infections, or hematologic disorders.

Hydronephrosis

Hydronephrosis is the abnormal dilation of the renal pelvis and renal calyces as a result of the obstruction of urinary flow. The obstruction can be caused by blockage from renal stones, a neoplasm (e.g., transitional cell carcinoma), compression from outside the system (from extrinsic tumors or fibrosis in the retroperitoneal cavity), or blood clots. Hydronephrosis can also be a congenital condition, as a result of an abnormal anatomy with strictured urethral valves or stenosis at the ureterovesical junction or ureteropelvic junctions. Hydronephrosis is often painless, unless a renal stone is present. Treatment is aimed at reversing the process that led to hydronephrosis and can include placement of tubes or stents to improve urinary outflow temporarily.

Renal cell carcinoma

Renal cell carcinoma is a malignancy that affects men (2:1 ratio) between the ages of 50–70 years. It is the most common cancer affecting the parenchyma of the kidney. Tobacco is a major risk factor. Other risk factors include adult polycystic disease, heavy metal (i.e., mercury, cadmium) exposure, and long-term dialysis. Presenting symptoms often include localized symptoms, such as flank pain, the presence of an abdominal mass, as well as systemic manifestations, including fever, hypertension, weight loss, polycythemia, and hematuria. Renal cell carcinoma can be associated with von Hippel–Lindau syndrome, an autosomal dominant condition, although most cases are sporadic.

Transitional cell carcinoma

Transitional cell carcinoma (also known as urothelial carcinoma) is the most frequently seen urinary tract malignancy and makes up the vast majority of bladder cancers in the United States. The incidence of transitional cell carcinoma is three times as high in men as in women and much more prevalent in older patients. Several chemicals and synthetic compounds have been implicated in the development of transitional cell carcinoma. A history of smoking cigarettes is the most common cause and is responsible for at least half of all newly diagnosed cases. Certain chemical carcinogens have also been linked to urothelial carcinoma, and these include paint components, polycyclic aromatic hydrocarbons, benzene, hair dyes, and diesel exhausts. High levels of arsenic in drinking water, chronic cystitis, and the chemotherapy agent, cyclophosphamide, have also been associated with a higher risk of urothelial bladder cancer. As with most disease processes and malignancies, genetic mutations and heredity also play a role in transitional cell carcinoma.

Wilms tumor

Wilms tumor is the most common cancer of the kidney in children and overall the fourth most common cancer in children. It is associated with several congenital syndromes, including Beckwith–Wiedemann syndrome and WAGR (i.e., Wilms tumor, aniridia, genitourinary anomalies, retardation). The pathologic error occurs during renal development with persistence of embryologic metanephric cells. Two genes that can mutate and give rise to Wilms tumor include WT1 gene on chromosome 11 and p53 gene on chromosome 17. While most cases are solitary in nature, approximately 5% of patients have bilateral lesions. Affected children most commonly are asymptomatic with an incidentally found abdominal mass, although other children can have abdominal pain, fever, hematuria, or hypertension. The differential diagnosis of Wilms tumor should include neuroblastoma, but usually these can be differentiated on computed tomography scan. Treatment is surgical resection, and further postoperative management depends on tumor stage.

Bladder cancer

The risk of developing bladder cancer increases as a patient gets older and is most pronounced after the age of 60. The vast majority of patients present with localized disease that has not yet invaded or metastasized. Most commonly, patients have hematuria that is gross, not microscopic, and painless. When pain is associated with bladder cancer, usually the tumor has invaded or metastasized. Diagnosis is usually made by evaluating urine cytology and by performing a transurethral biopsy. Staging is paramount. Depth of invasion can be determined by computed tomography or magnetic resonance imaging, specifically looking for tumor extension into the perivesical adipose tissue. Treatment is dependent on the depth of invasion and stage of disease. For superficial tumors, the treatment of choice is transurethral complete endoscopic resection. Patients with a high recurrence risk may receive intravesical bacillus Calmette-Guerin or mitomycin. For tumors that invade into the muscularis propria, the standard of care is radical cystectomy with a pelvic lymph node dissection.

Prostate cancer

Prostate cancer is the most common noncutaneous cancer diagnosed in men in the United States and the second most common cause of death in men. The main risk factor for prostate cancer is increasing age. Other risk factors include various environmental exposures, such as cadmium, race (e.g., Northern Europeans, Blacks), and family history. Some evidence suggests that dietary elements may be potential risk factors. Screening with prostate specific antigen (PSA) levels is controversial, and most urologists believe that a combination of PSA levels, risk factors, and exam findings should be taken into account when making a decision about performing a prostate biopsy. Localized disease can be observed in older men, whereas for high-risk individuals or younger men, the options include surgical prostatectomy, hormonal therapy, and radiation therapy.

Prerenal acute renal failure

Prerenal acute renal failure is caused by a decrease in glomerular blood flow due to a reduction in real or effective intravascular volume. Prerenal causes of acute renal failure can be detected in a history and physical examination in patients reporting symptoms related to volume depletion, such as recent diarrheal illness. Patients with congestive heart failure are at increased risk of prerenal acute renal failure due to a state of low renal blood flow. The major causes of prerenal acute renal failure are:
- Intravascular depletion, such as sepsis, hemorrhage, vomiting or diarrhea
- Decrease in the effective intravascular volume, such as with congestive heart failure, hepatorenal syndrome, and nephrotic syndrome
- Medications, such as angiotensin-converting enzyme inhibitors and nonsteroidal anti-inflammatory drugs

Management of prerenal acute renal failure involves the infusion of resuscitation fluid, either normal saline or lactated Ringer's solution. Patients with intravascular volume overload with congestive heart failure may benefit from a trial of diuretics. Inadequate or inappropriate response to diuretics may indicate the need for hemodialysis.

Acute renal failure

Acute renal failure is defined as an elevation in the serum creatinine level of more than 0.5 mg/dL over the patient's baseline level or as a drop in the glomerular filtration rate by half. Clinically, a hospitalized patient that is making less than 0.5 cc of urine x their weight in kilograms per hour is also considered to have oliguric acute renal failure. Nonoliguric renal failure is also possible but is more difficult to diagnose. The differential diagnosis when working up a patient with low urinary output or rising serum creatinine includes prerenal, intrinsic renal, and postrenal causes. When a hospitalized patient develops acute renal failure, their associated in-hospital mortality increases significantly. Patients may be asymptomatic if the acute renal failure is not severe, and the only manifestation may be a change in their serum chemistries, specifically their blood urea nitrogen and creatinine levels. However, other patients may present with signs and symptoms of worsening uremia, which include nausea, vomiting, altered mental status, anorexia, and an unusual metallic taste in their mouth.

Intrinsic renal causes

When a patient is diagnosed with acute renal failure, intrinsic renal causes are usually a diagnosis of exclusion after prerenal and postrenal causes have been ruled out. The causes of intrinsic acute renal failure are:

- Acute tubular necrosis caused by drugs and medications, intravenous contrast, myoglobin or hemoglobin, and ischemic conditions
- Glomerular diseases
- Vascular diseases, such as atheroembolic disease, thrombotic thrombocytopenic purpura, hemolytic-uremia syndrome, and HELLP syndrome (i.e., hemolysis, elevated liver enzymes, low platelet count)
- Interstitial diseases from drugs and medications, autoimmune diseases, or pyelonephritis

Intrinsic acute renal failure may be more likely in patients who have recently undergone an imaging study with intravenous contrast. Patients on medications with known nephrotoxicity are also more likely to have an intrinsic etiology. The diagnostic test of choice is a renal ultrasound, which can help define the size of the kidney, echogenicity, and adequacy of blood flow in the renal artery or vein. If the diagnosis is still unknown, a percutaneous or open kidney biopsy may be necessary.

Postrenal causes

Postrenal acute renal failure can be caused by several different etiologies, including: benign prostatic hypertrophy, an obstructing pelvic malignancy (i.e., gynecologic, rectal), or kidney stones. The other causes of postrenal acute renal failure are:

- Retroperitoneal pathology
- Obstructive processes at some level of the urinary tract (i.e., crystals, myeloma)
- Bladder cancer obstructing both ureteral orifices
- Dysfunctional bladder (neurogenic bladder)
- Strictures of the urethra due to instrumentation or another cause

A patient who has the acute onset of anuria after a period of normal urine output raises suspicion for postrenal acute renal failure. Damage to the kidney can occur if urinary obstruction is not relieved or bypassed. Renal ultrasound can be used to help make the diagnosis, but placement of a urinary catheter (especially in men) should be the first step in management.

Acute tubular necrosis

Acute tubular necrosis is a disease process in the kidney that results histologically in sloughing of the epithelial lining of the tubule with resulting occlusion due to casts and cellular debris. Many patients develop acute kidney injury in the hospital as a result of acute tubular necrosis. The major causes of acute tubular necrosis are:

- Renal ischemia: Patients with prerenal azotemia with episodes of hypotension or surgery are at risk for developing ischemic acute tubular necrosis.
- Sepsis/septic shock
- Nephrotoxic agents: Quite a few drugs are known to be toxic to the kidneys and result in acute tubular necrosis. The most common ones are aminoglycosides, cisplatin, hetastarch, and mannitol. Intravenous contrast dye is also known to produce renal injury in patients who are at risk.

The urinalysis in acute tubular necrosis classically demonstrates muddy brown casts and epithelial cells. Whereas prerenal azotemia responds quite well to fluid resuscitation within 24–48 hours, patients with acute tubular necrosis are relatively resistant and require more time to recover.

Chronic kidney disease

The diagnosis of chronic kidney disease is based on the presence of renal damage or dysfunction for a minimum of 3 months. This can be demonstrated through kidney biopsy or by an estimation of the glomerular filtration rate (GFR). Kidney damage is demonstrated through elevated levels of albuminuria, urinary sediment, or pathology showing glomerular, vascular, or tubulointerstitial disease. A GFR less than 60 mL/min is considered to be the threshold for the diagnosis of chronic kidney disease. Like acute renal failure, chronic kidney disease can result from a variety of causes, including diabetes, toxicity due to various drugs, autoimmune disease, or mechanical obstruction of the ureters or bladder.

Renal tubular acidosis (RTA)

There are three subsets of renal tubular acidosis (RTA): type 1 (distal), type 2 (proximal), and type 4 (hyperkalemia). These entities not only differ in their location in the nephron but also have diverse pathologic defects. Distal RTA occurs in the setting of impaired secretion of hydrogen ions (H+), either as a result of decreased proton pump activity or higher permeability of the luminal membrane to H+. The end result of this condition is a non-anion gap acidosis with low plasma bicarbonate concentrations (as low as 10 mEq/L). Hypokalemia is another manifestation of type 1 RTA.

Type 2 renal tubular acidosis (RTA) is characterized by a decrease in the ability of the proximal tubule to reabsorb bicarbonate. Hyperkalemic RTA occurs when there is a reduction in the reabsorption of sodium in the principal cells of the collecting duct. This eliminates the negative gradient across the tubular membrane, which significantly decreases the secretion of potassium. The result is hyperkalemia and metabolic acidosis.

Syndrome of inappropriate secretion of antidiuretic hormone

The syndrome of inappropriate secretion of antidiuretic hormone (SIADH) is caused by overproduction of antidiuretic hormone (ADH) that leads to excessive water retention and results in hyponatremia. Patients develop low serum osmolality with high urine osmolality and sodium concentration. Most often, patients present with asymptomatic hyponatremia. The SIADH may be caused by:
- Malignancies, such as small cell carcinoma, lymphoma, and sarcoma
- Tuberculosis
- Pneumonia
- Central nervous system disorders, such as meningitis, brain tumors, or head trauma
- Drugs, such as chemotherapy, antidepressants, antibiotics, and anti-epileptics

In addition to managing the underlying disorder, the SIADH is treated with free water restriction, increased salt intake, or vasopressin receptor antagonists. Limitations on water intake are first-line therapy. Patients are instructed to drink less than 1 L of water a day until serum sodium returns to the physiologic range. With severe symptoms, hypertonic solution may be infused to help normalize serum sodium.

Nephrogenic diabetes insipidus

Nephrogenic diabetes insipidus is a condition in which the kidney is unable to adequately concentrate urine, caused by resistance to the action of antidiuretic hormone (ADH). Production of ADH is unaffected. Nephrogenic diabetes insipidus may be inherited or acquired. There are a variety of inherited causes, but they most commonly include genetic mutations affecting ADH receptors. Acquired etiologies include drug toxicity from lithium, certain antiviral medications, and antibiotics. Hypercalcemia or hypokalemia may also lead to diabetes insipidus. Patients with acute or chronic renal failure can also develop this disorder. Patients develop increased urine output, especially at night, and increased thirst response. Urine osmolality is decreased, whereas serum osmolality and sodium are high; most patients present with hypernatremia. The diagnosis can be made with a water restriction test, which rules out primary polydipsia (pathologic excessive water intake that occurs in psychiatric conditions). Treatment involves correcting the underlying disorder or stopping the offending medication. If there is no response, a thiazide diuretic can be initiated, which will create a mildly volume-depleted state.

Nephrolithiasis

Nephrolithiasis (or kidney stones) occur as a result of an abnormal balance in the composition of salts and minerals in the urinary tract. There are four types:
- Calcium (radiopaque): These are the most common type of kidney stones, comprising up to 80% of stones. These can be either calcium phosphate or calcium oxalate and usually appear as radiopaque on radiologic imaging. Calcium stones occur due to a variety of different mechanisms, including milk-alkali syndrome and cancer.
- Struvite (radiopaque): These stones appear in the shape of a coffin (otherwise known as staghorn calculi) and are composed of magnesium ammonium phosphate. Alkaline urine (pH > 7) facilitates the formation of struvite stones. These tend to occur in patients with urinary tract infections with certain bacteria (i.e., *Klebsiella* or *Proteus* species), which produce urease, which alkalinizes the urine.

- Uric acid (radiolucent): Uric acid stones form in acidic urine and are more commonly found in patients with gout. These individuals produce high levels of uric acid and as a result have hyperuricemia.
- Cystine (radiolucent): These stones appear as crystals in the shape of a hexagon, which are identified in urine sediment.

Calcium oxalate or phosphate kidney stones

Calcium oxalate stones are the most common type of kidney stone and are responsible for 70%–80% of cases of nephrolithiasis. They occur in two main forms: monohydrate and dihydrate. The monohydrate crystals appear as dumbbell-shaped or needle-shaped, whereas the dihydrate crystals are envelope-shaped. The risk of calcium oxalate stone formation increases in patients with decreased urine output, high levels of calcium excretion, and low levels of citrate in the urine. The risk for calcium oxalate nephrolithiasis is independent of changes in urine pH. Calcium phosphate stones make up 15% of all cases of kidney stones. They can also occur in two main forms: apatite and hydrogen phosphate (brushite). Calcium apatite is the most common type of calcium phosphate stone. In addition to the risk factors for calcium oxalate stone formation, additional hazards for developing calcium phosphate stones include high urinary pH and elevated urine phosphate levels. Decreasing the urine pH lowers the chance of calcium phosphate nephrolithiasis.

Urate (uric acid) kidney stones

Uric acid stones are relatively rare, affecting only 8% of all cases of nephrolithiasis. They can also occur in combination with other types of stones, most often calcium oxalate crystals. These stones appear in a variety of different forms under the microscope, but most commonly take on a rhomboid or rosette appearance. Their color is characteristically yellow or red-brown. Sodium urate stones occur specifically in patients with gouty arthritis. There is an increased likelihood of uric acid stone formation in cases with decreased urine excretion, high levels of uric acid in the urine, and low urine pH. By alkalinizing the urine, the creation of uric acid stones should decrease significantly.

Struvite kidney stones

Struvite (also known as magnesium ammonium phosphate) stones form in the presence of specific bacteria in the urinary tract, specifically urease-producing bacteria. The most common example of urease-producing bacteria is *Proteus mirabilis*. Sediment analysis reveals "coffin-shaped" crystals. Struvite stones are rare, occurring in about 1% of cases of nephrolithiasis. Their production is higher in women because of their higher risk of urinary tract infections. The urease produced by bacteria cleaves urea into one carbon dioxide and two ammonia molecules, while producing a high urinary pH (between 8.5 and 9). These are usually very large stones that develop in the renal pelvis and are termed "staghorn" or branched calculi. Struvite stones very rarely pass spontaneously. Treatment, therefore, requires endoscopic or surgical intervention.

Renal artery stenosis

Renal artery stenosis mostly affects one kidney but can occur bilaterally, though rarely. Hypertension resulting from renal artery stenosis is exceedingly rare (less than 1% in patients with mild hypertension); it more commonly affects patients with refractory or acute cases of severe hypertension. There are two main causes of renal artery stenosis:

- Atherosclerotic disease usually affects older patients (> 45 years of age) and primarily at the proximal portion of the renal artery, where cholesterol deposits are more likely to build up.
- Fibromuscular dysplasia is much more common in young women (< 50 years of age) and impacts the renal artery more distally or even in the segmental branches of the renal artery.

The main treatment modality is medical therapy with antihypertensive agents. The best available agents are angiotensin-converting enzyme inhibitors and angiotensin II receptor blockers. These should only be used in unilateral disease and are contraindicated in bilateral renal artery stenosis. Certain select patients who are refractory to medical therapy may benefit from renal artery revascularization with angioplasty and stent placement.

Renal artery aneurysms

Renal artery aneurysms are most often found incidentally on imaging for other purposes with a less than 1% incidence in the general population. Based on their appearance and location, they can be categorized as saccular, fusiform, dissecting, or intrarenal. The most common type is saccular, making up over 75% of all renal artery aneurysms. Their location is variable, most often occurring extrarenally, but a small subset are within the parenchyma of the kidney. Fusiform aneurysms are the second most common and occur most often in young women. Histologically, renal artery aneurysms resemble fibromuscular dysplasia with weakness of the internal elastic lamina and increased collagen at the site. Complications, although rare, may include rupture, hypertension, thrombosis with renal infarction, embolization, and the spontaneous formation of an arteriovenous fistula. The larger the aneurysm, the more likely it is to rupture; generally, those greater than 4 cm have a statistically greater chance of rupture. Pregnant women are also at an increased risk of both developing an aneurysm and then subsequently developing a complication (i.e., rupture). In patients at high risk of rupture, treatment options include either open repair or more recently, endovascular stent or coil placement.

Renal vein thrombosis

Renal vein thrombosis can occur in patients after trauma or secondary to malignancy, but more recently it has been found in patients with nephrotic syndrome. Patients with nephrotic syndrome are believed to be hypercoagulable, putting them at higher risk of developing thrombosis. The hypercoagulability stems from both antithrombin deficiency and increased zymogen and fibrinogen levels but also platelet abnormalities. At the same time, it is believed that patients with nephrotic syndrome have a lower circulating plasma volume, increasing the risk of decreased flow through the renal vein. Acute cases of renal vein thrombosis present with an enlarged kidney and notching of the ureter on imaging. These patients have not had time to form collateral drainage from the kidney. Chronic cases are usually asymptomatic and found incidentally. Treatment is focused on anticoagulation with either heparin (initial therapy of choice) or warfarin (after 5–7 days of heparin).

Multiple myeloma

Multiple myeloma is a cancer of the blood, specifically the plasma cells. Approximately half of patients have evidence of renal disease at diagnosis, manifested by elevated serum creatinine. In some patients, renal failure is the presenting feature of the disease. The kidney can be affected at the level of the glomerulus, tubule, or interstitium. Glomerular disease can result from amyloidosis, deposition of monoclonal immunoglobulins (light chain or heavy chain), or cryoglobulinemia. Tubular disease can be due to "myeloma kidney" from light-chain cast nephropathy. Interstitial disease can be caused by infiltration by neoplastic plasma cells or by interstitial nephritis.

Myeloma cast nephropathy

Multiple myeloma can cause tubular disease of the kidneys, leading to acute or chronic renal failure, as a result of myeloma cast nephropathy. The pathogenesis is from monoclonal, light-chain immunoglobulins (i.e., Bence–Jones proteins) aggregating in the ascending loop of Henle and causing direct injury, obstruction to flow, and the formation of casts within the tubule when the proteins bind with another protein (i.e., Tamm–Horsfall mucoprotein) in the tubule. This process is exacerbated by dehydration, which causes a relative increase in the concentration of light chains. A negative urine dipstick for protein is falsely reassuring, because the urinary dipstick is meant for albumin protein detection, not light-chain detection. Instead, the serum should be checked for free light chains, which will be elevated, and serum protein electrophoresis will show a monoclonal gammopathy. A 24-hour urine protein electrophoresis will show monoclonal free light chains, also known as M-proteins.

Amyloidosis

Amyloidosis is a disease process that is characterized by immunoglobulin deposition in the extracellular space, eventually resulting in end-organ dysfunction. The immunoglobulins have a specific appearance under the microscope and appear apple-green birefringent when stained with Congo red. Renal involvement occurs in two types of amyloidosis: primary systemic amyloidosis and secondary amyloidosis (amyloid A). Patients with primary systemic amyloidosis present with proteinuria and nephrotic syndrome as a result of the deposition of amyloid fibrils in the glomerulus. They often develop fairly severe edema. Up to 20% of these patients develop end-stage renal disease. Secondary amyloidosis most often occurs in patients with chronic inflammation. Rheumatoid arthritis is the main etiology, but secondary amyloidosis can also be the result of ankylosing spondylitis, psoriatic arthritis, or inflammatory bowel diseases. In these conditions, hepatocytes produce significant amounts of amyloid A. The treatment of secondary amyloidosis revolves around management and control of the underlying chronic inflammatory condition.

Hyperkalemia

Hyperkalemia is a common clinical scenario, which can result from either a rise in potassium release from the intracellular compartment or a reduction in the excretion of potassium in the urine. Increased dietary intake of potassium is not sufficient enough to produce hyperkalemia in the absence of another cause. The causes that result from a rise in potassium release from the cells include the following: Pseudohyperkalemia is a spurious result that occurs most often secondary to mechanical trauma after venipuncture. Red blood cells are lysed and release potassium.

- Metabolic acidosis: In patients with acidemia, hydrogen ions move into cells in exchange for potassium moving out of cells.

- 313 -

- Insulin insufficiency: Insulin, in the normal physiologic state, promotes potassium movement into cells.
- Tissue catabolism: Breakdown of tissues leads to release of intracellular potassium.
- Nonselective beta-blockers: These drugs prevent the adrenergic-mediated uptake of intravascular potassium.

More commonly, hyperkalemia is a result of decreased excretion in the urine. The major causes include the following:
- Low levels of or resistance to aldosterone: This can be due to various drugs (i.e., potassium-sparing diuretics).
- Decrease in the delivery of sodium/water to the nephron: This is seen during states of low effective blood volume, congestive heart failure, and cirrhosis. Kidney disease (acute and chronic)

Sickle-cell disease

Sickle cell nephropathy results in a reduced ability to concentrate urine but a normal capacity to dilute urine. The inability to produce concentrated urine occurs as a result of a problem with the countercurrent exchange mechanism in the inner medulla. The vasa recta vessels in the juxtaglomerular apparatus are a common place for sickling to occur in patients with sickle cell disease. The relative hypoxia of the renal medulla and the elevated viscosity and decreased blood flow rate in the medulla are the major drivers.

Henoch–Schönlein purpura

Henoch–Schönlein purpura is one of the vasculitides that primarily affects small vessels (postcapillary venules). It appears microscopically very similar to immunoglobulin A (IgA) nephropathy with mesangial thickening and immune complex deposition. However, it exhibits several other features clinically that serve to differentiate it from IgA nephropathy. The additional signs and symptoms that are associated with Henoch–Schönlein purpura include the following:
- Purpuric rash distributed on the arms and legs
- Arthritis
- Intestinal complications
- Glomerulonephritis

Henoch–Schönlein purpura is most common in the first decade of life and rarely occurs in adults. It is a transient glomerulonephritis that is recognized soon after an upper respiratory infection. Patients almost always have the rash and arthritis, whereas only some patients get renal disease and intestinal bleeding. Treatment is usually not required for acute episodes, although steroids help manage the arthritis and abdominal symptoms.

Mixed cryoglobulinemia

Mixed cryoglobulinemia was described in the 1960s as a syndrome affecting multiple organ systems with symptoms of purpura, arthralgias, and proliferative glomerulonephritis. Now it is thought that there are two main subsets of patients with mixed cryoglobulinemia. One group has systemic involvement along with renal disease with a very aggressive course that results in death before the development of end-stage renal disease. The other patients with mixed cryoglobulinemia do not exhibit signs of systemic vasculitis and often do not progress to end-stage renal disease. More recently, an association between mixed cryoglobulinemia and hepatitis C virus (HCV) was discovered with the vast majority of patients testing positive for HCV RNA. Kidney involvement is more common in women. Patients with mixed cryoglobulinemia present with proteinuria with hematuria (microscopic) and can be found to have chronic renal disease. Hypertension is seen in most patients at the time of diagnosis. Treatment revolves around antiviral therapy (e.g., interferon, ribavirin) along with steroids for management of systemic symptoms.

Kidney diseases in HIV-infected patients

In the current era of highly active antiretroviral therapy (HAART), outcomes in patients with HIV and AIDS have improved dramatically. As a result, other chronic diseases have replaced progressive disease and opportunistic infections as the leading causes of morbidity and mortality. HIV-infected patients with renal disease have an increased risk of death compared to those without kidney failure. These patients are at high risk for developing acute renal failure or chronic kidney disease from a variety of causes, including nephrotoxicity secondary to HAART medications and HIV-associated nephropathy, among others. Protease inhibitors can cause crystalluria and resulting acute kidney injury. The other agents, including nucleoside reverse transcriptase inhibitors, antiviral medications, and antipneumocystis drugs, all have nephrotoxic potential and can cause acute kidney injury. All HIV patients should be screened, at least twice a year, for renal disease by frequently checking for proteinuria and reduced kidney function (elevated creatinine).

Idiopathic membranous nephropathy

Membranous nephropathy is a common cause of nephrotic syndrome. Drugs, bacteria, viruses, and other systemic diseases have been implicated as underlying causes, but in as many as 75% of cases, the etiology is unknown. Cases of idiopathic membranous nephropathy do not resolve when the "responsible" agent or underlying condition is treated. Clinical features for developing more severe renal disease in idiopathic membranous nephropathy include older age; male sex; elevated creatinine at baseline; and proteinuria (specifically 8–10 g/day), lasting at least 3 months. All patients should be put on an angiotensin-converting enzyme inhibitor or angiotensin-receptor blocker to help control blood pressure. In high-risk patients, immunosuppressive treatment should be initiated early to prevent progressive decline in renal function. Most nephrologists recommend a combination of glucocorticoids and cytotoxic agents, such as cyclophosphamide, although cyclosporine is another option.

Aminoglycoside antibiotics

Aminoglycoside antibiotics can freely cross the glomerular basement membrane and as a result, potentially achieve high concentrations in the renal tubule. After filtering through the glomerulus and into the proximal tubule, aminoglycosides can collect in the renal cortex at toxic levels. The result is acute kidney injury with elevations in plasma creatinine levels but with rare effects on urine output (nonoliguric renal failure). In fact, patients with aminoglycoside toxicity exhibit polyuria and hypomagnesemia as a result of excessive urinary losses. Other electrolyte abnormalities can occur but are less frequent, including hypokalemia, hypocalcemia, and hypophosphatemia. The renal injury caused by aminoglycosides is self-limited, and renal function usually recovers by 3 weeks after cessation of therapy. Some of the risk factors for developing nephrotoxicity from aminoglycosides are long duration of therapy, older age, multiple comorbidities, systemic infection, and frequent drug dosing.

Polycystic kidney disease

Polycystic kidney disease is an autosomal dominant genetic defect that generally presents for the first time in young (15–30 years of age) patients. It is the most common inherited kidney disorder in adults. Cystic abnormalities may affect the liver and other intra-abdominal organs. Nephrolithiasis also occurs at an increased rate. There is an increased risk of thoracic aortic aneurysms and berry aneurysms, one of the most dangerous complications of polycystic kidney disease. Berry aneurysms are vascular dilations that are found at branching points in the brain. Rupture is more common in patients with uncontrolled hypertension. Abdominal or flank pain are the most common presenting complaints. Other signs and symptoms may include hypertension, hematuria, palpable renal masses, and eventual progression to renal failure. Depending on the location of the renal cyst, rupture can cause complications, ranging from retroperitoneal hematoma to hematuria. Renal failure usually occurs in these patients by the age of 60.

Von Hippel–Lindau disease

Von Hippel–Lindau disease is an autosomal dominant cancer syndrome that affects multiple organ systems, including the eyes, brain, spinal cord, adrenals, pancreas, and kidneys. The genetic mutation is in a tumor-suppressor gene called VHL. In these patients, there is an increased rate of central nervous system and retinal hemangioblastomas, pheochromocytomas, pancreatic tumors, papillary cystadenomas of the broad ligament/epididymis, and clear cell renal cell carcinoma. Renal cell carcinoma is one of the most common cancers that develop in Von Hippel–Lindau disease, with most patients being affected by 60 years of age. These tumors are usually bilateral and multifocal. When compared to sporadic cases of renal cell carcinoma, patients with Von Hippel–Lindau disease have a better prognosis and survival as a result of a more benign histopathology. When these renal cell carcinomas metastasize, they are a major cause of death in these patients. Treatment is nephrectomy and can require bilateral nephrectomy and renal transplantation in patients with bilateral disease.

Alport's syndrome

Alport's syndrome is an inherited disorder (X-linked predominantly) that affects the basement membrane of the kidney, ears, and eyes. The genetic mutation is in the proteins that make up type IV collagen, the major building block of basement membranes. On pathologic examination, the glomerular basement membrane thickens or thins, with "basket weaving" and lamellar changes. Clinical manifestations are hematuria, acute renal failure due to nephritis, proteinuria, deafness (primarily sensorineural), and vision problems. Disease in men is much more severe than in women. The hematuria is mostly microscopic, but intermittently it becomes gross hematuria. This is a progressive disease that eventually leads to end-stage renal disease in all men but rarely in women. Other more rare manifestations of Alport's syndrome are leiomyomas of the esophagus and tracheobronchial tree, as well as thrombocytopenia in certain mutational variations of the disease. Kidney transplantation is the only treatment option for patients with Alport's syndrome and end-stage renal disease.

Fabry's disease

Fabry's disease is an X-linked congenital condition of abnormal lysosomal storage caused by lack of alpha-galactosidase A, resulting in lysosomal accumulation of globotriaosylceramide. Renal complications occur in about half of patients by adulthood, and the incidence continues to increase as patients age. Chronic renal failure develops from the abnormal accumulation of the globotriaosylceramide in glomeruli that initially causes proteinuria and polyuria. Renal sinus cysts may also develop. Accumulation of globotriaosylceramide in vascular endothelium can cause ischemia and infarction. Extrarenal manifestations can develop as well, including exercise-induced pain, neuropathic pain, heart failure, coronary artery disease, decreased sweating, stroke, or dermatologic manifestations like angiokeratomas or telangiectasias. Renal biopsy shows glycolipid deposits.

Proximal diuretics

The main action of diuretics is to block sodium reabsorption at various points along the tubule in the nephron. The net result is increased urinary sodium and urine output, which can be useful in several conditions plagued by volume overload. There are four main groups of diuretics, separated by the location of their action in the nephron: proximal tubule, loop, thiazide-type, and potassium-sparing diuretics. Diuretics like acetazolamide and mannitol exert their effect in the proximal tubule, albeit through different mechanisms. Acetazolamide is a carbonic anhydrase inhibitor, which causes net sodium chloride and bicarbonate loss. Mannitol is an osmotic diuretic that inhibits sodium and water uptake. Loop diuretics act at the thick ascending part of the loop of Henle through the inhibition of the Na^+-K^+-$2Cl^-$ transporter. Examples of loop diuretics include furosemide, bumetanide, torsemide, and ethacrynic acid. Thiazide diuretics prevent the reabsorption of sodium in the distal tubule and connecting segment by blocking the Na^+-Cl^- cotransporter. They have a much more modest effect on diuresis when compared to loop diuretics. The main drug in this class is hydrochlorothiazide. Potassium-sparing diuretics, such as spironolactone and eplerenone, act on aldosterone receptors in the collecting tubule. They prevent aldosterone from amplifying sodium retention and potassium secretion.

> ➤ **Review Video:** Diuretics
> *Visit **mometrix.com/academy** and enter **Code: 373276***

Acetazolamide

Acetazolamide blocks the activity of carbonic anhydrase, an enzyme located in the proximal tubule of the nephron, which converts water and carbon dioxide (CO_2) to bicarbonate (HCO_3^-) and hydrogen ions (H+). The net result of acetazolamide administration is increased secretion of sodium chloride (NaCl) and HCO_3^-. Given the proximal location of its action and the ability of other parts of the nephron to compensate, the net diuresis produced by acetazolamide is limited. The main indication for its administration is diuresis in patients with metabolic alkalosis, where bicarbonate loss in the urine is a useful side effect. Patients with chronic obstructive pulmonary disease and fluid overload who are prone to CO_2 retention and metabolic alkalosis greatly benefit from treatment with acetazolamide.

Furosemide

Furosemide is the most popular and well known of the loop diuretics. Its location of action is in the thick ascending limb of the loop of Henle where diuresis occurs through the inactivation of the Na^+-K^+-$2Cl^-$ carrier. It is believed that furosemide competes with the chloride ion to effectively block binding and subsequent transport of sodium (Na+) and potassium (K+). The net result is the excretion of 20%–25% of all the filtered Na+ coming through the nephron. This makes loop diuretics the most effective of all the diuretics administered to patients. A side effect of reducing Na+ reabsorption is the concurrent reduction in calcium uptake, which normally occurs passively

- 317 -

via the gradient created by the Na+-K+-2Cl⁻ carrier. Some of the known adverse effects with furosemide are ototoxicity, hyperuricemia (with resulting gout and kidney stones), and hyperglycemia.

Hydrochlorothiazide

Hydrochlorothiazide acts in the distal tubule and connecting segment between the distal tubule and the collecting duct. It inhibits the reabsorption of sodium (Na+) and chloride (Cl⁻) through competitive inhibition at the Cl⁻-binding site on the Na+-Cl⁻ co-transporter. While reducing Na+ uptake, thiazide diuretics increase the reabsorption of calcium in the distal tubule. A less important effect of hydrochlorothiazide occurs in the proximal tubule through the blockage of carbonic anhydrase. The net result of hydrochlorothiazide action is the excretion of 3%–5% of all filtered tubular Na+. Due to the only modest affect on diuresis, these agents are mostly used in the treatment of uncomplicated hypertension, rather than the management of fluid overload. Through a relatively unknown mechanism, hydrochlorothiazide seems to reduce systemic vascular resistance.

Potassium-sparing diuretics

The potassium- (K+-) sparing diuretics include amiloride, triamterene, spironolactone, and eplerenone. They act in the collecting duct, specifically involving aldosterone-sensitive sodium (Na+) channels in the principal cells. Normally, aldosterone activates these channels, thereby increasing the reabsorption of Na+ and facilitating the passive secretion of K+ down its gradient. The result is increased tubular Na+ and decreased K+ secretion with the potential to cause hyperkalemia and metabolic acidosis. Amiloride and triamterene block Na+-channel activity without impacting aldosterone receptors. Amiloride can be employed in the treatment of polyuria and polydipsia secondary to lithium-related diabetes insipidus. Conversely, spironolactone and eplerenone act directly on the aldosterone receptor and competitively inhibit its action. These agents are used in patients with primary aldosteronism or heart failure, specifically in those with cirrhotic livers.

Dialysis

Dialysis is a procedure that allows artificial filtration of the blood to substitute for chronic failing kidney function or to aid in fixing in acute bodily disturbances. Acute disturbances that require urgent dialysis include metabolic acidosis; uremia severe enough to cause pericarditis, gastrointestinal bleeding, pleuritis, and mental status changes; hyperkalemia; certain toxic ingestions, such as salicylic acid, lithium or ethylene glycol; and severe fluid overload. Indications for chronic dialysis include symptomatic renal disease, causing complications, such as hypertension, heart failure, encephalopathy, malnutrition, pruritus, electrolyte disturbances, or asymptomatic end stage renal disease with a glomerular filtration rate of 8–10 mL/min per 1.73 m².

Hemodialysis is the most commonly used form of dialysis. An external machine performs the job of filtration that the kidney would otherwise be performing, as blood is pumped from the vein, to the machine where it is exposed to a semipermeable membrane to filter out waste, and then returned back to the vein. Hemodialysis performed at a center is usually a 4-hour treatment three times a week; however, home hemodialysis can be performed 5 or more days a week overnight for 6–8 hours. Peritoneal dialysis makes use of the patient's peritoneum to act as the mode of filtration that the kidney is supposed to be doing. A catheter connects a dialysate solution from a bag to empty into the abdomen, where filtration occurs across the semipermeable peritoneal membrane, and then the fluid is drained back through the catheter. This is performed 4–5 times daily or once a day at night for 6–8 hours.

Hemodialysis requires an access point to the bloodstream. Temporary access can be achieved with a dialysis catheter, but for patients who will require chronic hemodialysis, access is attained via a primary arteriovenous (AV) fistula, a synthetic AV graft, or a tunneled catheter. Primary AV fistulas are the preferred method of access to the vasculature because they remain patent longer and have lower complication rates than the artificial fistulas or catheters; however, they require months to mature after surgery, during which time they cannot be used, so patients must be referred for this procedure approximately 6 months in advance of the requirement for dialysis. Synthetic AV grafts, made of polytetrafluoroethylene most often only require 2 weeks to mature; however, their rate of complications is higher than primary fistulas. Tunneled catheters also have higher complication rates, particularly infections, but can be used after placement without any delay; they tend to be used while awaiting the maturation of fistulas.

Agents or hormones that increase the glomerular filtration rate or renal perfusion

There are certain drugs or hormones that may produce a functional volume expansion, thereby increasing perfusion to the kidneys and raising the glomerular filtration rate (GFR). A reduction in the levels of angiotensin II and norepinephrine increase circulating volume by eliminating the stimulus for vasoconstriction. Elevated levels of dopamine and atrial natriuretic peptide also increase renal perfusion. Dopamine stimulates the afferent and efferent arterioles of the juxtaglomerular apparatus to dilate. This, in turn, increases blood flow to the kidney with minimal or no change in the GFR. Atrial natriuretic peptide works in a different way, dilating the afferent arteriole with concurrent constriction of the efferent arteriole. The net result is an increase in GFR and relatively no change in renal perfusion.

Dopamine

Dopamine can be produced both at distant sites and locally in the kidney, specifically in the proximal tubule. The actions of dopamine on the kidney are multiple but include both stimulating the excretion of sodium (Na+) and increasing renal perfusion. The major effect of dopamine on natriuresis occurs in the proximal tubule. Dopamine increases the production of cyclic-adenosine monophosphate, which decreases Na+ exchange by inhibiting the Na$^+$–H$^+$-exchange protein in the luminal membrane. It also blocks the Na$^+$–K$^+$ adenosine triphosphate pump both proximally and distally in the collecting tubule. In the collecting duct, it inhibits the reabsorption of sodium. At low doses, dopamine dilates both the afferent and efferent arterioles in the juxtaglomerular apparatus. The end result is an increase in renal perfusion with minimal affect on glomerular filtration rate. However, when the dose of dopamine is increased above 5 mcg/kg/min, it has the opposite effect and causes vasoconstriction in the kidney.

Fenoldopam

Fenoldopam is a selective dopamine receptor agonist that exerts most of its effects on the dopamine D$_1$ receptor. It serves to increase sodium excretion and renal perfusion. Fenoldopam can also act systemically and decrease peripheral vascular resistance, thereby producing relative hypotension. This action is rather limited at standard doses. Several studies have evaluated the benefit of fenoldopam. While some studies have shown that it significantly reduces the risk of acute kidney injury and in-hospital mortality, the current guidelines recommend not using it for the prevention of acute renal failure or acute kidney injury.

Immunosuppressive agents used for renal transplant patients

Kidney transplantation is the best available treatment for patients with end-stage renal disease. After undergoing renal transplantation, recipients must be followed closely by the transplant surgeon and nephrologist, as they usually require at least one immunosuppressive agent to prevent graft rejection. Immunosuppression can be divided into induction therapy and maintenance regimens. Induction therapy is started pretransplant or intraoperatively, whereas maintenance therapy is continued indefinitely for the life of the transplant. The various options for both include antibodies, calcineurin inhibitors, antimetabolites (i.e., antiproliferative agents), and glucocorticoids. While these agents have the benefit of maintaining graft function by preventing rejection, many of them have associated nephrotoxicity if their levels become too high. The newest antiproliferative drugs available for maintenance, mycophenolate mofetil or mTOR inhibitors (i.e., rapamycin), have no nephrotoxicity and very little bone marrow toxicity.

Drugs used for the management of benign prostatic hyperplasia

Benign prostatic hyperplasia (BPH) is enlargement of the prostate gland that generally occurs as men become older. Patients with BPH can be asymptomatic but can also suffer from urinary hesitancy, urgency, and nocturia, among other symptoms. Two main drug groups are available for the treatment of symptomatic BPH. Alpha-adrenergic antagonists are more effective for the treatment of the symptoms by acting on the smooth muscle in the neck of the bladder and the prostatic portion of the urethra. These agents relax the smooth muscle and allow urine to pass more easily through the urethra. Examples of alpha-adrenergic antagonists include tamsulosin, terazosin, and doxazosin. The other class of drugs is the 5-alpha-reductase inhibitors. These agents are more effective in reducing the volume of the prostate and decreasing the potential need for operative intervention by inhibiting the conversion of testosterone to dihydrotestosterone. Examples of 5-alpha-reductase inhibitors are finasteride and dutasteride.

Antibiotic options for the treatment of urinary tract infections

When deciding on an antibiotic choice for the treatment of cystitis or pyelonephritis, one must consider multiple factors. These include the efficacy, side effects, potential for resistance, cost, as well as ease of use. No study has ever shown one antibiotic to be superior to any other for the treatment of urinary tract infections. Furthermore, geographic differences in microbial resistance can complicate making any comprehensive guidelines. The antibiotics most commonly used in the treatment of urinary tract infections are:
- Nitrofurantoin: The efficacy of this agent for the treatment of uncomplicated urinary tract infections is between 90%–95% with minimal resistance or adverse effects. It is contraindicated in patients with reduced creatinine clearance.
- Trimethoprim-sulfamethoxazole (TMP-SMX): This drug is also very effective in standard urinary tract infections. However, the resistance to TMP-SMX is up to 20% in some parts of the country and should be avoided if it has been used in the prior 3 months.
- Fluoroquinolones: These agents are the only drugs currently recommended for the oral treatment of pyelonephritis as an outpatient. The bioavailability of intravenous and oral fluoroquinolones is equivalent. The current concern is that misuse of this class of antibiotics is leading to increased resistance in the community.

Renal transplantation

Kidney transplantation is the best treatment available for patients with end-stage renal disease on dialysis, as it both increases expected survival and improves quality of life. Currently, there is a lower than 5% expected mortality associated with renal transplantation. All potential transplant recipients must be formally evaluated at a transplant center, receive a complete history and physical examination, and have routine laboratory testing (e.g., serologies, electrolytes, liver function tests, urinalysis, electrocardiogram, chest x-ray). The absolute contraindications to renal transplantation are:
- Active infection/sepsis
- Current malignancy
- Drug dependence/substance abuse
- Medical comorbidities associated with short life expectancy (< 1–2 years)
- Liver cirrhosis

The relative contraindications, which previously were absolute, include: HIV infection, infection with hepatitis B and C, obesity, active peptic ulcer disease, age over 60 years, previous malignancy, and blood-group incompatibility.

Psychiatric illness in patients with end-stage renal disease

Unfortunately, mental disorders are very common among patients with end-stage renal disease on dialysis and other similar chronic illnesses. These include depression, dementia, alcoholism, schizophrenia, and personality disorders. Hemodialysis patients have a much higher rate of hospitalization for mental disease than do peritoneal dialysis patients. Depression is the most common psychiatric illness in this patient population, with an approximate 35% prevalence. Depression that presents at the beginning of dialysis therapy is the strongest indicator of the severity and lasting nature of the illness. Concurrent anxiety disorders are also common and have an adverse affect on quality of life. Many cases of depression in dialysis patients lead to increased morbidity and hospitalization and, in severe cases, lead to increased mortality. This underscores the importance of early diagnosis of mental disease in these patients and subsequent medical treatment and counseling.

Influence of socioeconomic factors on the maintenance of chronic kidney disease

Differences in kidney disease risk as a result of race are partly influenced by socioeconomic status as well. Socioeconomic disparities exert their effect on the incidence of chronic kidney disease through several factors:
- Low income and poverty
- Poor nutritional intake
- Lack of education
- Exposure to chemicals or heavy metals
- Drug abuse
- Inadequate access to health care and screening

Many of these variables are modifiable and, therefore, the focus of public health programs and interventions. It is believed that poor socioeconomic status can contribute up to 12% excess risk of developing chronic kidney disease. In a large-scale study called the Cardiovascular Health Study, rates of progressive chronic kidney disease had an inverse relationship with geographic area socioeconomic scores and individual incomes and education. The areas with the lowest socioeconomic status had 1.5 times the risk of progressive chronic kidney disease than the least impoverished locale.

Epidemiology of end-stage renal disease

The incidence of end-stage renal disease is 354 per 1 million people in the United States; however, it has been stable and is now decreasing in incidence over the last decade. This trend can be related to better medical control of blood pressure with angiotensin-converting enzyme inhibitors and other related agents. Additionally, better control of blood sugar in diabetics has improved outcomes in potential end-stage renal disease patients. More recently, the new diagnoses of end-stage renal disease cases have varied quite a bit between different patient populations. African-Americans have almost a four-fold increased incidence of developing renal failure when compared to whites. There are also higher rates in Asians and Hispanics, although the incidence is not as significantly elevated. When stratifying patients by age, the most rapid increase in end-stage renal disease cases is seen in patients 75 years of age and older.

Role of gender as a risk factor in developing chronic kidney disease

Men and women differ in several physiologic and anatomic characteristics, many of which determine their probability of developing certain diseases. The rate of progression to chronic kidney disease is dependent on several gender-specific variables, particularly differences in:
- Glomerular mass
- Hormone responsiveness
- Cytokine release
- Vasoactive/circulating factors
- Quantity of functional nephrons

Women have 10%–15% fewer functional glomeruli than men, although this may be more related to body surface area and weight. This does not translate to a divergent glomerular filtration rate, which is similar between the sexes. There is also thought to be some difference in the levels of circulating hormones and enzymes. Angiotensinogen, angiotensin II, prorenin, renin, angiotensin-converting enzyme, nitric oxide, and prostaglandin production varies among men and women. The net result of the differences in responses to stimuli may be a variable risk of developing chronic kidney disease.

Reproductive System

Early internal reproductive organ development

The reproductive system develops from the intermediate mesoderm. It is important to note that the development of the intestinal, urinary, and reproductive systems is closely related: The common opening in early embryonic development is referred to as the cloaca. The cloaca divides to become the urogenital sinus anteriorly and the rectum posteriorly. The urogenital sinus contains the mesonephric (Wolffian) duct, which forms the ureters (membranous/entire ureter in females, prostatic and membranous ureter in males) and plays an important role in male reproductive system development. Along the medial side of the mesonephric system, developing gonads form the gonadal ridge (identical at this stage for both males and females). Together, the mesonephric duct and gonads are called the urogenital ridge. Primordial germ cells differentiate in the yolk sac and migrate to the gonadal ridge, where they become surrounded by primitive sex cords. Sex differentiation begins around the seventh week of gestation.

Embryonic development of the internal reproductive organs

Male
The SRY gene on the Y chromosome contains the testis-determining factor (TDF) and is responsible for the development of the male reproductive system. The primitive sex cords form the medullary cords and testes. TDF triggers some epithelial cells of the sex cords to become Sertoli cells and some mesoderm cells between the cords to become interstitial cells of Leydig. Sertoli cells produce Müllerian-inhibiting substance (MIS), which prevents formation of the paramesonephric (Müllerian) ducts. Leydig cells produce testosterone, which signals the mesonephric ducts to give rise to the epididymis (stores mature sperm), ductus deferens (transports sperm during ejaculation), and seminal vesicles (create the majority of fluid in semen). The urethral epithelium distal to the bladder forms the prostate gland.

Female
Lack of the SRY gene, which is located on the Y chromosome, leads to the default development of the female reproductive system. Primitive sex cords degenerate and cortical cords form on the surface of the gonads. The absence of Müllerian-inhibiting substance (MIS) and testosterone causes the mesonephric ducts to degenerate and paramesonephric (Müllerian) ducts to develop. The upper portions of the ducts form the fallopian tubes. The lower portions of the ducts fuse to form the uterus and the upper part of the vagina. The pelvic portion of the urogenital sinus will form the urethra and also the lower portion of the vagina. The urethral epithelium distal to the bladder forms the urethral/paraurethral glands.

Descent of the testes and the formation of the tunica vaginalis

Like ovaries, the testes develop intra-abdominally and later descend into the scrotum. The gubernaculum, a band of mesenchyme tissue, connects the testes to the floor of the scrotum. The length of the gubernaculum does not increase, so as a male grows in size, the testes are "pulled" into the scrotum. In 97% of males, the testes are present in the scrotum at birth, 2% to 3% will descend by three months of age, and <1% will fail to descend (cryptorchidism). As the testes descend through the peritoneal cavity and through the inguinal canal, they take an outpouching of peritoneum called the processus vaginalis. The orifice of communication between the processus vaginalis and the peritoneal cavity closes, and the serous covering of the testes that results is known as the tunica vaginalis. Failure of the communication orifice to close can lead to an increased risk of hydrocele or hematocele in the future.

Development of external male and female genitalia

At the front of the cloacal folds that surround the cloaca, a genital tubercle forms. Cloacal folds separate into anal and urethral folds to surround the openings to the anal canal and urogenital sinus, respectively. Genital swellings develop lateral to the urethral folds. Sexual differentiation depends on the presence of testosterone or estrogen. Testosterone, converted to dihydrotestosterone (DHT), influences the development of the external male genitalia. The genital tubercle lengthens and becomes the penis. The urethral folds also extend with the penis, fusing along the ventral aspect of the penis to create the penile urethra. Genital swellings enlarge to become scrotal swellings, which fuse in the midline to form the scrotum. Estrogen directs the development of female external genitalia. The genital tubercle forms the clitoris. The urethral folds do not fuse; they form the labia minora on either side of the urethral and vaginal openings, collectively known as the vestibule. The genital swellings also stay separated and form the labia majora.

Gametogenesis

Male
The male form of gametogenesis is known as spermatogenesis, and the goal is to turn each diploid spermatogonium into four haploid mature sperm. Spermatogenesis is an ongoing process that begins at puberty and continues throughout the reproductive life of a male. Some spermatogonia go through mitosis to maintain the immature sperm in the testes. Other spermatogonia go through mitosis to become mature sperm. After mitosis, these immature sperm are called primary spermatocytes. To make mature sperm, each primary spermatocyte must go through two complete cycles of meiosis. After meiosis I, they are referred to as secondary spermatocytes. After meiosis II, they are referred to as spermatids. After completion of meiosis II, there are four mature haploid sperm that are ready to fertilize a female ovum.

Female
The female form of gametogenesis is known as oogenesis, and the goal is to turn one diploid oocyte into a single haploid ovum. It is believed that females are born with all the oocytes they will ever have. During fetal life, female germ cells (oogonia) enter meiosis but are arrested in prophase I until puberty. At this stage, the eggs are called primary oocytes. When puberty is reached, one primary oocyte per menstrual cycle completes meiosis I, resulting in one oocyte and one polar body. Immediately following completion of the first cycle of meiosis, the oocyte continues on to meiosis II and the polar body degrades. The second cycle of meiosis is halted at metaphase II until fertilization occurs. At this stage, the egg is referred to as a secondary oocyte. If fertilization occurs, meiosis II is completed and one ovum and one polar body are formed. The ovum continues on to implantation and the polar body degrades.

Ovaries

The ovaries are small, oval-shaped glands located on either side of the uterus, and they are the gonads of the female reproductive system. Ovaries produce hormones (estrogen, progesterone, and testosterone) and are responsible for producing an oocyte every menstrual cycle. The ovaries are secured to the uterus by the ovarian ligaments, to the peritoneal wall by suspensory ligaments, and to the body of the uterus by a part of the broad ligament called the mesovarium. Blood supply is via the ovarian artery and vein, which are contained in the suspensory ligaments. The ovarian arteries arrive directly from the aorta bilaterally. The right ovarian vein directly joins the inferior vena cava, and the left ovarian vein joins the left renal vein.

Fallopian tubes

The fallopian tubes (also known as uterine ducts or salpinges) extend from the superolateral portion of the uterus. Their open lateral ends are in very close proximity to the ovaries. The most lateral portion of the fallopian tube is called the infundibulum; it contains fingerlike fimbriae that "catch" the ovulated oocyte released from the ovary. The ampulla is just medial to the infundibulum, and it represents a slightly dilated portion of the tube. The majority of fertilizations occur in the ampulla of the fallopian tube. The remainder of the tube is referred to as the isthmus, and it connects medially to the uterus. The fallopian tube is lined with ciliated epithelium to aid in the movement of the oocyte to the uterus. The fallopian tubes are supplied with blood by the uterine and ovarian arteries.

Uterus

The uterus is a major organ in the female reproductive system. Distally, the cervix attaches to the vagina. The cervix is the site of cell collection during Pap smears to assess for cervical/uterine cancer. The body of the uterus is attached to the pelvic floor, fallopian tubes, and ovaries by the broad ligament. It is important to note that the broad ligament is not actually a ligament but a sheet of peritoneum. The cervix is attached to the ischial spines of the pelvis via the cardinal ligaments. The three layers of the uterus are the endometrium, myometrium, and perimetrium. The endometrium is built up during the menstrual cycle and is shed during menstruation if implantation does not occur. The myometrium is the smooth muscle of the uterus, and the perimetrium is the loose connective tissue surrounding the uterus. Blood supply to the uterus is by the ovarian and uterine arteries, which anastomose along the uterine walls. The uterine arteries arise from the internal iliac artery and are found within the cardinal ligaments.

External female genitalia

The vagina extends from the vulva to the cervix of the uterus. It is lined by rugae, which allow for expansion during coitus and childbirth. Blood supply is by the vaginal arteries, which are branches of the internal iliac artery. Like the uterus and fallopian tubes, innervation is largely autonomic but sensation is provided by the pudendal nerve. The external female genitalia consist of the labia majora, labia minora, Bartholin's glands, and the clitoris. The labia majora are the larger and more lateral of the two, and the labia minora are the smaller and more medial. Bartholin's glands are located on either side of the vaginal opening, and they provide lubrication. The clitoris is at the juncture of the labia minora and is the equivalent of the male penis. Similarly, it is very sensitive to stimulation.

Breasts

The breasts overlay the pectoralis major muscles of the chest wall and extend from the clavicle to the sternum and into the axilla. Female breasts contain multiple lactiferous lobes surrounded by adipose tissue. Lactiferous lobes contain lobules and ducts that terminate at the nipple. The nipple is surrounded by hyperpigmented skin called the areola. Estrogen maintains the glandular tissue of the breast, explaining the decrease in breast mass following menopause. Following labor and delivery, the sudden decrease in maternal progesterone induces lactation. Nerve stimulation caused by suckling increases oxytocin and prolactin. Oxytocin helps with milk letdown, and prolactin induces and maintains lactation.

Penis

The penis consists of three main muscles: two corpora cavernosa and one ventral corpus spongiosum. The corpora cavernosa contain erectile tissue, and the corpus spongiosum contains the urethra. The urethra functions to excrete urine during urination and also to eject semen during sexual intercourse (during erection, the urethra's connection to the bladder is closed, so the male is unable to urinate, and ejaculate is only able to go forward). The glans penis is formed by the distal extension of the corpus spongiosum. Blood supply to the penis is by the pudendal artery. Penile erection occurs when signaled by nitrous oxide (NO), which signals production of cyclic guanosine monophosphate (cGMP), which causes smooth-muscle relaxation. The relaxation of smooth muscle causes arterial/arteriolar dilatation, leading to increased blood flow into the penis. The sinusoids within the corpora cavernosa become distended with blood, and the venous complexes become compressed, decreasing blood outflow from the penis and resulting in erection.

Testis

The testes are the gonads of the male reproductive system, responsible for making testosterone and sperm. They are located within the scrotum and secured on either end by the spermatic cord. Seminiferous tubules are located within the testes and are the site of sperm production. The epididymis is located along the back of the testis, and it is responsible for storing sperm while they mature. The epididymis leads to the vas deferens, which transports the mature sperm in preparation for ejaculation. The vas deferens leads to the urethra, through which the sperm is ejaculated from the body. Prior to entering the penis, the urethra receives fructose-rich fluid from the seminal vesicles, designed to help support sperm, which makes up the majority of seminal fluid. The urethra also passes through the prostate, which contributes additional seminal fluid to support the sperm. The testes are supplied with blood via the testicular arteries that branch directly off of the aorta bilaterally. The pampiniform plexus, a collection of small veins that follows the spermatic cord, drains the testes, epididymis, and vas deferens. The plexus then merges into the testicular veins. The left testicular vein joins the left renal vein, and the right testicular vein joins directly to the inferior vena cava.

Scrotum

The scrotum is a pouch of loose skin that contains the testes. Its function is to maintain the temperature of the testes approximately 1° to 2° Celsius below core body temperature in order to sustain sperm vitality. The scrotum moves closer to the body in cases of cooler ambient temperature and further away from the body in cases of warmer temperatures. This is done by the cremasteric muscle, which surrounds the spermatic cord and testis. The cremasteric muscle contracts to bring the testes closer to the body and relaxes to let them fall further from the body. The cremasteric response (muscle contraction) can be elicited by lightly touching the skin of the inner thigh.

Stages of sexual response

The five stages of sexual response are 1. desire, 2. arousal, 3. plateau, 4. orgasm, and 5. resolution. Male and female arousal is caused by parasympathetic impulses from the sacral cord (S2-4), causing vasodilatation and increased blood flow/congestion to the respective organs. In males, the penis becomes erect during this stage. In females, the clitoris becomes erect and the Bartholin's glands produce mucous for vaginal lubrication. During the plateau phase, stimulation continues and characteristics of arousal are intensified. Orgasm is controlled by the sympathetic response (L1, L2). In males, this results in contraction that leads to emission and ejaculation of semen. In women, this leads to rhythmic contraction of the vagina and uterus. Resolution is defined as the return of the body to its normal state of functioning. It is followed by a refractory phase in males, which can range from minutes to days. It is important to note that although the refractory phase does increase with age, desire does not.

Female menstrual cycle

The female menstrual cycle lasts an average of 28 days, divided into ovarian and uterine cycles (day 1 = the first day of bleeding).

The ovarian cycle consists of the follicular phase, ovulation, and the luteal phase. During the follicular phase, follicular stimulating hormone (FSH) stimulates the maturation of a follicle to become a tertiary (Graafian) follicle, containing the secondary oocyte. The maturing follicle produces levels of estrogen that trigger a positive feedback loop to the hypothalamic-pituitary-gonadal axis, and a surge of leuteinizing hormone (LH) results (day 12). The LH spike causes the second phase, ovulation, when the oocyte is released from the follicle (day 14). During the luteal phase, the empty follicle becomes the corpus luteum, which produces progesterone that primes the uterus for implantation of a fertilized egg. Without implantation, the luteal phase lasts 14 days.

The uterine cycle is divided into menstruation, the proliferative phase, and the secretory phase. Menstruation occurs as a result of progesterone withdrawal if the corpus luteum is not sustained by human chorionic gonadotropin (hCG) (no pregnancy), and it lasts an average of 5 days. Menstruation overlaps with the ovarian follicular phase. Estrogen from the maturing follicle stimulates the second uterine phase, proliferation of the endometrium. The final secretory phase overlaps with the ovarian luteal phase. Progesterone from the corpus luteum primes the endometrium for implantation by increasing blood flow and uterine secretions. If an egg does not implant, the cycle starts over with menstruation.

Oligomenorrhea, polymenorrhea, metrorrhagia, menorrhagia, and menometrorrhagia

The average menstrual cycle lasts 28 days, but a cycle may range from 21 to 35 days. Oligomenorrhea is infrequent menstruation, defined as a menstrual cycle that is greater than 35 days long. Polymenorrhea is frequent menstruation, defined as a menstrual cycle that is less than 21 days long. Metrorrhagia is defined as frequent but irregular menstruation. Menorrhagia is defined as menstruation lasting longer than 8 days or with more than 80 mL of blood loss. Menometrorrhagia is defined as heavy and frequent/irregular menstruation. The menstruation pattern is an important part of the history in female patients because abnormalities in menstruation may lead to irregularity in/failure to ovulate or blood loss that leads to anemia.

Pregnancy, labor and delivery, and the post-gestational uterus

Term gestation is 37 to 40 weeks. A baby born before 37 weeks is considered preterm, and a baby born after 40 weeks is considered postterm. Labor and delivery is divided into three stages. The first stage of labor begins with cervical dilation and lasts until the cervix is fully dilated at 10 cm. The first stage includes latent labor (from onset of dilation until active labor) and active labor (accelerated cervical dilation beginning at 5 cm for multiparous women and 6 cm for nulliparous women). The second stage of labor begins when the cervix is completely dilated at 10 cm and ends when the baby is delivered. The third stage of labor begins after the delivery of the baby and ends with the delivery of the placenta. Following the delivery of the baby, the uterus begins to contract and decrease in size. It takes an average of 6 weeks for the uterus to return to prepregnancy size.

Androgens

Androgens include dihydrotestosterone (DHT), testosterone, and androstenedione (listed in order of potency, from the greatest to the least potent). When gonadotropin-releasing hormone (GnRH) is released from the hypothalamus, it triggers the release of leuteinizing hormone (LH) from the anterior pituitary. LH signals the interstitial cells of the testes to produce testosterone. Testosterone may then be converted to DHT by 5α-reductase. GnRH also signals the release of FSH from the anterior pituitary, which is crucial in initiating spermatogenesis. Testosterone has several important roles in male development, including the development of primary and secondary sex characteristics. If testosterone levels are low, GnRH will increase in an effort to increase production. If testosterone levels are high, there will be a negative feedback loop and GnRH will be inhibited. Exogenous testosterone administration will cause a decrease in GnRH, which will in turn lead to decreased intratesticular testosterone, decreased testicular size, and decreased sperm count. DHT plays a role in early differentiation of the penis, scrotum, and the prostate. Later in life, excess DHT may contribute to prostatic hyperplasia and male pattern baldness. Androstenedione is produced by the adrenal glands.

Estrogen

Estrogen is a critical factor in the female reproductive system. Estrogen is produced in the ovaries in the form of estradiol, by aromatization in the blood in the form of estrone, and by the placenta in the form of estriol (listed in order of potency, from the greatest to the least potent). Gonadotropin-releasing hormone (GnRH) from the hypothalamus triggers the release of leuteinizing hormone (LH) and follicle-stimulating hormone (FSH) from the anterior pituitary. LH activates 17α-hydroxylase, which converts cholesterol to androstenedione. FSH activates aromatase, which converts androstenedione to estrogen. Roles of estrogen include the development of primary and secondary sex characteristics, the growth of the follicle and endometrial proliferation during the menstrual cycle, and decreasing low-density lipoprotein (LDL)/increasing high-density lipoprotein (HDL). When estrogen levels are high, it can cause a negative feedback loop to decrease GnRH and subsequent FSH/LH levels. If estrogen levels are low, GnRH will increase in an effort to trigger the production of more FSH/LH and estrogen.

Menopause

Menopause is the end of female fertility and is associated with decreased estrogen levels. In an effort to increase estrogen, the hypothalamus will increase production of gonadotropin-releasing hormone (GnRH), which will cause an increase in leuteinizing hormone (LH) and follicle-stimulating hormone (FSH) from the anterior pituitary. However, due to the decrease in the number of follicles, the ovaries are not able to produce estrogen in response. The primary source of estrogen following menopause becomes peripheral aromatization. Menopausal symptoms such as hot flashes, vaginal dryness, and irritability are due to decreased estrogen. Diagnosis of menopause can be confirmed by laboratory tests, which will show decreased estrogen, increased GnRH, increased FSH, and increased LH. The average age of menopause is 53 years; menopause before the age of 40 is considered premature.

Progesterone

Progesterone is produced by the corpus luteum in the ovaries, the placenta during pregnancy and minimally by the testes. The main function of progesterone is to maintain pregnancy (progesterone = progestation) by increasing endometrial glandular secretions, increasing blood supply through spiral artery development, inhibiting gonadotropins (leuteinizing hormone [LH] and follicle-stimulating hormone [FSH]), and relaxing the uterine smooth muscle. During the menstrual cycle, progesterone is at its peak from 24 hours before ovulation until 24 hours after ovulation. During this time, progesterone will also cause a slight basal body temperature increase, which may be used to detect ovulation.

Changes in hormone production and their effects during pregnancy

Implantation of the fertilized ovum onto the endometrium of the uterus causes a production of human chorionic gonadotropin (hCG). This maintains the corpus luteum and its production of progesterone for the first trimester. By the second trimester, the placenta has developed and is able to produce its own estrogen and progesterone. If the corpus luteum is removed before this time, spontaneous abortion (miscarriage) may occur. Estrogens produced by the placenta differ from those produced by the ovary in that the placental estrogens are not produced over again but are formed from androgens formed by the adrenal glands of the mother and fetus. These estrogens cause continued enlargement of the mother's uterus, stimulate growth of the mother's breasts and ductal system, cause enlargement of the mother's external genitalia, and relax ligaments to create a more flexible pubic symphysis to aid in delivery of the fetus. Progesterone during pregnancy maintains a healthy decidual lining of the uterus, decreases contractility of the uterus to avoid preterm labor or spontaneous abortion, and helps estrogen stimulate the development of the mother's breasts.

Defense mechanism of the female reproductive system against infection

The female reproductive tract has special capabilities when it comes to defending against pathogens. The tight epithelial cell junctions create a physical barrier against infection. New evidence is also showing that the female reproductive tract is capable of presenting antigens and mounting its own immune response. Mucosal secretions from the female reproductive tract also contain several antimicrobial immunoglobulins, chemokines, and other endogenous microbicides. The lower female reproductive tract normal flora includes lactobacilli, which ferment glycogen and result in lower pH. The acidic vaginal pH inhibits other, possibly pathogenic, bacteria from inhabiting the tract.

Gonorrhea

Gonorrhea is caused by *Neisseria gonorrhoeae*, a gram-negative diplococcus. It can be grown on Thayer-Martin media, which is also known as VPN media because it contains vancomycin (to inhibit gram-positives), polymyxin (to inhibit gram-negatives), and nystatin (to inhibit fungi). It can cause urethritis, cervicitis, and pelvic inflammatory disease (PID) in females. It can lead to prostatitis and epididymitis in males. Gonorrhea is commonly associated with a purulent cervical/urethral discharge. If gonorrhea becomes disseminated, look out for systemic symptoms including fever and migratory polyarthritis. Disseminated gonorrhea is the most common cause of septic arthritis in the United States. The Centers for Disease Control and Prevention (CDC) treatment recommendation is combination therapy with ceftriaxone 250 mg IM plus either azithromycin 1 g po x 1 or doxycycline 100 mg po BID x 7 days.

Syphilis

Syphilis is caused by *Treponema pallidum*, a gram-negative spirochete. Primary syphilis presents as a single painless ulcer at the site of infection and may go unnoticed. Within three months of the primary infection, symptoms of secondary syphilis begin to develop, which consist of systematic symptoms (fever, chills, weight loss, etc.) and a distinct rash on the mucous membranes and skin (including palms of the hands/soles of the feet). Following secondary syphilis, the disease enters a latent phase that can last months to several years. Without treatment, 30% of patients will develop tertiary syphilis. Tertiary syphilis may manifest in the form of chronic gummas, neurosyphilis, or cardiovascular syphilis. Neurosyphilis appears in many forms including meningitis, general paresis, apathy, or seizure. A classic finding in neurosyphilis is Argyll Robertson pupils (pupils do not react to bright light but will accommodate when focusing on near objects). Syphilitic aortitis is the most common complication of tertiary syphilis and may result in aortitis/aneurysm formation. Treatment for syphilis is intramuscular penicillin G.

If syphilis is suspected, venereal disease research laboratory (VDRL) or rapid plasma reagin (RPR) testing are used for screening. It is important to realize that VDRL and RPR are good screening tests because of their high sensitivity, but they also have low specificity. VDRL detects antibodies that react with beef cardiolipin, which includes syphilis but also viruses such as mononucleosis and hepatitis; some drugs; rheumatic fever; systemic lupus erythema (SLE); and leprosy. Because of this low specificity, it is important to realize that there are many false positive when using VDRL. If the screening test is positive, confirm the diagnosis of syphilis with fluorescent treponemal antibody absorption (FTA-Abs), which has a high specificity for syphilis. Note that VDRL tests typically become negative again after successful treatment of syphilis; however, FTA-Abs will stay positive for life. Treponema does not show up on a Gram stain because it is too thin. To visualize treponema, darkfield microscopy or fluorescent antibody staining must be used.

Difference between chancroid, syphilis, and genital herpes

Chancroid is caused by *Haemophilus ducreyi*, a gram-negative coccobacillus. Chancroid is a very painful genital ulcer with exudate and may be associated with surrounding lymphadenopathy. The diagnosis is clinical because there is no standardized laboratory testing for *H. ducreyi* at this time. It is differentiated from syphilis by its extremely painful nature (syphilitic ulcers are painless). Chancroid is a common sexually transmitted disease in Africa and Southeast Asia, and it is usually only seen in the United States when the patient has traveled to one of these areas.

Genital herpes is caused by herpes simplex virus-2 (HSV-2). Genital herpes presents as multiple painful penile, vulvar, or cervical ulcers. It can also cause lymphadenopathy and systemic symptoms such as fever and myalgia. There is no cure for HSV-2 at this time, but symptoms and transmission rates may be reduced with antiviral therapy (i.e., acyclovir). The presence of herpetic genital ulcers at the time of delivery is an indication for a Cesarean section.

Chlamydia

Chlamydia is caused by *Chlamydia trachomatis*, a gram-negative rod or coccus (pleomorphic). It is best visualized by Giemsa stain because it is an obligate intracellular parasite and does not contain muramic acid in its cell wall. Chlamydia is the most common sexually transmitted disease in the

United States. Types D through K can produce urethritis and pelvic inflammatory disease (PID). Types L1, L2, and L3 can cause lymphogranuloma venereum, a sexually transmitted infection of the lymphatic system. It is more common in men, and the main risk factor is human immunodeficiency virus (HIV) infection. Lymphogranuloma venereum may present with a primary painless genital ulcer and inguinal lymphadenopathy. It can also cause rectal disease including rectal bleeding and tenesmus. Although it is rare in the United States, it is very important to recognize the features of lymphogranuloma venereum.

Difference between trichomoniasis, bacterial vaginosis, and candidiasis

Bacterial vaginosis (BV) is caused by *Gardnerella vaginalis*, a pleomorphic, gram-variable rod. BV causes a painless gray vaginal discharge. Although it is found in sexually active females, it is not considered a sexually transmitted disease. Diagnosis of BV is made by visualization of clue cells (vaginal epithelial cells covered with bacteria) under the microscope and/or a positive whiff test (production of a strong fishy odor with the addition of potassium hydroxide). BV is associated with an elevated vaginal pH (>4.5). Treatment of BV is metronidazole 500 mg po BID x 7 days.

Trichomoniasis is caused by the motile protozoan, *Trichomonas vaginalis*. It causes a green-yellow vaginal discharge in women and may cause nongonococcal urethritis in men, although it is frequently asymptomatic. Diagnosis is by wet mount, which will show mobile organisms. Trichomoniasis is associated with an elevated vaginal pH (>4.5). Treatment is metronidazole 50 mg po BID x 7 days.

Vaginal candidiasis is caused by *Candida albicans*, a yeast with buds and pseudohyphae. Symptoms include irritation and dysuria. On physical exam, a thick, curdy white discharge is seen. Candida is associated with a normal vaginal pH (3.5 to 4.5). Treatment for candidiasis is topical antifungals or fluconazole 150 mg po x 1 dose.

Condylomata acuminata

Condylomata acuminata are anogenital warts caused by human papilloma viruses (HPV) 6 and 11, which are sexually transmitted double-stranded DNA viruses. Certain strains of HPV predispose to malignancy; however, HPV 6 and 11 are considered among the least likely to lead to cancer. Risk factors for condylomata acuminata include smoking, oral contraceptive pills, multiple sexual partners, and sexual activity before the age of 18 years. Typical presentation is multiple warts that may be associated with pruritus, discharge, or bleeding. Most common locations of lesions are on the penis, vulva, or cervix. Diagnosis can be confirmed by Pap smear or acetowhitening (application of acetic acid causes whitening of lesions). Treatment includes cryotherapy, curettage, and surgical excision.

Pelvic inflammatory disease (PID)

PID is an infection of the uterus and fallopian tubes. The most common causative organisms are *Chlamydia trachomatis* and *Neisseria gonorrhoeae*. Risk factors include a history of sexually transmitted disease or previous PID. Patients with PID present with severe lower abdominal pain, fever, and cervical discharge. On physical exam, extreme cervical motion tenderness is often present (called the chandelier sign because patients jump to the ceiling during the pelvic exam). Complicated cases of PID may lead to Fitz-Hugh–Curtis syndrome, which is an extension of the infection to the liver capsule causing "violin-string" adhesions. PID is a risk factor for future ectopic pregnancy and infertility. Broad-spectrum antibiotics that cover both *N. gonorrhoeae* and *C.*

trachomatis are recommended in the treatment of PID (i.e., cefoxitin and doxycycline). Parenteral administration of antibiotics may be required initially, but patients may be switched to oral administration 24 hours after signs of improvement. It is important that total antibiotic coverage lasts 14 days.

Human immunodeficiency virus (HIV)

HIV is an enveloped, single-stranded, diploid RNA virus transmitted by the exchange of bodily fluids (sexual intercourse, blood transfusion, etc.). Envelope proteins are found on the surface of the virion and include gp120 and gp41. The capsid protein, p24, is found within the envelope. The matrix protein, p17, is found between the viral core and the viral envelope. HIV enters host cells by binding to CDXCR4 and CD4 on the surface of T cells and CCR5 and CD4 on the surface of macrophages. Once taken up by the host cell, there are three viral enzymes required for HIV survival: reverse transcriptase, integrase, and protease. Reverse transcriptase is used to synthesize double-stranded DNA (dsDNA) from the RNA. The dsDNA is then integrated into the host genome by integrase and replicated by host mechanisms. The new viral RNA is then removed from the host genome and used to make more immature HIV. The protease then cleaves the immature HIV genome in the right spot to create mature HIV.

Screening for HIV is performed with the enzyme-linked immunosorbent assay (ELISA). ELISA has high sensitivity for HIV antibodies but low specificity, resulting in a high false-positive rate, which means that the diagnosis of HIV should not be made until confirmed with Western blot assay. The Western blot has a high specificity for HIV antibodies but low sensitivity, resulting in a high false-negative rate. If both ELISA and the Western blot are positive, the diagnosis of HIV is made. It is very important to note that testing with ELISA and the Western blot depends on the presence of antibodies to HIV, which may not develop until one to three months following infection. This gap between infection and antibody formation, which may lead to inaccurate testing, is called the window period.

Treatment of HIV is very complicated and requires a combination of antiretrovirals from at least two different classes. This is referred to as highly active antiretroviral therapy (HAART). There is no cure for HIV, but appropriate use of HAART my lead to undetectable levels of HIV in the blood and increased survival. Different classes of antiretrovirals include protease inhibitors, fusion/entry inhibitors, integrase inhibitors, and reverse transcriptase inhibitors. Protease inhibitors prevent maturation of HIV particles by inhibiting the enzyme protease. Fusion/entry inhibitors interfere with the ability of HIV to bind with surface receptors on host cells. Integrase inhibitors block the integration of HIV genetic material into the host genome by inhibiting the enzyme integrase. Reverse transcriptase inhibitors interfere with the creation of double-stranded DNA (dsDNA) from HIV single-stranded RNA (ssRNA) by inhibiting reverse transcriptase.

Diagnostic process of AIDS and the importance of the CD4 count

The diagnosis of the acquired immunodeficiency syndrome (AIDS) is made when the CD4 count drops below 200, an HIV-positive patient contracts an AIDS-indicator condition, or the CD4:CD8 ratio is less than 1.5. Most commonly tested AIDS indicator conditions include esophageal candidiasis, disseminated histoplasmosis, Kaposi's sarcoma, Burkitt's lymphoma, extrapulmonary or disseminated *Mycobacterium avium*, *Pneumocystis carinii* pneumonia, and toxoplasmosis of the brain. The CD4 level is associated with a risk of developing certain infections. Below a CD4 count of 400, patients are at risk for developing oral thrush, tinea pedis, reactivation varicella zoster virus, reactivation tuberculosis, and recurrent bacterial infection. A count of less than 200, patients are at risk for developing reactivation herpes simplex virus, cryptosporidiosis, isosporiasis, disseminated coccidioidomycosis, and *P. carinii* pneumonia. To prevent these infections, it is recommended that patients with a CD4 count of less than 200 begin prophylactic therapy with sulfamethoxazole/trimethoprim or dapsone. When the CD4 count is less than 100, the patient is at risk for developing candidal esophagitis, toxoplasmosis, and histoplasmosis. At this point, it is recommended that patients add azithromycin to their prophylactic regimen. At a CD4 count of less than 50, patients are at high risk of developing cytomegalovirus (CMV) retinitis/esophagitis, disseminated *M. avium*, and cryptococcal meningoencephalitis. With a CD4 of less than 50, patients should add antifungals.

Opportunistic infections

Eye
The most common opportunistic infection of the eye is cytomegalovirus (CMV) retinitis. Some people with CMV retinitis may be asymptomatic, but symptoms include blind spots, floaters, and blurry vision. Without treatment, it can lead to blindness or retinal detachment. Patients with CD4 counts of less than 100 should have regular ophthalmic exams to screen for CMV retinitis. A dilated funduscopic exam will show retinal necrosis and white lesions along retinal vessels described as "pizza pie." Treatment consists of antivirals, which should be continued as long as the CD4 counts are less than 100, in addition to lifelong highly active antiretroviral therapy (HAART).

Brain in HIV
Opportunistic infections of the brain include cryptococcal meningitis, toxoplasmosis, cytomegalovirus (CMV) encephalopathy, and pro-gressive multifocal leukoencephalopathy (PML). Cryptococcal menin-gitis is a fungal infection caused by *Cryptococcus neoformans*. Neuroimaging shows gray matter lesions that resemble soap bubbles. Diagnosis is by cerebrospinal fluid (CSF) analysis/culture, India ink stain, and cryptococcal antigen testing. Treatment consists of amphotericin and flucytosine therapy until the CD4 counts are greater than 100. Toxoplasmosis is caused by the parasite *Toxoplasmosis gondii*. Neuroimaging shows multiple ring-enhancing lesions. Diagnosis can be confirmed with cerebrospinal fluid (CSF) testing; however, lumbar puncture is often contraindicated due to elevated intracranial pressure. Diagnosis is often based on improve-ment with empiric treatment of pyrimethamine, sulfadiazine, and folic acid. Alternative therapy is trimethoprim-sulfamethoxazole. Suppressive therapy should be continued until CD4 counts are greater than 200. CMV encephalopathy is caused by cytomegalo-virus. Diagnosis is by CSF analysis/culture and polymerase chain reaction (PCR). Neuroimaging shows large ventricles and ring-enhancing lesions. Treatment is with antivirals until the CD4 counts are greater than 100. PML is a demyelinating disease of the CNS caused by human papovavirus. Diagnosis is by PCR of the CSF. Neuroimaging shows multiple white matter lesions. There is no standardized treatment for PML. Lifelong HAART therapy is advised.

Mouth and throat in HIV
Opportunistic infections of the mouth and throat include candidiasis, cytomegalovirus (CMV), and oral hairy leukoplakia. Oral and esophageal candidiasis are caused by the yeast *Candida albicans*. It is a white pseudomembrane that is easily scraped off. Treatment is antifungal therapy. Oral CMV ulcers appear as necrotic lesions with white halos and are usually associated with systemic disease. Diagnosis is confirmed with biopsy. Treatment is of the systemic infection with ganciclovir. Oral hairy leukoplakia is caused by the Epstein–Barr virus. It is a corrugated white lesion on the lateral margins of the tongue and is not removable. Diagnosis is made with biopsy. Treatment is not required as it is asymptomatic, but may be given with antivirals. It is recommended that HIV patients with opportunistic infections continue lifelong HAART therapy.

<u>Gastrointestinal tract in HIV</u>
Opportunistic infections of the gastrointestinal tract include cryptosporidiosis, *Mycobacterium avium-intracellulare* complex (MAC), cytomegalovirus (CMV) colitis, and isosporiasis. Cryptosporidiosis is caused by the protozoan *Cryptosporidium*. A cause of diarrhea in children, cryptosporidiosis can cause severe, prolonged diarrhea and acalculous cholecystitis in HIV. Treatment includes antiparasitics and cholecystectomy in cases of cholecystitis. Disseminated MAC can cause abdominal pain and diarrhea. Diagnosis is made by culture or biopsy. Treatment consists of antibiotic therapy, and prophylaxis with azithromycin or clindamycin continuing until CD4 counts are >50. CMV colitis can present with a range of symptoms including abdominal pain, diarrhea, and peritoneal signs in severe cases. With immunohistochemical stain-ing, cells with an "owl's-eye" appearance are seen. Imaging and colonoscopy may show bowel wall thickening and mucosal ulcerations. Treatment consists of antivirals and continuation of ganciclovir until CD4 counts are >50. Patients with ischemia or uncontrolled bleeding may require surgical resection. Isosporiasis is caused by the protozoan *Isospora belli*. Usually transient in immuno-competent patients, isosporiasis can lead to chronic diarrhea in patients with HIV. Peripheral eosinophilia and stool ova and parasite studies are important in diagnosis. Treatment is with antiparasitics and supportive care, also lifelong suppressive treatment with trimethoprim-sulfamethoxazole. Lifelong HAART therapy is advised.

Neoplasms associated with HIV

Neoplasms associated with HIV include Kaposi's sarcoma and central nervous system (CNS) lymphoma. HIV-related Kaposi's sarcoma is a very aggressive spindle cell cancer. It usually presents with cutaneous lesions that can go on to involve the oral mucosa, lymph nodes, gastrointestinal (GI) tract, and lungs. Skin lesions tend to be brown or red, on lower extremities or the head/neck, and appear in a symmetrical distribution along Langer's lines. Diagnosis is confirmed by biopsy. Treatment includes HAART therapy in addition to chemotherapy for metastatic disease and surgical excision for local disease. CNS lymphoma is a large cell non-Hodgkin lymphoma associated with Epstein–Barr virus. Neuroimaging shows a single ring-enhancing lesion, although multiple lesions may be present. Biopsy is often necessary to differentiate from toxoplasmosis. There is no standardized treatment for CNS lymphoma, but survival can be greatly prolonged with combination radiation and chemotherapy. It is important to note that patients with HIV also have a higher risk of invasive cervical cancer and non-Hodgkin's lymphoma.

Acute mastitis

Acute mastitis is an infection of the breast that is most commonly seen in breast-feeding women. The risk for mastitis is increased during breast-feeding due to exposure to the infant's oral flora and engorgement. Frequent, complete emptying of the breasts can reduce the risk of mastitis by preventing engorgement. *Staphylococcus aureus* is the most common causative organism. Patients present with engorged, red, painful breasts and there may be associated systemic symptoms such as fever and malaise. Treatment of acute mastitis is continuation of breast-feeding (or pumping of breast milk if breast-feeding is too painful) and oral antibiotics that cover *S. aureus* (i.e., amoxicillin/clavulanate, ciprofloxacin, and clindamycin). Untreated mastitis may lead to the formation of a breast abscess.

Acute prostatitis

Acute prostatitis is a bacterial infection of the prostate. The majority of cases of acute prostatitis are caused by the same organisms responsible for most urinary tract infections (UTIs). These include *Escherichia coli, Proteus mirabilis, Klebsiella, Enterobacter, Pseudomonas aeruginosa,* and *Serratia*. Similar to UTIs, *E. coli* is the most common pathogen. *Staphylococcus aureus* may be the cause of acute prostatitis when associated with indwelling catheters. Acute prostatitis usually presents as dysuria, fever, and perineal or rectal pain. Physical exam will show an enlarged, tender prostate. Urine studies will show bacteria and leukocytes, urine culture will be positive, and prostate-specific antigen will be elevated. A computed tomography (CT) scan and ultrasound may show a prostatic abscess. Treatment consists of antibiotics and surgical drainage if an abscess is present. Initial antibiotic therapy should target gram-negative bacteria (i.e., trimethoprim-sulfamethoxazole), but it should be adjusted based on the culture results.

Erectile dysfunction

Erectile dysfunction (ED) is the inability to obtain or maintain an erection. Causes of ED can be divided into organic (vascular insufficiency, diabetes, neurologic injury, hypogonadism, hypopituitarism, etc.), psychogenic (depression, anxiety, etc.), or secondary to a medication (beta-blockers, SSRIs, etc.). Differentiation of the cause of ED relies on a thorough history and physical examination. Psychogenic causes of ED are often distinguished by the ability to obtain a physiologic erection (e.g., morning erection). A thorough history and physical examination are necessary for diagnosis, and treatment of underlying disorders is recommended. Phosphodiesterase type 5 (PDE-5) inhibitors, such as sildenafil and tadalafil, are the most common treatment for ED. The mechanism of action of PDE-5 inhibitors is by preventing the breakdown of cyclic guanosine monophosphate (GMP), which causes vasodilation. The use of PDE-5 inhibitors is strictly contraindicated in patients using nitroglycerin due to the risk of potentially fatal vasodilation and hypotension. Less common treatment options include prostaglandin-E1 injections, constriction devices, vacuum devices, and penile implants.

Varicocele, hydrocele, and hematocele

Common causes of enlarged scrotum include varicoceles, hydroceles, and hematoceles. A varicocele is the dilatation of the pampiniform plexus within the scrotum, seen in approximately 20% of the male population. While varicoceles do not cause infertility in all men, 40% of men who are infertile have varicoceles. Infertility in these cases is thought to be due to the interference with testicular thermal control. The dilated pampiniform plexus is palpable on physical exam, often described as a "bag of worms." Varicoceles are easily correctable by surgical repair if pain or infertility is a concern. A hydrocele is a collection of fluid within the tunica vaginalis of the scrotum. On physical exam, hydroceles can be transilluminated with light (homogeneous glow with no internal shadows). A hematocele is a collection of blood within the tunica vaginalis, often associated with trauma. Hematoceles are not transilluminated with light.

Testicular torsion

Testicular torsion is the torsion of the spermatic cord structures (ductus deferens and associated vessels and nerves, testicular artery, pampiniform plexus, genital branch of the genitofemoral nerve), resulting in loss of testicular blood supply. It causes severe, sudden onset of pain followed by scrotal swelling. It is often associated with abdominal pain, nausea, and vomiting. Testicular torsion is most commonly seen in neonates and children, but it may be associated with malignancy or trauma in the adult. This is a urologic emergency that requires immediate detorsion. Manual detorsion may be done by externally rotating the testis; however, surgical detorsion is the definitive treatment. Detorsion within 6 to 8 hours of presentation is associated with testicular salvage, with the risk of necrosis becoming significant if more than 12 hours pass. Patients often require surgical fixation of the testes to prevent recurrence.

Polycystic ovarian syndrome

Polycystic ovary syndrome is caused by an increase in leuteinizing hormone (LH). The elevated levels of LH cause increased ovarian stromal stimulation, leading to overproduction of androgen by the ovaries, followed by peripheral conversion of androgen to estrogen, which causes increased pituitary sensitivity to LH releasing factor, which leads to increased release of LH. The elevated LH level leads to enlarged, bilateral cystic ovaries. As a result of the hormone imbalances, these patients present with amenorrhea, infertility (due to anovulation), obesity, insulin resistance, and hirsutism. Diagnosis can be confirmed with laboratory testing, which shows increased LH, decreased FSH (the LH-to-FSH ratio is greater than 2:1), and increased testosterone. Due to increased estrogen exposure, these patients are at increased risk of endometrial cancer. Treatment includes weight loss and oral contraceptive pills. Gonadotropin analogs and clomiphene can be used to treat infertility. Metformin is used to treat insulin resistance, and spironolactone is used to treat hirsutism.

Ovarian cancer

Ovarian cancer is the most common cause of gynecologic cancer death in the United States. Most primary ovarian cancer can be divided into three types: epithelial ovarian carcinoma, germ cell tumors, and sex cord stromal tumors. Epithelial ovarian carcinoma comprises the majority of ovarian cancer (70%). Germ cell tumors are most common in adolescents. Symptoms that point to ovarian cancer include abdominal and pelvic pain, abdominal distension, and early satiety. Risk factors for ovarian cancer are nulliparity, family history of ovarian cancer, personal history of breast cancer, being *BRCA1* or *BRCA2* positive, and a history of hormone replacement therapy. Oral contraceptive pills have been found to be protective against ovarian cancer.

Ovarian dysgerminoma

Ovarian dysgerminomas are a type of malignant germ cell tumor that accounts for less than 2% of all ovarian cancer. However, dysgerminomas make up 65% of ovarian cancer in women younger than 20 years old. Five percent of dysgerminomas are seen in patients with dysgenetic gonads, such as streak ovaries in Turner (XO) syndrome. Dysgerminomas are associated with elevated lactate dehydrogenase (LDH), human chorionic gonadotropin (hCG), and inhibin. The majority (>75%) of dysgerminomas present as stage I and can be treated with surgical resection and unilateral salpingectomy, which preserves future fertility. Patients who present with more advanced stages of dysgerminoma require adjunct chemotherapy or radiation therapy.

Ovarian choriocarcinoma

Ovarian choriocarcinoma can be divided into the gestational or nongestational type. Gestational ovarian choriocarcinoma is caused by metastasis from primary uterine choriocarcinoma (a type of gestational trophoblastic neoplasia), or it may be primarily in the ovary as a result of ectopic pregnancy in the ovary. Nongestational ovarian choriocarcinoma is a very rare form of germ cell tumor. All forms of ovarian choriocarcinoma are highly malignant. Gestational choriocarcinoma is most common in women older than age 40 and is associated with hydatidiform moles. Nongestational choriocarcinoma is typically seen in younger women. Diagnosis is confirmed by elevated human chorionic gonadotropin (hCG) in the absence of pregnancy and the presence of placental trophoblastic cells on biopsy. Gestational choriocarcinoma of the ovary is treated with combination chemotherapy. Nongestational choriocarcinoma is so rare that there is no standardized treatment at this time.

Yolk sac tumors

Yolk sac tumors, also known as endodermal sinus tumors, are highly malignant germ cell tumors found in ovaries and testes. Yolk sac tumors are the most common testicular neoplasm in prepubertal males. Pure yolk sac tumors are associated with elevated α-fetoprotein levels (AFP), which are directly related to prognosis (AFP <1,000 ng/mL = good prognosis, AFP 1,000–10,000 ng/mL = intermediate prognosis, AFP >10,000 ng/mL = poor prognosis). Diagnosis can be confirmed with biopsy, which shows pathognomonic Schiller–Duval bodies in the majority of cases. Schiller–Duval bodies are perivascular formations of eosinic globules that also contain AFP. Most yolk sac tumors are discovered in their early stages before metastasis, but without treatment, these tumors are very aggressive and will lead to death. Yolk sac tumors are resistant to radiation therapy but are known to respond well to chemotherapy, accounting for the high cure rate.

Teratomas

Teratomas are germ cell tumors that consist of cells from more than one germ layer. Germ cells of the teratoma are able to differentiate into any tissue of the body, commonly including hair, teeth, and endocrine tissue. There are many different types of teratomas, ranging from mature teratomas that are benign to immature teratomas that are highly malignant. Struma ovarii is a rare form of teratoma that consists of thyroid tissue and can present as hyperthyroidism. The most common locations for teratomas are sacrococcygeal (57%) and in the gonads (30%). The most common gonadal location for teratomas is the ovary, very rarely occurring in testes. When teratomas do occur in the testes, they are most often malignant. Complications of ovarian teratoma include torsion (most common), rupture, and infection. Treatment of teratomas is by surgical removal.

Ovarian epithelial tumors

Epithelial tumors comprise 80% of all ovarian malignancies, arising from the epithelium covering the ovaries. Ovarian epithelium is derived from the same embryologic line of cells responsible for the fallopian tubes, uterus, and cervix. Thus, the two main types of ovarian epithelial tumors are serous (resembling cervical epithelium), and mucinous (resembling fallopian tube epithelium). Serous and mucinous cystadenomas are benign tumors; serous and mucinous cystadenocarcinomas are malignant tumors. Serous cystadenomas and cystadenocarcinomas tend to be bilateral. Classic histologic findings of serous cystadenocarcinoma are psammoma bodies. Metastatic disease is most commonly seen on peritoneal surfaces (i.e., the omentum and liver). A ruptured mucinous cystadenocarcinoma (either from ovary or appendix) may lead to a rare condition known as pseudomyxoma peritonei, which is a widespread intraperitoneal accumulation of mucinous material that leads to fibrosis and organ dysfunction.

Sex cord tumors

Sex cord tumors are also known as stromal tumors. The most common sex cord tumors in females are ovarian, derived from granulosa cells (granulosa cell tumors) or fibroblasts (fibromas). Rarely,

Sertoli or Leydig cell tumors may be seen in females, leading to hirsutism secondary to excess androgen production. Granulosa cell tumors produce excess estrogen and often lead to pseudoprecocious puberty in prepubescent girls. Call–Exner bodies, small follicles filled with eosinophilic material, are a classic histologic finding in granulosa cell tumors. Meigs syndrome is a triad of ascites, pleural effusion, and ovarian cancer (most commonly fibromas). Treatment of Meigs syndrome is symptomatic. Fibromas are benign, but their mitotically active counterparts, fibrosarcomas, are malignant.

Sex cord tumors in males are found in the testes, composed of Sertoli cells (Sertoli cell tumors) or Leydig cells (Leydig cell tumors). Rarely, granulosa cell tumors may be seen in males. Sertoli cell tumors arise from abnormal Sertoli cells native to the seminiferous tubule. These tumors are more commonly estrogenic than androgenic, resulting in gynecomastia and impotence. Sertoli cell tumors are all benign, and treatment is through orchiectomy. Leydig cell tumors are derived from testicular Leydig cells that produce testosterone. The excess testosterone is converted peripherally to estrogen, and it may lead to hirsutism in boys and gynecomastia in both boys and adult males. Leydig cell tumors tend to be benign in children, but they carry a small risk of malignancy in adults.

Gestational trophoblastic disease

Gestational trophoblastic disease originates in the placenta and can be classified into hydatidiform moles (partial or complete), invasive moles, and choriocarcinoma. Complete hydatidiform moles contain no fetal tissue, usually result from two identical paternal chromosomes, and are almost always 46, XX. Partial hydatidiform moles contain fetal tissue, result from fertilization of an ovum by two sperm, and may be 69, XXX or 69, XXY. Hydatidiform moles can present with vaginal bleeding, hyperemesis, and signs/symptoms of hyperthyroidism. There are no fetal heart tones, ultrasonography shows the classic snowstorm pattern, and human chorionic gonadotropin (hCG) levels are greater than 100,000 mIU/mL. Invasive moles and choriocarcinomas are categorized as gestational trophoblastic neoplasia. Invasive moles are diagnosed in the presence of myometrial invasion or pulmonary metastasis. Choriocarcinomas are rare trophoblastic malignancies developing from hydatidiform moles (50%), abortion (25%), full-term pregnancy (22%), or ectopic pregnancy (3%). They are comprised of sheets of large trophoblasts and hemorrhage. Hydatidiform moles are treated by careful suction and curettage. Treatment of invasive moles or choriocarcinoma may also include chemotherapy or hysterectomy. Response to therapy is monitored by measuring hCG levels.

Endometrial hyperplasia and endometrial carcinoma

Endometrial hyperplasia is caused by excess unopposed estrogen. The increased estrogen stimulation leads to abnormal endometrial gland proliferation and manifests as postmenopausal vaginal bleeding. Risk factors for endometrial hyperplasia are those that increase estrogen exposure, including hormone replacement therapy, polycystic ovarian syndrome, nulliparity, early menarche, late menopause, and granulosa cell tumors. These patients are at increased risk for endometrial carcinoma. Endometrial carcinoma is the most common malignancy of the female reproductive system, typically preceded by endometrial hyperplasia. In addition to risk factors for endometrial hyperplasia, risk factors for endometrial carcinoma include tobacco use, obesity (increased peripheral conversion of androgen to estrogen), diabetes, hypertension, and family history. Premenopausal oral contraceptive pills are protective against both endometrial hyperplasia and carcinoma. A postmenopausal female with vaginal bleeding should undergo an endometrial biopsy to test for hyperplasia or carcinoma. Treatment of endometrial hyperplasia is progestin (oral, intramuscular, or intrauterine). Treatment for endometrial carcinoma is hysterectomy.

Uterine leiomyoma and leiomyosarcoma

Uterine leiomyomas, also known as uterine fibroids, are benign tumors of the uterine smooth muscle. They occur more commonly in black than white women, with the peak incidence at 20 to 40 years of age. Leiomyomas present with changes in menstrual patterns, abdominal/pelvic pain and pressure, dyspareunia, miscarriage, or infertility. Malignant transformation is very rare. Diagnosis is usually by physical exam and ultrasonography. Treatment is with constant gonadotropin-releasing hormone (GnRH). Uterine leiomyosarcoma is a highly malignant cancer of the uterine smooth muscle. It does not arise from leiomyomas. It also occurs more commonly in black than white women, with the peak incidence in middle-aged women. Leiomyosarcoma is very aggressive with a high rate of recurrence. Treatment is with hysterectomy.

Human papilloma virus (HPV), cervical carcinoma in situ (CIS), and cervical cancer

Cervical cancer is the third most common malignancy in women but the leading cause of cancer-related deaths in women. For this reason, cytologic screening with Pap smear is recommended for all women 21 years and older with the option of additional human papillomavirus (HPV) testing for women 30 years and older. Virtually all cervical cancer is caused by HPV, specifically HPV 16, 18, and 45. The risk of cervical cancer increases with the use of oral contraceptives for five years or longer, tobacco use, family history, HIV infection, and risky sexual behavior (due to increased risk of HPV infection). Cervical dysplasia (carcinoma in situ–CIS) is classified as cervical intraepithelial neoplasia (CIN) 1, CIN 2, or CIN 3. On Pap smear, dysplasia is characterized by the presence of koilocytes. If left untreated, it can progress to invasive cervical cancer. Cervical CIS is usually asymptomatic; cervical cancer may present as postcoital bleeding, vaginal discomfort, vaginal discharge, and dysuria. Treatment of CIS depends on the degree of CIN, but it includes getting rid of abnormal cells by methods of cryosurgery, laser therapy, loop electrosurgical excision procedure, or cone biopsy. Treatment of cervical cancer usually consists of hysterectomy with or without radiation and chemotherapy.

Vaginal carcinoma

Primary vaginal carcinoma is very rare. The most common type of vaginal carcinoma is squamous cell carcinoma, which is found in the upper third of the vagina. Risk factors for primary vaginal carcinoma include human papillomavirus (HPV), history of cervical carcinoma, in-utero exposure to diethylstilbestrol (DES), prior hysterectomy, and tobacco use. Sarcoma botryoides (also known as embryonal rhabdomyosarcoma) is the most common type of vaginal cancer among children. The classic presentation of sarcoma botryoides is vaginal bleeding in a female younger than eight years old. On physical exam, the typical appearance is of a friable "bunch of grapes."

Benign breast tumors

Benign breast tumors include fibroadenoma, intraductal papilloma, and phyllodes tumor. Fibroadenomas are benign stromal tumors and are the most common cause of a breast mass in women younger than 25 years old. On physical exam, fibroadenomas are small, mobile masses that may increase in size and tenderness with estrogen exposure during pregnancy and menstruation. Fibroadenomas are not associated with an increased risk of malignancy. Intraductal papillomas are tumors of the lactiferous ducts, typically beneath the areola. They are the most common cause of

- 339 -

bloody nipple discharge in women younger than 50 years old. Intraductal papillomas are associated with a slightly increased risk of malignancy. Phyllodes tumors, in contrast to fibroadenomas and intraductal papillomas, are most common in elderly women. On histology, they have leaflike projections. Phyllodes tumors may become malignant.

Malignant breast cancer

Malignant breast tumors are most common in postmenopausal women. They can arise from mammary duct epithelium (ductal cancer) or lobular glands (lobular cancer). Risk factors include family history (*BRCA1* or *BRCA2*), increased estrogen exposure (early menarche, nulliparity, or late first birth, etc.), and obesity (increased peripheral conversion of androgen to estrogen). Types of breast cancer include infiltrating ductal carcinoma, lobular carcinoma in situ (LCIS), infiltrating lobular carcinoma, medullary carcinoma, ductal carcinoma in situ (DCIS), and Paget disease (listed in order of occurrence, most common to least common). Infiltrating ductal carcinoma presents as a "rock-hard" mass and is the most aggressive type of breast cancer. LCIS is always estrogen receptor/progesterone receptor (ER/PR) positive, and histology shows signet ring cells. Infiltrating lobular carcinoma often presents with multiple, bilateral lesions. Medullary carcinoma typically presents in younger women and has a good prognosis. A subtype of DCIS is comedocarcinoma, which has necrotic centers. Mammary Paget disease is an eczematous condition on the skin of the areola and nipple that indicates underlying breast carcinoma. ER-/PR-positive cancers are responsive to tamoxifen and raloxifene. Cancers that express Her1/ErbB2 are responsive to trastuzumab.

Benign prostatic hyperplasia (BPH)

BPH is an enlargement of the prostate that compresses the urethra and causes symptoms of urinary frequency, urgency, hesitancy, incomplete bladder emptying, and dribbling. BPH is seen in 90% of men by the age of 85 years. The enlargement of the prostate is caused by increased dihydrotestosterone (DHT), which is metabolized from testosterone by 5-α reductase. DHT binds to androgen receptors in the prostate, which results in increased growth and hyperplasia. Diagnosis can be made by presentation, digital rectal exam, and elevated prostate-specific antigen (PSA). Complications include urinary retention, renal insufficiency, recurrent urinary tract infections, gross hematuria, and bladder calculi. BPH is not considered a precursor to prostate cancer. Medication treatment options include α-1-receptor blockers, α-adrenergic receptor blockers, phosphodiesterase-5 enzyme inhibitors, 5-α reductase inhibitors, and anticholinergic agents. Surgical treatment options include transurethral resection of the prostate (TURP) and prostatectomy.

Prostate cancer

Prostate cancer is the most common noncutaneous cancer in males, and it is the second most common cause of cancer-related death in males. It commonly presents with urinary retention, back pain, and hematuria. Symptoms of advanced disease may include bone pain (due to metastasis to the bone), venous thrombosis, and cachexia. Diagnosis of prostate cancer is confirmed by biopsy. While an elevated prostate-specific antigen (PSA) level may point toward a diagnosis of prostate cancer, a low or normal PSA level does not exclude the diagnosis. Digital rectal exams may be helpful in diagnosis, but many patients with prostate cancer have normal exams. Treatment of localized prostate cancer includes radical prostatectomy, radiation therapy, and antiandrogen therapy. Metastatic prostate cancer has a very low cure rate, and management is based on palliation.

Testicular lymphoma

Testicular lymphoma is a type of non-Hodgkin lymphoma, usually found in a single testicle. It is the most common type of testicular cancer in older men. It most commonly presents with testicular enlargement. During evaluation, it is important to evaluate both testes with ultrasonography. The standard of treatment for testicular lymphoma is orchiectomy followed by chemotherapy and/or radiation therapy.

Testicular cancer

The risk of testicular cancer goes up significantly in patients with cryptorchidism (undescended testis). Orchiopexy, the surgical fixation of the testicle in the scrotum, allows for earlier detection of testicular cancer but does not decrease the risk of developing cancer. Testicular cancer can be divided into germ cell tumors and non-germ cell tumors. Non-germ cell tumors consist of Leydig cell tumors, Sertoli cell tumors, and testicular lymphoma (all discussed elsewhere). Testicular germ cell tumors account for the majority of cases and include seminomas, embryonal carcinomas, teratomas, choriocarcinomas, and yolk sac tumors. Testicular seminomas are the most common type of germ cell tumor and also the most common malignancy in men ages 15 to 35 years. Patients with seminoma typically present with a painless testicular lump, which can lead to infertility and hydrocele. Histology shows large cells with watery cytoplasm that have a "fried-egg" appearance. Treatment includes radical orchiectomy; radiation therapy; and, in cases of advanced disease, chemotherapy. Prognosis is very good overall.

Prenatal and perinatal counseling and screening

Prenatal and perinatal counseling and screening are encouraged for future parents with a known family history of inheritable diseases or increased risk of genetic abnormality. Women 35 or more years old are considered of advanced maternal age and should be counseled before pregnancy on increased risk of pregnancy-related hypertension, gestational diabetes, abnormal placental location that may require Cesarean section (i.e., placenta previa, placenta accreta), miscarriage, and chromosomal abnormalities. While all women are usually offered prenatal screening and more invasive diagnostic testing for chromosomal abnormalities, it is especially important to offer these tests to women of advanced maternal age. If either parent has a family or personal history of genetic diseases, they should be counseled on the risk of inheritance and offered specific testing (i.e., achondroplasia, neurofibromatosis, and cystic fibrosis).

Chromosomal screening and diagnostic testing options during pregnancy

The rate of Down syndrome (trisomy 21) and other trisomic disorders goes up significantly with maternal age. For example, the rate of Down syndrome is 1:1,667 in 20-year-old women, but it goes up to 1:385 in 35-year-old women and 1:107 in 40-year-old women. However, even with the higher risk, only 20% of all babies with trisomy 21 are born to women older than 35 years. First-trimester screening options for trisomy 21 are combined screening and quadruple screening. Quadruple screening is also used to detect Edwards' syndrome (trisomy 18) and Patau's syndrome (trisomy 13). Diagnostic tests include amniocentesis and chorionic villus sampling (CVS) but are more invasive and carry a small risk of miscarriage (less than 1%).

Interpretation of combined screening for trisomy 21 and quadruple screening for trisomy 21, 18, and 13

Combined screening for Down syndrome (trisomy 21) includes nuchal translucency testing by ultrasound, pregnancy-associated plasma protein A (PAPP-A), and human chorionic gonadotropin (hCG). The rate of detecting Down syndrome with nuchal translucency alone is approximately 70%. By combining the nuchal translucency results with PAPP-A and hCG, the detection rate improves to almost 85%. In a positive combined screen for trisomy 21, nuchal translucency thickness will be increased, hCG will be increased, and PAPP-A will be decreased. Quadruple screening for Down syndrome, Edwards' syndrome (trisomy 18), and Patau's syndrome (trisomy 13) includes α-fetoprotein (AFP), hCG, estriol, and inhibin A. Quadruple screening has a detection rate of about 80%. In trisomy 21, AFP will be decreased, hCG will be increased, estriol will be decreased, and inhibin A will be increased. In trisomy 18, AFP, estriol, hCG, and inhibin will all be decreased. In trisomy 13, AFP is typically high but hCG, estriol, and inhibin A may all be normal.

Autoimmune disease and recurrent pregnancy loss

Several autoimmune diseases are linked with recurrent spontaneous abortion (miscarriage) or fetal death. These include antiphospholipid antibody syndrome (APS), systemic lupus erythematosus (SLE), and autoimmune thyroid disorders. APS, also known as lupus anticoagulant syndrome or Hughes syndrome, is associated with anticardiolipin, lupus anticoagulant, and anti-β_2 glycoprotein I antibodies. SLE is associated with antinuclear antibody (ANA), anti-double-stranded DNA (dsDNA) antibody, and anticardiolipin antibody. Autoimmune thyroid disorders include Hashimoto's disease and Grave's disease, which are associated with thyroid-specific autoantibodies. Many patients with pregnancy loss due to thyroid disease are otherwise asymptomatic. Due to these risks, it is important to counsel patients with autoimmune disease when planning a pregnancy.

Spontaneous abortion

Abortion is the spontaneous or induced loss of an early pregnancy, defined as the period of pregnancy prior to fetal viability outside the uterus (less than 20 weeks of gestation). Spontaneous abortion may also be called miscarriage. Miscarriage can be classified as complete miscarriage, incomplete miscarriage, missed (threatened) miscarriage, or inevitable miscarriage. A complete miscarriage presents with vaginal bleeding and abdominal pain, which subsides following passage of tissue. On physical exam, the cervix is closed. An incomplete miscarriage presents with vaginal bleeding and abdominal pain. On physical exam, the cervix is open and products of conception are present. A missed miscarriage presents with vaginal bleeding and abdominal pain. On physical exam, the cervix is closed and there is no presence or history of passing tissue. An inevitable miscarriage presents with vaginal bleeding. On physical exam, the cervix is dilated and the products of conception are still in the uterus. Many missed miscarriages and almost all inevitable miscarriages go on to complete loss of pregnancy. The most common cause of miscarriage in the first trimester is chromosomal abnormality. The most common cause of miscarriage in the second trimester is maternal factors (i.e., insulin-dependent diabetes mellitus, hypertension, systemic lupus erythematosus, thyroid disorder, and maternal infection).

Placental complications of pregnancy

The most common placental complications include abnormal location (placenta previa), abnormal attachment (placenta accreta, placenta increta, and placenta percreta), and abruptio placentae. Placenta previa is when the placenta is implanted over the internal cervical os. It is the leading cause of hemorrhage in the third trimester, presenting with painless vaginal bleeding. Risk factors for placenta previa include history of Cesarean section. Patients with placenta previa require Cesarean section at the time of delivery. Placenta accreta is when the placenta is attached too deeply to the surface of the uterine wall, placenta increta is when the placenta has invaded the uterine myometrium, and placenta percreta is when the placenta has grown through the uterine wall. The biggest risk factor for abnormal placental attachment is prior Cesarean section. Patients with placenta accreta, increta, or percreta require Cesarean section at the time of delivery, and they often require hysterectomy. Abruptio placentae is the premature separation of the placenta from the uterus. Risk factors include maternal hypertension (most common), trauma, and cocaine use. Abruptio placentae presents as sudden onset vaginal bleeding and abdominal pain, often accompanied by fetal distress. If the mother or fetus becomes unstable, immediate delivery by Cesarean section is required.

Hypertension during pregnancy

Hypertension during pregnancy can be due to chronic hypertension, preeclampsia, eclampsia, or gestational hypertension (also known as pregnancy-induced hypertension). Chronic hypertension is defined as preexisting hypertension that continues during pregnancy. It is often diagnosed before 20 weeks of gestation. Preeclampsia is the new onset of hypertension after 20 weeks of gestation and proteinuria. Other symptoms may include visual disturbances, headache, right-upper-quadrant abdominal pain (due to liver swelling), hyperreflexia, and peripheral edema. Delivery is recommended at 37 weeks for mild preeclampsia and 34 weeks for severe preeclampsia. Preeclampsia may develop into eclampsia or HELLP syndrome. Eclampsia is new-onset grand mal seizure or unexplained coma in a patient with history of preeclampsia. Use prophylaxis against or treat seizures with intravenous magnesium sulfate. HELLP syndrome is a complication of eclampsia that consists of hemolysis, H, elevated liver enzymes, EL, and low platelets, LP. The only definitive treatment for eclampsia and HELLP syndrome is delivery. Gestational hypertension is defined as new-onset hypertension after 20 weeks without symptoms of preeclampsia. In gestational hypertension, blood pressure normalizes following delivery. Preferred agents for management of hypertension during pregnancy are methyldopa or nifedipine. Angiotensin-converting enzyme inhibitors (ACEIs) and angiotensin II receptor blockers (ARBs) are contraindicated during pregnancy due to teratogenicity.

Postpartum hemorrhage

Postpartum hemorrhage is defined as greater than 500 mL of blood loss following vaginal delivery and greater than 1,000 mL of blood loss following Cesarean section. It is the leading cause of maternal mortality worldwide. The most common cause of postpartum hemorrhage is uterine atony. Other causes include retained placenta, genital tract trauma, and thrombosis. Complications include hemorrhagic shock and potential death. Treatment includes management of shock (i.e., intravascular volume replacement) and treatment of the underlying cause. Oxytocin is used to treat uterine atony, manual removal of tissue is used to treat retained placenta, repair of lacerations is used in cases of trauma, and blood products are indicated in thrombosis. In some cases, surgery may be required for arterial ligation or hysterectomy.

Ectopic pregnancy

An ectopic pregnancy is a pregnancy that occurs outside of the endometrial cavity. The most common location for an ectopic pregnancy is in the ampulla of the fallopian tubes. The classic presentation for ectopic pregnancy is abdominal pain and vaginal bleeding in a patient with a

- 343 -

history of sexual activity and secondary amenorrhea. Diagnosis is confirmed with elevated serum human chorionic gonadotropin (hCG) levels and ultrasound. Risk factors for ectopic pregnancy include history of pelvic inflammatory disease, previous ectopic pregnancy, and tobacco use. Treatment options include expectant management (monitor hCG levels), methotrexate (abortifacient), and surgical removal. Methotrexate is the treatment of choice for unruptured ectopic pregnancies. If the patient is unstable, immediate surgical exploration is required for presumed ruptured ectopic pregnancy.

Polyhydramnios and oligohydramnios

Amniotic fluid is crucial to proper growth and development of the fetus. Polyhydramnios is an abnormally high level of amniotic fluid, and oligohydramnios is an inadequate volume of amniotic fluid. Amniotic fluid is composed mainly of fetal urine and is reduced by fetal swallowing. Thus, polyhydramnios may indicate an abnormality in fetal swallowing and oligohydramnios may indicate an abnormality in the fetal urinary tract. Complications of polyhydramnios include preterm labor and delivery, premature rupture of membranes, abruptio placenta, malpresentation, and postpartum hemorrhage. Polyhydramnios is also associated with an increased risk of fetal congenital anomaly. Complications of oligohydramnios include poor fetal lung development, fetal heart conduction abnormalities, umbilical cord compression, and fetal acidosis.

Premature ovarian failure

Premature ovarian failure is also known as primary ovarian insufficiency. It is defined as the failure of the ovary to function properly in a woman younger than 40 years old. It is caused by a complete loss of primordial follicles. It presents with secondary amenorrhea, hypoestrogenism, and elevated follicle stimulating hormone (FSH). Similar changes in a woman older than 40 years of age are considered to be the beginning of menopause. There is no treatment for primary premature ovarian failure. Ovarian insufficiency may also be secondary, caused by inadequate gonadotropin stimulation of the ovary. Important causes of secondary ovarian insufficiency include prolactinomas and Cushing syndrome. Secondary ovarian insufficiency may be corrected by treating the underlying causes.

Endometriosis and adenomyosis

Endometriosis is the presence of endometrial tissue in locations other than the uterine cavity. The most common sites of endometriosis are, in descending order, the ovaries, the posterior cul-de-sac, and the broad ligament. Adenomyosis, a subtype of endometriosis, is the presence of endometrial tissue within the uterine myometrium. Clinical features of endometriosis include dysmenorrhea, pelvic pain, dyschezia, and dyspareunia. It can also contribute to infertility. Diagnosis is one of exclusion, but it can be confirmed with laparoscopy and visualization of endometriosis. Medical treatment of endometriosis consists of combination oral contraceptive pills, danazol, and gonadotropin-releasing hormone analogs. Surgical treatment consists of removal of the abnormally located endometrial tissue.

Drugs that have adverse effects on the reproductive system

There are many drugs with known adverse sexual effects. Gynecomastia, the enlargement of breast tissue in males, can be caused by spironolactone, digitalis, cimetidine, chronic alcohol use, estrogens, ketoconazole, and marijuana. Hot flashes can be caused by tamoxifen and clomiphene. Trazodone, a tetracyclic antidepressant, can cause priapism (persistent erection). Antipsychotics such as haloperidol, thioridazine, and chlorpromazine can cause hyperprolactinemia, leading to galactorrhea. Many antidepressants such as selective serotonin reuptake inhibitors (SSRIs), selective norepinephrine reuptake inhibitors (SNRIs), tricyclic antidepressants (TCAs), and monoamine oxidase inhibitors (MAOIs) can cause sexual dysfunction (i.e., erectile dysfunction, anorgasmia). This is a common cause of poor medication adherence. It is important to discuss nonadherence in these cases and come up with alternatives. Antidepressants with the least risk of sexual adverse effects are bupropion (increases norepinephrine and dopamine) and mirtazapine (tetracyclic antidepressant).

Teratogenic drugs

Teratogenic effects of phenytoin include craniofacial anomalies (broad nasal bridge, cleft palate, microcephaly). Valproic acid is a folic acid antagonist that can lead to fetal neural tube defects. Angiotensin-converting enzyme (ACE) inhibitors and angiotension II receptor blockers (ARBs) have been shown to cause renal dysplasia. Lithium leads to Ebstein's anomaly of the heart (atrialization of right ventricle). Many antibiotics should be avoided during pregnancy, including sulfonamides (kernicterus), aminoglycosides (ototoxicity), fluoroquinolones (cartilage damage), tetracyclines (discolored teeth), ribavirin (teratogenic), griseofulvin (teratogenic), chloramphenicol ("gray baby"), and metronidazole (teratogenic if given in first trimester).

Klinefelter syndrome

Klinefelter syndrome occurs in 1 out of every 850 males and is also referred to as XXY syndrome. Patients are male but have an extra X chromosome in the form of a Barr body (inactive). Patients with Klinefelter syndrome have testicular atrophy and are typically taller than their peers and have long extremities. Atrophic testes produce abnormally low levels of testosterone and inhibin, resulting in increased levels of follicle-stimulating hormone (FSH), leuteinizing hormone (LH), and estrogen. This alteration in hormones leads to gynecomastia, female hair distribution, eunuchoid body shape, and infertility. Klinefelter syndrome is associated with learning disabilities including delayed speech and language skills, but affected males may have normal intelligence.

Turner syndrome

Turner syndrome occurs in 1 out of every 3,000 females and is also referred to as XO syndrome. Patients are female but only have one X chromosome and are missing the second X chromosome, the Barr body. Patients with Turner syndrome have short stature, cystic hygroma (webbing of posterior neck), low hairline at the back of the neck, and lack of secondary sexual characteristics. These patients also have ovarian dysgenesis, leading to dysfunctional ovaries composed of fibrous tissue (streak ovaries on ultrasonography). This condition results in decreased estrogen, leading to increased leuteinizing hormone (LH) and follicle-stimulating hormone (FSH). Turner syndrome is the most common cause of primary dysmenorrhea. Cardiac complications include coarctation of the aorta or aortic valve abnormalities.

Hermaphroditism, pseudohermaphroditism, and androgen insensitivity syndrome

True hermaphroditism is when both ovarian and testicular tissue are present, causing ambiguous genitalia. It is very rare. Pseudohermaphroditism is when the female or male internal reproductive organs do not match the external genitalia. In female pseudohermaphrodites, the genotype is XX and there are ovaries; however, external genitalia are virilized or ambiguous. This can be caused by inappropriate exposure to androgens during early fetal development. In male pseudohermaphrodites, the genotype is XY and there are testes present; however, the external genitalia are female or ambiguous. This can be caused by various mechanisms, but the most common cause is androgen insensitivity syndrome. Androgen insensitivity syndrome is also known as testicular feminization. It occurs when an XY male with testes has defective androgen receptors. There are no internal female reproductive organs, but the defective receptors lead to external female genitalia, a rudimentary vagina, and lack of sexual body hair. The condition is often discovered at the time of puberty, when testes descend and appear as masses in the labia majora. This condition results in increased testosterone, estrogen, and leuteinizing hormone (LH).

Female fertility drugs

The most common fertility drug is clomiphene, which is a selective estrogen receptor modulator (SERM). It is an oral pill that acts by binding to estrogen receptors in the hypothalamus, interfering with the normal negative feedback loop. The inhibition of the negative feedback loop leads to increased levels of gonadotropin-releasing hormone (GnRH), which leads to increased release of leuteinizing hormone (LH) and follicle-stimulating hormone (FSH) from the pituitary. Elevated LH levels force ovulation in women who are not ovulating normally. Other options for treatment of female infertility include injectable forms of human chorionic gonadotropin (hCG), FSH, or GnRH. These hormones will also stimulate ovulation.

Contraception

There are many different types of contraceptives available, including hormones (estrogen and/or progesterone), physical barrier methods (condoms, etc.), and intrauterine devices (IUDs). Definitive forms of contraception include fallopian tube ligation and vasectomy. Oral contraceptive pills come in the form of progestin-only pills (POPs) or combination progesterone and estrogen pills. Progestin-only contraception is a form of contraception that is good for women who are not able to take estrogen (i.e., those with a history of deep venous thrombosis or lactating women). POPs work by suppressing ovulation and thickening cervical mucus, which inhibits sperm motility. Other progestin-only contraception includes implants, intramuscular injections, and intrauterine devices. The main mechanism of combination progesterone and estrogen oral contraception is the inhibition of ovulation. The reliability of ovulation suppression is much higher in combination oral contraception than POPs due to the synergistic effect of estrogen and progesterone. Constant low-level estrogen and progesterone prevent ovulation by suppressing the leuteinizing hormone (LH) surge. The two main types of IUDs are progesterone IUDs (effective for 5 years) and copper IUDs (effective for 10 years). IUDs work by thickening cervical mucus and inhibiting sperm motility. There is also a component of mechanical barrier because the IUD blocks the entrance to the fallopian tubes. The most effective reversible forms of contraception are combination oral contraception pills and IUDs.

Progesterone therapy

Progesterone is an important hormone during the menstrual cycle that is responsible for preparing the uterus for pregnancy by increasing endometrial vascularization. Progesterone from the corpus luteum is also important in maintaining early pregnancies. During pregnancy, progesterone helps prepare the breasts for milk production and lactation. Progesterone agonists (or analogs) may be used to help maintain early pregnancy, as contraceptives (either alone or in combination with estrogen), or to treat secondary amenorrhea (withdrawal causes menstruation). Progesterone decreases endometrial growth, so it may be added during hormone therapy to decrease risk of endometrial cancer with unopposed estrogen. It may also be used alone in the prevention or as part

- 346 -

of the treatment for endometrial hyperplasia. Adverse effects of progesterone include headache, nausea, and breast tenderness.

Estrogen agonists

Estrogen agonists (also known as analogs) include ethinyl estradiol, diethylstilbestrol (DES), and mestranol. Their mechanism of action is by binding to and activating estrogen receptors. Estrogen analogs are indicated in the treatment of ovarian failure, menstrual abnormalities (i.e., dysmenorrhea), and postmenopausal symptoms (hormone replacement therapy) in women. In men, estrogen analogs may be used to help treat androgen-dependent prostate cancer. Although hormone replacement therapy is protective against osteoporosis and can alleviate postmenopausal symptoms (i.e., hot flashes), it is very controversial because unopposed estrogen is associated with an increased risk of breast cancer, uterine cancer, heart disease, and stroke. Other adverse effects of estrogen analogs include postmenopausal vaginal bleeding, and thrombosis. In-utero exposure to DES is associated with an increased risk of developing adenocarcinoma of the vagina. Estrogen analogs are strictly contraindicated in patients with history of estrogen-receptor-positive breast cancer or deep venous thrombosis.

Selective estrogen receptor modulators (SERMs)

SERMs act as partial estrogen agonists or antagonists, binding only to certain estrogen receptors and thus having different effects. Clomiphene binds to estrogen receptors in the hypothalamus, preventing the normal feedback inhibition loop. This leads to an uninhibited release of gonadotropin releasing hormone (GnRH) from the hypothalamus and subsequent pituitary release of leuteinizing hormone (LH) and follicle-stimulating hormone (FSH), which stimulate ovulation. Clomiphene can be used in cases of polycystic ovarian syndrome and infertility to induce ovulation. Adverse effects of clomiphene include hot flashes, visual disturbances, and multiple gestation. Tamoxifen is a SERM that works as an antagonist on estrogen receptors in the breast and as an agonist on receptors in the uterus. Tamoxifen can be used to treat and prevent estrogen-receptor-positive breast cancer; however, it may also be associated with an increased risk of uterine cancer. Raloxifene acts as an estrogen agonist in bone, which decreases bone resorption and can be used to treat or prevent osteoporosis. An adverse effect of raloxifene is an increased risk for venous thrombosis.

Stimulants used for induction of labor

Oxytocin is a hormone secreted by the posterior pituitary that increases intracellular calcium and causes contraction of the uterus. Uterine oxytocin receptors increase 300-fold in preparation for labor and delivery. Oxytocin may be given intravenously to stimulate uterine contractions and induce labor. It can also be used following delivery to treat postpartum hemorrhage.
Cervical ripening (softening) precedes delivery and is caused by an increase in cyclooxygenase-2, which causes an increase in prostaglandin in the cervix. This causes cervical ripening through a series of effects including small-vessel dilation, collagen degradation, increased hyaluronic acid and glycosaminoglycans, and interleukin-8 release. Prostaglandin agonists such as dinoprostone (suppository) and misoprostol (suppository or oral pill) can be given to soften the cervix and induce labor.

Inhibitors of labor

Tocolytics are medications that are used to stop uterine contractions and are indicated in the treatment of preterm labor. Tocolytics include magnesium sulfate, ritodrine, terbutaline, nifedipine, and indomethacin. The exact mechanism of magnesium sulfate on the uterus is unknown, but tocolysis is thought to be achieved through calcium inhibition. Ritodrine and terbutaline are beta$_2$ agonists that result in uterine smooth muscle relaxation. Nifedipine and indomethacin may be used for tocolysis but are considered second-line treatment options. Nifedipine is a calcium channel blocker that inhibits uterine smooth-muscle contraction. Indomethacin is a prostaglandin inhibitor, which decreases prostaglandin activity that may soften the cervix and induce labor.

Stimulators and inhibitors of lactation

Two essential hormones in lactation are prolactin and oxytocin. Prolactin is secreted from the anterior pituitary and stimulates mammary gland growth and initiates milk synthesis. Prolactin secretion is both positively and negatively regulated, but dopamine plays a key role in prolactin inhibition. Oxytocin is released from the posterior pituitary in response to stimulation by the infant's suckling. Oxytocin causes smooth-muscle contraction of the lactiferous ducts, leading to milk extraction. Bromocriptine is a dopamine analog that works to inhibit lactation by inhibiting prolactin. Antidopaminergic agents such as metoclopramide may help to induce lactation, but this is still being studied.

Male infertility

Causes of male infertility include endocrinopathies (i.e., hypogonadotropic hypogonadism, hyperprolactinemia, congenital adrenal hyperplasia [CAH]) and antisperm antibodies. Hypogonadotropic hypogonadism is caused by low levels of gonadotropin-releasing hormone (GnRH), which leads to low follicle stimulating hormone (FSH), leuteinizing hormone (LH), and androgen production. Many of these patients respond to treatment with GnRH replacement. Hyperprolactinemia can be treated with bromocriptine, a dopamine antagonist that inhibits prolactin. CAH may respond to therapy with glucocorticoids or testosterone replacement. Antisperm antibodies are a rare cause of infertility and may be treated with immunosuppression using cyclic steroids.

Androgen agonists and antagonists

Testosterone is the naturally occurring androgen in the male. It may be given exogenously to act as an androgen agonist. It is used to treat hypogonadism (low testosterone levels) and sexual dysfunction in males. In females, it may be used to treat postmenopausal symptoms (i.e., hot flashes) and sexual dysfunction. Testosterone therapy is controversial due to adverse effects, which include the potential for increased risk of prostate cancer, hirsutism, and cardiovascular disease.

Androgen antagonists include 5-α-reductase inhibitors and competitive inhibitors. 5-α-reductase is responsible for the conversion of testosterone to the more potent dihydrotestosterone (DHT). The most common 5-α-reductase inhibitor is finasteride. Finasteride may be used to treat benign prostatic hyperplasia and male pattern baldness, conditions that result from elevated levels of DHT. Competitive androgen receptor inhibitors include flutamide and spironolactone. Flutamide is indicated in the treatment of prostate carcinoma (in combination with continuous leuprolide). Spironolactone is a common antiandrogen used in the treatment of polycystic ovarian syndrome to prevent hirsutism. Adverse effects of antiandrogens include gynecomastia and amenorrhea.

Gonadotropin-releasing hormone (GnRH) agonist and antagonist agents

In normal physiology, GnRH is released in a pulsatile pattern from the hypothalamus. This pulsatile release stimulates release of leuteinizing hormone (LH) and follicle-stimulating hormone (FSH) from the anterior pituitary. If GnRH is continuously present at high levels, it inhibits gonadotropin (LH and FSH) release. Due to the difference in the pulsatile and continuous effects of GnRH, GnRH analogs can be used as both agonists and antagonists. The most common GnRH analog is leuprolide. If leuprolide is given to mimic the physiologic pulsatile GnRH release, it can be used to treat infertility. If given continuously, leuprolide can be used to help treat prostate cancer or uterine fibroids. The adverse effects of leuprolide include nausea, vomiting, hot flashes, and emotional lability.

Abortifacients

Abortifacients are used to cause loss of pregnancy, both elective and medically indicated. They include mifepristone and methotrexate. Mifepristone is a progesterone antagonist, and it works via competitive inhibition of the progesterone receptor. By blocking progesterone, the early pregnancy is no longer supported and is lost. Methotrexate is an antimetabolite that blocks dihydrofolate reductase, which is responsible for folate production and required for DNA synthesis in replicating cells. By blocking folate production, methotrexate inhibits the growth of the early trophoblastic cells and the pregnancy is lost. The abortifacients are followed by misoprostol, a prostaglandin that softens the cervix in preparation to pass the products of conception. Methotrexate is the medical treatment for nonruptured ectopic pregnancies.

Antineoplastic drugs used in the prevention or treatment of breast cancer

Tamoxifen and raloxifene are selective estrogen receptor modulators (SERMs) that may be used to prevent or treat estrogen receptor (ER)-positive breast cancer. Both tamoxifen and raloxifene act as estrogen antagonists in the breast. However, tamoxifen works as an estrogen agonist on the uterine endometrium and may increase the risk of uterine cancer. Raloxifene is not associated with an increased risk of uterine cancer.

Anastrozole and exemestane are aromatase inhibitors that can be used to treat breast cancer. Aromatase is an enzyme responsible for the peripheral conversion of androgen to estrogen. By competitively inhibiting aromatase, these medications can decrease the progression of estrogen-sensitive breast cancers.

Emotional and behavioral factors that may influence lactation

Maternal stress and fatigue can adversely affect milk production and lactation. An important hormone in lactation is prolactin, produced and secreted by the anterior pituitary. Inhibitors of prolactin include dopamine and norepinephrine, which increase naturally with stress. Thus, a relaxed maternal state is very important for breastfeeding women. This can be quite difficult for new mothers due to the many social and emotional changes with which childbirth are associated, but lactation counseling and support groups may help in this process.

High-risk sexual behaviors and their associated risks

High-risk sexual behavior includes unprotected sexual intercourse (without a condom), unprotected mouth-to-genital contact, early sexual activity (younger than 18 years old), multiple sexual partners, having a high-risk sexual partner, anal sex, sex with an intravenous drug user, and sex in exchange for money. Patients should be counseled on the health dangers of high-risk sexual behavior including sexually transmitted diseases, HIV, and unplanned pregnancy. Patients participating in such activities should be offered resources such as counseling or social work for counseling, safe housing options, legal support, etc.

Family planning and pregnancy

Family planning should be encouraged for every patient. Planned pregnancy and childbirth can ease the process and decrease complications associated with labor, deliver, and the care of newborns. Education of potential parents should include family history/genetic risk, health education during pregnancy, education regarding labor and delivery, and education about infant care. Regular and consistent prenatal care should be available. Routine prenatal testing includes rubella, syphilis (rapid plasma reagin), varicella, group-B streptococcus (GBS), HIV, hepatitis B and C, and ABO and Rh screening. Patients who are GBS-positive should be treated with penicillin during labor and delivery. Pregnant women should be routinely screened for gestational diabetes. Screening for Down syndrome is recommended, especially for women older than age 35.

Appropriate response to minors requesting abortions or contraception

Patients younger than 18 years do not require parental permission when requesting contraception or abortion. Patients younger than 18 years who are pregnant are considered adults. In these cases, the patients are able to make their own medical decisions. If the parents of the patient request information regarding their child, a medical professional must first receive permission from the patient before providing any information.

Traumatic stress syndrome, violence, and rape and the appropriate response

A history of traumatic stress syndrome or personal violence such as rape and physical or emotional abuse can have a significant effect on patient health. It is important to provide a safe environment for victims to receive more treatment. Patients suffering from traumatic stress syndrome should be referred to receive consistent counseling from a trained professional. Patients who have been victims of sexual violence should be seen by a medical provider and receive a rape kit, and law enforcement should be contacted.

Endocrine System

Pancreas

Two outpouchings of the foregut portion of the duodenum known as pancreatic buds give rise to the pancreas. The dorsal pancreatic bud is the larger of the two buds and will form the body and tail of the pancreas. The smaller ventral bud rotates to fuse with the dorsal pancreatic bud and forms the head of the pancreas and the uncinate process. As the two buds fuse, the duct of the ventral bud connects to the distal portion of the duct in the dorsal bud, thus forming the pancreatic duct. While the proximal portion of the dorsal duct does not usually persist throughout development, it is maintained as an accessory pancreatic duct in some individuals. Rarely, the ventral bud may be divided into two lobes, which can aberrantly wrap around the duodenum. This abnormality results in the development of an annular pancreas and can obstruct the duodenum.

Gonads

The gonads, which begin to develop during the fifth week, originate as a thickening of mesothelium and its underlying mesenchyme on the mesonephros, an embryonic excretory structure. This thickening grows to form the gonadal ridge. Finger-like extensions of epithelial tissue eventually extend into the mesenchyme of the gonadal ridge and are referred to as gonadal cords. The primordial germ cells are migratory, and though derived from the wall of the umbilical vessel, they make their way to the gonadal ridge and ultimately enter gonadal cords. At this stage, the primitive gonad is indifferent, consisting of a cortex and a medulla. After week 7, changes are sex specific. Embryos possessing two X chromosomes will develop ovaries, which are primarily derived from cortex of the indifferent gonad. In XY embryos, on the other hand, development of the medulla predominates and gives rise to the testes.

Testes

After week 7, male-specific development begins and is initiated by the action of the SRY gene, which directs the synthesis of a transcription factor known as testis determining factor (TDF). TDF promotes a number of changes, beginning with branching and subsequent fusion of gonadal cords extending into the medulla to form the rete testis. More peripheral gonadal cords form the seminiferous tubules, which contain both spermatogonia derived from primordial germ cells and Sertoli cells. Mesenchyme surrounding the seminiferous tubules form Leydig cells, which importantly secrete the testosterone that directs male-specific changes of the Wolffian duct. In response to testosterone, the Wolffian duct differentiates into the vas deferens, the seminal vesicle, and the epididymis. The fetal testes also secretes anti-Müllerian hormone during fetal development. This hormone inhibits differentiation of female reproductive structures, including the uterus and oviducts. During testicular development, a fibrous casing surrounding the testes forms, called the tunica albuginea.

The testes comprise highly coiled seminiferous tubules and clusters of endocrine cells in the space surrounding the tubules, Leydig cells. The seminiferous tubule is the site of spermatogenesis, and the developing sperm cells are arranged concentrically with the least mature cells located at the periphery of the tubule and late spermatids near the lumen. The seminiferous tubules also contain large Sertoli cells, which stretch across the radius of the tubule and nourish the developing sperm cells. The Leydig cells outside of the table are the site of testosterone production. In addition to promoting the development of male secondary sex characteristics, testosterone acts to promote spermatogenesis. It exerts negative feedback on the hypothalamus and anterior pituitary, thereby reducing levels of LH and FSH and tempering its own production.

The testes are controlled by the hypothalamus, which produces gonadotropin-releasing hormone (GnRH). GnRH signals to the gonadotropes within the anterior pituitary, stimulating these cells to secrete follicle stimulating hormone (FSH) and luteinizing hormone (LH). FSH promotes the action of Sertoli cells, cells that are present within the seminiferous tubule and that function to nourish developing sperm cells. Spermatogenesis also requires testosterone, which is secreted by Leydig cells outside of the seminiferous tubules in response to LH. The levels of both FSH and LH are modulated by negative feedback mechanisms. Sertoli cells release the peptide hormone inhibin, which prevents secretion of FSH from the pituitary gland. Testosterone inhibits both the hypothalamus and the pituitary, thereby reducing the secretion of GnRH and LH.

Hypothalamus

The hypothalamus is derived from the anterior end of the diencephalon, and thus comprises nervous tissue. The tissue is organized into a variety of nuclei. Several of these nuclei contain cell bodies whose axons extend to the posterior pituitary via the hypothalamo-hypophyseal tract. Although the anterior pituitary is also closely associated with the hypothalamus, the linkage is vascular rather than cellular. The portal hypophyseal vessel joins a plexus of capillaries on the ventral surface of the hypothalamus to a plexus of capillaries within the anterior pituitary. Because blood travels through both capillary beds in succession, this portal venous system allows the hypothalamus to send chemical signals directly to the anterior pituitary. The anterior pituitary has five distinct types of secretory cells: somatotropes, lactotropes, corticotropes, thyrotropes, and gonadotropes.

The hypothalamus directs the action of both the anterior and posterior pituitary. Since several of the hypothalamic nuclei contain cell bodies that extend into the posterior lobe of the pituitary gland, the hormones secreted by the posterior pituitary are actually synthesized in the hypothalamus. They then travel to the posterior lobe of the pituitary in secretory granules that move along the length of the axons in the hypothalamo-hypophyseal tract. By contrast, the hypothalamus exerts hormonal control over the anterior pituitary, which is itself a glandular structure. The hypothalamus produces a variety of releasing hormones, which travel to the anterior lobe of the pituitary through the portal hypophyseal vessel. These hypothalamic hormones regulate the release of anterior pituitary hormones.

Meningitis, Langerhans cell histiocytosis, and sarcoidosis may cause hypothalamic dysfunction. The most common clinical finding of hypothalamic dysfunction is central diabetes insipidus, which occurs because no ADH is synthesized by the hypothalamus. Signs of hypopituitarism may also be evident, because releasing hormones are not made and released by the hypothalamus, which causes dysregulation of the anterior pituitary that may result in increased or decreased hormone production. For example, decreased synthesis of corticotropin-releasing hormone (CRH) from the hypothalamus results in decreased release of ACTH from the anterior pituitary because CRH stimulates ACTH release. However, dopamine from the hypothalamus normally inhibits prolactin release by the anterior pituitary; therefore, pathology causing decreased dopamine synthesis in the hypothalamus results in hyperprolactinemia.

Ovaries

Females lack a Y chromosome and therefore the SRY gene that directs the formation of male-specific gonadal development. In its absence, both autosomal and X-linked genes promote ovarian organogenesis. These genes stimulate the gonadal cords in the indifferent gonad to form both the rudimentary rete ovarii, which breaks down, and cortical cords. The cortical cords take in migratory primordial germ cells and increase in size before separating themselves into distinct primordial follicles at approximately 16 weeks. Each primordial follicle contains one oogonium derived from a primordial germ cell. The oogonia eventually turn into primary oocytes, and females are born with approximately 2 million of these egg precursor cells. Postnatal formation of additional primary oocytes does not occur. During ovarian development, a fibrous casing surrounding the ovaries forms, called the tunica albuginea.

During the follicular phase of the menstrual cycle, the ovary contains many primordial follicles, one of which becomes dominant as nearby follicles undergo atresia. The follicle consists of the immature ovum surrounded by layers of cells known as the theca externa, the theca interna, and the granulosa. The cells of the granulosa secrete estrogen, which stimulates thickening of the uterine lining. The low levels of estrogen present early in the follicular phase inhibit FSH and LH. However, a surge in estrogen at the end of the follicular phase exerts positive feedback on FSH and LH, which in turn leads to ovulation. The luteal phase follows, during which the granulosa cells and theca cells divide to form the corpus luteum. Luteal cells produce estrogen and progesterone, which act to further thicken and maintain the endometrium. Together, estrogen and progesterone also lead to a decrease in FSH and LH. This decrease prompts the degeneration of the corpus luteum, a sharp decline in estrogen and progesterone levels, and breakdown of the endometrium.

Pituitary gland

The two parts of the pituitary gland are derived from ectoderm. The anterior pituitary (adenohypophysis) begins to form at week 3 when ectoderm on the roof of the pharynx evaginates, forming a pouch known as the hypophyseal diverticulum or Rathke's pouch. This pouch separates from the oral cavity by the eighth week and contacts an outpouching of the ventral ectodermal wall of the diencephalon, the neurohypophyseal diverticulum. The cells of the hypophyseal diverticulum proliferate to form the anterior lobe of the pituitary, which is glandular. The cells of the neurohypophyseal diverticulum proliferate to gives rise to the posterior pituitary (neurohypophysis); therefore, this portion of the pituitary is comprised of nervous tissue.

The hormones secreted by the posterior pituitary are synthesized in hypothalamic nuclei. The hormones are carried via secretory granules through the axons that extend into the posterior pituitary, where they are secreted into the bloodstream. The supraoptic nuclei synthesize ADH, a hormone that regulates blood osmolarity. ADH targets cells lining the late distal tubules and collecting ducts, promoting transport of aquaporins to the cell membranes. These aquaporins allow for the reabsorption of water, thereby decreasing blood osmolarity. The paraventricular nuclei produce oxytocin, which targets breast and uterine tissues. Oxytocin stimulates milk release by promoting contraction of myoepithelial cells in the breast. Oxytocin also has a role in promoting the progression of labor. Uterine smooth muscle cells have increased sensitivity to oxytocin due to the upregulation of oxytocin receptors. Furthermore, oxytocin secretion is increased during labor and acts to stimulate uterine contractions.

Causes of posterior pituitary dysfunction include infections such as meningitis, sarcoidosis, and Langerhans cell histiocytosis. The posterior pituitary releases ADH (vasopressin) into the bloodstream, which regulates blood osmolarity by promoting reabsorption of water in the distal tubules and collecting ducts of nephrons. Posterior pituitary dysfunction occurs when not enough ADH is secreted and the body's ability to concentrate urine is impaired, resulting in central diabetes insipidus. Central diabetes insipidus is characterized by polydipsia, polyuria, and hypernatremia with inappropriately hypotonic urine. Diabetes insipidus can also occur when the kidneys do not respond to secreted ADH, termed nephrogenic diabetes insipidus. Causes of nephrogenic diabetes insipidus include chronic renal disease, drugs such as lithium and demeclocycline, and aquaporin gene mutations.

Syndrome of inappropriate ADH secretion (SIADH) has a variety of causes, including infection (pneumonia or tuberculosis), drugs (such as carbamazepine), trauma and stress. Tumors, most commonly small cell lung cancer, may also secrete an ADH-like substance and cause SIADH. Excessive circulating ADH causes the retention of free water through stimulating the production of more aquaporin channels in the distal convoluted tubules and collecting ducts of the nephron. Therefore, urine concentration is inappropriately high. This results in hyponatremia (typically Na less than 130 mEq/L), which leads to brain swelling, altered mental status, and even seizures. Treatment of SIADH is water restriction. Refractory cases may be treated with demeclocycline, a nephrotoxic antibiotic that decreases the kidney's response to ADH.

The anterior pituitary gland has five distinct types of secretory cells: somatotropes, lactotropes, corticotropes, thyrotropes, and gonadotropes. The somatotropes secrete growth hormone (GH), which targets the liver and directs it to synthesize insulin-like growth factor (IGF). In addition to its tropic effects, GH can also directly induce bone growth. The lactotropes secrete prolactin, which targets mammary tissue and promotes milk production. The corticotropes secrete ACTH, a tropic hormone that targets the three zones of the adrenal cortex, which in turn produce a variety of steroid hormones. Thyrotropes secrete thyroid-stimulating hormone (TSH), a hormone that promotes the action of the thyroid gland. Gonadotropes release follicle-stimulating hormone (FSH) and luteinizing hormone (LH). These gonadotropins target the ovaries and testes, influencing gametogenesis and hormone production within the gonads.

The hypothalamus regulates the action of the anterior pituitary by producing a variety of releasing hormones, also known as hypophysiotropic hormones. These hormones travel to the anterior lobe of the pituitary through the portal hypophysial vessel. The releasing hormones include:
- Corticotropin-releasing hormone (CRH) is a peptide hormone. Involved in the stress response, it stimulates the secretion of ACTH and β-LPH.
- Dopamine (prolactin-inhibiting factor or PIH) is a catecholamine. Although it also acts as a neurotransmitter within the nervous system, its secretion from the hypothalamus inhibits the secretion of prolactin.
- Gonadotropin-releasing hormone (GnRH) is a peptide hormone that stimulates the secretion of luteinizing hormone (LH) and follicle-stimulating hormone (FSH).
- GH-releasing hormone, a peptide hormone, directs the secretion of growth hormone.
- Somatostatin (GH-inhibiting hormone) prevents the secretion of both growth hormone and TSH.
- Thyrotropin-releasing hormone (TRH) is a tripeptide that stimulates the secretion of TSH and prolactin.

Thyroid gland

At 24 days of gestation, the development of the thyroid gland begins when endodermal tissue on the floor of the pharynx thickens. The endodermal thickening descends into the neck, and the resulting pouch, the thyroid diverticulum, is connected to the pharynx via the thyroglossal duct. This duct typically degenerates prior to the seventh week of gestation. The foramen cecum, a remnant of the thyroglossal duct's entry point to the pharynx, is a small invagination found at the back of the tongue that persists throughout development. If the thyroglossal duct degeneration is incomplete, a thyroglossal duct cyst forms and presents as a mass on the neck that moves upon swallowing.

The thyroid gland has two lobes joined by the thyroid isthmus. It is composed of multiple follicles, each of which consists of a ring of epithelial cells surrounding a lumen filled with protein known as the colloid. The colloid contains the glycoprotein thyroglobulin, which plays a key role in the synthesis the primary hormones secreted by the thyroid gland, T_3 (triiodothyronine) and T_4 (thyroxine). Thyroglobulin is secreted into the colloid by the follicle cells. These cells also transport iodide into the colloid, where it is oxidized and used to iodinate thyroglobulin during thyroid hormone synthesis. When stimulated by TSH, the follicle cells endocytose iodinated thyroglobulin. T_3 and T_4 are then uncoupled from thyroglobulin and released outside the follicle, a region that is richly vascularized. This region also contains parafollicular cells, which release calcitonin. T_3 and T_4 have a variety of functions and are involved in regulating growth, CNS development, and metabolism. Calcitonin acts to decrease blood calcium levels.

There are several types of thyroiditis. Acute and subacute thyroiditis is associated with thyroid gland tenderness. Acute thyroiditis is usually bacterial in origin (*S. aureus*) and associated with enlarged cervical lymph nodes. Subacute thyroiditis (de Quervain thyroiditis) is viral in origin, most commonly after an upper respiratory tract infection, and does not have enlarged cervical lymph nodes. A third type, Riedel thyroiditis, results in hypothyroidism due to progressive fibrosis of the thyroid gland, which is nontender.

The most common types of autoimmune thyroid pathology are Hashimoto thyroiditis and Graves disease, both caused by IgG autoantibodies for the TSH receptor. Hashimoto thyroiditis is caused by IgG autoantibodies that block the TSH receptor, which results in decreased thyroid hormone production. Antimicrosomal and antithyroglobulin antibodies (which can be tested for to diagnose Hashimoto) are then made by the body due to thyroid inflammation and destruction, since the contents of thyroid follicles are no longer separated from the blood and immune system. Symptoms initially simulate thyroid hormone overproduction due to the release of thyroid hormones into the blood during gland destruction. This is followed by hypothyroidism.

Graves disease is the result of IgG autoantibodies that stimulate the TSH receptor, causing thyroid gland growth and increased thyroid hormone secretion. Antimicrosomal and antithyroglobulin antibodies may also be present due to a hypersensitivity reaction within the thyroid gland. In addition to signs of hyperthyroidism, Graves disease can cause exophthalmos (proptosis with ocular muscle swelling and weakness) and rarely pretibial myxedema (infiltrative disorder causing edema and skin discoloration, most pronounced over the shins and dorsum of the feet).

Parathyroid gland

Humans usually have four parathyroid glands, which are embedded on the posterior surface of the thyroid gland. However, the number and locations of the parathyroid glands are variable. The parathyroid glands comprise two cell types: chief cells and oxyphil cells. The chief cells are the smaller of the two cell types and are present throughout an individual's lifetime. Because of their function in secreting parathyroid hormone (PTH), these cells are richly filled with components of the endomembrane system. Secreted PTH is released into a highly vascularized environment, thus facilitating transport of PTH systemically. PTH plays an important role in calcium homeostasis and functions to increase blood calcium through a variety of mechanisms. Oxyphil cells are the larger of the two cell types and usually first appear during puberty. They have many mitochondria, but the function of oxyphil cells is not understood.

The parathyroid glands are derived from the third and fourth pharyngeal pouches. The dorsal portion of the third pharyngeal pouch gives rise to the inferior parathyroids, while the dorsal portion of the fourth pharyngeal pouch gives rise to the superior parathyroids. Although the third pharyngeal pouch is initially closer to the head, its resulting parathyroid glands migrate to a position below the parathyroid glands derived from the fourth pouch. Since the inferior parathyroid glands migrate further during development, their location is more variable. Failure of the third and fourth pouches to differentiate results in DiGeorge syndrome. Not only do individuals with DiGeorge syndrome have hypocalcaemia due to a parathyroid deficiency, but, because the ventral portion of the third pouch gives rise to the thymus, these individuals also present with a T-cell deficiency. This deficiency results in an increased susceptibility to infection.

Parathyroid hormone (PTH)

Target tissues for PTH include bone and kidney.

Bone: PTH promotes the action of osteoclasts, which mobilize Ca^{2+} from bone and thereby increase Ca^{2+} levels in the extracellular fluid.

Kidney: PTH has several roles, including the following:
- It promotes reabsorption of Ca^{2+} in the distal tubule of nephrons thus inhibiting calcium excretion.
- It prevents reabsorption of phosphate in the proximal tubule. Renal excretion of phosphates is thus increased, preventing phosphates from binding with calcium within the body.
- It increases the activity of 1α-hydroxylase in the kidney, the enzyme that catalyzes the formation of 1,25-dihydroxycholecalciferol (the active form of vitamin D) from 25-hydroxycholecalciferol. 1,25-dihydroxycholecalciferol promotes calcium absorption in the intestine.

Together, these actions of PTH increase serum levels of elemental calcium. PTH directly affects calcium bone resorption and calcium reabsorption from the kidney. It also works indirectly on the intestine via the action of vitamin D.

Parathyroid cells have a calcium-sensing G protein-coupled receptor on their surfaces. The receptor becomes activated in response to Ca^{2+}, which in turn inhibits PTH secretion. When serum calcium levels are low, the inactive receptor permits secretion of PTH. Prior to its secretion from chief cells, PTH is processed into an 84-amino-acid polypeptide. Although this 84-amino-acid form of PTH is active, it is transported to Kupffer cells in the liver, where it is cleaved to produce amino-terminal and carboxyl-terminal fragments. The carboxyl-terminal fragment is biologically inactive. However, the amino-terminal fragment has the same targets and effects of the fully intact polypeptide. Both the intact form and the amino-terminal fragments have a short half-life of only approximately 5 minutes. Coupled with the extraordinary sensitivity of the calcium-sensing G protein-coupled receptors to even slight reductions in serum calcium levels, this short half-life ensures precise control of calcium homeostasis.

Hyperthyroidism

Transient hyperthyroidism can occur due to thyroiditis, hyperfunctioning thyroid adenomas, toxic multinodular goiter (Plummer disease), and Graves disease. Symptoms include fatigue, weight loss (despite good appetite), heat intolerance, diarrhea, anxiety, and palpitations. Clinical signs of hyperthyroidism include tachycardia, increased reflexes, and a fine tremor.

Thyroid adenomas are focal tissue nodules that are hyperfunctioning. If an adenoma becomes autonomous and releases thyroid hormones independent of TSH level, it is termed a toxic thyroid nodule. A final example of thyroid pathology is a goiter, which is diffuse enlargement of the thyroid gland, most commonly either caused by iodine deficiency or associated with Graves disease.

Laboratory findings include low TSH and high T4. A normal TSH level in the presence of an elevated T4 level is concerning for hypothalamic or pituitary pathology. If low TSH and high T4 levels are found, the next step is an iodine-131 uptake scan. Decreased iodine-131 uptake is consistent with thyroiditis. Increased iodine-131 uptake throughout the whole thyroid gland most likely represents Graves disease, while increased iodine-131 uptake in a small section likely indicates a toxic adenoma.

The treatment of hyperthyroidism depends on the cause. Graves disease may be treated in 3 ways. Thiocarbamide drugs (most commonly propylthiouracil and methimazole) block thyroid peroxidase activity, thus inhibiting the formation of T_4 and T_3. Since some patients may experience spontaneous remission of Graves disease, these drugs are often the first-line treatment. Side effects include rash, arthralgias, and agranulocytosis (rarely). Beta-blockers can be used when initiating therapy to decrease tremors, tachycardia, and hypertension. Radioactive iodine ablation with iodine-131 may also be considered (at a significantly decreased dose compared with ablation therapy for thyroid tumors). Lastly, thyroidectomy or subtotal thyroidectomy can be performed, with care not to remove parathyroid glands and damage the recurrent laryngeal nerves.

Treatment of toxic multinodular goiter is most often radioiodine ablation with iodine-131.

> ➢ **Review Video:** 7 Symptoms of Hyperthyroidism
> *Visit **mometrix.com/academy** and enter **Code: 923159***

Adrenal gland

The adrenal cortex and medulla have distinct developmental origins. The rudimentary cortex first appears at gestational week 6, arising from cells lining the posterior abdominal wall. The embryonic cortex eventually differentiates into three zones: the zona glomerulosa and zona fasciculata are present at birth, whereas the zona reticularis is not fully formed until 4 years of age. As the three zones differentiate, the embryonic cortex obliterates, and the resulting mature adrenal gland is smaller than its fetal counterpart. The adrenal medulla arises from neural crest cells that migrate to the site of the developing cortex, which begins to encapsulate the medulla by the eighth week of development.

Adrenal cortex

The adrenal cortex is the outer portion of the adrenal gland, which accounts for 72% of the gland's mass. It produces steroid hormones. Thus, its cells are rich in endoplasmic reticulum, where steroid hormones form. These cells are organized into three functionally distinct regions: the zona glomerulosa in the periphery, the zona fasciculata, and the zona reticularis (the innermost layer). The cells of the zona glomerulosa produce aldosterone, a hormone that functions to promote renal reabsorption of Na^+, K^+, H^+, and water, thereby increasing blood pressure. Interestingly, cells of the zona glomerulosa have regenerative capacities that give rise to new cortical cells. Cells of the zona fasciculata primarily function to produce glucocorticoids, such as cortisol and corticosterone. While corticosterone gets converted to aldosterone, cortisol enables the body to respond to stress by promoting gluconeogenesis and by suppressing activity of the immune system. The zona reticularis produces androgens, dehydroepiandrosterone and androstenedione, that have weak androgenic activity. Androstenedione may be converted to testosterone in the testes or estradiol in the ovary.

The adrenal cortex consists of three zones, the zona glomerulosa, the zona fasciculata, and the zona reticularis, which produce aldosterone, glucocorticoids, and androgens, respectively. All three zones have receptors for ACTH, which stimulates the production of cAMP. This in turn activates protein kinase A, which phosphorylates cholesteryl ester hydrolase (CEH). CEH mobilizes cholesterol stored in lipid droplets, making it available for conversion to steroid hormones. ACTH also activates cholesterol desmolase, an enzyme that catalyzes the formation of pregnenolone from cholesterol. Pregnenolone is the major precursor that gives rise to the three major groups of steroid hormones. Production of aldosterone and cortisol require 21β-hydroxylase. Both also possess a 2-carbon side chain at position 17, making them 21-carbon steroids. A hydroxylation event at position 17 produces cortisol. Steroids hydroxylated at position 17 can alternatively undergo a cleavage event that leads to removal of the 2-carbon side. This cleavage yields dehydroepiandrosterone or androstenedione, 19-carbon steroids that may be further processed in the testes or ovaries to generate testosterone or estradiol.

Adrenal medulla

The adrenal medulla is the inner portion of the adrenal gland and accounts for 28% of the gland's mass. It is made up of neuroendocrine cells known as chromaffin cells, and it is heavily innervated by the sympathetic nervous system to help regulate the body's response to stress. The chromaffin cells produce epinephrine, norepinephrine, and dopamine, all of which have varying effects to create a sympathetic response. In addition to their adrenal production, norepinephrine and dopamine are also largely present as neurotransmitters in the central nervous system. By contrast, epinephrine is almost entirely synthesized in the adrenal medulla for systemic effect via the bloodstream.

Pancreatic islets

The pancreas has both endocrine and exocrine functions. As an endocrine gland, its primary role is to regulate blood glucose levels. The endocrine cells compose just 1% to 2% of the pancreas by mass and are organized in clusters known as islets, which are scattered throughout the pancreas. Each islet has multiple cell types including α cells, β cells, and δ cells. α cells produce glucagon and are found predominantly on the periphery of the islets. Glucagon acts to increase blood glucose levels by stimulating the breakdown of glycogen in the liver and the subsequent release of glucose into the bloodstream. β cells comprise 65% to 75% of an islet and are clustered in its center. β cells generate insulin, which opposes the effects of glucagon by promoting cellular uptake of glucose. δ cells are less numerous than α cells but are also found towards the periphery of islets. They produce somatostatin, a hormone that decreases secretion of both insulin and glucagon.

Adipose tissue

The adipose tissue is an important endocrine structure and generates hormones collectively known as adipokines. Well-known adipokines include leptin, adiponectin, resistin, and TNF-α. Leptin is a peptide hormone that is produced in response to food intake and low energy expenditure. It signals to the hypothalamus and promotes satiety by decreasing the synthesis of the appetite stimulant neuropeptide Y, and by increasing the synthesis of α-MSH, a hunger suppressant. Leptin deficiencies lead to increased caloric intake and obesity. However, these deficiencies are rare and account for only a small number of obesity cases. Most obese individuals actually have increased serum leptin levels. All four adipokines have been linked to insulin resistance and are purported to play a role in metabolic syndrome. Both leptin and adiponectin act to decrease insulin resistance, while TNF-α and resistin promote insulin resistance.

Prolactin

Prolactin is a peptide hormone that shares sequence homology with growth hormone. It functions to promote milk secretion and breast development. Produced by the anterior pituitary gland, prolactin's release is regulated by the hypothalamus. The hypothalamus exerts a tonic inhibitory effect on prolactin secretion through its release of prolactin-inhibiting hormone (dopamine). Thyrotropin-releasing hormone (TRH) and TSH promote the release of prolactin, whose levels peak at parturition (childbirth). Because prolactin itself signals to the hypothalamus to increase dopamine secretion, it tempers its own production in a negative feedback loop. Prolactin's levels are highest during parturition. The high levels of prolactin inhibit the production and release of gonadotropins, which in turn prevents ovulation.

ACTH

ACTH is a peptide hormone. Its precursor molecule, pro-opiomelanocortin (POMC), is synthesized by the corticotropes in the anterior pituitary gland. Subsequent hydrolysis of POMC yields ACTH, β-LPH, and β-endorphin. In the intermediate-lobe cells, which also produce POMC, processing can yield α-MSH and β-MSH, neither of which are ultimately secreted in adults. ACTH secretion is stimulated by corticotropin-releasing hormone that travels from the hypothalamus to the anterior pituitary gland via the portal hypophyseal vessel. ACTH targets all three zones of the adrenal cortex, leading to an increase in the synthesis of aldosterone, glucocorticoids, and androgens. ACTH also acts to heighten the sensitivity of the adrenal cortex to its own action by promoting the production of its receptor.

Growth hormone

Growth hormone (somatotropin) is a peptide hormone with structural homology to prolactin. In response to hypothalamic growth hormone–releasing hormone (GHRH), growth hormone is synthesized by somatotropes in the anterior pituitary. It consists of 191 amino acids and contains two disulfide bridges. Growth hormone has both tropic and nontropic effects. As a tropic hormone, it acts on the liver, directing it to produce insulin-like growth factors (IGFs), which are also known as somatomedins. IGFs in turn induce growth of bone, muscle, and cartilage growth by stimulating protein synthesis. As a nontropic hormone, GH has a variety of metabolic effects. GH antagonizes the action of insulin, preventing cellular glucose uptake. It is thus diabetogenic. GH also increases protein synthesis in muscle and circulating levels of free fatty acids (FFA).

Growth hormone (GH) levels are tightly regulated through a variety of mechanisms. Growth hormone–releasing hormone (GHRH) from the hypothalamus is carried to the anterior pituitary via the portal hypophyseal vessel. Once in the anterior pituitary, it stimulates the release of GH from somatotropes. GHRH exerts negative feedback on the hypothalamus, decreasing its own secretion. Like GHRH, GH also tempers its own production. This negative feedback is mediated by GH's action on the hypothalamus, where it promotes the synthesis of somatostatins. Somatostatins impair the ability of the anterior pituitary to respond to GHRH. Somatomedins (insulin-like growth factors), which are produced in GH target tissues in response to GH, also promote somatostatin release. Moreover, they directly inhibit GH production in the anterior pituitary.

Antidiuretic hormone

Antidiuretic hormone (ADH), or vasopressin, is a peptide hormone synthesized in the supraoptic nuclei of the hypothalamus. ADH secretion is promoted by an increase in blood osmolarity, vomiting, low plasma and interstitial fluid volume, and pain. Once ADH is released from the posterior pituitary, it acts on the V_2 receptors (a G-protein coupled receptor) of epithelial cells that line the lumen of the collecting duct. Activation of V_2 receptors leads to increased levels of the second messenger cyclic adenosine monophosphate (cAMP). This increased cAMP stimulates fusion of aquaporin-containing vesicles with the cell membrane, thereby increasing the cells' permeability to water. Water is reabsorbed, decreasing blood osmolarity. ADH also promotes vasoconstriction by acting on V_{1A} receptors, which in turn promote IP_3-mediated Ca^{2+} release.

Follicle-stimulating hormone (FSH) and luteinizing hormone (LH)

FSH and LH are synthesized by the gonadotropes within the anterior pituitary gland. Both are glycoproteins consisting of an α and β subunit. They are structurally similar to thyroid-stimulating hormone (TSH), which is secreted by the nearby thyrotropes. The α subunit of all three of these glycoprotein hormones is derived from a single gene and varies only in its carbohydrate moiety. The synthesis of the β subunits is directed by distinct genes; it is the β subunit that confers the unique properties of these hormones. FSH and LH are secreted in response to gonadotropin-releasing hormone from the hypothalamus. In females, FSH and LH target the ovary. FSH stimulates the growth of follicles, which nourish developing oocytes and produce estrogen. LH promotes ovulation and the subsequent development of the corpus luteum. LH also stimulates the secretion of estrogen and progesterone from the corpus luteum. In males, FSH and LH target the testes. FSH promotes spermatogenesis, while LH directs the synthesis and secretion of testosterone from Leydig cells.

Insulin

Insulin is a peptide hormone that consists of an A chain and a B chain covalently linked by two disulfide bridges. The mature molecule is a product of the proteolytic cleavage of a longer single-chain peptide, proinsulin. In proinsulin, the A and B chains are linked via the connecting peptide (C-peptide). The C-peptide is necessary for proper folding of the molecule but is removed by two proteases once folding and disulfide bond formation is complete. The mature molecule is stored in secretory granules, which release insulin in response to increased blood glucose levels. When glucose levels are high, glucose enters β-cells via the Glut 2 receptor, and its catabolic breakdown elevates cytoplasmic ATP. ATP in turn acts to close K^+ channels, impairing K^+ movement out of β-

- 360 -

cells. K+ retention in the cytoplasm depolarizes the cell, stimulating voltage-gated Ca^{2+} channels in the cell membrane to open. The influx of Ca^{2+} into the β-cells causes insulin-containing granules to fuse with the cell membrane, thereby releasing insulin.

Insulin target tissues, which include muscle, adipose, and liver, possess the insulin receptor, a receptor tyrosine kinase (RTK) consisting of two extracellular α subunits and two transmembrane β subunits. Binding of insulin to the α subunits stimulates the tyrosine kinase activity of the β subunits, which autophosphorylate. The downstream cell signaling events that ensue culminate in activation of phosphatidylinositol 3-kinase (PI3K), which promotes the movement of vesicles containing GLUT4 to the cell membrane. The increased permeability of the membrane to glucose facilitates glucose entry into cells, decreasing blood glucose levels. In muscle and liver, the glucose is incorporated into glycogen for storage, while gluconeogenesis is inhibited. In addition to affecting glucose metabolism, insulin also influences lipid and protein metabolism. It increases protein and lipid synthesis, while inhibiting catabolic breakdown of these molecules. Finally, insulin activates the Na^+-K^+ pump, and the resulting active transport of K^+ into cells decreases blood K^+ concentration.

Glucagon

Glucagon is a peptide hormone produced in the α cells of the pancreas. It is produced in response to hypoglycemia. Its target tissues include adipose tissue and the liver. In adipose tissue, glucagon stimulates lipolysis, which in turn increases production of acetyl coenzyme A (CoA) and ketones. In the liver, glucagon stimulates glycogenolysis and gluconeogenesis. Acting on G protein-coupled receptors, glucagon increases levels of the second messenger cAMP within hepatic cells. The resulting activation of protein kinase A in turn activates glycogen phosphorylase. Glycogen breakdown ensues, elevating blood glucose levels. Protein kinase A (PKA) also inhibits two steps in glycolysis: the conversion of phosphoenolpyruvate to pyruvate and the production of fructose 2,6-bisphosphate. This inhibition of glycolysis diverts substrate to gluconeogenesis instead of glucose breakdown.

Melanocyte-stimulating hormone

Melanocyte-stimulating hormones, including α-MSH and β-MSH, are formed in the intermediate-lobe cells of the pituitary gland. They are peptide hormones derived from the precursor pro-opiomelanocortin (POMC), which also gives rise to ACTH. In a variety of organisms including fish, reptiles, and amphibians, α-MSH and β-MSH promote skin color changes by stimulating movement of the pigment melanin within cells known as melanophores. In humans, the roles of α-MSH and β-MSH are not clear since the intermediate lobe is rudimentary and these hormones do not enter circulation. However, humans possess cells known as melanocytes, which increase melanin secretion in response to MSHs. α-MSH has also been linked to appetite and serves to decrease food intake.

Calcitonin

Calcitonin is produced in the parafollicular cells within the thyroid gland. It is a peptide hormone consisting of 32 amino acids and is produced in response to an increase in blood calcium levels. Accordingly, it acts to reduce the serum concentrations of calcium and phosphate. It functions antagonistically to parathyroid hormone (PTH) and vitamin D, both of which increase calcium and phosphate levels through a variety of mechanisms. Calcitonin's target tissues include bone and kidney, where it acts on G protein-coupled receptors. In the bone, calcitonin stimulates resorption of calcium and phosphate, while in the kidney, it promotes Ca^{2+} excretion in the urine.

Vitamin D

Vitamin D is a group of related sterols. The active form of vitamin D, 1,25-(OH)2-cholecalciferol, acts to increase levels of Ca^{2+} and phosphate within the extracellular fluid. 1,25-(OH)$_2$-cholecalciferol is produced in a series of reactions occurring successively in the skin, liver, and kidney. In the skin, 7-dehydrocholesterol is converted to cholecalciferol, a step that requires sunlight. Cholecalciferol can also be ingested in the diet. After its transport to the liver, cholecalciferol is converted to 25-OH-cholecalciferol, which in turn travels to the kidney. In the kidney, the enzyme 1α-hydroxylase catalyzes the formation of 1,25-(OH)2-cholecalciferol. This active form of vitamin D acts to increase intestinal and renal absorption of Ca^{2+} and phosphate, and to promote resorption of Ca^{2+} and phosphate from bone.

Glucocorticoids

Glucocorticoids are prescribed for their anti-inflammatory effect. Common examples include severe asthma and inflammatory bowel disease. Glucocorticoids suppress the immune system primarily through the suppression of phospholipase A_2; therefore, they inhibit the formation of arachidonic acid. By contrast, NSAIDs block the reaction of arachidonic acid into prostaglandins. Glucocorticoids exert a more powerful anti-inflammatory effect than NSAIDs because preventing the formation of arachidonic acid inhibits for production of both prostaglandins and leukotrienes.

Glucocorticoids have additional effects that should be monitored, such as increased gluconeogenesis in the liver and resulting hyperglycemia. Glucocorticoids also demarginalize leukocytes from the walls of arteries, causing an apparent spike in serum white blood cells after administration. Hypertension also follows the administration of glucocorticoids, likely due to increased sensitivity to endogenous norepinephrine. Long-term glucocorticoid administration is the leading cause of Cushing syndrome.

Glucocorticoids are steroid hormones produced in the zona fasciculata of the adrenal cortex. Like other steroids, glucocorticoids have a central cyclopentanoperhydrophenanthrene nucleus. They are 21-carbon steroids, each possessing a two-carbon side chain and a hydroxyl group at position 17. Although other glucocorticoids are produced in the cortex, cortisol is one of the only glucocorticoids that circulate in the bloodstream. Its secretion follows biorhythms with levels peaking in the morning prior to waking and reaching its lowest point in the evening. Its secretion is also controlled by the hypothalamus, which secretes corticotropin-releasing hormone (CRH). CRH acts on the corticotrophs within the anterior pituitary, promoting the corticotrophs to release ACTH. ACTH in turn stimulates the synthesis and release of cortisol.

Cortisol has a number of effects that enable the body to respond to stress. Cortisol's action leads to:
- mobilization of energy stores. Cortisol increases catabolism of both proteins and lipids, and the resulting breakdown products are used in the liver for gluconeogenesis.
- repression of the immune system. Cortisol affects the immune system by reducing inflammatory responses. This reduction is achieved via inhibition of histamine release, inhibition of interleukin-2 production, and promotion of lipocortin synthesis. Lipocortin impairs the activity of phospholipase A_2. Since phospholipase A_2 promotes the production of two potent inflammatory agents, prostaglandins and leukotrienes, the inhibition of phospholipase A_2 activity mediated by cortisol reduces inflammation.

- an increase in blood pressure. Cortisol works synergistically with norepinephrine to increase blood pressure. Cortisol induces the production of α_1 receptors on arterioles. This heightens the effect of norepinephrine on these blood vessels, enhancing vasoconstriction.

Secretion of glucocorticoids (cortisol)

Secretion of glucocorticoids, namely cortisol, from the zona fasciculata of the adrenal cortex is controlled by the hypothalamus and the anterior pituitary. The hypothalamus secretes corticotropin-releasing hormone (CRH) from its paraventricular nuclei. CRH moves to the corticotrophs in the anterior pituitary via the hypophyseal vessel. The corticotrophs respond to CRH by upregulating pro-opiomelanocortin (POMC), which is subsequently processed into adrenocorticotropic hormone (ACTH). Once released, ACTH binds to receptors present in all three zones on the adrenal cortex, including the zona fasciculata. Receptor activation promotes formation of the second messenger cAMP, which ultimately frees cholesterol from lipid droplets and enables its use in the synthesis of cortisol. ACTH also leads to activation of cholesterol desmolase, an enzyme that catalyzes the first step in the conversion of cholesterol into cortisol. Because ACTH promotes production of its own receptor within the cortex, it acts to heighten the ACTH-driven response. Cortisol modulates its own secretion through negative feedback and inhibits the secretion of CRH and ACTH.

Androgens

Androgens are a group of 19-carbon steroid hormones, including testosterone, dihydrotestosterone, and androstenedione. Androstenedione serves as a precursor for testosterone synthesis and can be produced by the zona reticularis of the adrenal gland or by Leydig cells in the testes. The Leydig cells can synthesize testosterone from cholesterol or from adrenal-derived androstenedione. Testosterone is the primary androgen that enters circulation. Once at its target tissue, it may get converted to dihydrotestosterone, a reaction catalyzed by 5α-reductase. Both testosterone and dihydrotestosterone influence development of the male reproductive structures and of secondary sex characteristics. Testosterone induces the differentiation the epididymis, vas deferens, and seminal vesicles. It also promotes enlargement of the penis and seminal vesicles, deepening of the voice, and increased muscle mass, which occur at puberty. Throughout adulthood, testosterone promotes spermatogenesis. Dihydrotestosterone has related effects and induces the differentiation of the penis, scrotum, and prostate. It also promotes sebaceous gland secretion and hair growth.

Estrogens and progesterone

Theca cells and granulosa cells in the ovarian follicles produce estrogens, which are 18-carbon steroids. The theca cells first produce testosterone from cholesterol, which subsequently diffuses into nearby granulosa cells. Within granulosa cells, aromatase catalyzes the conversion of testosterone to 17β-estradiol. Aromatase is also present within fatty tissue. The synthesis of progesterone, a 21-carbon steroid, increases after the development of the corpus luteum in the menstrual cycle, which is its primary site of production. It is also made as a precursor in other steroid-secreting glands. Estrogens and progesterone have a variety of effects. Estrogens play a role in the development of secondary sex characteristics and in the maturation of reproductive structures, including the uterus, oviducts, cervix, and vagina. During the menstrual cycle, estrogens promote the development of the endometrial lining, coordinating its proliferation with oocyte maturation and release. Progesterone works in conjunction with estrogen to promote breast development. It also targets the uterus, inducing further thickening and maintenance of the endometrium. This maintenance is required to sustain pregnancy.

The ovaries are controlled by the hypothalamus, which produces gonadotropin-releasing hormone (GnRH). GnRH signals to the gonadotropes within the anterior pituitary, stimulating these cells to secrete follicle-stimulating hormone (FSH) and luteinizing hormone (LH). During the follicular phase of the menstrual cycle, low levels of FSH and LH promote follicular development. The resulting estrogen from the growing follicle exerts negative feedback on the anterior pituitary, thereby tempering FSH and LH secretion. Once the follicle begins secreting high levels of estrogen, its effect on the anterior pituitary reverses. Positive feedback due to large amounts of estrogen leads to a surge in LH, which in turn prompts ovulation. After ovulation, the corpus luteum develops from the ovarian follicle and secretes both estrogen and progesterone. The combination of both hormones leads to negative feedback that once again decreases levels of FSH and LH. Consequently, the corpus luteum degenerates. Without the estrogen and progesterone from the corpus luteum, the uterine lining is shed. Alternatively, in the event of a pregnancy, embryo-derived human chorionic gonadotropin (hCG) maintains the corpus luteum. Estrogen and progesterone levels remain high, keeping the uterine lining intact.

Aldosterone synthesis

Aldosterone production is regulated by renin and angiotensin. Renin is a glycoprotein produced in the juxtamedullary apparatus of the kidney in response to a decrease in blood pressure. Its protease activity stimulates the cleavage of a liver-derived precursor protein, angiotensinogen, yielding the decapeptide angiotensin I. Angiotensin I is further processed by angiotensin-converting enzyme (ACE), and the resulting angiotensin II has a variety of effects. In addition to its role as a potent vasoconstrictor, angiotensin II induces the secretion of aldosterone from the adrenal cortex. Within the adrenal cortex, angiotensin II binds to G protein-coupled receptors located in cells of the zona glomerulosa. This binding leads to downstream activation of phospholipase C, which in turn facilitates the conversion of cholesterol to pregnenolone. Pregnenolone undergoes a series of conversions, yielding the 21-carbon steroid hormone aldosterone. Together, angiotensin II and aldosterone work to increase blood volume and blood pressure. Drugs that prevent the action of angiotensin-converting enzyme, known as ACE inhibitors, are effective in the treatment of high blood pressure.

The renin-angiotensin-aldosterone system is activated in response to a decrease in blood pressure. Angiotensin II and aldosterone are the biologically active mediators of this system and act coordinately to increase blood volume and blood pressure. Angiotensin II promotes sodium reabsorption in the proximal convoluted tubules of the nephron. It is also a potent vasoconstrictor and targets the brain to increase thirst. Angiotensin II's direct actions complement its indirect effects through its promotion of aldosterone secretion from the zona glomerulosa of the adrenal cortex. Aldosterone targets the distal convoluted tubule of nephrons and the collecting duct, where it enters principal cells and binds to an intracellular aldosterone receptor. Receptor activation rapidly prompts insertion of epithelial sodium channels (ENaCs) into the cell membrane and activates Na^+-K^+ exchangers. Thus, the reabsorption of Na^+ is increased, while the activated exchanger leads to K^+ secretion. In addition to these rapid effects, aldosterone promotes changes in gene expression within the principal cells, including upregulation of ENaCs.

Thyroid hormone synthesis

Thyroid hormone secretion is regulated by the hypothalamus and the anterior pituitary. Thyrotropin-releasing hormone (TRH) produced in the hypothalamus travels via the hypophyseal vessels to the thyrotropes in the anterior pituitary. In response to TRH, the thyrotropes secrete thyroid-stimulating hormone (TSH), which in turn stimulates increased secretion of T_3 and T_4 from the thyroid gland. T_3 exerts negative feedback on the anterior pituitary, where it decreases TRH receptor expression. The reduced number of TRH receptors prevents TSH secretion, thereby modulating thyroid hormone production. T_3 has more biological activity than T_4 and binds to intracellular receptors that act as transcription factors when associated with T_3. During development, thyroid hormone is required for bone growth and proper CNS maturation. Throughout the lifespan, thyroid hormones are important regulators of metabolism. Thyroid hormones promote O_2 consumption and increase basal metabolic rate. Accordingly, thyroid hormones also increase catabolism of various nutrients, including proteins, glycogen, and lipids. The increased O_2 demands are supported by thyroid hormone's ability to increase heart rate by promoting expression of β_1-andrenergic receptors in myocytes.

The thyroid gland produces thyroxine (T_4) and triiodothyronine (T_3). Both are tyrosine-based hormones that require iodine for their synthesis. Spatially, thyroid hormone synthesis takes place in the colloid and its surrounding thyroid cells. The thyroid cells collect iodide and oxidize it to iodine, a reaction catalyzed by peroxidase enzyme. The thyroid cells secrete this iodine and a tyrosine-containing protein, thyroglobulin, into the colloid. Within the colloid, tyrosines on thyroglobulin react with iodine to form monoiodotyrosine (MIT) and diiodotyrosine (DIT). Subsequent coupling of two DIT molecules yields T_4, while coupling of MIT and DIT produces T_3. In response to thyroid-stimulating hormone (TSH), thyroid cells endocytose thyroglobulin and the attached T_3 and T_4 moieties. Lysosomal enzymes release the T_3 and T_4 from thyroglobulin, thereby freeing these thyroid hormones to enter circulation. T_3 exerts more biological activity than T_4; however, T_3 conversion to T_4 may take place in peripheral tissues.

Catecholamines

Catecholamines are derived from the amino acid tyrosine and include epinephrine, norepinephrine, and dopamine. In addition to their production within the nervous system, catecholamines are also produced in the chromaffin cells of the adrenal medulla. The synthesis of catecholamines involves the addition of a hydroxyl group and the removal of a carboxyl group from tyrosine, which yields dopamine. Production of dopamine occurs within the cytoplasm of chromaffin cells. Further processing of dopamine takes place in granulated vesicles, which contain dopamine β-hydroxylase (DBH). DBH catalyzes the conversion of dopamine to norepinephrine, a step involving the addition of another hydroxyl group. A second enzyme, phenylethanolamine-N-methyltransferase, adds a methyl group to norepinephrine, yielding epinephrine. The adrenal medulla is controlled by the sympathetic nervous system, which promotes the release of catecholamines in response to stress.

Epinephrine and norepinephrine

Epinephrine and norepinephrine are released from the adrenal medulla in response to stress and act to modulate metabolism, heart rate, blood pressure, and alertness. They act on G protein-coupled receptors, which are grouped into two classes: α- and β-adrenergic receptors. Epinephrine and norepinephrine promote catabolic activities including glycogen breakdown and lipolysis. Their effects on glucose metabolism are mediated both through α- and β-adrenergic receptors. Epinephrine and norepinephrine also exert effects on the circulatory system. By binding with β-

adrenergic receptors in cardiomyocytes, epinephrine and norepinephrine act to increase heart rate and force of contraction. They also direct blood flow to skeletal muscle and the liver, while decreasing blood flow to other tissues, including the small intestine. This is accomplished through epinephrine binding to β-adrenergic receptors on skeletal muscle and liver blood vessels, which leads to vasodilation, and through norepinephrine action on α-adrenergic receptors on blood vessels that service tissues such as the small intestine, which leads to vasoconstriction. Both epinephrine and norepinephrine increase alertness, anxiety, and fear.

Changes in hormone levels

In the United States, boys typically undergo puberty between 9 and 14 years of age. Changes are initiated by pulsatile secretion of GnRH. The increased GnRH stimulates gonadotropes in the anterior pituitary to release luteinizing hormone (LH), which targets the Leydig cells within the testes. LH binds to G protein-coupled receptors on Leydig cells, initiating a signal transduction pathway that culminates in the conversion of cholesterol to pregnenolone, the first step in testosterone production. The increase in testosterone observed at puberty promotes the development of secondary sex characteristics. Both internal and external genitalia, including the penis, testes, seminal vesicles, prostate, and seminal vesicles, enlarge. The larynx also enlarges, producing a deeper voice. Hair growth patterns change; an increase in facial, axillary, and pubic hair is observed, while scalp hair may actually decrease. Body shape changes because of increased muscle development. During puberty, secretion of follicle-stimulating hormone (FSH) from the anterior pituitary also increases because of the action of GnRH. FSH targets Sertoli cells, thereby promoting spermatogenesis.

During childhood, levels of circulating gonadotropin-releasing hormone (GnRH) are low; it is produced but not secreted. The onset of puberty occurs between the 8 and 13 years of age in females and is characterized by pulsatile release of GnRH, which stimulates the gonadotropes within the anterior pituitary to release FSH and LH. These hormones in turn signal to the ovary, stimulating estrogen production. The increase in estrogens is responsible for many of the changes associated with puberty. Adrenal androgen secretion also contributes. Female puberty consists of three stages, including thelarche, pubarche, and menarche. Thelarche, or the start of breast development, typically occurs first. This is primarily controlled by estrogens, though progesterone also participates in breast enlargement. Thelarche, the first appearance of pubic hair, occurs next and is controlled by androgens. It is prominent in the axilla and on the labia. Approximately 2 years after thelarche, menarche ensues. The menstrual periods within the first year may not be accompanied by ovulation.

Menopause typically occurs in women between 45 and 55 years of age. It is initiated by a sharp decrease in the release of estrogen and progesterone from the ovaries. This decrease occurs as the number of primary follicles diminishes with advancing age. Because estrogen and progesterone exert negative feedback on the anterior pituitary, high plasma levels of FSH and LH are observed in menopausal women. The dysregulation of the hormone cycles leads to irregular menstrual cycles that ultimately cease altogether; menopause has occurred when menstrual periods have been absent for 12 consecutive months. Menopause may be accompanied by vaginal atrophy and hot flashes.

Increased levels of parathyroid hormone (PTH) are observed in elderly patients, and the effect is more pronounced in women. This increase may be related to the impaired ability of the kidney to reabsorb calcium.

The levels of several hormones decline with age. Hormones whose levels decrease include:
- Growth hormone (GH)
- Renin/aldosterone
- Estrogen and progesterone
- Testosterone

Decreased levels of GH may account for the degeneration of muscle, bone, and skin in older patients. Although blood pressure tends to rise with age, renin and aldosterone levels decline and are not responsible for this tendency. The loss of estrogen and progesterone secretion from the ovary leads to menopause, which typically occurs between 45 and 55 years of age. Although men experience declining levels of testosterone as they age, the ability to produce and release functional gametes remains intact.

Waterhouse-Friderichsen syndrome

Waterhouse-Friderichsen syndrome is bilateral adrenal hemorrhage causing acute adrenocortical hypofunction, typically due to overwhelming sepsis from *Neisseria meningitidis. Neisseria* are gram-negative encapsulated bacteria that contain lipooligosaccharide (LOS) within the outer membrane, a polysaccharide that acts as an endotoxin when the bacterial capsule and cell membranes are lysed. Infections may begin as meningitis, but can become disseminated infections associated with a petechial rash and disseminated intravascular coagulation (DIC). DIC may then lead to hemorrhagic infarction of both adrenal glands, leading to extreme hypotension due to lack of glucocorticoids.

Hypophysectomy (transection of the pituitary stalk)

Traumatic transection of the pituitary stalk may be due to trauma or may be iatrogenic (for example, during surgery for a craniopharyngioma). This results in dysregulation of the anterior pituitary gland, because releasing hormones are not made and released by the hypothalamus, which may result in increased or decreased hormone production. For example, decreased synthesis of corticotropin-releasing hormone (CRH) from the hypothalamus results in decreased release of ACTH from the anterior pituitary because CRH stimulates ACTH release. However, dopamine from the hypothalamus normally inhibits prolactin release by the anterior pituitary; therefore, pathology causing decreased dopamine synthesis in the hypothalamus results in hyperprolactinemia. Hypophysectomy also results in loss of posterior pituitary hormone production (ADH and oxytocin).

Neoplastic thyroid pathology

There are four main types of primary thyroid cancer. (1) Papillary adenocarcinoma comprises about 80% of thyroid cancers and typically affects middle-age women. The most important risk factor is prior exposure to ionizing radiation. Papillary adenocarcinoma spreads via the lymphatic system. (2) Follicular carcinoma is also typically seen in females and is more aggressive than papillary tumors, typically spreading via the vascular system to the lungs and skeletal system. Thus, metastases may be detected before the primary thyroid tumor is detected. (3) Medullary carcinoma arises from calcitonin-producing parafollicular cells and is more aggressive than papillary and follicular tumors. High calcitonin levels are usually present. The familial form of medullary carcinoma is associated with the *RET* proto-oncogene mutation, and may also be associated with MEN IIa and MEN IIb syndromes. (4) Lastly, anaplastic thyroid cancer is the most aggressive of all and occurs in elderly patients. Lymphoma may also involve the thyroid gland.

Neoplastic disorders of the hypothalamus

The most common cause of hypothalamic pathology is children is a craniopharyngioma, which is a benign tumor derived from the hypophyseal diverticulum (Rathke pouch). This tumor is usually located above the sella turcica and can compress the optic chiasm, causing bitemporal hemianopsia. Other primary (for example, dermoid) and metastatic brain tumors can also cause hypothalamic dysfunction. These tumors may cause panhypopituitarism if the tumor involves the anterior pituitary gland. Signs of hypopituitarism may also be present if only the hypothalamus is involved because releasing hormones are not made and released by the hypothalamus, which causes dysregulation of the anterior pituitary that may result in increased or decreased hormone production. For example, decreased synthesis of corticotropin-releasing hormone (CRH) from the hypothalamus results in decreased release of ACTH from the anterior pituitary, because CRH stimulates ACTH release. However, dopamine from the hypothalamus normally inhibits prolactin release by the anterior pituitary; therefore, pathology causing decreased dopamine synthesis in the hypothalamus results in hyperprolactinemia.

Hyperfunctioning pituitary adenomas

Prolactinoma is the most common pituitary adenoma and leads to hyperprolactinemia. Notably, hyperprolactinemia can also result from the lack of inhibitory dopamine from the hypothalamus. In both males and females, increased prolactin may result in galactorrhea. Because prolactin inhibits gonadotropin synthesis and release, females may present with amenorrhea while males may experience impotence and hypogonadism. These symptoms resolve when prolactin levels are decreased, which can be achieved with bromocriptine or cabergoline, both dopamine agonists (which inhibit prolactin secretion by the anterior pituitary). The second most common pituitary adenoma is a growth hormone (GH) adenoma. Elevated GH stimulates increased IGF-1 secretion from the liver, which in turn promotes bone and cartilage growth. Because IGF-1 also promotes gluconeogenesis, high levels of growth hormone are associated with hyperglycemia. Therefore, children develop gigantism and adults develop acromegaly.

Hypofunctioning pituitary adenomas can be associated with multiple endocrine neoplasia type 1 (MEN I) syndrome, which is an association of pituitary adenomas, parathyroid adenoma (hyperparathyroidism), and pancreatic islet cell tumors (gastrin- or insulin-secreting tumors).

Pancreatic neuroendocrine (islet cell) tumors

There are 5 major types of pancreatic neuroendocrine tumors (PNETs) based on the hormone secreted. Neuroendocrine tumors may be benign or malignant. A well-known type of PNET is a gastrin-producing islet cell tumor, resulting in Zollinger-Ellison syndrome. The gastrin stimulates increased hydrochloric acid production by gastric parietal cells, which leads to peptic ulcers, diarrhea, and indigestion.

The most common type of PNET is insulinoma, which is a benign insulin-secreting tumor that can cause severe hypoglycemia. C-peptide levels are high because this is endogenously produced insulin. The majority of patients with insulinomas have MEN I syndrome.

Other types of PNETs include glucagonoma (high glucagon levels cause hyperglycemia and necrolytic migratory erythema), VIPoma (vasoactive intestinal peptide that causes diarrhea), and somatostatinoma. Since somatostatin is usually an inhibitory hormone, this tumor has a wide variety of effects due to decreased inhibition of gastrin (leads to achlorhydria), cholecystokinin (leads to cholestasis and cholelithiasis), and gastric inhibitory peptide (causes diabetes mellitus).

Multiple endocrine neoplasias (MEN)

The multiple endocrine neoplasia (MEN) syndromes are patterns of endocrine tumors that tend to occur in the same patients. These are autosomal dominant disorders. MEN IIa and IIb are associated with the *RET* oncogene.

- MEN I: Parathyroid adenoma, pancreatic neuroendocrine (islet cell tumor), and pituitary adenomas. The most common pancreatic neuroendocrine tumor in this syndrome is insulinoma. The pituitary adenomas most common secrete prolactin or growth hormone.
- MEN IIa: Parathyroid adenoma, medullary thyroid carcinoma, and pheochromocytoma.
- MEN IIb: Medullary thyroid cancer, pheochromocytoma, and mucosal neuromas (oral or intestinal ganglioneuromas).

Common adrenal tumor

The most common adrenal tumor in adults is pheochromocytoma, which arises from the adrenal medulla and produces catecholamines, such as epinephrine. Therefore, symptoms of pheochromocytoma correlate with a state of increased sympathetic tone: hypertension, palpitations and tachycardia, anxiety, and drenching sweats. Pheochromocytomas are commonly taught to follow the rule of 10s: 10% are benign, 10% involve both adrenal glands, and 10% are located outside the adrenal gland (in the organ of Zuckerkandl near the aortic bifurcation). Pheochromocytoma may be seen in MEN IIa and MEN IIb syndromes, neurofibromatosis, and von Hippel-Lindau disease.

Diagnosis is made using a 24-hour urine collection, which shows increased metanephrine and vanillylmandelic acid (VMA), both metabolites of epinephrine and norepinephrine.

The most common adrenal tumor in children is neuroblastoma, which most commonly presents as a palpable abdominal mass in children younger than 5 years. Since the tumor arises from the adrenal medulla, increased catecholamine production is usually present, although the signs of high sympathetic tone are more difficult to identify in young children. However, like pheochromocytoma in adults, urine levels of metanephrines and vanillylmandelic acid (VMA) are present. Neuroblastoma is associated with amplified *N-MYC* oncogene. The staging of neuroblastoma is interesting—like most tumors, increased stage of disease (and poor prognosis) is due to larger tumor size, lymph node involvement, and metastasis. However, a special grouping is made for infants younger than 1 year (stage 4S) who have a good prognosis despite widely metastatic disease.

Hypocalcemia

There are many causes of hypocalcemia, including hypoparathyroidism and pseudohypoparathyroidism. Disorders in the production of 1,25-dihydroxycholecalciferol (active vitamin D) can cause hypocalcemia, and longstanding decreased vitamin D levels leads to rickets. Liver and renal failure can both lead to low vitamin D levels because both organs are needed in the synthesis of the active form of vitamin D.

Both high and low levels of magnesium can lead to hypocalcemia. Since both magnesium and calcium are divalent cations, magnesium can mimic calcium in a negative feedback capacity to inhibit PTH production. Paradoxically, hypomagnesemia both inhibits PTH production and blocks the action of PTH in bones and in the kidney, also resulting in hypocalcemia.

Low albumin levels in the blood, which can be caused by malnutrition or nephrotic syndrome, lead to low total calcium levels but normal serum ionized calcium levels.

Lastly, medications (such as bisphosphonates), hyperphosphatemia, pancreatitis, and sepsis also cause hypocalcemia.

Hyperparathyroidism

Hyperparathyroidism is characterized by high serum PTH and is categorized into primary, secondary, and tertiary hyperparathyroidism. Primary hyperparathyroidism is most often caused by a parathyroid adenoma that continues to secrete PTH despite high serum calcium levels. This leads to further hypercalcemia that can cause renal calculi (calcium oxalate stones), reduced bone mineralization due to increased osteoclastic activity (osteitis fibrosa cystica), and reduced renal function. Parathyroid adenomas may be associated with MEN I or MEN II syndromes.

Secondary hyperparathyroidism is the result of parathyroid hyperplasia in the setting of low Vitamin D levels from renal failure (the kidneys do not synthesize 1,25-dihydroxycholecalciferol, active vitamin D). Serum calcium in this case is decreased since the kidneys cannot retain calcium. Tertiary hyperparathyroidism may occur as a consequence of longstanding secondary hyperparathyroidism, and is the result of parathyroid cells gaining autonomous function and no longer responding to serum calcium levels.

Causes of disrupted calcium metabolism

1. Low PTH and low serum calcium: If serum calcium is low, the PTH level should be high, so this is a case of inappropriately low PTH or hypoparathyroidism. Causes of hypoparathyroidism include iatrogenic (inadvertent surgical removal), autoimmune, or agenesis (DiGeorge syndrome). Hypomagnesemia can also cause this clinical scenario, since low serum magnesium also inhibits PTH synthesis and prevents PTH effects in the kidney and bones, thus causing a picture of hypoparathyroidism.
2. Low PTH and high serum calcium: The most common cause of hypercalcemia in hospitalized individuals is malignancy. Hypercalcemia of malignancy is associated with squamous cell carcinomas, renal and ovarian carcinomas, and lymphomas. Hypercalcemia is the result of release of PTH-related peptide (PTHrP), which has the same actions as PTH but is not inhibited by high serum calcium levels. In this case, low PTH is the result of the normal inhibitory effect of high serum calcium levels on the parathyroid glands.
3. High PTH and low serum calcium: In this case, a low serum calcium level is causing the parathyroid glands to release high amounts of PTH. The most common cause of this situation occurs in cases of low levels of vitamin D, typically in the setting of renal failure (secondary hypoparathyroidism). The kidneys do not reabsorb calcium (an effect of vitamin D) and therefore serum calcium levels remain low despite high PTH levels.
4. High PTH and high serum calcium: High serum calcium levels are not having the normal inhibitory effect on parathyroid gland secretion of PTH. This is likely caused by a parathyroid adenoma.

Cushing syndrome

Cushing syndrome is characterized by abnormally elevated levels of cortisol. The most common cause is iatrogenic chronic corticosteroid therapy (for Crohn disease, for example). Other causes include an anterior pituitary adenoma (high ACTH and high cortisol), an adrenal cortex adenoma (low ACTH and high cortisol), or ectopic production of ACTH by a neoplasm (high ACTH and high cortisol). Signs and symptoms of Cushing syndrome include central weight gain (characteristically moon facies or buffalo hump), abdominal striae, hirsutism, muscle weakness in the arms and legs, and osteoporosis. Hyperglycemia and hypertension are typically present. Diagnosis can be made by measuring urine free cortisol and by conducting a high-dose dexamethasone suppression test. High-dose dexamethasone has negative feedback on pituitary ACTH production from a pituitary adenoma, causing transient low levels of cortisol hours later; dexamethasone administration will not affect cortisol levels from other etiologies of Cushing syndrome.

The amount of cortisol secreted throughout the day varies, with peak serum cortisol levels occurring in the early morning. Serum cortisol levels then quickly dissipate; evening serum cortisol levels greater than 50% of morning levels are indicative of Cushing syndrome. Dexamethasone is a potent glucocorticoid that laboratories are able to differentiate from cortisol. A high-dose dexamethasone suppression test is the most helpful test in diagnosing Cushing syndrome. A baseline serum cortisol level is drawn on day 1. Dexamethasone is administered during the evening of day 1, and serum cortisol is measured the morning of day 2. In a normal patient, dexamethasone suppresses ACTH secretion from the anterior pituitary gland, and thus serum cortisol levels are low (less than 50% of baseline day 1 level). High-dose dexamethasone can suppress cortisol in Cushing disease (pituitary adenoma); ACTH is normal to elevated but serum cortisol levels on day 2 of the suppression test are decreased. An MRI should then be ordered to evaluate the pituitary gland. Serum cortisol levels are essentially unchanged if the cause of Cushing syndrome is from an adrenal adenoma or neoplastic syndrome.

Hyperaldosteronism

Primary hyperaldosteronism (Conn's syndrome) is characterized by hypertension, muscle weakness, and headaches. High serum aldosterone causes hypernatremia, hypokalemia (inappropriately elevated exchange of sodium for potassium or hydrogen ions in the proximal convoluted tubule of the kidney), and metabolic alkalosis. As more severe hypokalemia develops, more hydrogen ions are excreted as sodium is retained, leading to progressive metabolic alkalosis. This causes paresthesia, tetany, and, in severe cases, intermittent paralysis.

Hyperaldosteronism is most commonly caused by a functional adrenal cortical adenoma. Less common causes include bilateral adrenal hyperplasia and adrenal carcinoma. Secondary hyperaldosteronism may be seen in heart failure due to low cardiac output, low renal blood flow, and chronic activation of the renin-angiotensin-aldosterone system.

Chronic adrenal insufficiency

Chronic adrenal insufficiency (Addison's disease) has a variety of causes, all leading to a clinical picture of hypotension, weakness, and hyperpigmented skin. Hypotension is due to a deficiency in aldosterone, which leads to hyponatremia, hyperkalemia, and normal anion gap metabolic acidosis. Hyperpigmented skin is due to increased ACTH levels from the anterior pituitary that stimulate melanocytes in the skin. Secondary adrenal insufficiency is due to deficient anterior pituitary function (low ACTH), and is not associated with skin hyperpigmentation.

The most common cause of primary Addison's disease in developed countries is autoimmune destruction of the adrenal glands. The most common cause in undeveloped countries is tuberculosis. Histoplasmosis (fungal) infection, metastatic cancer to the adrenal gland (most commonly lung cancer or melanoma), and congenital adrenal hyperplasia symptoms also can cause Addison's disease.

Vascular disorders affecting the pituitary gland

An important cause of hypopituitarism is Sheehan syndrome, which is caused by ischemic necrosis of anterior pituitary gland tissue due to hypovolemia and blood loss. While this can occur after severe trauma, the most common cause is peripartum or postpartum hemorrhage because the anterior pituitary gland enlarges during pregnancy, and therefore is more sensitive to decreased blood flow. This ischemic necrosis causes decreased prolactin release, which results in loss of ability to lactate.

Type I diabetes mellitus

Type I diabetes mellitus is the result of autoimmune-mediated destruction of pancreatic beta cells, resulting in a lack of insulin production and secretion. This typically affects younger individuals (younger than 20 years). Clinical signs include polyuria, polydipsia, and weight loss, despite increased oral intake (polyphagia). In about 25% of patients, these symptoms go undiagnosed and patients may present in diabetic ketoacidosis. Diabetic ketoacidosis is characterized by severe hyperglycemia leading to volume depletion (hyperglycemia causes an osmotic diuresis with loss of sodium and water). Ketones are formed due to the breakdown of fatty acids into acetyl-CoA (hormone-sensitive lipase is not inhibited since insulin levels are low), which is converted to acetone, acetoacetic acid, and ß-hydroxybutyric acid.

Latent autoimmune diabetes (diabetes mellitus type 1.5) occurs in adults and has the same symptoms as type I diabetes mellitus. Glutamic acid decarboxylase (GAD) antibodies are present. For the diagnosis of diabetes mellitus, a hemoglobin A_{1c} level more than 6.5 is now commonly used. Fasting blood glucose levels more than 126 mg/dL, random blood glucose level more than 200 mg/dL with symptoms of diabetes mellitus, or blood glucose levels more than 200 mg/dL 2 hours after a 75 g glucose load are also diagnostic.

Type II diabetes mellitus

Type II diabetes mellitus (DM) is much more common than type I DM. Type II DM is typically seen in overweight adults (30 years and older). Native Americans and African Americans also have an increased incidence compared with other races. The result of progressive insulin resistance, symptoms are related to hyperglycemia. But in contrast to the rapid onset of type I DM, type II DM has an slowly progressive onset, and symptoms are typically the result of end-organ dysfunction: changes in vision, chronic kidney disease, neuropathy, and infections.

Since insulin is present, type II DM individuals do not typically develop diabetic ketoacidosis. Instead, chronic severe hyperglycemia may result in hyperosmolar nonketotic (HONK) syndrome, characterized by severe dehydration due to osmotic diuresis associated with hyperglycemia, but no ketoacids are formed because of the presence of insulin (which inhibits hormone-sensitive lipase and breakdown of fatty acids).

For the diagnosis of diabetes mellitus, a hemoglobin A_{1c} level more than 6.5 is now commonly used. Fasting blood glucose levels more than 126 mg/dL, random blood glucose level more than 200 mg/dL with symptoms of DM, or blood glucose levels more than 200 mg/dL 2 hours after a 75 g glucose load are also diagnostic.

Diabetes insipidus

Diabetes insipidus may be divided into central diabetes insipidus (inadequate ADH secretion) and nephrogenic diabetes insipidus (failure of kidneys to respond to secreted ADH). These two entities can be distinguished from primary polydipsia via the water deprivation test. A normal response to water deprivation is to concentrate urine to an osmolality higher than that of plasma and to decrease urine output. A normal response is seen in patients with primary polydipsia. Patients with diabetes insipidus are unable to concentrate urine, and urine output remains high while urine osmolarity remains inappropriately low. Central and nephrogenic etiologies can be distinguished by measuring serum ADH levels (high in nephrogenic diabetes insipidus) or by giving DDAVP (a synthetic ADH). DDAVP should cause decreased urine output and increased urine concentration in central diabetes insipidus, while having almost no effect on nephrogenic diabetes insipidus.

DDAVP (also called desmopressin) is a synthetic ADH that can also be used to treat central diabetes insipidus. Nephrogenic diabetes insipidus is treated by limiting salt intake and by giving thiazide diuretics, which, when used together, cause a relative volume depletion and increase water reabsorption in the proximal tubules of the nephron.

Hyperglycemia

The most common organs affected by hyperglycemia are the eyes, nerves, and kidneys. Retinopathy is the result of osmotic-mediated death of pericyte cells (which control the permeability of retinal blood vessels), which leads to increased retinal vessel permeability and aneurysm formation. Neuropathy is the result of osmotic damage to the Schwann cells of the peripheral nervous system, leading to demyelination. Long nerves, such as the nerves heading to the hands and feet, are typically affected first. Neuropathy may also occur in the autonomic nervous system, leading to delayed gastric emptying and delayed intestinal motility. Nephropathy is also the result of osmotic damage to vessel walls, resulting in increased collagen formation in the basement membrane of small blood vessels. This leads to altered vessel permeability and abnormal filtration within the glomeruli. Microvascular changes also result in increased atherosclerotic disease and risk of stroke and myocardial infarction.

Metabolic syndrome

Metabolic syndrome, also known as syndrome X, is a combination of clinical and laboratory test findings that are all related to the presence of insulin resistance. There are various definitions of the syndrome depending on the source group. A commonly used definition in the United States is defined by the American Heart Association:
1. abdominal obesity (waist circumference more than 40 inches in men or more than 35 inches in women)
2. hypertriglyceridemia (triglycerides more than 150 mg/dL)
3. low HDL (less than 40 mg/dL in men or less than 50 mg/dL in women),
4. hypertension (systolic blood pressure greater than 130 mm Hg or diastolic blood pressure greater than 85 mm Hg)
5. hyperglycemia (fasting glucose more than 100 mg/dL)

- 373 -

Hypothyroidism

Primary causes of hypothyroidism include autoimmune (Hashimoto), iodine deficiency, and drugs (lithium and amiodarone). Secondary hypothyroidism occurs due to hypothalamic or anterior pituitary dysfunction. Clinical signs of adult hypothyroidism include decreased metabolism (weight gain and fatigue), dry and brittle hair, cold intolerance, constipation, cognitive slowing, and periorbital edema. Proximal muscle atrophy can also occur, resulting in increased serum creatine kinase (CK) levels. Physical exam may reveal delayed reflexes and bradycardia. Laboratory tests demonstrate high TSH (or low TSH if there is anterior pituitary dysfunction) with low total and free T4. Other findings may include high cholesterol, elevated CK, and anemia.

Longstanding severe hypothyroidism can lead to myxedema coma, which includes hypothermia, weakness, and a stuporous state.

Hypothyroidism during pregnancy can result in congenital hypothyroidism (cretinism), characterized by intellectual disability, feeding problems, and edema. Hypothyroidism after birth may be the result of thyroid gland agenesis or hypoplasia, which results in learning disabilities, short stature, and delayed puberty. The degree of these symptoms depends on the level of residual thyroid function and how quickly thyroid replacement therapy is initiated.

Hypothyroidism is treated with oral levothyroxine, which is a synthetic form of T_4. T_4 is converted to the more active T_3 by cells throughout the body. Levothyroxine is well tolerated, and side effects are generally due to overreplacement of T_4. Therefore, symptoms of treatment toxicity are the same as the symptoms of hyperthyroidism (palpitations, tremors, feeling of nervousness or anxiety, diarrhea). Treatment dose should be titrated by measuring TSH (goal is generally TSH between 0.5 and 2 mIU/L). Patients with pituitary or hypothalamic dysfunction will not have TSH levels that respond to therapy, and thus free T_4 must be measured and used to adjust levothyroxine dose. Use of IV levothyroxine is rare and used only for myxedema coma.

Developmental thyroid pathology

Developmental thyroid pathology results from failure of the thyroid tissue to correctly descend into the neck during fetal development, and includes lingual thyroid tissue (which can cause dysphagia) and thyroglossal duct cyst (midline cyst in the neck). Thyroglossal duct cysts may not be identified unless they become infected. Lingual or other ectopic thyroid tissue (for example, in the chest/anterior mediastinum) can be identified using iodine-131 uptake scans.

Hypoparathyroidism pathology

The most common cause of hypoparathyroidism is iatrogenic: accidental removal during thyroid or other neck surgery. Hypoparathyroidism may also be autoimmune in nature, either with autoantibodies directly targeting the parathyroid glands or due to surrounding inflammation from autoimmune thyroid disease.

DiGeorge syndrome is a type of congenital immunodeficiency disorder characterized by failure of the third and fourth pharyngeal pouches to develop, resulting in agenesis of the thymus and parathyroid glands. The abnormality has been localized on chromosome 22, and is associated with midline facial anomalies (such as cleft palate), cardiac defects, and opportunistic infections due to the absent thymus. The lack of parathyroid glands results in hypocalcemia and tetany.

Laboratory findings in hypoparathyroidism include low serum ionized calcium and inappropriately low serum PTH. Elevated phosphate levels and low vitamin D levels will also likely be present, since PTH normally facilitates renal excretion of phosphate and stimulates the activation of vitamin D in the liver and kidney.

Pseudohypoparathyroidism occurs when a genetic mutation causes PTH receptors to be resistant to PTH. This is most commonly part of Albright syndrome, a hereditary osteodystrophy.

Congenital adrenal hyperplasia (adrenogenital syndrome)

Congenital adrenal hyperplasia, also known as adrenogenital syndromes, is a group of autosomal recessive disorders caused by deficiency of a key enzyme within the adrenal cortex. Knowledge of adrenocortical hormone synthesis pathways is required to fully understand these syndromes, since lack of a single enzyme will shunt substrates into other pathways. Adrenal hyperplasia is due to a lack of cortisol production, with subsequent increase in ACTH that causes hyperplasia of the adrenal cortex as well as skin hyperpigmentation. Abnormal levels of mineralocorticoids may cause hypertension (high aldosterone level) or hypotension along with hyponatremia and hyperkalemia (low aldosterone level). Increased androgens, such as testosterone, lead to precocious puberty in males and ambiguous genitalia in females. The most common enzyme deficiency is 21-hydroxylase deficiency, which leads to abnormally low aldosterone and cortisol levels and increased androgen levels. Thus, symptoms are hypotension and ambiguous genitalia in females or precocious puberty in males.

Zollinger-Ellison syndrome

Zollinger-Ellison syndrome is caused by a gastrin-secreting neuroendocrine tumor, most often located in the pancreas. If a gastrin-secreting tumor is suspected, it can usually be located using somatostatin-receptor scintigraphy (a nuclear medicine imaging method). If the tumor is able to be surgically resected (no distant metastases), surgical removal is the best treatment. Proton pump inhibitors should be prescribed before surgery to inhibit hydrochloric acid secretion by the gastric parietal cells. Surgical removal is the treatment of choice for other pancreatic neuroendocrine tumors as well, such as insulinomas (the most common type).

Somatostatin may also be used to treat neuroendocrine tumors, most commonly carcinoid tumors. Somatostatin is an inhibitory hormone normally produced by the anterior pituitary, and a synthetic form can be administered to counteract the hypersecretion of GI hormones such as secretin, vasoactive intestinal peptide (VIP), and motilin. This can help relieve symptoms of chronic abdominal pain, cramping, and diarrhea that are often associated with carcinoid tumors.

Antiobesity agents

First-line treatment of obesity is behavior modification, including exercise, nutrition, and lifestyle changes. If this is not successful, bariatric surgery (gastric bypass or gastric banding) may be considered for morbidly obese patients.

There are several anti-obesity agents. Orlistat (tetrahydrolipstatin) inhibits pancreatic lipase, thereby limiting ingested fat breakdown and absorption. Since ingested fats are not absorbed, the major side effect is steatorrhea. Phentermine is a stimulant that was used during the 1970s and 1980s as a weight-loss aid. It worked primarily by increasing norepinephrine secretion by the adrenal medulla. Major side effects include arrhythmias, restlessness, and insomnia. However, phentermine was removed from the market after being associated with heart valvular damage.

Hypocalcemia

The treatment of low serum calcium levels depends on the underlying cause. Since there is no FDA-approved synthetic PTH hormone, first-line treatment for hypoparathyroidism is often large daily doses of calcium and vitamin D in an attempt to induce hyperabsorption in the small intestine. This is likely to cause hypercalciuria (and renal calculi), so a thiazide diuretic can also be added to stimulate calcium reabsorption in the proximal tubules. Conversely, loop diuretics (like furosemide) can cause hypocalcemia and should be stopped when trying to correct serum calcium levels.

If high phosphate levels are present, this must be corrected first because giving calcium may cause calcium phosphate crystals to form in the blood and soft tissues. Hyperphosphatemia is corrected acutely through dialysis, and on a more long-term basis by using phosphate binders (sevelamer) and limiting dietary phosphate. Hypomagnesemia may be corrected by giving IV magnesium.

Hypercalcemia

The treatment of high serum calcium depends on the underlying cause. In the acute setting, large amounts of IV fluid are usually given to increase the amount of extracellular fluid to dilute the concentration of calcium. In severe cases, intranasal calcitonin can be given. Loop diuretics (like furosemide) can be given to encourage calcium excretion through the kidneys. Medications like thiazide diuretics should be stopped. Cancer-related hypercalcemia improves with antineoplastic therapy. Dietary calcium and vitamin D should be limited. Last, if increased bone resorption is present, bisphosphonates should be given to inhibit osteoclast function.

Insulin

Insulin and dietary adjustment (low-glycemic foods and carbohydrate counting) are used in the treatment of type I diabetes and also in type II diabetes when blood glucose levels remain uncontrolled on other medications. Synthetic insulin causes the same effects as endogenous insulin: increased glucose uptake by cells and decreased glycogen breakdown in the liver. Insulin is injected subcutaneously, and various types of insulin are available depending on how quickly they are absorbed by the body. In general, the dose of long-acting insulin is titrated to cover metabolic glucose production. The dose of short-acting insulins is titrated from meal to meal based on the carbohydrate content of the meal.
- Rapid-acting insulin (Insulin Lispro or Aspart) begins to work within minutes and lasts for less than 5 hours.
- Short-acting insulin (regular insulin) beings to work within 20 minutes and lasts 6 to 8 hours.
- Intermediate-acting insulin (Insulin NPH) begins to work in 1 to 2 hours and lasts about 18 hours.
- Long-acting insulin (Insulin Glargine, Ultralente, or Detemir) are administered once daily, begin to work in 3 to 4 hours, and last 24 hours. These insulins have no time of peak effect.

While tight glucose control has been shown to prevent or delay end-organ damage, tight glucose control may result in hypoglycemia.

Noninsulin antihyperglycemic therapy

Metformin is generally the first-line agent for treating type II diabetes. Metformin works by inhibiting gluconeogenesis in the liver and by enhancing glucose uptake in cells elsewhere in the body. The most common adverse effects are nausea and diarrhea (due to decreased sugar absorption). A noteworthy adverse effect is the potential for lactic acidosis if metformin is given in the setting of kidney failure.

Sulfonylureas (Glipizide, Glyburide) stimulate insulin secretion from the pancreas. The major side effect is that these drugs may cause hypoglycemia.

Alpha-glucosidase inhibitors (acarbose, miglitol) inhibits alpha-glucosidase enzyme in the small intestine, limiting absorption of carbohydrates. The most common adverse effects are bloating, cramping, and diarrhea.

Thiazolidinediones (rosiglitazone, pioglitazone) are peroxisome proliferator-activated receptor gamma (PPAR-gamma) agonists, which are insulin sensitizers that aid in peripheral glucose uptake. A major toxicity is the potential for liver damage, and liver function tests should be monitored every few months.

Diabetic ketoacidosis

Diabetic ketoacidosis (DKA) generally has a precipitating factor, such as viral illness, that increases the body's sensitivity to lack of circulating insulin. This leads to hyperglycemia, ketoacid formation, and hypovolemia (due to diuresis). The most important treatment of DKA is volume resuscitation. A continuous insulin drip (IV insulin) is also administered; blood glucose levels are checked at least every 30 minutes. Both insulin and fluids are continued until the anion gap has normalized (remember, anion gap is calculated as sodium – [chloride + bicarbonate]).

Electrolyte replacement is also imperative. Insulin normally leads to closing of a potassium channel, preventing potassium from leaving the cell. Since no insulin is present, insulin leaks from cells into the blood. Therefore, even if a DKA patient's serum potassium is within the normal range, total body potassium is low and must be replaced.

Thyroid tumors

Thyroid nodules may be detected on physical exam or incidentally on imaging studies for other purposes. An ultrasound can be performed to characterize the nodule and determine its size. Fine needle aspiration biopsies can be performed for concerning nodules, usually greater than 1 cm or 1.5 cm in size. Or, an iodine-131 scan can be used to determine if the nodule is "hot" (increased iodine uptake associated with benign nodules) or "cold" (decreased iodine uptake more concerning for tumor).

Small nodules can be resected, but typically tumors require total thyroidectomy and limited lymph node dissection. Patients with large nodules or at risk of metastatic disease may then undergo radioablation therapy with iodine-131 (the same substance used for iodine-131 scans, but at more than 30 times the dose to induce local radiation damage and cell death). Patients with total thyroidectomies must then receive thyroid replacement therapy for the rest of their lives. Since no thyroid tissue should be present, serum thyroglobulin levels can be checked for cancer surveillance: a rise in serum thyroglobulin levels indicates that recurrent/metastatic thyroid tissue is present and an iodine-131 scan may be able to localize the recurrent tumor. Medullary cancers are treated with surgery only, since the parafollicular cells do not take up iodine. Anaplastic cancers may also be treated with radiation therapy.

Pituitary prolactinoma

The increased endogenous prolactin from prolactinomas causes menstrual cycle irregularities and impotence in women, and causes decreased libido and impotence in men. Normally, the hypothalamus regulates the secretion of prolactin by the anterior pituitary gland via dopamine (also known as prolactin-inhibiting hormone). Therefore, dopamine agonists such as bromocriptine and cabergoline may be used to decrease prolactin levels in patients suffering from hyperprolactinemia; the goal is usually to restore fertility and gonadal dysfunction. If dopamine agonist therapy is unsuccessful, transsphenoidal surgery may be performed to remove the prolactinoma. During this procedure, the surgeon will access the pituitary gland through the nose and by breaking through the sphenoid sinuses.

Risk factors for developing type 2 diabetes

Type 2 diabetes is a multifactorial disease, brought on by a combination of environmental and genetic risk factors. Over 80% of patients with type 2 diabetes exhibit visceral obesity. The distribution of fat is an important predictor of diabetes with abdominal fat putting individuals at higher risk than peripheral fat depots. Because inactivity and high caloric intake are associated with obesity, these can also be considered risk factors for type 2 diabetes. Strong genetic influences also play a role. Twin studies have shown a disease concordance rate of 35% to 60% in identical twins, with about half this rate observed in dizygotic twins. Furthermore, genome-wide association studies have recently unveiled over a dozen loci associated with type 2 diabetes. Race is also an important consideration; blacks, Hispanics, Asian-Americans, and American Indians are at a higher risk for type 2 diabetes than whites. Although the risk of type 2 diabetes increases with age, it is becoming more common in children and adolescents.

Risk factors for developing thyroid diseases

In general, autoimmune thyroid disorders (Graves and Hashimoto diseases) are associated with a gender predilection towards females. The female-to-male ratio for Graves disease is about 8:1 and for Hashimoto is almost 15:1. Both affect younger women, typically 20 to 50 years of age.

The most important risk factor for most types of thyroid cancer is exposure to radiation. This is why thyroid shields are worn during interventional procedures using fluoroscopy.

Papillary and follicular thyroid carcinomas comprise about 95% of all thyroid cancers. Both have a strong female predilection (female to male ratio of 3:1) and also occur more commonly in Caucasians than African Americans. Anaplastic thyroid carcinoma (1% of thyroid cancers) also has a strong female predilection. Medullary thyroid carcinoma and lymphoma are not associated with a strong gender bias.

Immune System

B-cell development

Precursors to B lymphocytes (pre–B lymphocytes begin their development in the bone marrow as lymphoid stem cells and continue to divide under the control of certain hormones. B lymphocytes, which display each possible antigen the host may encounter, are formed. During an infection, the B cells interact with the antigen in the lymph nodes or spleen. Cells displaying the correct receptor against the invading antigen begin to proliferate, creating B-cell clones and antibodies against the pathogen. B cells are responsible for the humoral immune response.

T-cell development

Precursors to T lymphocytes (pre–T lymphocytes) develop in the bone marrow and migrate to the thymus. While in the thymus, the lymphocytes are exposed to a variety of possible antigens. Lymphocytes with receptors to each of those possible antigens are produced. They exit the thymus as mature, but undifferentiated T lymphocytes. During an infection, the T cells interact with the antigen in the peripheral lymph tissue. T cells displaying the correct receptor against the antigen proliferate and begin the process of cell-mediated immunity. T-cell development occurs in the thymus and is greatest during early childhood and in the fetal period. The thymus shrinks after puberty.

Positive selection

Positive selection of T cells occurs deep in the thymic cortex. Immature T lymphocytes, expressing both CD4 and CD8, move into the cortex during development and are presented with self-antigens. Only cells that are capable of interacting appropriately with the major histocompatibility complex (MHC) molecules (either I or II) survive, while cells that interact either too strongly or too weakly die off. In fact, most lymphocytes do not receive this survival signal and eventually die. T cells that interact well with MHC-II molecules become CD4 cells, and T cells that interact well with MHC-I molecules become CD8 cells.

Negative selection

Negative selection occurs in the medulla of the thymus and checks for T cells that have too strong an affinity for self-antigens. While in the medulla of the thymus, they are presented with self-antigens on the major histocompatibility complex of specialized thymic cells. T cells that react too strongly with these self-antigens undergo apoptosis. The goal of this process is to increase immune tolerance of the self and to prevent the lymphocytes from directly attacking the host's own cells.

Granulocytes

There are two classifications of white blood cells, or leukocytes: granulocytes and agranulocytes. Granulocytes are characterized by the presence of many granules, which are bound by a membrane, in their cytoplasm. These granules contain specialized enzymes and cellular mediators that are designed to destroy macrophages and trigger other inflammatory processes. These mediators can also break down intracellular debris, resulting from injury or infection. The enzymes and chemical mediators are released from the granules as a result of specific stimuli. They are also released by all granulocytes during apoptosis. Granulocytes include the neutrophils, eosinophil's, and basophils.

Natural killer cells

Natural killer (NK) cells are specialized lymphocytes, similar to T cells. They do not have antigen-specific receptors and cannot bind antigens during an immune response. This means that they do not proliferate or clone as a result of their interaction with an antigen. The NK cells can recognize changes (nonantigenic) on the surface of infected cells and can act like a cytotoxic T cell, directly killing the infected or malignant cells. The NK cells also participate in antibody-dependent cellular cytotoxicity, meaning they have an Fc receptor, allowing the NK cells to bind to Fc regions on infected cells coated with antibody.

Macrophages

Macrophages are a type of white blood cell, or leukocyte, and are actually quite large (20–40 µm). They are agranulocytes, meaning they do not contain membrane-bound granules in the cytoplasm. Macrophages appear at the site of injury or inflammation a few days after the initial injury but may appear as early as 24 hours. They are typically associated with chronic inflammation, not an acute infection. Macrophages serve several important functions in the immune response: they assist with antigen processing and presentation to lymphocytes and the secretion of colony-stimulating factors, and they assist with tissue repair. They respond to lymphokines and also produce substances that encourage the growth, development, and maturation of other immune cells.

Mast cells

Mast cells are large cells that have granules in their cytoplasm. These granules contain proteins and cell mediators involved in the immune response. Histamine is one such mediator that is in particular abundance in the granules of mast cells. However, the mediators found in mast cells work with many different types of cells, including nerves, smooth muscle cells, and vascular endothelial cells. Mast cells are found in the connective tissue, mucous membranes, and dermis. When released, these mediators cause nearby blood vessels to become more permeable, or leaky. Mast cells are active during chronic inflammation, wound healing, and other processes.

Dendritic cells

Dendritic cells, or antigen-presenting cells, process antigens and present them to the T cells. These cells are present in the skin and the mucosal membrane of the nose, stomach, and lungs. Immature forms of these cells can be found in the blood, which then migrate to the lymph nodes when activated. Once in the lymph nodes, they interact with other cells of the immune system, namely the B cells and T cells, to present their antigens and initiate an immune response. They are similar in appearance to the dendrites of the neurological system; that is, central cells with long projections that extend from the main cell body.

Cell receptors

Cell receptors are proteins found inside or on the surface of cells that receive signals from outside the cell and transmit that signal into or throughout the cell through electrical stimulation (or other means). They can also be found in the nucleus or on the nuclear membrane. Receptors are a specific shape, and only molecules that are complementary to that shape will fit in and activate the receptor.

T-lymphocyte receptors

T-cell receptors (TCRs) are found on the surface of T cells. Their primary function is to recognize major histocompatibility complex (MHC) antigens. They are not specific and, as a result, can recognize many different MHC antigens. The TCRs are composed of two protein chains: an alpha chain and a beta chain. Each chain contains two regions: a variable, or V region, and a constant, or C region. The constant region attaches the TCRs to the membrane, and the V region attaches the TCRs to the MHC antigen. Each variable region on both the alpha and beta chains has three complementary determining regions (CDRs): CDR1 interacts with the antigenic peptide; CDR2 recognizes MHC; and CDR3 is the main region that recognizes antigens.

T-cell activation and proliferation

Lymphocytes exit the thymus as mature but undifferentiated T lymphocytes. There are two signals required for activation of the T cells. The first occurs when an antigen on the surface of a dendritic cell or B lymphocyte activates the T-cell receptors. The second signal is activated by a co-stimulatory molecule, most commonly CD28. Once activated, the T cells proliferate and differentiate into helper

T cells and cytotoxic T cells specific to the antigen originally presented by the major histocompatibility complex. The T cells also encourage secretion of cytokines.

Cytotoxic T cells

Cytotoxic T cells are also known as CD8 cells and are directly involved in the destruction of tumor cells and cells infected by viruses. They may also be involved in the processes associated with transplant rejection. The CD8 cells work with major histocompatibility complex class I (MHC I) molecules to recognize and process antigens. If the T-cell receptor (TCR) on a cytotoxic T cell is specific to and recognizes the antigen expressed on the MHC I molecule of an infected cell, it will bind to it and directly kill the cell. The glycoprotein CD8 is required to bind to the C region of the MHC I molecule, which is why cytotoxic T cells are called CD8. In addition to the interaction between the MHC I and the TCR, a second signal is required for activation of cytotoxic T cells. This is usually CD80 or CD86 expressed by the antigen-presenting cell.

Memory T cells

The primary function of memory T cells is to proliferate and spread throughout the body after an infection has already resolved. This helps the immune system "remember" the infection and rapidly respond to future infections by the same antigen. Memory T cells can cause a stronger and more effective response during subsequent infections than they did with the first infection. There are multiple types of memory T cells, including central-memory T cells and effector-memory T cells. Central-memory T cells secrete interleukin-2. Effector-memory T cells secrete interferon gamma and interleukin-4.

B-lymphocyte receptors

The B-lymphocyte receptors (BCRs) are proteins that are found on the outer membrane of B cells. On the first encounter with an antigen, B cells rapidly proliferate and differentiate into memory B cells and effector B cells. In addition to processing the antigen and assisting in generating the immune response, B cells play a crucial role in presenting the antigen to helper T cells. There are two regions of the BCRs: the ligand-binding moiety and the signal-transduction moiety. The ligand-binding moiety contains one of five different types of immunoglobulins. The signal-transduction moiety extends through the plasma membrane.

B-lymphocyte activation and growth

Under hormonal guidance, B cells circulate through the human bursa-equivalent tissue where they proliferate and gain the ability to interact with foreign antigens and to create antibodies. Before moving through the human bursa-equivalent tissue, B cells are not able to interact with antigen, nor produce antibodies. According to the clonal selection theory, a large number of B cells with the potential to respond to all possible antigens, are produced during early development, though each cell is only able to respond to one specific antigen. When an activated B cell encounters an antigen for the first time, the appropriate antibody receptors undergo differentiation and proliferation. They are then called plasma cells and are found in the blood and lymph circulation.

Immunoglobulins

There are five types of immunoglobulins: IgA, IgD, IgE, IgG, and IgM. Immunoglobulin A is found in normal body secretions in the form of IgA2, while IgA1 is usually found circulating in the blood. Immunoglobulin E is the immunoglobulin usually associated with allergies, allergic conditions, and asthma. Immunoglobulin D is found in the blood, and more specifically, on the surface of developing B cells. Its exact function is unclear. Immunoglobulin G is the most common immunoglobulin and is responsible for many immune and antibody functions, including complement activation, agglutination, and antibody precipitation. Immunoglobulin M is the first immunoglobulin produced during the initial immune response to an antigen.

Antibody

Antibodies are Y-shaped glycoproteins produced by plasma cells to disable foreign material in the body. Immunoglobulin is the generic term for this class of molecules, whereas antibodies are immunoglobulins against a specific antigen. The two tips of the "Y" are called antigen-binding fragments (Fab fragments), and they bind the antigen to the antibody with "lock and key" specificity. The tail of the "Y" is called the crystalline fragment (Fc fragment) and is the biologically active portion of the molecule. The Fc fragment is composed of two heavy chains that, depending on the class of immunoglobulin, contain several constant domains, allowing the antibody to produce the appropriate immune response.

Antibody diversity

Immunoglobulins are Y-shaped molecules that contain two heavy chains and two light chains of many amino acids. Each chain (both heavy and light) has both a constant region and a variable region. There are two types of light chains (i.e., lambda, kappa) and five classes of heavy chains (i.e., IgA, IgD, IgE, IgG, IgM,). The variety of DNA segments that code for the different regions on the heavy and light chains leads to an incredible diversity of antibodies against 15,000,000 antigens or more.

Memory B lymphocytes

During the initial exposure to an antigen, two types of B lymphocytes are produced: memory B cells and plasma B cells. Memory B cells are produced immediately after an infection and remain in circulation in the body. If that antigen reappears in the body, the memory B cells are able to mount an immune response that is much quicker and more effective than the initial response. With each subsequent infection or exposure to the antigen, more and more memory B cells are produced, and a stronger response occurs. This is called a secondary immune response.

Lymph nodes

Lymph nodes are found throughout the body and are connected by lymphatic vessels. They are shaped like small, oval beans with an inner medulla and an outer cortex surrounding the medulla, except at the hilum of the node. Thin fibers of elastin and reticulin form a reticular network inside, where the white blood cells are tightly packed. There are also lymph sinuses where the lymph fluid is able to flow through the node. Afferent lymph vessels bring the lymph into the node, and efferent vessels transport the lymph out of the lymph node. The lymph nodes trap and filter foreign material from the lymph fluid and also activate the immune response.

Normal host immune mechanisms

Normal host immune mechanisms include a combination of both an innate, or nonspecific, immune system and an adaptive, or antigen-specific, immune system. The innate immune system includes physical barriers, like the skin and mucous membranes, chemical membranes, like the enzymes secreted by the gastrointestinal and respiratory tracts, and general immune processes, like inflammation and complement. Cells of the immune system are also found throughout the body and can respond to invading pathogens in a nonspecific manner. These cells include macrophages, dendritic cells, natural killer cells, and leukocytes. The adaptive immune system allows for a more antigen-specific response and includes the B and T lymphocytes, antibodies, and the process of immunological memory. When a foreign body enters the body, these cells are able to launch a direct attack on the foreign antigen. Memory cells are also produced so that subsequent infections can cause a more effective response.

Barriers to infection

There are many natural barriers to infection within the body. Physical barriers include the skin and mucous membranes, which prevent invading bacteria and other pathogens from entering the body; innate mechanisms help to expel antigens that have already entered the body, like sneezing, coughing, and the flushing action of tears and urine. Mucus in the respiratory and gastrointestinal tracts also trap bacteria and flush them out of the body. There are multiple chemical barriers at work within the immune system as well. Enzymes and antimicrobial proteins are secreted in body fluids and help to break down pathogens by altering the pH or by direct enzymatic action. Within the gastrointestinal and genitourinary tracts, there is a population of normal flora that competes with pathogenic bacteria. Without this normal flora, abnormal bacteria would be able to proliferate and cause infection.

Mucosal immunity

The mucous membranes provide both a physical barrier and a chemical barrier to infection. The mucous membranes in the nose and airway provide a means of preventing invading bacteria and other pathogens from entering the body and have innate mechanisms (i.e., sneezing) for expelling antigens that have already entered the body. Mucus also acts to trap bacteria and other debris and keep it from entering the body or causing infection. Finally, there are enzymes and other antimicrobial proteins secreted by the mucous membranes that directly attack and kill invading pathogens.

Immunogenetics

Immunogenetics explores how immunology and genetics are related. Researchers specializing in this field do research on autoimmune disorders, abnormalities in immune function, and the heritability of normal immunity. They also look at developing new treatment modalities that aim to treat or cure previously incurable diseases. For example, some autoimmune diseases or other immune deficiencies are caused by abnormalities in a patient's DNA or genetics. Studying how these diseases are inherited can help researchers develop new therapies for these conditions.

ABO and Rh blood types

Blood type is the result of a group (or lack of a group) of antigens found on the surface of red blood cells. There are two types of antigens: A and B. People with blood type A have the A antigen present on their red blood cells. They also produce antibodies against the B antigen. People with blood type B have the B antigen present and produce anti-A antibodies. People with AB blood type have both A and B antigens on their red blood cells and do not produce either anti-A or anti-B antibodies. People with O blood type do not have any antigens present but produce anti-A and anti-B antibodies. Rh type is also determined by the presence or absence of the rhesus antigen. There are several rhesus antigens, but the most significant one is the D group because it is most likely to cause an immune reaction. Individuals with a Rh-positive blood type have the rhesus antigen on their blood cells; those with a Rh-negative blood type do not.

Histocompatibility complex class I molecules

Major histocompatibility complex class I (MHC I) is one of the two main classes of the MHC molecules. These MHC I molecules are found on almost every cell in the body that contains a nucleus. They display pieces of cellular proteins to T cells to help the immune system determine which cells are foreign and which are not. These proteins are usually fragments of proteins found within the cytoplasm of the cell. If the cell has pieces of bacteria or viruses in the cytoplasm after cellular infection, the MHC I molecules will display those fragments, alerting the immune system to the infection. When these viral fragments are displayed, apoptosis induced by the cell-mediated immune system occurs. Many viruses, however, have undergone evolutionary changes that enable them to inactivate the MHC I molecules in order to evade detection. Natural killer (NK) cells, which are normally deactivated in the presence of normally operating MHC I molecules, will destroy the virus-infected cells, because the NK cells have not been given the deactivation signal by the MHC I molecules, which have been inactivated by the virus.

Major histocompatibility complex

Major histocompatibility complex genes are inherited as a group of genes on chromosome 6, one from the mother and one from the father. Each group contains three class I and three class II loci from each parent, totaling twelve altogether. The class I loci are B, C, and A; the class II loci are DP, DQ, and DR. Each of these loci code for the expression of different histocompatibility antigens, meaning that there are twelve different antigens involved.

Major histocompatibility complex class II molecules

Major histocompatibility class II (MHC II) molecules are the second of the two main classes of the MHC molecules. Unlike the MHC I molecules, these antigens are only found on antigen-presenting cells and B cells. The antigens expressed by this class of molecules are found in the extracellular fluid, not in the cytoplasm. These extracellular proteins are taken into the cell by phagocytosis, digested in the lysosomes, and then the peptide fragments are subsequently loaded into the MHC II molecules and moved to the surface of the cell. The MHC II molecules interact primarily with the CD4, or helper T cells.

Adaptive immune response

The adaptive immune system allows for a more antigen-specific response and includes the B and T lymphocytes, antibodies, and the process of immunological memory. When a foreign body enters the body, these cells are able to launch a direct attack on the foreign antigen. Memory cells are also produced so that subsequent infections can cause a larger, more effective reaction. Regulatory T cells help suppress over-responses of the immune system and prevent the development of autoimmune disease.

Pathways for complement activation

There are three different pathways that activate the complement system: the classical pathway, the alternative pathway, and the lectin pathway. The classical pathway is activated when an antibody binds to its specific antigen, known as an immune complex. Each antibody has multiple antigen-binding sites; for example, when the Fc regions of an antibody are close together, production of complement is activated when C1 binds to these adjacent Fc regions. A cascade of enzymatic reactions occur that activate other forms of complement, which, in turn, activate inflammatory processes, vasodilation, and mast-cell degranulation. The alternative pathway is activated through several different mechanisms: antigen opsonization, endotoxin secreted by bacterial cell walls, inflammation, and anaphylaxis. The lectin pathway is very similar to the classical pathway, except that substances other than C1 (i.e., opsonin, mannose-binding lectin, ficolins) activate the pathway.

Complement

Complement is a part of the innate immune system that complements, or assists, the immune response. It helps antibodies and other cells to clear foreign invaders from the body. There are four main functions of complement: opsonization, the process of making an antigen more susceptible to phagocytosis; chemotaxis, the process of attracting macrophages and other leukocytes; lysis, the process of causing cell-membrane rupture of foreign cells; and the clumping of immune complexes for processing.

Opsonization

Opsonization is the process of optimizing phagocytosis of an antigen. This occurs when opsonins bind to the surface of the antigen, so that they are "marked" and more easily identified. Antibodies and complement factors C3b and C4b are the most common opsonins. Once these antigens are marked, they are targeted by the immune system for destruction by either phagocytosis or antibody-dependent cellular toxicity. In antibody-dependent cellular toxicity, granulocytes are attracted to the antigen and subsequently release toxic substances surrounding the foreign material. While this causes cell death of the pathogen, it also causes cell death of the normal host tissue, causing inflammation and tissue damage.

Cytokines

Cytokines are a class of small proteins that are produced by macrophages as well as by a number of other cells that are responsible for cell signaling. Cytokines include chemokines, interferons, lymphokines, tumor necrosis factor, and interleukins. They bind to specialized receptors on cells in the immune system and are actively involved in maintaining the balance between humoral and cell-based immunity. They are also responsible for the responsiveness and growth of immune cells. They are distributed widely throughout the body. Interleukin-12 secretion occurs after an infected macrophage displays the antigen on its surface, which causes the proliferation of helper T cells. Macrophages also secrete cytokines to aid in wound healing a few days after the initial injury. In addition to secreting cytokines, macrophages also have receptors for lymphokines.

Interleukins

Interleukins are cytokines produced by immune cells and play a role in enhancing the immune response. Interleukin-1 is produced by antigen-presenting cells and assists the T cells in their immune response. Interleukin-2 is secreted by natural killer cells and the helper T cells to encourage growth and maturation of helper T cells into mature T cells. Interleukin-4 is secreted primarily by T lymphocytes and mast cells to encourage growth and proliferation of T cells, active B cells, and macrophages. Interleukin-6 is secreted by both T and B cells to aid in B-cell proliferation and hematopoiesis; it also increases the inflammatory response. Interleukin-10 is produced by helper T cells and decreases proliferation of helper T cells and increases cytotoxic T-cell production; it also decreases cytokine production. Interleukin-12 is secreted by macrophages to increase the production of helper T cells and other lymphocytes.

Interferons

Interferons are small proteins produced by virally infected cells to help prevent viral infection of other cells. They are cytokines that can alert other cells about potential threats. They do not kill viruses, but they prevent infection of cells by viruses by binding to receptors on other nearby cells. If they are unaffected by the virus, binding of interferon encourages the cell to pump out antiviral proteins.

Tumor necrosis factor

Tumor necrosis factor (TNF) is a cytokine produced by the monocytes, macrophages, natural killer cells, and lymphocytes. When secreted, it produces a cytotoxic effect, causing apoptosis in targeted cells. Its primary function is to regulate the growth and activation of immune cells and can cause fever, cachexia, and inflammation. Abnormal TNF production has been investigated as a potential causal factor for cancer, Alzheimer's disease, and other immune disorders.

Selective immunoglobulin A deficiency

Selective immunoglobulin A (IgA) deficiency is a genetic condition found in approximately 1 in 300 people. People with this condition completely lack IgA, an immunoglobulin found in the mucous membranes of the digestive and respiratory tracts. Although most people with this condition are asymptomatic, they are often prone to infection, especially in the respiratory and genitourinary tracts. These infections are most often mild, although some people have severe anaphylactic reactions to blood transfusions or immunoglobulin infusions because of IgA in the product. There is no cure for this condition; treatment instead focuses on quickly identifying and treating infections. Measures to prevent infection are also stressed.

Common variable immunodeficiency

Common variable immunodeficiency is genetically linked although the exact relationship has not been determined, and is one of the most common primary immunodeficiencies; that is, it is not an acquired deficiency as from an infection. People with this condition do not produce adequate levels of antibodies, despite having normal B-cell counts. This means that their immune system is not able to protect them adequately from invading pathogens and infections. As a result, patients are susceptible to severe recurring infections, although they usually respond to antibiotics or antivirals. Other symptoms include enlarged lymph nodes, enlarged spleen, fatigue, gastrointestinal symptoms, muscle and joint pain, and failure to thrive. Diagnosis is made by exclusion, when other causes for these symptoms cannot be found. People with this condition also tend to have low levels of immunoglobulins. Treatment is infusion of immunoglobulin to strengthen the immune response.

Ataxia-telangiectasia

Ataxia-telangiectasia is a rare genetic disorder that affects not only the immune system but also the nervous system. The first symptoms occur in early childhood, usually in toddlers. Affected children have difficulty walking and standing still, often stumbling or wobbling. As time passes, they have difficulty moving their eyes from one side to the other and eventually develop difficulty speaking and swallowing. Children with this condition are prone to upper respiratory infections and chronic telangiectasia, or redness of the blood vessels in the sclera of the eyes. They are also significantly more likely to develop cancer, especially lymphoma and leukemia. Finally, many people with this condition have low levels of immunoglobulins and lymphocytes, which can sometimes be treated by immunization. Diagnosis is usually made from steadily increasing blood levels of alpha-fetoprotein. The average life expectancy is approximately 25 years of age. The ataxia-telangiectasia mutated gene is thought to be causative.

Natural killer cells

Natural killer– (NK-) cell deficiency is a genetic condition where there is a complete absence of NK cells. There are many different genes that contribute to this condition. A child must inherit two mutated genes, one from each parent, in order to have the condition. People with this condition have extremely low or a complete lack of NK cells, making sufferers very susceptible to infections; patients are also at an increased risk of developing cancer. There is no cure for NK-cell deficiency so the focus is on preventing and managing infection.

Leukocyte-adhesion deficiency

Leukocyte-adhesion deficiency (LAD) is an extremely rare genetic disorder where a patient's leukocytes are unable to produce a protein called CD18 in sufficient quantity or quality. Normal leukocytes, when they detect an infection, adhere to the wall of the blood vessel. They then slowly roll over to the site of the infection and begin to process the antigen. In patients with LAD, their leukocytes are able to detect the infection but are not able to adhere to the vessel wall so they can start dealing with the antigen. There are four subtypes of this condition: type 1, classical; type 1, novel; type 2; and type 3. Symptoms vary, depending on the type of LAD, but in general, they include recurrent skin and other internal infections, gum disease, leukocytosis, an increased number of yeast infections, and abnormal wound healing. Patients with novel type 1 may also have an enlarged spleen and muscle tenderness. Treatment includes aggressively managing infections with antibiotics (oral and intravenous) and, in severe cases, transfusions with white blood cells and stem cells.

Chediak-Higashi syndrome

Chediak-Higashi syndrome is a rare genetic disorder. It is inherited as an autosomal recessive condition. People with this condition have improperly functioning lysosomes, so phagocytosed bacteria and debris are not properly discarded within the cell. Patients also have cells characterized by large lysosomes and vesicles within the cytoplasm and abnormalities in nuclear structure; they exhibit partial albinism and sensitivity to light, especially the sun. They are susceptible to frequent infections in the skin, mucous membranes, and respiratory tract. The prognosis for people with this condition is poor; few people live to adulthood because of serious infection. In the accelerated form, white blood cells (WBCs) divide abnormally and rapidly. These abnormal WBCs invade the tissues and act almost like a severe lymphoma, causing bleeding, fever, and organ failure. There is no cure for Chediak-Higashi syndrome; management involves treating and preventing infection. Bone marrow transplants have been successful in some patients.

Chronic granulomatous disease

Chronic granulomatous disease (CGD) is actually a group of immune diseases where certain immune cells are unable to produce superoxide radicals that are necessary to kill phagocytosed pathogens. As a result, granulomas (i.e., a small nodule or collection of macrophages) are formed in many different organs. Symptoms include recurrent infection, especially pneumonia and skin abscesses. People with CGD are also more likely to contract atypical infections, from *Staphylococcus aureus*, *Serratia marcescens*, and *Listeria*, among others. It is a genetic condition, and most cases are the result of mutations on the X chromosome. There is no cure, but treatment focuses on preventing and managing infections. Interferon has been approved by the Food and Drug Administration for treatment of CGD, namely by reducing the number and severity of infections.

C1 esterase-inhibitor deficiency

The C1 esterase-inhibitor deficiency, also known as hereditary angioedema, is a rare genetic disorder that is characterized by episodes of edema in the hands, feet, and face. Edema also occurs in the throat, which can be life-threatening, and in the intestines, which can lead to severe pain, nausea, and vomiting. The C1 esterase inhibitor is a protein in the complement system, responsible for regulating inflammation and coagulation. Without it, fluid and electrolyte imbalances occur, causing fluid to leak from the capillaries into the surrounding tissues. This is what causes the swelling. There are many potential triggers, including certain medications, especially angiotensin-converting enzyme inhibitors; hormonal changes, such as pregnancy and menstruation; and increases in activity and stress. Treatment includes managing the acute edema and preventing future attacks with the use C1 esterase inhibitors, such as Cinryze and Berinert; a kallikrein inhibitor, ecallantide (Kalbitor); and a bradykinin-receptor antagonist, icatibant injection (Firazyr).

C3 deficiency

A C3 deficiency is an extremely rare genetic condition, inherited in an autosomal recessive manner; C3 plays a crucial role in activating the immune and inflammatory response. As a result, people with this condition are at risk for severe infections due to their extremely impaired immune response. In addition, patients are at risk for many lupus-like conditions, vasculitis, and glomerulonephritis. A C3 deficiency causes poor opsonization, leading to ineffective processing of antigens and pathogens. Screening for this condition is very easy; a simple blood test is able to detect levels of C3. There is no treatment or cure for this condition; instead, treatment focuses on preventing and managing acute infections.

C4 deficiencies

The peptide C4 is crucial to the lectin and classical pathways for complement activation and inflammation. Deficiency of C4 has been associated with severe infections, especially bacterial meningitis. A C4 deficiency can be either genetic or acquired, usually the result of infections, like kidney disease, chronic hepatitis, and childhood diabetes. Levels of C4 can be measured in the blood; low levels can indicate a systemic lupus flare.

Decay-accelerating factor

Decay-accelerating factor (DAF) is a protein that regulates the complement system. It is found on the cell membranes and recognizes the components formed during all three pathways of complement activation. When activated, DAF prevents the conversion of C2 and factor B to their more active forms, activating the rest of the complement cascade and ultimately blocking the formation of the membrane attack complex.

X-linked agammaglobulinemia (Bruton's disease)

The X-linked agammaglobulinemia (XLA), or Bruton's disease, is an X-linked recessive disorder, meaning that men tend to inherit this condition more frequently than women. People with this condition do not have an adequate number of B cells, antibodies, or immunoglobulins. Children tend to be healthy at birth because they are protected by maternal antibodies acquired during the neonatal period. After this time, however, these infants start having serious and recurrent bacterial infections. The most common infections that plague patients with XLA include sinusitis, pneumonia, otitis, conjunctivitis, and intestinal infections causing severe diarrhea. There is no cure for XLA, but treatment focuses on treating infections early and aggressively. Methods for preventing infection should be stressed to patients and their family. Depending on the clinical situation, antibody replacement through an intravenous infusion of intravenous immunoglobulin may be indicated.

DiGeorge syndrome

DiGeorge syndrome is a genetic disorder caused by an abnormality on chromosome 22. Patients with this condition inherit cardiac defects, cleft palate, behavioral problems, immune dysfunction, and abnormal electrolyte levels. Symptoms include cyanosis, fatigue, failure to thrive or weight gain, shortness of breath, frequent infections, developmental and speech delays, and particular facial features (i.e., small, low-set ears; wide, hooded eyes; long face). There is no cure for DiGeorge syndrome. Treatment focuses on interventions for the associated sequelae: correcting electrolyte disturbances, repairing a cleft palate, surgery to repair cardiac defects, occupational and speech therapy, and in some cases, early intervention programs.

Autosomal dominant hyper-immunoglobulin E (hyper-IgE) syndrome (Job syndrome)

Autosomal dominant hyper-immunoglobulin E (hyper-IgE) syndrome, also known as Job syndrome, is an extremely rare autosomal dominant genetic disorder. People with this condition have an increased production of IgE, causing frequent skin infections, usually caused by bacteria or fungi. In addition to skin infections, patients with this condition are also more prone to eczema, staphylococcal infections, failure to lose primary teeth, osteoporosis, conjunctivitis, lymphadenitis, lung infections, fever, and reduced bone density. Diagnosis is usually made after measuring an elevated serum IgE level, in conjunction with the clinical history. Treatment involves treating and preventing infections with antibiotics and good skin care. Sometimes intravenous immunoglobulin is indicated for managing severe eczema.

Chronic mucocutaneous candidiasis

Chronic mucocutaneous candidiasis is a genetic condition that causes an abnormality of the T cells. As a result, the patient suffers from chronic *Candida* infections of the skin and mucous membranes. These *Candida* infections are most common in the mouth and mucous membranes, the head and scalp, the skin, and the vagina. In most cases, the rest of the immune system is functioning well, so the body is able to fight off infections. In some cases, however, antibodies are also affected, which makes patients susceptible to other severe infections. While annoying, patients with this condition do not typically suffer from severe, life-threatening infections or from a shortened lifespan. Treatment is long-term antifungal creams applied to the skin or affected areas. If topical creams do not treat the infection, systemic drugs like fluconazole (Diflucan) can be used.

Severe combined immunodeficiency

Severe combined immunodeficiency (SCID) is a primary immune deficiency affecting primarily the T and B cells. This leads to severe infections, starting at birth. Children with this condition are even susceptible to diseases found in live-virus vaccines. This condition is often called the "bubble-boy disease" because affected children must be protected from all infections. Inheritance of this condition varies; the most common is X-linked, though some cases are the result of autosomal recessive inheritance or a spontaneous genetic mutation. There is no cure for this condition, but infection prevention is a priority. Treatment is early and aggressive treatment of all infections.

Hyperimmunoglobulin M (hyper-IgM) syndrome

Hyperimmunoglobulin M (hyper-IgM) syndrome is a genetic disorder where immunoglobulin M antibodies are overproduced. In normal circumstances, during an initial exposure to an antigen, IgM is the primary immunoglobulin produced; however, after the initial exposure, IgM production wanes, and other immunoglobulins are produced in high numbers. Patients with hyper-IgM syndrome just keep pumping out IgM, leading to an underproduction of the rest of the antibodies needed for immune function. There are five types. In hyper-IgM syndrome, type 1, T cells are unable to communicate with the B cells to tell them to switch immunoglobulin classes. In hyper-IgM syndrome, type 2, B cells are not able to make the genetic changes necessary for production of other immunoglobulins. In hyper-IgM syndrome, type 3, B cells are unable to receive the message from T cells needed to switch immunoglobulins. In hyper- IgM syndrome, types 4 and 5, more complex genetic changes occur, preventing the necessary class-switch.

Wiskott-Aldrich syndrome

The Wiskott-Aldrich syndrome is a very rare X-linked genetic disorder. Patients with this condition tend to have abnormal platelet production, leading to thrombocytopenia. In addition, patients with this condition also have decreased antibody production and poorly functioning T cells. The combination of these factors causes patients to be more likely to contract routine infections of the ear and sinuses. Symptoms include increased bleeding, eczema, and bacterial infections, starting during infancy, and splenomegaly. Most patients also have autoimmune disorders and are at an increased risk for developing cancer. There is no cure; treatment is palliative and is focused on managing symptoms. Transfusions, intravenous immunoglobulin, and stem-cell transplants may be indicated, depending on the clinical situation.

Hashimoto's disease

Hashimoto's disease is an autoimmune condition where the thyroid gland is attacked by multiple components of the immune system. In most patients, antibodies against thyroid peroxidase, thyroglobulin, and thyroid-stimulating hormone receptors are present. Cytotoxic T cells and macrophages are recruited, as a result of the activation of helper T cells, destroying thyroid tissue. This condition is diagnosed by testing for levels of these antithyroid antibodies in conjunction with the clinical presentation. Symptoms include those of hypothyroidism but progress to a large, painless thyroid goiter and periorbital myxedema. Treatment involves replacing thyroid hormone in the form of levothyroxine. Periodic thyroid levels should be taken to ensure that supplementation is adequate.

Systemic lupus erythematosus

Systemic lupus erythematosus (SLE) is an autoimmune disorder that affects the entire body. The disease is characterized by periods of active disease, called flares, and periods of remission. It is a type II and a type III hypersensitivity reaction that causes tissue damage to the cardiopulmonary system, the skin, liver, kidneys, joints, and nervous system. A single distinct cause has not yet been identified, but there are thought to be both genetic links and environmental triggers. In addition, some medications can induce an SLE-like reaction that is not permanent. In patients with SLE, a large number of antibodies against host tissues are produced, most commonly against the patient's own DNA and other nucleic material. Immune complexes containing these antibodies are deposited in the joints, kidneys, and elsewhere, causing the chronic inflammation that occurs with SLE. Symptoms include joint pain, distinct butterfly rash on the face, kidney disease, blood abnormalities, cardiac disease, fatigue, and photosensitivity.

Graves' disease

Graves' disease is an autoimmune disease primarily affecting the thyroid gland. In this condition, antibodies to the receptors for thyroid-stimulating hormone (TSH), T3 and T4, are produced. These antibodies bind to the receptors for TSH and cause chronic overstimulation of the gland, leading to overproduction of TSH and hyperthyroidism. Symptoms include exophthalmos (i.e., bulging wide eyes), nonpitting edema (i.e., pretibial myxedema), increased heartbeat, hyperactivity, hair loss, weight loss, muscle weakness, insomnia, and irritability. People with this condition also tend to have a large goiter (enlarged thyroid gland). This disease is easily diagnosed by a simple blood test for TSH. Treatment includes antithyroid drugs, medications that minimize thyroid hormone secretion. It can take up to 2 years for the medication to be effective. Radioiodine therapy or surgery may also be indicated for some patients.

Rheumatoid arthritis

Rheumatoid arthritis is an autoimmune disease that causes system-wide inflammation, though it affects primarily the synovial membrane of the joints. This inflammation can also affect the pleura of the lungs, the white of the eye, and the pericardium. It is believed that abnormal communication between B and T cells is partially responsible for the disease. Cytokine and tumor necrosis factor secretion by the lymphocytes drives inflammation in the joints and other membranes throughout the body. Diagnosis is made by a combination of clinical data, x-rays, and blood tests for rheumatoid factor and erythrocyte sedimentation rate. Symptoms include painful and stiff joints, fatigue, fever, and malaise. There are multiple lifestyle changes that can be made, as well as medications (e.g., a class of drugs called disease-modifying antirheumatic drugs) to treat the symptoms and improve joint function. There is no cure for rheumatoid arthritis.

Scleroderma

Scleroderma is a chronic autoimmune disease that is characterized by hardening of the skin, primarily on the upper extremities and face. There are two forms of this condition: limited scleroderma and diffuse scleroderma. Symptoms of limited scleroderma include calcinosis, Raynaud's phenomenon, esophageal dysfunction, skin thickening on the fingers, and telangiectasias. Diffuse scleroderma is a more systemic and more severe form of the condition. It affects the skin and internal organs, usually the lungs, heart, or kidneys. The exact cause is unknown, but it is known that there is an overabundance of collagen production, leading to sclerosis formation on the skin and organs. There is no cure; the goal of treatment is symptom relief. In addition, immunosuppressants are sometimes indicated.

Ankylosing spondylitis

Ankylosing spondylitis is a chronic disease, involving inflammation of the axial skeleton. Chronic inflammation in the spine and pelvis causes the bones to fuse. There is strong evidence that genetics plays a role in the transmission of this disease. There are several cytokines and antibodies that have been associated with ankylosing spondylitis, including tumor necrosis factor–alpha, interleukin-1, and antineutrophil cytoplasmic antibodies. There is no diagnostic testing that can be used to diagnosis ankylosing spondylitis. Instead, magnetic resonance imaging, which is used to show characteristic changes in the bones of the spine and pelvis, and blood testing, which looks for the genetic markers, are the two preferred tests. There is no cure for ankylosing spondylitis. Medications, lifestyle changes, and physical therapy can reduce the severity of symptoms and improve functioning.

Type I diabetes

Type I diabetes, which is also known as juvenile insulin-dependent diabetes, is caused by the immune system attacking the beta cells of the pancreas. This results in a complete lack of insulin production, meaning that blood glucose levels rise to very high levels. Primary symptoms are frequent urination, increased hunger and thirst, and weight loss. Type I diabetes is diagnosed by glucose and hemoglobin A1c blood testing. Patients with this condition must take insulin supplementation for the rest of their lives, usually with every meal. Patients should also monitor their blood sugar frequently.

Immune function in the neonate

The fetus and early neonate depend on maternal antibodies circulating through the placenta and secreted through breast milk for immunity. During the last trimester, the fetus is capable of producing a primary immune response with the production of immunoglobulin M only but is not able to produce immunoglobulin G. There is a layer of trophoblasts that separate maternal blood from fetal blood. Maternal antibodies are not able to cross that membrane directly but instead are transported across by trophoblast cells. After birth, maternal antibodies begin to break down, causing a decrease in immune function. Infants are born with very immature immune systems, lacking many of the antibodies and immune activity, especially phagocytic and complement activity, required to fight infection.

Immune function in the elderly population

Immune function (especially hypersensitivity reactions), T-cell responses and activity, and antibody responses, decrease in elderly individuals. There is, however, an increase in the number of antibodies and immune complexes circulating throughout the body. The thymus has reached its maximal growth by puberty and decreases in size through old age. In addition, thymus hormone secretion decreases.

Type I hypersensitivity

Type I hypersensitivity is also known as an allergic response, usually to an environmental allergen. During this type of reaction, an antigen is presented to the helper T cells and B cells in the same manner as the normal immune response. The main difference is that immunoglobulin E (IgE) is produced instead of immunoglobulins A, G, or M. The first exposure to an antigen is called sensitization; IgE antibodies bind to the Fc receptors on mast cells and basophils. A second exposure to that same antigen causes the IgE antibodies to crosslink. This results in mast cell and basophil degranulation and the production of histamine, leukotriene, and prostaglandin. The production of these cell mediators causes the symptoms of an allergy, such as smooth muscle contraction and vasodilation, especially in the mucous membranes.

Type II hypersensitivity disorders

Type II hypersensitivity is also known as tissue-specific hypersensitivity. Certain tissues or cells within the body have antigens present on their plasma membranes that are specific to that type of cell and are not found on any other cell within the body. These are known as tissue-specific antigens. Type II hypersensitivity reactions affect only these tissue-specific antigens. There are four mechanisms by which these reactions occur: (1) cell lysis mediated by complement, (2) phagocytosis by macrophages, (3) antibody-dependent, cell-mediated toxicity, and (4) blockage of receptors on the cell membrane.

Type III hypersensitivity disorders

Type III hypersensitivity reactions are also known as immune complex–mediated reactions. These reactions are caused by the deposition of immune complexes that are not adequately cleared and are subsequently inserted into small blood vessels, joints, and the kidneys. This activates the inflammatory response and the complement cascade. Neutrophils attempt to phagocytize the immune complex but are often unable to ingest the complex, causing degranulation. Degranulation of the mast cells also occurs, and the recruitment of other immune and inflammatory cells heightens the reaction.

Type IV hypersensitivity disorders

Type IV hypersensitivity reactions are also known as the cell-mediated tissue reactions and the delayed-type hypersensitivity because the reaction occurs several days after the exposure. This type of reaction is mediated by the T cells, not antibodies as the other types of hypersensitivity. Helper T cells recognize antigen that is bound to the major histocompatibility complex class II. Macrophages secreting interleukin-12 and interferon are the primary antigen-presenting cells. This activates CD8 T cells, which destroy the target cells. Many autoimmune disorders, like diabetes type 1, multiple sclerosis, Crohn's disease, and contact dermatitis are examples of type IV hypersensitivity reactions. In addition, the Mantoux test, which is used to diagnose tuberculosis, is based on type IV hypersensitivity, which is why it takes several days for the induration to show up if exposure to the tuberculosis bacterium has occurred.

Organ transplantation

Though life-saving, organ transplantation is a risky procedure. In addition to surgical complications, there is a risk of the recipient contracting an infection from the donor, although this is rare. All tissue donors are carefully screened for serious infections, like hepatitis B, hepatitis C, and human immunodeficiency virus, but rarely, these infections remain undetected in the donors and are passed to the recipients. There is also a risk of infection from the immunosuppressant medications that recipients are required to take for the rest of their lives to prevent organ rejection. Finally, there is a risk for rejection of the organ by the immune system, meaning that the immune cells destroy the transplanted tissue.

Graft-versus-host disease

Graft-versus-host disease (GVHD) is a transplant rejection reaction where the white blood cells of the donated tissue recognize the transplant recipient's tissues as foreign material and then attack the host cells. According to the Billingham Criteria, there are three factors that must be in place for a diagnosis of GVHD to be made: an immunocompetent organ was transplanted with functioning immune cells, the donor and recipient are histoincompatible, and the recipient has a compromised immune system. The T cells in the donated tissue express a number of cytokines and other cell mediators, which can all cause the immune reaction. There are several antigens that trigger this response, the most important being the human leukocyte antigens. There are two types of GVHD: acute and chronic. The acute form begins within the first 100 days after the transplant and is likely caused by memory T cells that were in the graft. The acute form begins over 100 days after the transplant. Clinical symptoms include liver damage, skin and mucous membrane rash, pneumonia, and intestinal inflammation, causing diarrhea, pain, nausea, and vomiting. Patients may also suffer from damage to the mucous membranes, both in the mouth and in the vagina, which can cause scarring and severe pain.

Allergic reactions during a blood transfusion

Allergic reactions to donated blood or blood products are common complications. These reactions usually occur when the recipient of the donated blood has built up antibodies to chemicals, drugs, or food in the donor blood. Symptoms include itching, hives, edema, and dizziness. If not treated quickly, the reaction can progress to anaphylaxis or shock. At the first sign of an allergic reaction, the transfusion should be stopped and the patient treated with hydrocortisone or epinephrine, if appropriate. The physician should then evaluate the patient to see if it is safe to resume the transfusion.

Anaphylaxis

Anaphylaxis is a serious blood transfusion reaction that usually starts within the first hour after starting the transfusion. It is caused by immunoglobulin E antibodies in the patients reacting with the allergen (i.e., food, drugs, chemicals) in the transfused blood. Anaphylaxis can also occur when immunoglobulin A (IgA) is transferred to a patient with an IgA deficiency or when the patient has antibodies to other components in the donor blood, such as immunoglobulin G, transferrin, complement, or other cytokines. Patients having an anaphylactic reaction present with hypotension, cough, bronchospasm, laryngospasm, edema, itching, and hives. At the first sign of a reaction, the transfusion should be stopped. Epinephrine, antihistamines, and steroids should be administered as indicated. A hematologist should be consulted before administering another transfusion.

Febrile nonhemolytic transfusion reaction

Febrile nonhemolytic transfusion reaction (FNHTR) is a transfusion reaction where a fever occurs, but there is no hemolysis. It is thought that this reaction is leukocyte driven, because either contaminated leukocytes in the donor blood accumulate in the blood during storage or because the recipient has antibodies against leukocytes in the donor blood. Symptoms usually start within the first hour after the transfusion begins and include chills, elevated temperature, headache, nausea, and vomiting. The transfusion should be stopped, and the patient should be evaluated promptly for evidence of more severe reactions. Antipyretics and meperidine (Demerol) should be administered for management of fever and severe rigors, as needed.

Organ rejection

Transplant rejection is also known as host-versus-graft disease and is a serious complication of organ transplant. It occurs when the immune system perceives the new organ as foreign based on mismatched human leukocyte antigens. The immune system then attacks the transplanted organ and may cause the organ to fail. There are three types of rejection: hyperacute, acute, and chronic. A hyperacute reaction occurs within minutes after the transplant. The transplanted organ must be removed immediately to prevent death of the recipient. An acute reaction occurs after the first week up until 3 months after. This type of rejection reaction is extremely common, and in fact, most recipients have some degree of acute rejection. A chronic rejection reaction occurs after 3 months and can take place over many years. To prevent and treat rejection reactions, the patient must take immunosuppressant medications.

Acute hemolytic transfusion reaction

An acute hemolytic transfusion reaction is a reaction that occurs within the first 24 hours after a blood transfusion and is a medical emergency. It is most frequently caused by ABO incompatibility and takes place when the host antibodies destroy the donor red blood cells. There are two types: immune mediated and nonimmune mediated. Immune-mediated transfusion reactions occur when anti-A, anti-B, both anti-A and anti-B, or other antibodies are formed in the host. If blood with these same antigens is administered to the host, severe hemolysis can occur and is mediated by tumor necrosis factor, interleukin-8, and interleukin-1.

A nonimmune-mediated reaction occurs when the transfused red blood cells are damaged or hemolyzed before the transfusion even occurs. Symptoms include anxiety, a feeling that something is wrong, hypotension, fever, and red-colored urine. As the reaction progresses, a worsening of hypotension and disseminated intravascular coagulation (DIC) can occur. The transfusion should be discontinued immediately. The physician should also anticipate and plan for renal failure (i.e., low-dose dopamine, hydration, mannitol), severe hypotension, and DIC (transfusion of frozen plasma or platelets). This can be fatal if not properly treated.

Hemolytic disease of the newborn

Hemolytic disease of the newborn (HDN) is also called erythroblastosis fetalis. This condition occurs during the fetal period and is caused by blood type incompatibility between the mother and her infant. Because it is easily preventable, HDN is fairly uncommon, but it is more likely to occur during a second or later pregnancy. Hemolytic disease of the newborn can happen from either ABO incompatibility or more commonly, Rh incompatibility. When an Rh-negative mother becomes pregnant with the infant from an Rh-positive father, it is possible that the infant will also be Rh positive. This becomes problematic if the infant's red blood cells (RBCs) enter the maternal bloodstream. The mother's blood identifies the Rh antigen as foreign and develops antibodies against it.

During subsequent pregnancies (if the infant is also Rh positive), those antibodies cross the placenta and attack the fetal RBCs, causing hemolysis and anemia in the infant. The infant tries to compensate by quickly making more blood cells, but the immature blood cells are not as effective as mature red blood cells. In addition, bilirubin is formed by the liver as the RBCs break down, causing hyperbilirubinemia.

Jarisch-Herxheimer disorder

Jarisch-Herxheimer disorder is a reaction that occurs after the administration of antibiotics. As the medications begin to work and the bacteria begin to die, they release endotoxins that cause the reaction. Symptoms include fever, muscle pain, tachycardia, headache, chills, hypotension, anxiety, and hyperventilation. It usually starts pretty quickly after the first dose is administered and is self-limited. Anti-inflammatories, like aspirin (if clinically appropriate) or prednisone can be used, and the patient should be monitored closely. This reaction is commonly seen in the treatment of syphilis with penicillin, or when treating other spirochete-causing infections (e.g., Lyme disease, leptospirosis).

Active immunity

Active immunity is when the immune system is exposed to a pathogen or antigen and generates its own antibodies against that antigen. There are two forms of active immunity: natural immunity and vaccine-induced immunity. Natural immunity occurs when the body is exposed to the actual illness and creates antibodies against the pathogen. Vaccine-induced immunity results from vaccination; an attenuated or inactivated portion of the virus is injected into the body to stimulate the immune system. Active immunity lasts a long time.

Passive immunity

Passive immunity is when someone is given the antibodies to a disease, rather than creating them on their own. There are two forms of passive immunity: natural and acquired. Natural passive immunity is the transfer of maternal antibodies during the prenatal period or during breastfeeding. Acquired passive immunity is the administration of immunoglobulin or antibodies against a specific disease administered through a blood product. In both cases, passive immunity lasts only weeks or months.

Live, attenuated vaccines

Live, attenuated vaccines are viruses that are grown in cell cultures or in animal embryos. Each time the virus is passed into a different embryo, it loses a little of its ability to replicate in a human cell. The process continues until the virus is completely unable to replicate (or replicate well) in a human cell, losing its ability to cause an infection. The virus is, however, still able to elicit an immune response. It can take up to 200 different cell cultures or animal embryos before the virus is vaccine ready. There is a concern that the virus can revert to a form that can be harmful to the human host and cause disease. While rare, it is actually relatively common with the oral polio vaccine, which is why inactive polio vaccine replaced the oral form on the immunization schedule. Live, attenuated vaccines include the measles, mumps, and rubella vaccine; varicella vaccine; influenza nasal spray; and rotavirus vaccine.

Inactivated or killed vaccines

Killed or inactivated vaccines include the polio and hepatitis A vaccines. These viruses are killed or inactivated by either heat or chemicals like formaldehyde. This keeps the virus intact and able to be recognized by the immune system but destroys the virulent part of it so that the virus is unable to replicate. These vaccines are unable to cause disease in any way. They tend to be less effective in the long run and may require booster vaccinations in the future.

Human immunodeficiency virus

Human immunodeficiency virus (HIV) is a virus transmitted by sexual contact or contact with certain body fluids of an infected person. It cannot be transmitted through contact with saliva, tears, or mucus; transmission is primarily through sexual contact, blood transfusions, sharing needles, intravenous drug paraphernalia, and breastfeeding. The HIV virus invades and destroys

CD4 cells, meaning that as the virus progresses, patients are increasingly unable to fight infections. Once the CD4 count falls below 200 or the patient experiences one of the AIDS-specific infections (i.e., pneumocystic pneumonia, cytomegalovirus, tuberculosis, toxoplasmosis, cryptosporidiosis) they are officially diagnosed with AIDS. Diagnosis is made by finding antigens produced in response to the HIV virus; thus, it can take up to 3 months before there is a sufficient level of HIV antigens in the blood for a diagnosis. Once the diagnosis has been confirmed, a CD4 count and viral load should determine the disease severity and its likely progression.

The primary method of human immunodeficiency virus (HIV) prevention is avoiding exposure to potentially infectious body fluids. There should be no unprotected sex (i.e., without a condom or other barrier method) and avoidance of contact with blood or breast milk. This includes not sharing needles and avoiding needle sticks in the health care setting. If unexpected contact occurs, testing for HIV should occur for both parties for several months after the exposure. Sometimes prophylactic antiviral medications are indicated. Treatment involves a combination of antiretroviral medications that help to reduce viral replication and can ward off serious infection and progression to full-blown AIDS. Frequently used drug classes include protease inhibitors, non-nucleoside reverse transcriptase inhibitors, nucleoside-reverse transcriptase inhibitors, fusion and entry inhibitors, and integrase inhibitors. Usually, prescribers use a combination of two or three medications in different drug classes.

Nucleoside reverse transcriptase inhibitors

Nucleoside reverse transcriptase inhibitors (NRTIs) are a class of medications called antiretrovirals that are used to treat human immunodeficiency virus (HIV) infections. The NRTIs are very similar structurally to the deoxynucleotides used to synthesize viral DNA, and, therefore, compete to get incorporated into the DNA chain. The main difference is that NRTIs lack an important hydroxyl group, which prevents the next deoxynucleotide from extending the chain, essentially ending the DNA chain. There are strains of HIV that are resistant to certain NRTIs, leading to the need for multiple agents for optimal effectiveness.

Non-nucleoside reverse transcriptase inhibitors

Non-nucleoside reverse transcriptase inhibitors (NNRTIs) are a class of antiretroviral medications used to treat human immunodeficiency virus (HIV) infections. This particular class of drugs will only work against HIV-1 and has no effect on HIV-2. The NNRTIs bind directly to the active site of reverse transcriptase, an enzyme that is used to create complementary DNA from RNA. This process is essential in the lifecycle of HIV, so disrupting it helps to prevent the progression of HIV infection. The activity of NNRTIs is altered (additively or synergistically) by other antiretroviral drugs, so this must be taken into account when using NNRTIs in combination with protease inhibitors especially.

Protease inhibitors

Protease inhibitors are a class of drugs widely used in the treatment of human immunodeficiency virus (HIV) and hepatitis C infections. They bind to and block viral protease, which (when blocked) prevents the cleavage of protein precursors that are used in the production of virus particles. Protease inhibitors act against specific enzymes, and there is a risk of the virus becoming resistant to certain drugs. Protease inhibitors are used in combination with other medications for the most effective treatment. There are many protease inhibitors on the market: saquinavir (Invirase) and ritonavir (Norvir) were the first two developed. In addition, indinavir (Crixivan), nelfinavir

(Viracept), amprenavir (Agenerase), lopinavir (ABT-378), atazanavir (Reyataz), fosamprenavir (Lexiva), tipranavir (Aptivus), and darunavir (Prezista) are also protease inhibitors.

Integrase inhibitors

Integrase inhibitors are a class of drugs known as antiretroviral drugs. They block integrase, a crucial enzyme that is involved in the insertion of the human immunodeficiency virus (HIV) genome into the host cell DNA. Blocking this step helps prevent the spread of the virus to other cells. Integrase inhibitors are used in combination with drugs of other classes in the treatment of HIV. They can also be used in patients whose virus has become resistant to other medications. There are two integrase inhibitors currently available for use in the United States: elvitegravir (Stribild) and dolutegravir (Tivicay).

Fusion inhibitors

Fusion inhibitors are also called entry inhibitors and are a class of antiretroviral drugs. They are used in combination with other medications for the treatment of human immunodeficiency virus (HIV). These drugs block HIV from entering into a cell, which is a crucial step in HIV infection. These drugs are especially helpful in preventing the progression of HIV into full-blown AIDS. In the United States, there are two approved fusion inhibitors: selzentry (Maraviroc) and enfuvirtide (Fuzeon). There are many new fusion inhibitors in the research phase.

Alemtuzumab (Campath)

Alemtuzumab (Campath) is a monoclonal antibody used to treat B-cell chronic lymphocytic leukemia. It attaches to the CD52 protein found on all B and T lymphocytes and attracts other immune cells to the area to kill the cells. As a result, this medication can suppress the immune system and platelets. Patients taking this medication should be cautioned regarding infection prevention and when to call the physician. They should also be warned about the possibility of bleeding and the risk of taking certain other medications (e.g., other blood thinners, nonsteroidal anti-inflammatory drugs, vitamin E) with alemtuzumab. It is given as a venous infusion over 2 hours.

Cetuximab (Erbitux)

Cetuximab (Erbitux) is a monoclonal antibody that is an epidermal growth factor receptor inhibitor. It is used in the treatment of metastatic colorectal or non–small cell lung cancers, and head/neck cancer. It works by binding to epidermal growth factor receptors that are mutated and send signals to divide uncontrollably. There is another protein in the pathway that epidermal growth factor receptors signal through, called KRAS, which if also mutated, indicates that cetuximab will not be effective. Practitioners should test for a KRAS mutation before prescribing cetuximab. This drug is administered through the intravenous route over about 2 hours.

Rituximab (Rituxan)

Rituximab (Rituxan) is a monoclonal antibody against CD20, a protein found on the surface of B cells. This drug is used to treat diseases where there are an excessive number of normal or abnormal B cells, including lymphoma, leukemia, and certain autoimmune disorders (e.g., rheumatoid arthritis, multiple sclerosis, systemic lupus erythematosus). It does not distinguish between normal or abnormal B cells, just destroying any cell that expresses CD20 on its membrane.

It can also be used (in an off-label manner) as an antirejection agent for kidney transplant patients. Rituximab has been associated with some serious adverse effects, including cardiac arrest, tumor lysis syndrome, pulmonary toxicity, bowel obstruction and perforation, and progressive multifocal leukoencephalopathy.

Trastuzumab (Herceptin)

Trastuzumab (Herceptin) is a monoclonal antibody used in the treatment of breast, stomach, and esophageal cancer. It binds to human epidermal growth factor receptor 2 (HER2) receptors and attracts other immune cells to them to destroy them. Certain breast and stomach cancers have a higher than normal number of these receptors on their surfaces. It is important to verify that a breast or stomach cancer is HER2 positive before initiating trastuzumab therapy. Use of this drug in combination with other chemotherapeutic agents may have a damaging effect on the heart, so the physician should verify all medications that the patient is taking. It should be administered via an intravenous infusion over about 90 minutes. If tolerated well, the next dose can be given over 30 minutes, instead of 90.

Cyclosporine (Sandimmune)

Cyclosporine (Sandimmune) is a potent immunosuppressant that is used as part of the antirejection medication regimen for patients who have received a kidney, heart, or liver transplant. It reduces T-cell activity, lymphokine production, and interleukin secretion. Cyclosporine can also be used to treat active rheumatoid arthritis or plaque psoriasis, when other treatments have failed or in patients who cannot tolerate other systemic medications.

There are many potential drug interactions, so the physician should be sure to get a full medication history before prescribing this drug. It is available in either an oral or intravenous form. Renal function may need to be evaluated periodically. Finally, the patient is at an increased risk of developing an infection or cancer and should be informed of infection prevention techniques and instructed to call the physician with early signs or symptoms of infection.

Tacrolimus (Prograf)

Tacrolimus (Prograf) and is an immunosuppressive medication used after organ transplant to minimize the risk of rejection. It has been approved for use after heart, kidney, lung, liver, small bowel, pancreas, skin, bone marrow, and cornea transplants by the Food and Drug Administration. A topical preparation can be used for atopic dermatitis. It works by suppressing an enzyme called calcineurin. This enzyme plays a key role in the division of T cells.

Blood tests should be done periodically to monitor the level of tacrolimus in the blood, and the dose is adjusted accordingly. Patients should be counseled to take this medication with food to avoid stomach pain, avoid grapefruit juice when taking this drug, and take it consistently to avoid swings in blood levels. Live virus vaccines should be avoided, and the physician should take a thorough medication history because of the possibility of serious drug interactions.

Sirolimus or rapamycin (Rapamune)

Sirolimus or rapamycin (Rapamune) is an immunosuppressant drug used to prevent rejection in patients who have had an organ transplant. It is most effective in kidney transplant patients. It works by inhibiting the response of T and B cells to interleukin-2, thus preventing their activation.

Sirolimus has low renal toxicity, which is an advantage over other immunosuppressant drugs. Adverse effects include lung toxicity, interstitial pneumonitis, and the increased risk of cancer or infection.

Azathioprine (Imuran)

Azathioprine (Imuran) is an immunosuppressant drug that is used to prevent rejection after kidney transplant. It can also be used to treat patients with rheumatoid arthritis or other autoimmune diseases, who have not tolerated other medications. It works by inhibiting an enzyme required for DNA synthesis in rapidly dividing cells, like the B and T cells. It can also cause profound bone marrow suppression. This drug is listed as a carcinogen by the International Agency for Research on Cancer, and patients should be advised of the increased risk of cancer with its use.

Glucocorticoids

Glucocorticoids are steroids that play a role in the regulation of glucose metabolism. They are synthesized in the adrenal glands. Glucocorticoids play an important role in the feedback system regulating immunity. They can be used to suppress the immune system in diseases of overactive immunity, like allergies, autoimmune disease, and sepsis. When they bind to the glucocorticoid receptor, glucocorticoids increase the expression of anti-inflammatory proteins and decrease the expression of proinflammatory proteins. Finally, they are known to be involved in T-cell development.

Bevacizumab (Avastin)

Bevacizumab (Avastin) is a monoclonal antibody that inhibits vascular endothelial growth factor A (VEGFA). The VEGFA plays a crucial role in the development of new blood vessels (a process known as angiogenesis), especially in metastasizing cancers. Bevacizumab inhibits VEGFA and thus helps slow the spread of aggressive and metastasizing cancers. It is most frequently used in colon cancer but is also used in cancer of the lungs, breast, brain, kidneys, and ovaries.

Basiliximab (Simulect)

Basiliximab (Simulect) is a monoclonal antibody used to prevent organ rejection after transplant. This drug is most often used for kidney transplant patients. It works as an antagonist at the interleukin-2 receptor on the surface of activated T cells. Patients taking basiliximab should be advised of the increased risk for developing a severe infection and counseled appropriately. Patients should also be advised that they should avoid live vaccinations while taking this medication. Finally, basiliximab has been shown to elevate blood sugar levels.

Monoclonal antibodies

Monoclonal antibodies are therapeutic antibodies that can be specifically created for almost any cell-surface target. When the antibody binds to its target cell, the immune system is stimulated to attack and destroy the cell. Monoclonal antibodies are used therapeutically for many different conditions: cancer, rheumatoid arthritis, Crohn's disease, and ulcerative colitis.

There are two types of monoclonal antibodies: naked and conjugated. Naked monoclonal antibodies work by themselves and do not require an adjunctive drug or radioactive material. These antibodies attach directly to antigens on the cancer cells and either target the cell for destruction or block antigens used as signals for cell growth. Conjugated monoclonal antibodies are attached to a medication, toxin, or radioactive particle. They are used to bring that conjugate directly to the target cell, which helps to minimize damage to normal cells.

Polyclonal antibodies

Polyclonal antibodies are antibodies created from many different B cells or B-cell lines. These antibodies are all specific to the same antigen, but each has a different epitope. The two most commonly used polyclonal antibodies are digoxin immune Fab (Digibind), which is the antidote for digoxin toxicity, and rho(D) immune globulin (RhoGAM), which is used to prevent hemolytic disease of the newborn. Rho(D) immune globulin is administered to women who are Rh negative and who have had a child who is Rh positive. When an Rh-negative mother becomes pregnant with the infant from an Rh-positive father, it is possible that the infant will be Rh positive. The mother's blood treats the Rh antigen as foreign and develops antibodies against it. During subsequent pregnancies (if the infant is also Rh positive), those antibodies cross the placenta and attack the fetal red blood cells. Rho(D) immune globulin is a collection of Rh antibodies and is used to provide passive immunity, preventing the maternal immune response against the fetus.

Denosumab (Prolia)

Denosumab (Prolia) is a monoclonal antibody, used to treat osteoporosis, bone metastases, and other bone cancers and disorders. RANKL is a protein that activates cell surface receptors on preosteoclasts, precursors to osteoclasts. They act as a signal for bone removal; they act abnormally in many bone-loss conditions. When these surface receptors are activated, the preosteoclasts mature into osteoclasts and begin to break down bone. Denosumab works to inhibit this ligand and prevent further bone loss.

Digoxin immune Fab (Digibind)

Digoxin immune Fab (Digibind) is the antidote for digitalis toxicity or overdose. It is only used for a severe overdose. It is a polyclonal antibody that is synthesized from antidigoxin immunoglobulins found in sheep's blood. These sheep are first immunized with a derivative of digoxin to get them to create the antibodies. Digoxin immune Fab is given intravenously, and as the antibodies circulate, they bind to the molecules of digoxin, rendering them useless. The digoxin fragments are then excreted by the kidney.

Omalizumab (Zolair)

Omalizumab (Zolair) is a monoclonal antibody that helps patients with severe allergies or asthma reduce their sensitivity to allergens. This drug is especially useful in patients who are highly sensitive to their allergen but who cannot tolerate corticosteroids well. It binds to free immunoglobulin E (IgE) in the blood and interstitial fluid. It also binds to membrane-bound IgE on the surface of B cells. It is administered as a subcutaneous injection, every 2–4 weeks.

Palivizumab (Synagis)

Palivizumab (Synagis) is a monoclonal antibody used to treat respiratory syncytial virus (RSV) infections. These infections are life-threatening for high-risk infants and young children with congenital heart disease. Indications for immunization with palivizumab include prematurity and age at start of the RSV season, history of lung disease of prematurity, a history of congenital heart disease, patients who are immunocompromised, or patients who have cystic fibrosis. This drug targets a protein on the RSV virus, which prevents it from entering the cell. It is given as an intramuscular injection once a month throughout the RSV season.

Disease prevention and treatment

Before diagnosis, patients experiencing autoimmune diseases can experience frustration or conflict with family members or their physician. Many of the symptoms of several autoimmune diseases can be vague, such as fatigue, pain, and weight gain. Patients often feel frustrated that their concerns are not taken seriously or are minimized by loved ones or by their physician. Patients also may feel frustrated that they are chronically ill and want to get back to their life before they became ill. Chronic illness can also impact a person's ability to work or fully participate in their life.

Occupation can play a role in disease prevention and treatment. Working with certain populations (e.g., in the prison system, working with young children) increases a person's risk of infection. Daily exposure to some pollutants or environmental toxins can cause genetic mutations, increasing a person's risk of cancer or of developing allergies. For example, people who work with dry cleaning chemicals are at an increased risk of getting bladder cancer. Treatment is also impacted by a person's occupation. A person may not be able to take time off to see a physician, or they may not have health insurance to pay for their treatment. This can delay or even prevent treatment and worsen the disease.

Emotional and psychological stress play an important role in immune disorders. When feeling pressured, stress hormones, like epinephrine, are released. These hormones increase blood pressure and heart rate to prepare for the flight or fight response, but they also decease the strength and effectiveness of the immune response. People with chronic stress tend to suffer from more colds and infections. In addition, people who are depressed or who have poor coping mechanisms tend to a have poorer quality of life during and after cancer treatment. On the other hand, patients who actively seek ways to manage stress and reduce anxiety have lower rates of depression and fewer symptoms of their cancer and treatment. Patients who are expressing or describing extreme stress levels should be referred to the appropriate resources, including a psychologist or support group.

Women are significantly more likely than men to develop an autoimmune disease, like scleroderma or rheumatoid arthritis. Men, however, are at a higher risk for non-Hodgkin's lymphoma. Ethnicity also plays a role in immune function and the development of immune disorders. For example, Caucasians are significantly more likely to get non-Hodgkin's lymphoma or type I diabetes, especially in the United States and Europe. Lupus tends to be more prevalent in the African-American and Hispanic populations.

Behavioral factors affecting immunity

There are several factors that are known to decrease immune function, including quality and quantity of sleep, exercise habits, diet, stress, and sense of humor. There are studies that have shown that a chronic lack of sleep can suppress the immune system, leading to more infections and illnesses. In addition, lack of exercise and poor dietary habits, leading to poor nutrition can also lower the immune response. A diet that is high in sugar or low in vitamins and minerals decreases the immune response. People with high stress have higher levels of stress hormones, like epinephrine and norepinephrine. These hormones not only increase blood pressure and heart rate to prepare for the flight or fight response, but they also decrease the strength and effectiveness of the immune response. People with chronic stress tend to suffer from more colds and infections. Finally, laughter has been shown to decrease stress hormones and boost lymphocyte levels. People who laugh frequently and have a strong connection to family and friends tend to have stronger immune systems and get fewer illnesses.

Secret Key #1 - Time is Your Greatest Enemy

Pace Yourself

Wear a watch. At the beginning of the test, check the time (or start a chronometer on your watch to count the minutes), and check the time after every few questions to make sure you are "on schedule."

If you are forced to speed up, do it efficiently. Usually one or more answer choices can be eliminated without too much difficulty. Above all, don't panic. Don't speed up and just begin guessing at random choices. By pacing yourself, and continually monitoring your progress against your watch, you will always know exactly how far ahead or behind you are with your available time. If you find that you are one minute behind on the test, don't skip one question without spending any time on it, just to catch back up. Take 15 fewer seconds on the next four questions, and after four questions you'll have caught back up. Once you catch back up, you can continue working each problem at your normal pace.

Furthermore, don't dwell on the problems that you were rushed on. If a problem was taking up too much time and you made a hurried guess, it must be difficult. The difficult questions are the ones you are most likely to miss anyway, so it isn't a big loss. It is better to end with more time than you need than to run out of time.

Lastly, sometimes it is beneficial to slow down if you are constantly getting ahead of time. You are always more likely to catch a careless mistake by working more slowly than quickly, and among very high-scoring test takers (those who are likely to have lots of time left over), careless errors affect the score more than mastery of material.

Secret Key #2 - Guessing is not Guesswork

You probably know that guessing is a good idea. Unlike other standardized tests, there is no penalty for getting a wrong answer. Even if you have no idea about a question, you still have a 20-25% chance of getting it right.

Most test takers do not understand the impact that proper guessing can have on their score. Unless you score extremely high, guessing will significantly contribute to your final score.

Monkeys Take the Test

What most test takers don't realize is that to insure that 20-25% chance, you have to guess randomly. If you put 20 monkeys in a room to take this test, assuming they answered once per question and behaved themselves, on average they would get 20-25% of the questions correct. Put 20 test takers in the room, and the average will be much lower among guessed questions. Why?
1. The test writers intentionally write deceptive answer choices that "look" right. A test taker has no idea about a question, so he picks the "best looking" answer, which is often wrong. The monkey has no idea what looks good and what doesn't, so it will consistently be right about 20-25% of the time.
2. Test takers will eliminate answer choices from the guessing pool based on a hunch or intuition. Simple but correct answers often get excluded, leaving a 0% chance of being correct. The monkey has no clue, and often gets lucky with the best choice.

This is why the process of elimination endorsed by most test courses is flawed and detrimental to your performance. Test takers don't guess; they make an ignorant stab in the dark that is usually worse than random.

$5 Challenge

Let me introduce one of the most valuable ideas of this course—the $5 challenge:

You only mark your "best guess" if you are willing to bet $5 on it.
You only eliminate choices from guessing if you are willing to bet $5 on it.

Why $5? Five dollars is an amount of money that is small yet not insignificant, and can really add up fast (20 questions could cost you $100). Likewise, each answer choice on one question of the test will have a small impact on your overall score, but it can really add up to a lot of points in the end.

The process of elimination IS valuable. The following shows your chance of guessing it right:

If you eliminate wrong answer choices until only this many remain:	Chance of getting it correct:
1	100%
2	50%
3	33%

However, if you accidentally eliminate the right answer or go on a hunch for an incorrect answer, your chances drop dramatically—to 0%. By guessing among all the answer choices, you are GUARANTEED to have a shot at the right answer.

That's why the $5 test is so valuable. If you give up the advantage and safety of a pure guess, it had better be worth the risk.

What we still haven't covered is how to be sure that whatever guess you make is truly random. Here's the easiest way:

Always pick the first answer choice among those remaining.

Such a technique means that you have decided, **before you see a single test question**, exactly how you are going to guess, and since the order of choices tells you nothing about which one is correct, this guessing technique is perfectly random.

This section is not meant to scare you away from making educated guesses or eliminating choices; you just need to define when a choice is worth eliminating. The $5 test, along with a pre-defined random guessing strategy, is the best way to make sure you reap all of the benefits of guessing.

Secret Key #3 - Practice Smarter, Not Harder

Many test takers delay the test preparation process because they dread the awful amounts of practice time they think necessary to succeed on the test. We have refined an effective method that will take you only a fraction of the time.

There are a number of "obstacles" in the path to success. Among these are answering questions, finishing in time, and mastering test-taking strategies. All must be executed on the day of the test at peak performance, or your score will suffer. The test is a mental marathon that has a large impact on your future.

Just like a marathon runner, it is important to work your way up to the full challenge. So first you just worry about questions, and then time, and finally strategy:

Success Strategy

1. Find a good source for practice tests.
2. If you are willing to make a larger time investment, consider using more than one study guide. Often the different approaches of multiple authors will help you "get" difficult concepts.
3. Take a practice test with no time constraints, with all study helps, "open book." Take your time with questions and focus on applying strategies.
4. Take a practice test with time constraints, with all guides, "open book."
5. Take a final practice test without open material and with time limits.

If you have time to take more practice tests, just repeat step 5. By gradually exposing yourself to the full rigors of the test environment, you will condition your mind to the stress of test day and maximize your success.

Secret Key #4 - Prepare, Don't Procrastinate

Let me state an obvious fact: if you take the test three times, you will probably get three different scores. This is due to the way you feel on test day, the level of preparedness you have, and the version of the test you see. Despite the test writers' claims to the contrary, some versions of the test WILL be easier for you than others.

Since your future depends so much on your score, you should maximize your chances of success. In order to maximize the likelihood of success, you've got to prepare in advance. This means taking practice tests and spending time learning the information and test taking strategies you will need to succeed.

Never go take the actual test as a "practice" test, expecting that you can just take it again if you need to. Take all the practice tests you can on your own, but when you go to take the official test, be prepared, be focused, and do your best the first time!

Secret Key #5 - Test Yourself

Everyone knows that time is money. There is no need to spend too much of your time or too little of your time preparing for the test. You should only spend as much of your precious time preparing as is necessary for you to get the score you need.

Once you have taken a practice test under real conditions of time constraints, then you will know if you are ready for the test or not.

If you have scored extremely high the first time that you take the practice test, then there is not much point in spending countless hours studying. You are already there.

Benchmark your abilities by retaking practice tests and seeing how much you have improved. Once you consistently score high enough to guarantee success, then you are ready.

If you have scored well below where you need, then knuckle down and begin studying in earnest. Check your improvement regularly through the use of practice tests under real conditions. Above all, don't worry, panic, or give up. The key is perseverance!

Then, when you go to take the test, remain confident and remember how well you did on the practice tests. If you can score high enough on a practice test, then you can do the same on the real thing.

General Strategies

The most important thing you can do is to ignore your fears and jump into the test immediately. Do not be overwhelmed by any strange-sounding terms. You have to jump into the test like jumping into a pool—all at once is the easiest way.

Make Predictions

As you read and understand the question, try to guess what the answer will be. Remember that several of the answer choices are wrong, and once you begin reading them, your mind will immediately become cluttered with answer choices designed to throw you off. Your mind is typically the most focused immediately after you have read the question and digested its contents. If you can, try to predict what the correct answer will be. You may be surprised at what you can predict.

Quickly scan the choices and see if your prediction is in the listed answer choices. If it is, then you can be quite confident that you have the right answer. It still won't hurt to check the other answer choices, but most of the time, you've got it!

Answer the Question

It may seem obvious to only pick answer choices that answer the question, but the test writers can create some excellent answer choices that are wrong. Don't pick an answer just because it sounds right, or you believe it to be true. It MUST answer the question. Once you've made your selection, always go back and check it against the question and make sure that you didn't misread the question and that the answer choice does answer the question posed.

Benchmark

After you read the first answer choice, decide if you think it sounds correct or not. If it doesn't, move on to the next answer choice. If it does, mentally mark that answer choice. This doesn't mean that you've definitely selected it as your answer choice, it just means that it's the best you've seen thus far. Go ahead and read the next choice. If the next choice is worse than the one you've already selected, keep going to the next answer choice. If the next choice is better than the choice you've already selected, mentally mark the new answer choice as your best guess.

The first answer choice that you select becomes your standard. Every other answer choice must be benchmarked against that standard. That choice is correct until proven otherwise by another answer choice beating it out. Once you've decided that no other answer choice seems as good, do one final check to ensure that your answer choice answers the question posed.

Valid Information

Don't discount any of the information provided in the question. Every piece of information may be necessary to determine the correct answer. None of the information in the question is there to throw you off (while the answer choices will certainly have information to throw you off). If two seemingly unrelated topics are discussed, don't ignore either. You can be confident there is a relationship, or it wouldn't be included in the question, and you are probably going to have to determine what is that relationship to find the answer.

Avoid "Fact Traps"

Don't get distracted by a choice that is factually true. Your search is for the answer that answers the question. Stay focused and don't fall for an answer that is true but irrelevant. Always go back to the question and make sure you're choosing an answer that actually answers the question and is not just a true statement. An answer can be factually correct, but it MUST answer the question asked. Additionally, two answers can both be seemingly correct, so be sure to read all of the answer choices, and make sure that you get the one that BEST answers the question.

Milk the Question

Some of the questions may throw you completely off. They might deal with a subject you have not been exposed to, or one that you haven't reviewed in years. While your lack of knowledge about the subject will be a hindrance, the question itself can give you many clues that will help you find the correct answer. Read the question carefully and look for clues. Watch particularly for adjectives and nouns describing difficult terms or words that you don't recognize. Regardless of whether you completely understand a word or not, replacing it with a synonym, either provided or one you more familiar with, may help you to understand what the questions are asking. Rather than wracking your mind about specific detailed information concerning a difficult term or word, try to use mental substitutes that are easier to understand.

The Trap of Familiarity

Don't just choose a word because you recognize it. On difficult questions, you may not recognize a number of words in the answer choices. The test writers don't put "make-believe" words on the test, so don't think that just because you only recognize all the words in one answer choice that that answer choice must be correct. If you only recognize words in one answer choice, then focus on that one. Is it correct? Try your best to determine if it is correct. If it is, that's great. If not, eliminate it. Each word and answer choice you eliminate increases your chances of getting the question correct, even if you then have to guess among the unfamiliar choices.

Eliminate Answers

Eliminate choices as soon as you realize they are wrong. But be careful! Make sure you consider all of the possible answer choices. Just because one appears right, doesn't mean that the next one won't be even better! The test writers will usually put more than one good answer choice for every question, so read all of them. Don't worry if you are stuck between two that seem right. By getting down to just two remaining possible choices, your odds are now 50/50. Rather than wasting too much time, play the odds. You are guessing, but guessing wisely because you've been able to knock out some of the answer choices that you know are wrong. If you are eliminating choices and realize that the last answer choice you are left with is also obviously wrong, don't panic. Start over and consider each choice again. There may easily be something that you missed the first time and will realize on the second pass.

Tough Questions

If you are stumped on a problem or it appears too hard or too difficult, don't waste time. Move on! Remember though, if you can quickly check for obviously incorrect answer choices, your chances of guessing correctly are greatly improved. Before you completely give up, at least try to knock out a couple of possible answers. Eliminate what you can and then guess at the remaining answer choices before moving on.

Brainstorm

If you get stuck on a difficult question, spend a few seconds quickly brainstorming. Run through the complete list of possible answer choices. Look at each choice and ask yourself, "Could this answer the question satisfactorily?" Go through each answer choice and consider it independently of the others. By systematically going through all possibilities, you may find something that you would otherwise overlook. Remember though that when you get stuck, it's important to try to keep moving.

Read Carefully

Understand the problem. Read the question and answer choices carefully. Don't miss the question because you misread the terms. You have plenty of time to read each question thoroughly and make sure you understand what is being asked. Yet a happy medium must be attained, so don't waste too much time. You must read carefully, but efficiently.

Face Value

When in doubt, use common sense. Always accept the situation in the problem at face value. Don't read too much into it. These problems will not require you to make huge leaps of logic. The test writers aren't trying to throw you off with a cheap trick. If you have to go beyond creativity and make a leap of logic in order to have an answer choice answer the question, then you should look at the other answer choices. Don't overcomplicate the problem by creating theoretical relationships or explanations that will warp time or space. These are normal problems rooted in reality. It's just that the applicable relationship or explanation may not be readily apparent and you have to figure things out. Use your common sense to interpret anything that isn't clear.

Prefixes

If you're having trouble with a word in the question or answer choices, try dissecting it. Take advantage of every clue that the word might include. Prefixes and suffixes can be a huge help. Usually they allow you to determine a basic meaning. Pre- means before, post- means after, pro - is positive, de- is negative. From these prefixes and suffixes, you can get an idea of the general meaning of the word and try to put it into context. Beware though of any traps. Just because con- is the opposite of pro-, doesn't necessarily mean congress is the opposite of progress!

Hedge Phrases

Watch out for critical hedge phrases, led off with words such as "likely," "may," "can," "sometimes," "often," "almost," "mostly," "usually," "generally," "rarely," and "sometimes." Question writers insert these hedge phrases to cover every possibility. Often an answer choice will be wrong simply because it leaves no room for exception. Unless the situation calls for them, avoid answer choices that have definitive words like "exactly," and "always."

Switchback Words

Stay alert for "switchbacks." These are the words and phrases frequently used to alert you to shifts in thought. The most common switchback word is "but." Others include "although," "however," "nevertheless," "on the other hand," "even though," "while," "in spite of," "despite," and "regardless of."

New Information

Correct answer choices will rarely have completely new information included. Answer choices typically are straightforward reflections of the material asked about and will directly relate to the question. If a new piece of information is included in an answer choice that doesn't even seem to relate to the topic being asked about, then that answer choice is likely incorrect. All of the information needed to answer the question is usually provided for you in the question. You should not have to make guesses that are unsupported or choose answer choices that require unknown information that cannot be reasoned from what is given.

Time Management

On technical questions, don't get lost on the technical terms. Don't spend too much time on any one question. If you don't know what a term means, then odds are you aren't going to get much further since you don't have a dictionary. You should be able to immediately recognize whether or not you know a term. If you don't, work with the other clues that you have—the other answer choices and terms provided—but don't waste too much time trying to figure out a difficult term that you don't know.

Contextual Clues

Look for contextual clues. An answer can be right but not the correct answer. The contextual clues will help you find the answer that is most right and is correct. Understand the context in which a phrase or statement is made. This will help you make important distinctions.

Don't Panic

Panicking will not answer any questions for you; therefore, it isn't helpful. When you first see the question, if your mind goes blank, take a deep breath. Force yourself to mechanically go through the steps of solving the problem using the strategies you've learned.

Pace Yourself

Don't get clock fever. It's easy to be overwhelmed when you're looking at a page full of questions, your mind is full of random thoughts and feeling confused, and the clock is ticking down faster than you would like. Calm down and maintain the pace that you have set for yourself. As long as you are on track by monitoring your pace, you are guaranteed to have enough time for yourself. When you get to the last few minutes of the test, it may seem like you won't have enough time left, but if you only have as many questions as you should have left at that point, then you're right on track!

Answer Selection

The best way to pick an answer choice is to eliminate all of those that are wrong, until only one is left and confirm that is the correct answer. Sometimes though, an answer choice may immediately look right. Be careful! Take a second to make sure that the other choices are not equally obvious. Don't make a hasty mistake. There are only two times that you should stop before checking other answers. First is when you are positive that the answer choice you have selected is correct. Second is when time is almost out and you have to make a quick guess!

Check Your Work

Since you will probably not know every term listed and the answer to every question, it is important that you get credit for the ones that you do know. Don't miss any questions through careless mistakes. If at all possible, try to take a second to look back over your answer selection and make sure you've selected the correct answer choice and haven't made a costly careless mistake (such as marking an answer choice that you didn't mean to mark). The time it takes for this quick double check should more than pay for itself in caught mistakes.

Beware of Directly Quoted Answers

Sometimes an answer choice will repeat word for word a portion of the question or reference section. However, beware of such exact duplication. It may be a trap! More than likely, the correct choice will paraphrase or summarize a point, rather than being exactly the same wording.

Slang

Scientific sounding answers are better than slang ones. An answer choice that begins "To compare the outcomes..." is much more likely to be correct than one that begins "Because some people insisted..."

Extreme Statements

Avoid wild answers that throw out highly controversial ideas that are proclaimed as established fact. An answer choice that states the "process should used in certain situations, if..." is much more likely to be correct than one that states the "process should be discontinued completely." The first is a calm rational statement and doesn't even make a definitive, uncompromising stance, using a hedge word "if" to provide wiggle room, whereas the second choice is a radical idea and far more extreme.

Answer Choice Families

When you have two or more answer choices that are direct opposites or parallels, one of them is usually the correct answer. For instance, if one answer choice states "x increases" and another answer choice states "x decreases" or "y increases," then those two or three answer choices are very similar in construction and fall into the same family of answer choices. A family of answer choices consists of two or three answer choices, very similar in construction, but often with directly opposite meanings. Usually the correct answer choice will be in that family of answer choices. The "odd man out" or answer choice that doesn't seem to fit the parallel construction of the other answer choices is more likely to be incorrect.

Special Report: How to Overcome Test Anxiety

The very nature of tests caters to some level of anxiety, nervousness, or tension, just as we feel for any important event that occurs in our lives. A little bit of anxiety or nervousness can be a good thing. It helps us with motivation, and makes achievement just that much sweeter. However, too much anxiety can be a problem, especially if it hinders our ability to function and perform.

"Test anxiety," is the term that refers to the emotional reactions that some test-takers experience when faced with a test or exam. Having a fear of testing and exams is based upon a rational fear, since the test-taker's performance can shape the course of an academic career. Nevertheless, experiencing excessive fear of examinations will only interfere with the test-taker's ability to perform and chance to be successful.

There are a large variety of causes that can contribute to the development and sensation of test anxiety. These include, but are not limited to, lack of preparation and worrying about issues surrounding the test.

Lack of Preparation

Lack of preparation can be identified by the following behaviors or situations:

- Not scheduling enough time to study, and therefore cramming the night before the test or exam
- Managing time poorly, to create the sensation that there is not enough time to do everything
- Failing to organize the text information in advance, so that the study material consists of the entire text and not simply the pertinent information
- Poor overall studying habits

Worrying, on the other hand, can be related to both the test taker, or many other factors around him/her that will be affected by the results of the test. These include worrying about:

- Previous performances on similar exams, or exams in general
- How friends and other students are achieving
- The negative consequences that will result from a poor grade or failure

There are three primary elements to test anxiety. Physical components, which involve the same typical bodily reactions as those to acute anxiety (to be discussed below). Emotional factors have to do with fear or panic. Mental or cognitive issues concerning attention spans and memory abilities.

Physical Signals

There are many different symptoms of test anxiety, and these are not limited to mental and emotional strain. Frequently there are a range of physical signals that will let a test taker know that he/she is suffering from test anxiety. These bodily changes can include the following:

- Perspiring
- Sweaty palms
- Wet, trembling hands
- Nausea
- Dry mouth
- A knot in the stomach
- Headache
- Faintness
- Muscle tension
- Aching shoulders, back and neck
- Rapid heart beat
- Feeling too hot/cold

To recognize the sensation of test anxiety, a test-taker should monitor him/herself for the following sensations:

- The physical distress symptoms as listed above
- Emotional sensitivity, expressing emotional feelings such as the need to cry or laugh too much, or a sensation of anger or helplessness
- A decreased ability to think, causing the test-taker to blank out or have racing thoughts that are hard to organize or control.

Though most students will feel some level of anxiety when faced with a test or exam, the majority can cope with that anxiety and maintain it at a manageable level. However, those who cannot are faced with a very real and very serious condition, which can and should be controlled for the immeasurable benefit of this sufferer.

Naturally, these sensations lead to negative results for the testing experience. The most common effects of test anxiety have to do with nervousness and mental blocking.

Nervousness

Nervousness can appear in several different levels:

- The test-taker's difficulty, or even inability to read and understand the questions on the test
- The difficulty or inability to organize thoughts to a coherent form
- The difficulty or inability to recall key words and concepts relating to the testing questions (especially essays)
- The receipt of poor grades on a test, though the test material was well known by the test taker

Conversely, a person may also experience mental blocking, which involves:

- Blanking out on test questions
- Only remembering the correct answers to the questions when the test has already finished.

Fortunately for test anxiety sufferers, beating these feelings, to a large degree, has to do with proper preparation. When a test taker has a feeling of preparedness, then anxiety will be dramatically lessened.

The first step to resolving anxiety issues is to distinguish which of the two types of anxiety are being suffered. If the anxiety is a direct result of a lack of preparation, this should be considered a normal reaction, and the anxiety level (as opposed to the test results) shouldn't be anything to worry about. However, if, when adequately prepared, the test-taker still panics, blanks out, or seems to overreact, this is not a fully rational reaction. While this can be considered normal too, there are many ways to combat and overcome these effects.

Remember that anxiety cannot be entirely eliminated, however, there are ways to minimize it, to make the anxiety easier to manage. Preparation is one of the best ways to minimize test anxiety. Therefore the following techniques are wise in order to best fight off any anxiety that may want to build.

To begin with, try to avoid cramming before a test, whenever it is possible. By trying to memorize an entire term's worth of information in one day, you'll be shocking your system, and not giving yourself a very good chance to absorb the information. This is an easy path to anxiety, so for those who suffer from test anxiety, cramming should not even be considered an option.

Instead of cramming, work throughout the semester to combine all of the material which is presented throughout the semester, and work on it gradually as the course goes by, making sure to master the main concepts first, leaving minor details for a week or so before the test.

To study for the upcoming exam, be sure to pose questions that may be on the examination, to gauge the ability to answer them by integrating the ideas from your texts, notes and lectures, as well as any supplementary readings.

If it is truly impossible to cover all of the information that was covered in that particular term, concentrate on the most important portions, that can be covered very well. Learn these concepts as best as possible, so that when the test comes, a goal can be made to use these concepts as presentations of your knowledge.

In addition to study habits, changes in attitude are critical to beating a struggle with test anxiety. In fact, an improvement of the perspective over the entire test-taking experience can actually help a test taker to enjoy studying and therefore improve the overall experience. Be certain not to overemphasize the significance of the grade - know that the result of the test is neither a reflection of self worth, nor is it a measure of intelligence; one grade will not predict a person's future success.

To improve an overall testing outlook, the following steps should be tried:

- Keeping in mind that the most reasonable expectation for taking a test is to expect to try to demonstrate as much of what you know as you possibly can.
- Reminding ourselves that a test is only one test; this is not the only one, and there will be others.
- The thought of thinking of oneself in an irrational, all-or-nothing term should be avoided at all costs.
- A reward should be designated for after the test, so there's something to look forward to. Whether it be going to a movie, going out to eat, or simply visiting friends, schedule it in advance, and do it no matter what result is expected on the exam.

Test-takers should also keep in mind that the basics are some of the most important things, even beyond anti-anxiety techniques and studying. Never neglect the basic social, emotional and biological needs, in order to try to absorb information. In order to best achieve, these three factors must be held as just as important as the studying itself.

Study Steps

Remember the following important steps for studying:

- Maintain healthy nutrition and exercise habits. Continue both your recreational activities and social pass times. These both contribute to your physical and emotional well being.
- Be certain to get a good amount of sleep, especially the night before the test, because when you're overtired you are not able to perform to the best of your best ability.
- Keep the studying pace to a moderate level by taking breaks when they are needed, and varying the work whenever possible, to keep the mind fresh instead of getting bored.
- When enough studying has been done that all the material that can be learned has been learned, and the test taker is prepared for the test, stop studying and do something relaxing such as listening to music, watching a movie, or taking a warm bubble bath.

There are also many other techniques to minimize the uneasiness or apprehension that is experienced along with test anxiety before, during, or even after the examination. In fact, there are a great deal of things that can be done to stop anxiety from interfering with lifestyle and performance. Again, remember that anxiety will not be eliminated entirely, and it shouldn't be. Otherwise that "up" feeling for exams would not exist, and most of us depend on that sensation to perform better than usual. However, this anxiety has to be at a level that is manageable.

Of course, as we have just discussed, being prepared for the exam is half the battle right away. Attending all classes, finding out what knowledge will be expected on the exam, and knowing the exam schedules are easy steps to lowering anxiety. Keeping up with work will remove the need to cram, and efficient study habits will eliminate wasted time. Studying should be done in an ideal location for concentration, so that it is simple to become interested in the material and give it complete attention. A method such as SQ3R (Survey, Question, Read, Recite, Review) is a wonderful key to follow to make sure that the study habits are as effective as possible, especially in the case of learning from a textbook. Flashcards are great techniques for memorization. Learning to take good notes will mean that notes will be full of useful information, so that less sifting will need to be done to seek out what is pertinent for studying. Reviewing notes after class and then again on occasion will keep the information fresh in the mind. From notes that have been taken summary sheets and outlines can be made for simpler reviewing.

A study group can also be a very motivational and helpful place to study, as there will be a sharing of ideas, all of the minds can work together, to make sure that everyone understands, and the studying will be made more interesting because it will be a social occasion.

Basically, though, as long as the test-taker remains organized and self confident, with efficient study habits, less time will need to be spent studying, and higher grades will be achieved.

To become self confident, there are many useful steps. The first of these is "self talk." It has been shown through extensive research, that self-talk for students who suffer from test anxiety, should be well monitored, in order to make sure that it contributes to self confidence as opposed to sinking the student. Frequently the self talk of test-anxious students is negative or self-defeating, thinking that everyone else is smarter and faster, that they always mess up, and that if they don't do well, they'll fail the entire course. It is important to decreasing anxiety that awareness is made of self talk. Try writing any negative self thoughts and then disputing them with a positive statement instead. Begin self-encouragement as though it was a friend speaking. Repeat positive statements to help reprogram the mind to believing in successes instead of failures.

Helpful Techniques

Other extremely helpful techniques include:

- Self-visualization of doing well and reaching goals
- While aiming for an "A" level of understanding, don't try to "overprotect" by setting your expectations lower. This will only convince the mind to stop studying in order to meet the lower expectations.
- Don't make comparisons with the results or habits of other students. These are individual factors, and different things work for different people, causing different results.
- Strive to become an expert in learning what works well, and what can be done in order to improve. Consider collecting this data in a journal.
- Create rewards for after studying instead of doing things before studying that will only turn into avoidance behaviors.
- Make a practice of relaxing - by using methods such as progressive relaxation, self-hypnosis, guided imagery, etc - in order to make relaxation an automatic sensation.
- Work on creating a state of relaxed concentration so that concentrating will take on the focus of the mind, so that none will be wasted on worrying.
- Take good care of the physical self by eating well and getting enough sleep.
- Plan in time for exercise and stick to this plan.

Beyond these techniques, there are other methods to be used before, during and after the test that will help the test-taker perform well in addition to overcoming anxiety.

Before the exam comes the academic preparation. This involves establishing a study schedule and beginning at least one week before the actual date of the test. By doing this, the anxiety of not having enough time to study for the test will be automatically eliminated. Moreover, this will make the studying a much more effective experience, ensuring that the learning will be an easier process. This relieves much undue pressure on the test-taker.

Summary sheets, note cards, and flash cards with the main concepts and examples of these main concepts should be prepared in advance of the actual studying time. A topic should never be eliminated from this process. By omitting a topic because it isn't expected to be on the test is only setting up the test-taker for anxiety should it actually appear on the exam. Utilize the course syllabus for laying out the topics that should be studied. Carefully go over the notes that were made in class, paying special attention to any of the issues that the professor took special care to emphasize while lecturing in class. In the textbooks, use the chapter review, or if possible, the chapter tests, to begin your review.

It may even be possible to ask the instructor what information will be covered on the exam, or what the format of the exam will be (for example, multiple choice, essay, free form, true-false). Additionally, see if it is possible to find out how many questions will be on the test. If a review sheet or sample test has been offered by the professor, make good use of it, above anything else, for the preparation for the test. Another great resource for getting to know the examination is reviewing tests from previous semesters. Use these tests to review, and aim to achieve a 100% score on each of the possible topics. With a few exceptions, the goal that you set for yourself is the highest one that you will reach.

Take all of the questions that were assigned as homework, and rework them to any other possible course material. The more problems reworked, the more skill and confidence will form as a result. When forming the solution to a problem, write out each of the steps. Don't simply do head work. By doing as many steps on paper as possible, much clarification and therefore confidence will be formed. Do this with as many homework problems as possible, before checking the answers. By checking the answer after each problem, a reinforcement will exist, that will not be on the exam. Study situations should be as exam-like as possible, to prime the test-taker's system for the experience. By waiting to check the answers at the end, a psychological advantage will be formed, to decrease the stress factor.

Another fantastic reason for not cramming is the avoidance of confusion in concepts, especially when it comes to mathematics. 8-10 hours of study will become one hundred percent more effective if it is spread out over a week or at least several days, instead of doing it all in one sitting. Recognize that the human brain requires time in order to assimilate new material, so frequent breaks and a span of study time over several days will be much more beneficial.

Additionally, don't study right up until the point of the exam. Studying should stop a minimum of one hour before the exam begins. This allows the brain to rest and put things in their proper order. This will also provide the time to become as relaxed as possible when going into the examination room. The test-taker will also have time to eat well and eat sensibly. Know that the brain needs food as much as the rest of the body. With enough food and enough sleep, as well as a relaxed attitude, the body and the mind are primed for success.

Avoid any anxious classmates who are talking about the exam. These students only spread anxiety, and are not worth sharing the anxious sentimentalities.

Before the test also involves creating a positive attitude, so mental preparation should also be a point of concentration. There are many keys to creating a positive attitude. Should fears become rushing in, make a visualization of taking the exam, doing well, and seeing an A written on the paper. Write out a list of affirmations that will bring a feeling of confidence, such as "I am doing well in my English class," "I studied well and know my material," "I enjoy this class." Even if the affirmations aren't believed at first, it sends a positive message to the subconscious which will result in an alteration of the overall belief system, which is the system that creates reality.

If a sensation of panic begins, work with the fear and imagine the very worst! Work through the entire scenario of not passing the test, failing the entire course, and dropping out of school, followed by not getting a job, and pushing a shopping cart through the dark alley where you'll live. This will place things into perspective! Then, practice deep breathing and create a visualization of the opposite situation - achieving an "A" on the exam, passing the entire course, receiving the degree at a graduation ceremony.

On the day of the test, there are many things to be done to ensure the best results, as well as the most calm outlook. The following stages are suggested in order to maximize test-taking potential:

- Begin the examination day with a moderate breakfast, and avoid any coffee or beverages with caffeine if the test taker is prone to jitters. Even people who are used to managing caffeine can feel jittery or light-headed when it is taken on a test day.
- Attempt to do something that is relaxing before the examination begins. As last minute cramming clouds the mastering of overall concepts, it is better to use this time to create a calming outlook.
- Be certain to arrive at the test location well in advance, in order to provide time to select a location that is away from doors, windows and other distractions, as well as giving enough time to relax before the test begins.
- Keep away from anxiety generating classmates who will upset the sensation of stability and relaxation that is being attempted before the exam.
- Should the waiting period before the exam begins cause anxiety, create a self-distraction by reading a light magazine or something else that is relaxing and simple.

During the exam itself, read the entire exam from beginning to end, and find out how much time should be allotted to each individual problem. Once writing the exam, should more time be taken for a problem, it should be abandoned, in order to begin another problem. If there is time at the end, the unfinished problem can always be returned to and completed.

Read the instructions very carefully - twice - so that unpleasant surprises won't follow during or after the exam has ended.

When writing the exam, pretend that the situation is actually simply the completion of homework within a library, or at home. This will assist in forming a relaxed atmosphere, and will allow the brain extra focus for the complex thinking function.

Begin the exam with all of the questions with which the most confidence is felt. This will build the confidence level regarding the entire exam and will begin a quality momentum. This will also create encouragement for trying the problems where uncertainty resides.

Going with the "gut instinct" is always the way to go when solving a problem. Second guessing should be avoided at all costs. Have confidence in the ability to do well.

For essay questions, create an outline in advance that will keep the mind organized and make certain that all of the points are remembered. For multiple choice, read every answer, even if the correct one has been spotted - a better one may exist.

Continue at a pace that is reasonable and not rushed, in order to be able to work carefully. Provide enough time to go over the answers at the end, to check for small errors that can be corrected.

Should a feeling of panic begin, breathe deeply, and think of the feeling of the body releasing sand through its pores. Visualize a calm, peaceful place, and include all of the sights, sounds and sensations of this image. Continue the deep breathing, and take a few minutes to continue this with closed eyes. When all is well again, return to the test.

If a "blanking" occurs for a certain question, skip it and move on to the next question. There will be time to return to the other question later. Get everything done that can be done, first, to guarantee all the grades that can be compiled, and to build all of the confidence possible. Then return to the weaker questions to build the marks from there.

Remember, one's own reality can be created, so as long as the belief is there, success will follow. And remember: anxiety can happen later, right now, there's an exam to be written!

After the examination is complete, whether there is a feeling for a good grade or a bad grade, don't dwell on the exam, and be certain to follow through on the reward that was promised and enjoy it! Don't dwell on any mistakes that have been made, as there is nothing that can be done at this point anyway.

Additionally, don't begin to study for the next test right away. Do something relaxing for a while, and let the mind relax and prepare itself to begin absorbing information again.

From the results of the exam - both the grade and the entire experience, be certain to learn from what has gone on. Perfect studying habits and work some more on confidence in order to make the next examination experience even better than the last one.

Learn to avoid places where openings occurred for laziness, procrastination and day dreaming.

Use the time between this exam and the next one to better learn to relax, even learning to relax on cue, so that any anxiety can be controlled during the next exam. Learn how to relax the body. Slouch in your chair if that helps. Tighten and then relax all of the different muscle groups, one group at a time, beginning with the feet and then working all the way up to the neck and face. This will ultimately relax the muscles more than they were to begin with. Learn how to breathe deeply and comfortably, and focus on this breathing going in and out as a relaxing thought. With every exhale, repeat the word "relax."

As common as test anxiety is, it is very possible to overcome it. Make yourself one of the test-takers who overcome this frustrating hindrance.

Additional Bonus Material

Due to our efforts to try to keep this book to a manageable length, we've created a link that will give you access to all of your additional bonus material.

Please visit http://www.mometrix.com/bonus948/usmle1 to access the information.